Nutritional and Integrative Strategies in Cardiovascular Medicine

Nutritional and Integrative Strategies in Cardiovascular Medicine

Edited by

Stephen T. Sinatra
University of Connecticut School of Medicine
Farmington, Connecticut, USA

Mark C. Houston
Vanderbilt University School of Medicine
Nashville, Tennessee, USA

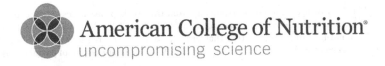

American College of Nutrition®
uncompromising science

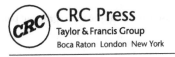

CRC Press
Taylor & Francis Group
Boca Raton London New York

CRC Press is an imprint of the
Taylor & Francis Group, an **informa** business

CRC Press
Taylor & Francis Group
6000 Broken Sound Parkway NW, Suite 300
Boca Raton, FL 33487-2742

First issued in paperback 2021

© 2015 by Taylor & Francis Group, LLC
CRC Press is an imprint of Taylor & Francis Group, an Informa business

No claim to original U.S. Government works

Version Date: 20150211

ISBN 13: 978-1-03-209873-9 (pbk)
ISBN 13: 978-1-4665-7226-3 (hbk)

Visit the Taylor & Francis Web site at
http://www.taylorandfrancis.com

and the CRC Press Web site at
http://www.crcpress.com

Contents

Introduction

Stephen T. Sinatra

It gives me great pleasure to offer *Nutritional and Integrative Strategies in Cardiovascular Medicine* as an in-depth communication offering vital information in the diagnosis and management of atherosclerotic cardiovascular disease. Despite 40 years of aggressive pharmaceutical and surgical interventions,[1] coronary artery disease (CAD) remains the number one killer of women and men in Western civilization. Although urgent use of percutaneous coronary artery intervention (PCI) can be lifesaving in acute myocardial infarction, the elective use of these procedures offers minimal protection from future cardiovascular events or even longevity.[2] Clearly, when it comes to CAD, "prevention is easier than cure" and if CAD does present itself, a combination of conventional and alternative methodologies can truly make a difference in people's lives. Nutritional interventions with both appropriate noninflammatory diets and targeted nutraceutical supports are simple and basic strategies to prevent as well as help manage CAD.

In an ideal world, we would eat all the nutrients necessary to sustain and protect our health. In reality, however, most of us do not eat a nutritious diet full of fruits and vegetables, healthy fats, and lean protein. Instead, we too frequently eat on the basis of convenience and price, and that means more processed foods that are high in calories and low in nutrients.

Even if we do manage to eat healthy foods most of the time, our diets probably do not contain therapeutic amounts of antioxidants, vitamins, and minerals necessary to help prevent cancer, cardiovascular disease, and other degenerative diseases, and which contribute to premature aging. Behind these conditions is inflammation. And what drives inflammation are out-of-control free radicals, molecular fragments produced by natural metabolism, foods, transfats, sugar, environmental toxins, and radiation, to mention a few. As our bodies contain limited amounts of enzymes that neutralize free radicals, we need to look for antioxidants from outside sources.

Today, we realize that vast numbers of people eat poorly and do not get proper nutrition from their diets that their bodies need to sustain good health. Moreover, a global wave of revealing nutritional research has rendered the conventional viewpoint on supplementation utterly obsolete. Hundreds of published studies have shown that individual nutrients at doses higher than those usually present in food have a significant preventive and therapeutic effect on one's health.

Targeted nutraceuticals are not a substitute for good nutrition, but they provide the kind of support that can help prevent inflammatory damage and boost energy production in the body. Knowing which nutrients are best for you individually, as well as in what amounts, can help you nurture yourself appropriately. For example, supplementing with nutrients designed to facilitate and stimulate energy substrate production is the basis of metabolic cardiology.

The combination of targeted supplements and a healthy diet has been the cornerstone of the nutritional strategy that I applied for decades to help my patients with heart disease and many other maladies. I used this approach therapeutically as well as preventively to heal and create optimum health. Most doctors today prescribe drugs for specific effects, such as lowering cholesterol, blood pressure, and blood sugar.

When pharmaceutical drugs do not work in restoring blood flow, surgeons may be called in to perform lifesaving bypasses or heart transplants. In integrative medicine, we use or recommend these methods as well. But we have learned to do something extra, something normally ignored, absolutely simplistic, and bargain-basement cheap compared to dazzling, big-ticket technology. We optimize your nutritional status with vitamins, minerals, antioxidants, and other natural substances—by doing that we optimize your healing and health. In the fight against disease, we do not fight the enemy with limited weapons. We use many. We use what works best, whether the weapons are conventional, natural, or complementary.

Before 1990, vitamins and minerals were seen by most physicians as substances in food that prevented nutritional deficiency states such as scurvy, beriberi, rickets, and pellagra. Mainstream medicine viewed supplementation as unnecessary because, supposedly, "we get all the nutrition we need from our diet." For decades, only a small minority of nutritionally oriented physicians recommended supplements for serious diseases and not just for serious deficiency states.

The wealth of research has greatly influenced the way I perceive healing. A comprehensive targeted nutritional supplement program in combination with a noninflammatory diet is a major part of a preventive and therapeutic intervention. The supplements address specific cardiovascular shortcomings and simultaneously strengthen overall physiology to thwart off infection, inflammation, and plaque while attenuating oxidative lipid issues and blood pressure problems.

Sick people need this nutritional upgrade. They benefit magnificently. It often keeps them out of the hospital. Sometimes supplements work rapidly like magic. Patients suddenly become rejuvenated as their nutritionally starved bodies respond to healing nutrients that were missing for years. Other times, we see a steady but remarkable return to health by patients who previously sputtered along on near-empty tanks. Now, with their tanks full, they move actively forward in life, feeling better than they have felt in years.

In this book, a list of talented authors offers discussions and therapeutic options highlighting their expertise in cardiovascular disease. An in-depth evaluation of fats and lipids as well as alternative and integrative options are offered in the management of lipid disorders and high blood pressure. Other than cigarette smoking, hypertension remains the second most significant risk factor in both men and women. The management of hypertension with diet and targeted nutritional supports is thoroughly presented by several authors. Detoxification, Lyme disease (a serious microbe threat to the heart), and the enormous importance of dental considerations are presented to the reader. The discussion on metabolic syndrome is extremely timely given the fact that this inflammatory metabolic problem is affecting millions of our youth. A naturopathic approach to cardiovascular disease highlighting the value of detoxification is introduced in the care and the management of cardiovascular patients. Hormonal bioidentical interventions and the special concerns of heart disease in women are highlighted with a gender-specific focus. The impact of emotional stress on the heart and the poorly understood association regarding pharmaceutical drugs' influence on nutrient depletion are also presented.

Multiple authors have their own way of telling their stories while offering valuable information. Some of the chapters are conversational, others are like reading a scientific journal, and still others reflect personal observations in the care of their patients. Multiple styles of writing offer the reader creative ways of assimilating the information. Although you may find some duplication of the content, the reader is offered multiple choices in the search for treatments and solutions.

This textbook was designed to help health professionals utilize natural healing foods, as well as nutritional supports and other valuable interventions in the battle against cardiovascular disease. This book was written for doctors who want to know about the most leading and cutting-edge integrative advances that will benefit their patients. In the final analysis, we physicians and health professionals want to reduce the suffering of our patients while extending quality of life at the same time. The contents of *Nutritional and Integrative Strategies in Cardiovascular Medicine* are a testimony to the integrative care of the patient.

I want to thank all the authors for their hard work and contribution to the subject matter and especially Dr. Mark Houston for assisting me with the editing process. I would also like to thank the American College of Nutrition for their willingness to review this book and place their seal of approval on its contents.

REFERENCES

1. Roger VL, Go AS, Lloyd-Jones DM et al. American Heart Association Statistics Committee and Stroke Statistics Subcommittee Executive summary: Heart disease and stroke statistics—2012 update: A report from the American Heart Association. *Circulation* 2012;125:188–197.
2. Boden WE, O'Rourke RA, Teo KK et al. COURAGE Trial Research Group. Optimal medical therapy with or without PCI for stable coronary disease. 2007;356:1503–1516.

Editors

Dr. Stephen T. Sinatra is a board-certified cardiologist with over 40 years of experience in treating cardiovascular disease. He is presently an assistant clinical professor of medicine at the University of Connecticut School of Medicine in Farmington, Connecticut, and a clinical assistant professor of family medicine at the University of New England College of Osteopathic Medicine in Biddeford, Maine. Certified as a bioenergetic psychotherapist and nutrition and antiaging specialist, he integrates psychological, nutraceutical, and energy medicine/electroceutical therapies in the matrix of healing.

Dr. Sinatra is the founder of www.heartmdinstitute.com, an informational website dedicated to promoting public awareness of integrative medicine. He is also a fellow in the American College of Cardiology and the American College of Nutrition. He was the former chief of cardiology (8 years) and director of medical education (19 years) at Manchester Memorial Hospital in Manchester, Connecticut.

Dr. Sinatra has written over 30 peer-reviewed medical publications and has done extensive research on coenzyme Q10 in human, rodent, and equine models. He has written multiple chapters in medical textbooks as well as several book introductions and prefaces for other authors. He has written 18 books including *The Great Cholesterol Myth, The Sinatra Solution/Metabolic Cardiology* and *Earthing: The Most Important Health Discovery Ever, Heartbreak and Heart Disease,* and *Reverse Heart Disease Now.*

Dr. Sinatra feels that his greatest contributions to health and healing include his research on metabolic cardiology and earthing's beneficial relationship to zeta potential, blood thinning, and blood viscosity.

Dr. Sinatra has also appeared on many TV shows including *Dr. Oz, The Doctors, The Today Show, The 700 Club, Fox on Health, MSNBC,* and *Your Health.* He has also been the recipient of numerous awards in the integrative medical field, including excellence in health journalism. Since 1995, Dr. Sinatra has formulated over a hundred nutraceutical products for Healthy Directions, LLC, and he continues to speak at multiple medical conferences teaching integrative and metabolic cardiology.

Dr. Mark Houston is an associate clinical professor of medicine at Vanderbilt University School of Medicine, director of the Hypertension Institute and Vascular Biology, and medical director of the Division of Human Nutrition at Saint Thomas Medical Group, Saint Thomas Hospital and Health Services in Nashville, Tennessee. He is also on the faculty of the American Academy of Anti-Aging Medicine (A4M) for the Fellowship in Anti-Aging and Regenerative Medicine (FAARM) and the University of South Florida (USF), the Institute for Functional Medicine (IFM) and the Metabolic Medicine Institute (MMI) and George Washington University (GWU). He is one of the opinion leaders and faculty for the Personalized Lifestyle Medicine Institute (PLMI).

Dr. Houston was selected as one of the top physicians in hypertension in the United States in 2008–2014 by the Consumer Research Council, and by *USA Today* as one of the most influential doctors in the United States in both hypertension and hyperlipidemia twice in 2009 and 2010. He was selected for The Patient's Choice Award in 2010–2012 by *Consumer Reports USA.*

Dr. Houston is triple board certified by the American Board of Internal Medicine (ABIM), the American Society of Hypertension (ASH), and the American Board of Anti-Aging and Regenerative Medicine (ABAARM). He holds two masters in human nutrition (University of Bridgeport) and in metabolic and nutritional medicine (University of South Florida-Tampa). He is a fellow of the American College of Physicians (ACP), the American Heart Association (AHA), American Society of Hypertension (ASH), American College of Nutrition (ACN), and American Academy of Anti-Aging and Regenerative Medicine (AARM).

Dr. Houston graduated with highest honors (summa cum laude) and the Alpha Omega Alpha (AOA) honorary society distinction from Vanderbilt Medical School and completed his medical internship and residency at the University of California, San Francisco (UCSF). He then returned to Vanderbilt Medical Center where he was chief resident in medicine and served as full-time faculty.

Dr. Houston has presented over 10,000 lectures, nationally and internationally, and published over 250 medical articles, scientific abstracts in peer-reviewed medical journals, books, and book chapters. He is on the consulting editorial board for many medical journals and was previous editor-in-chief for *Journal of the American Nutraceutical Association (JANA)*. He is an author and teacher, and is active in clinical research. Six books that he has authored are the *Handbook of Antihypertensive Therapy, Vascular Biology for the Clinician, What Your Doctor May Not Tell You about Hypertension, Hypertension Handbook for Students and Clinicians,* and *The Hypertension Handbook*. His latest book, *What Your Doctor May Not Tell You about Heart Disease*, is a best seller.

Dr. Houston is one of the founding members and director of the International Society of Integrative Metabolic and Functional Cardiovascular Medicine (ISIMFC) founded in 2012.

Dr. Houston is one of the most sought-after lecturers in the United States on the medical topics of hypertension, dyslipidemia, vascular aging, vascular biology, metabolic and functional medicine, and integrative and preventive cardiovascular medicine. He has an active clinical practice, teaches, and does clinical research at Saint Thomas Hospital in Nashville, Tennessee, and is on the medical faculty at Vanderbilt University School of Medicine.

Contributors

Jonny Bowden, PhD, CNS
Board Certified Nutrition Specialist
Woodland Hills, California

Ryan Bradley, ND, MPH
National College of Natural Medicine
School of Research and Graduate Studies
Helfgott Research Institute
Portland, Oregon

and

School of Pharmacy
University of Washington
Seattle, Washington

and

Guarneri Integrative Health
La Jolla, California

Mark A. Breiner, DDS, FAGD, FIAOMT
Breiner Whole-Body Health Center
Fairfield, Connecticut

Benjamin Brown, ND
The UK College of Nutrition and Health (BCNH)
London, England

Dallas Clouatre, PhD, FACN
Glykon Technologies
Seattle, Washington

William Lee Cowden, MD, MD(H)
Academy of Comprehensive Integrative Medicine
Panama City, Republic of Panama

Richard Delany, MD, FACC
Personalized Preventive Medicine
Milton, Massachusetts

Mimi Guarneri, MD, FACC
Integrative Medicine Atlantic Health System Morristown
Morristown, New Jersey

Mark Houston, MD, MS, FACP, FAHA, FACN
Hypertension Institute of Nashville

and

Vanderbilt University School of Medicine

and

Saint Thomas Medical Group and Health Services
Nashville, Tennessee

James B. LaValle, RPh, CCN
University of South Florida School of Medicine
Tampa, Florida

and

School of Integrative Medicine
George Washington University
Washington, DC

Deanna Minich, PhD, FACN, CNS
University of Western States
Portland, Oregon

and

Personalized Lifestyle Medicine Institute
Seattle, Washington

and

Institute for Functional Medicine
Federal Way, Washington

Harry G. Preuss, MD, MACN, CNS
Georgetown University Medical Center
Washington, DC

Drew Sinatra, ND, LAc, MSA
Focus Health Clinic
Sausalito, California

**Stephen T. Sinatra, MD, FACC,
    FACN, CNS**
University of Connecticut School of
    Medicine
Farmington, Connecticut

Pamela Smith, MD, MPH, MS
Morsani College of Medicine
University of South Florida
Tampa, Florida

Beverly B. Teter, PhD, MACN, FACN, CNS
Department of Animal and Avian Sciences
University of Maryland
College Park, Maryland

1 Myths of Cholesterol
Rethinking a Paradigm

Jonny Bowden and Stephen T. Sinatra

CONTENTS

In this opening chapter, we will present the case for a reevaluation of some of the most widely held beliefs about cholesterol and saturated fat. We will argue that the cholesterol hypothesis—at least the version that most people continue to cling to—is seriously flawed and deserves a reassessment.

We believe that a thorough examination of the mechanisms by which cholesterol is presumed to cause heart disease is long overdue and that an objective reexamination of the evidence will reveal that cholesterol is being wrongly blamed for crimes that it does not—and never did—commit. Cholesterol is found at the scene of the crime, but it is not the perpetrator, and may well turn out to be a marker for other variables. Blaming cholesterol for plaque and heart disease is a bit like blaming the St. Bernard for the avalanche. And, despite massive efforts by the *Big Pharma* to convince us otherwise, the evidence for cholesterol lowering as an effective strategy for preventing or reducing heart disease is actually pretty flimsy.

In 2012, the two of us came together to write a book, *The Great Cholesterol Myth*, the purpose of which was to educate the public about what really causes heart disease and to suggest some practical and effective tips for reducing risk above and beyond the rather myopic focus on cholesterol numbers. The reaction to the book was somewhat unprecedented. Although it garnered hundreds of glowingly positive reviews on Amazon (many of them from physicians) and spent 6 months in the number one slot in the heart disease category, it also generated enough vitriol and anger from some members of the medical establishment to suggest that the subject of cholesterol has become extremely polarized and sclerotic. The hysteria generated by the book—indeed, by all books that have questioned cholesterol orthodoxy*—suggests that it might be time to take a step back and reexamine the evidence. The great nutritionist, Robert Crayhon, once famously said that there are two problems with nutrition: thinking that it cannot do *anything* and thinking that it can do *everything*. The exact same words could be said about cholesterol.

For decades, we—doctors and patients alike—collectively believed that cholesterol was the most important marker for cardiovascular risk, and billions of dollars have been spent bolstering that notion and developing and promoting treatments based on it. Our collective, single-minded focus on lowering cholesterol has several consequences, none of them good. It has caused us to pay relatively *less* attention to likely promoters of heart disease such as sugar, oxidative damage, inflammation, and emotional stress.

---

* *The Cholesterol Myths: Exposing the Fallacy that Saturated Fat and Cholesterol Cause Heart Disease* by Swedish researcher Uffe Ravnskov, MD, PhD, was one of the first books to seriously and scientifically question the cholesterol paradigm—it was literally burned on television in Finland in 1992.

The demonization of cholesterol has also resulted in a corresponding (and unjustified) demonization of saturated fat in the diet. As we will see, a considerable body of emerging research shows no linkage between dietary saturated fat and heart disease. The wrongful indictment of fat—and saturated fat in particular—led to dietary recommendations that we believe deserve a big part of the blame for the current epidemics in diabetes and obesity.[1]

It has also resulted in a vast amount of overprescribing for cholesterol-lowering drugs to patients that may not need them, and may even, in many cases, be harmed by them—all at an enormous cost.

Although we remain "cholesterol skeptics," our view is not quite as extreme as some critics have suggested. It can be summed up as follows:

1. Cholesterol is a *player* in heart disease, but not in the way (nor to the extent) that is widely believed.
2. The standard cholesterol test—given as part of a standard sequential multiple analysis computer (SMAC) profile—is out of date and obsolete. We are measuring cholesterol in the crudest of ways, and are not looking at the data that could actually provide useful information about risk and treatment (i.e., particle *number*, particle size and pattern, Lp[a], apoB [apolipoprotein, a lipid marker of very low density lipoprotein and low density lipoprotein [LDL]; when elevated, considered a marker of inflammation]).
3. According to the discussion in point 2, we are treating many people who are *not* at risk with powerful drugs (purely on the basis of low-density lipoprotein cholesterol [LDL-C] numbers), and we are missing many people who *are* at risk.
4. The dietary recommendations we have been given for the past 40 years, based largely on the fear of cholesterol and saturated fat, are out of date and counterproductive. Saturated fat does *not* cause heart disease, and its effect on cholesterol is far more nuanced than we have been led to believe. Meanwhile, the very foods that have been directly or indirectly recommended to us for so many years as replacements for the saturated fat—margarine, cereal, pasta, bread, potatoes, refined vegetable oils, and many grain products—actually contribute to heart disease (as well as obesity and diabetes) in a number of insidious ways.
5. Regarding heart disease, the true demon in the diet is not—and never has been—fat. It is *sugar.*
6. Cholesterol in the blood never becomes a problem until it is oxidized.
7. Our efforts at prevention should focus on reducing oxidation, inflammation, and stress—three major promoters of cardiovascular disease (CVD).
8. Statin drugs are being widely overprescribed, particularly in situations where the evidence for benefit is slim to none (primary prevention), populations where there is not sufficient evidence that they do much good (women, the elderly) and populations in which there is reasonable evidence that they may be doing great harm (children).
9. The significant side effects of these expensive and overprescribed drugs are hugely underreported and underpublicized. People are being prescribed powerful medicines that they believe will extend their lives, oblivious of the fact that research shows clearly that they do no such thing.

(We will discuss points 8 and 9 in Chapter 3.)

IN SEARCH OF A NEW PARADIGM

In philosophy 101, we learn of "the black swan theory"—an unexpected event that appears to be an exception to a widely accepted rule (all swans are white) causing a reevaluation of the original rule, and often a rationalization that allows the believer to hold on to the original hypothesis (i.e., "it had to be a white swan that flew into some paint").

The problem with the belief that cholesterol is the main player in heart disease is that there is not just *one* black swan exception, there are many. More than a few studies have shown little relationship between cholesterol and heart disease. In the Lyon Diet Heart Study,[2] the intervention group experienced a 70% reduction in all-cause mortality without any change in their cholesterol levels. A 1994 study published in *JAMA* found no association between cholesterol and coronary heart disease mortality and morbidity and all-cause mortality in persons older than 70.[3] The Framingham study, which as of this writing, is on its third generation of participants, did demonstrate an inverse relationship between high-density lipoprotein cholesterol (HDL-C) and coronary heart disease (CHD), as well as positive associations between high blood pressure and smoking.[4] But though the Framingham study is often cited as "proof" of the lipid hypothesis, senior investigator William Castelli, MD, apparently had serious doubts. In a much-quoted article in *JAMA Internal Medicine* he wrote the following:

> Most of what we know about the effects of diet factors, particularly the saturation of fat and cholesterol, on serum lipid parameters derives from metabolic ward-type studies. Alas, such findings, within a cohort studied over time have been disappointing, indeed the findings have been contradictory. For example, in Framingham, Mass., the more saturated fat one ate, the more cholesterol one ate, the more calories one ate, the lower the person's serum cholesterol. The opposite of what one saw in the 26 metabolic ward studies, the opposite of what the equations provided by Hegsted et al. and Keys et al.[5]

At least three major review[6–8] studies have shown no relationship between saturated fat in the diet and heart disease, and certainly no advantage in swapping carbohydrate for saturated fat. In fact, just the opposite is the case. Mozaffarian et al.[9] actually showed that risk factors for heart disease go *up* when you substitute carbohydrates for saturated fat. Jakobsen et al.[10] compared the association between saturated fats and carbohydrates with ischemic heart disease (IHD) risk among 53,644 men and women in a Danish cohort of the Diet, Cancer, and Health Study and found that saturated fat intake was not associated with risk of myocardial infarction (MI) compared with carbohydrate consumption, leading to an editorial in the *American Journal of Clinical Nutrition* by Frank Hu, entitled "Are refined carbohydrates worse than saturated fat?"[11]

The hypothesis that cholesterol and saturated fat are major promoters of heart disease has had more than its fair share of black swan-type studies, and yet, the establishment continues to dismiss these studies as either anomalies or outliers. In some cases, they simply ignore them. The cholesterol establishment at this point is so entrenched and has so many tentacles into industry, government, and medicine (Big Food and it is "low-fat" products, the incredibly sophisticated and extremely well-funded marketing machine of the pharmaceutical industry, the National Cholesterol Education Program, the American Heart Association), that "rapid response" teams are able to effectively marginalize any studies whose results call into question the basic tenants of cholesterol dogma. (How do we explain away a study showing no benefit to lowering cholesterol? Simple: they did not lower it *enough*!).

An example of this kind of thinking about fat and cholesterol can be seen in something known as "the French Paradox." For years, we were taught that the French had lower rates of heart disease *despite* the fact that they consumed copious amounts of saturated fat, a puzzlement no one could apparently figure out. So we were taught to think of this as a *paradox* (the secular version of a *miracle*) because we could not bring ourselves to rethink the *paradigm* that saturated fat causes heart disease. Given the massive cognitive dissonance engendered by these conflicting "truths"—*saturated fat causes heart disease, the French eat a ton of saturated fat, the French have low rates of heart disease*—we "reconciled" them in the only way possible: we called it a "paradox." Of course, if one of those accepted "truths" is wrong—i.e., if saturated fat does *not* cause heart disease in the first place—there is no paradox at all. The French eat a lot of fat, they do not have much heart disease, so what? (It is only a paradox if both premises are true.) But to consider this possibility would require what Thomas Kuhn, in his classic book, *The Structure of Scientific Revolutions*, called a "paradigm shift."[12]

We think a paradigm shift is exactly what is needed when it comes to thinking about cholesterol.

The case against cholesterol was made in the middle of the twentieth century, became the "accepted wisdom" in the mid-1980s, and in the ensuing years has become a petrified, sclerotic dogma. The current paradigm—that cholesterol is measured in an accurate and meaningful way, that it is the major initiator of heart disease, and that reducing it will lower the incidence of heart disease—is simply no longer supportable by the available evidence. Cardiologist Laura Corr of Guys and St. Thomas' Hospitals, writing in the *European Heart Journal*,[13] put it best:

> The commonly-held belief that the best diet for prevention of coronary heart disease is a low saturated fat, low cholesterol diet is not supported by the available evidence from clinical trials. In primary prevention, such diets do not reduce the risk of myocardial infarction or coronary or all-cause-mortality. Cost-benefit analyses of the extensive primary prevention programs, which are at present vigorously supported by Governments, Health Departments and health educationalists, are urgently required.

The case against cholesterol and saturated fat deserves to be reopened.

A LITTLE HISTORY

The cholesterol hypothesis—the general name for two distinct but related theories called the "diet-heart hypothesis" and the "lipid hypothesis"—had its nascent beginnings around the turn of the century. And it all started with rabbits.

In 1913, a Russian experimenter named Nikolai Anichkov discovered that when you fed rabbits large amounts of cholesterol, they developed atherosclerosis. As Konstantinov et al. point out in an article in the *Texas Heart Institute Journal*,[14] Anichkov's classic experiments literally paved the way to our current beliefs about the role of cholesterol in CVD. Anichkov's work was considered so important that in 1958—in an editorial in *Annals of Internal Medicine* no less—it was compared to the discovery of the tubercle bacillus by Robert Koch.[15]

But rabbits are, after all, vegetarians, and their bodies have no idea what to do with an animal product like cholesterol. (Dogs and baboons, for example, do not respond the same way to cholesterol feeding as rabbits do.) Putting aside the question of whether cholesterol-fed rabbits are the best choice for demonstrating metabolic mechanisms in humans, Anichkov's work actually raises a couple of other interesting points about cholesterol and heart disease.

One: the cholesterol-fed rabbits *did* develop atherosclerosis—but they did *not* get heart attacks. This is important. One of the main determinants of plaque rupture is the balance between collagen synthesis and collagen degradation, a process that requires vitamin C.[16] The most abundant amino acids in collagen are proline and lysine, and when collagen is damaged, these two amino acids become exposed. Lipoprotein(a)—a highly atherogenic cholesterol particle—is attracted to both lysine and proline, and will attach itself to the now exposed and damaged strands of collagen. "It is an attempt by the body to repair damage to the collagen of the artery walls in the absence of adequate levels of vitamin C," writes Andrew W. Saul, PhD.[17]

> Unfortunately the repair is not ideal and over many years repeated deposits can cause the artery to become narrow and inflamed. Heart attack or stroke is likely to follow (usually caused by a clot forming at the site of the narrowed artery, or by a piece of plaque breaking off and blocking a smaller vessel downstream). When vitamin C levels are low, the body manufactures more cholesterol, especially Lp(a). Conversely, when vitamin C levels are high the body makes less cholesterol.

"If high blood cholesterol were the primary cause of heart disease, all bears and other hibernating animals would have become extinct long ago," writes Dr. Saul. "They naturally have high cholesterol levels. One reason bears are still with us is simple: they produce large amounts of vitamin C in their bodies, which stabilizes the artery walls, and there is therefore no tendency to develop cholesterol deposits or plaque." Guinea pigs, like humans, cannot make their own vitamin C, and if you deprive a guinea pig of vitamin C it develops damage to the arteries within a few short weeks. A 1992 review of the literature on vitamin C and CVD in the *Journal of the American College of Nutrition* found that "Evidence linking vitamin C to human CVD is largely circumstantial, but taken in total, is suggestive of an association" and called for further examination of the relationship.[18] Further examination is exactly what was done in 2011, when a study in the *American Heart Journal* found that plasma vitamin C did indeed predict incident heart failure in both men and women.[19]

The second thing Anichkov demonstrated was that when cholesterol was *injected* into the rabbits, rather than fed to them, no atherosclerosis was found. This should immediately raise some eyebrows. Ingest arsenic orally or inject it into the bloodstream, either way you wind up dead. But the fate of *injected* cholesterol and *ingested* cholesterol in the body are quite different. When eaten, cholesterol is packaged by the liver into carriers known as lipoproteins. (That does not happen when you *inject* cholesterol.) So when we are "measuring cholesterol" we are actually measuring *lipoproteins*, an important distinction. Let us not forget that cholesterol is a *passenger* on the lipoprotein boat, but the boat *itself*—the lipoprotein—also has activities and characteristics that need to be examined.

Nonetheless, the idea that cholesterol and atherosclerosis were somehow related in a causal way remained in the scientific ether, to be resurrected with a vengeance in the mid-twentieth century. Here is how it happened.

It was the middle of the twentieth century. Young men were returning from the front lines of the war and were inexplicably showing signs of heart disease. Remember that heart disease, as we know it today, was far less common in the beginning of the twentieth century—in fact, the very term for a specialist in heart disease—"cardiologist"—was hardly used at all till the second decade of the century.[20] So, for apparently healthy young men to suddenly be showing signs of CVD at unprecedented rates was a remarkable and alarming phenomenon.

There was a demand for explanations, and an even stronger demand for action. What was causing this "epidemic" of heart disease, and, more importantly, what could be done about it? The McGovern Select Committee on Nutrition had been formed in 1968 under President Nixon, largely to deal with food insecurity and hunger, and by 1974—3 years before it was disbanded—the committee decided to expand its focus to include the nation's nutrition policy. Hard to imagine now, but the nascent belief that diet could be a factor in disease, including heart disease, was very far from universally accepted. For the government to make dietary recommendations as a public health measure was pretty radical. Still, there was a feeling among the committee members that before going off into the sunset, they ought to do it.

Enter a physiologist named Ancel Keys.

Keys was a respected researcher who invented the K-rations used by the U.S. Army, and did research on the physiology of starvation in the Minnesota Starvation Experiment.[21] He was well aware of the previous work on cholesterol-fed rabbits, and was convinced that diet played a major role in heart disease. Specifically, he believed that saturated fat in the diet raised cholesterol in the blood, which in turn put one at great risk for heart disease (this was called "the diet-heart hypothesis"). (Interestingly, he never believed that cholesterol in the *diet* mattered a whit.)

When stationed in Pioppi, Italy, in the 1940s, Keys chatted with doctors from the Mediterranean regions who pointed out that heart disease was rare in the area, and Keys came to believe that the main reason this was so was because they ate less saturated fat. He postulated a connection between cholesterol in the blood, saturated fat in the diet, and higher rates of heart disease, and designed his classic study—the Seven Countries Study[22]—to demonstrate just that. We will return to Keys in just a moment.

This is an excellent place to discuss the actual Mediterranean diet that Keys became so enamored of. What we call "the Mediterranean Diet" seems to be the only dietary pattern nearly everyone in the field of nutrition agrees is "good," even though it is extremely hard to get a solid, specific definition of what the Mediterranean diet *is*, and even harder to get agreement on what elements in the diet—or the Mediterranean lifestyle in general—is responsible for the benefits. Understanding how we think about the Mediterranean diet will actually help us understand some of the flaws in our thinking about cholesterol and saturated fat.

What we know as "The Mediterranean Diet" is actually inspired by traditional patterns of eating in Greece, Spain, and Southern Italy. Though there are many more versions of Mediterranean eating than you might imagine, the pattern is generally characterized by large amounts of olive oil, unrefined cereals, vegetables, fruits, nuts, fish, poultry, moderate wine, and moderate dairy with relatively small amounts of red meat.

A meatless, low-fat diet is hardly typical of all Mediterranean cuisine. Lamb is widely eaten—though it is almost always grass-fed, an enormous distinction that too often goes unnoticed. Lard and butter are commonly used in Northern Italy, and, with some exceptions, sheep's tail fat and rendered butter (samma) are traditional staple fats in North Africa and the Middle East.[23] Though much of the world believes—wrongly, we feel—that the benefits of the Mediterranean diet accrue because it is low in meat and saturated fat, an equally good case can be made that the benefits accrue because it is low in sugar.

That there is a robust association between what we know as the Mediterranean pattern of eating and better health is not in question. However, as mentioned above, the *reason* for that association is not nearly as clear. Keys began his research convinced that the culprit in the American diet was saturated fat, and he was able to find data that seemed (if you did not look too carefully) to confirm that. (Neuroeconomists would call this "confirmation bias"—the tendency to read the evidence in a way that confirms what you already believe). But there is a lot more to the Mediterranean diet than a comparatively low intake of saturated fat.

The Mediterranean diet pattern is startlingly low in sugar and in highly processed carbs. Those in the Mediterranean region rarely snack, and hardly ever on the processed snack foods that are endemic in the United States. But the diet is characterized not just by what they eat *less* of, but what they eat *more* of: nuts, vegetables, fiber, and high-antioxidant oils. According to Walter Willett, MD, whose research at Harvard was in part responsible for the acceptance of the Mediterranean eating plan by virtually everyone as the poster-diet for healthy eating, traditional Mediterranean diets used plenty of fruits and vegetables, are higher in fat, and are relatively low in easily digested carbohydrates. Because of this, they also have a relatively low impact on blood sugar.[24]

To attribute their lower rates of heart disease to a lower level of saturated fat in the diet is a faith-based attribution. It is not justified by science, and it is in no way supported by actual evidence. What we have in the Mediterranean region is a multifactorial lifestyle that involves a host of variables including activity, community, sunlight, snacking behavior, sugar consumption, sleep patterns, and more options for dealing with stress and isolation, a vastly different picture from the one we see in the United States. Yet, we continue to cling to the dogma that there is less heart disease in the Mediterranean because they eat less red meat and saturated fat.

The idea of a multifactorial design producing a result, which is then attributed to one factor in the design, is something that has been seen before in what has become an increasingly partisan war over the role of fat and cholesterol in heart disease. One of the most glaring examples of this is the famous "reversing heart disease" study by one of the biggest proponents of the low-fat diet, Dean Ornish, MD.

Ornish's reputation—and much of the public's faith in the low-fat diet approach—was fueled by his famous 5-year intervention study (the Lifestyle Heart Trial), which demonstrated that intensive lifestyle changes may lead to regression of CHD.[25] Ornish took 48 middle-aged white men with moderate to severe CHD and assigned them to two groups. One group received "usual care," and the other group received a special, intensive five-part lifestyle intervention consisting of (1) aerobic exercise, (2) stress management training, (3) smoking cessation, (4) group psychological support, and (5) a strict vegetarian diet that itself had several subcharacteristics including a high amount of fiber, almost no sugar, a large amount of natural anti-inflammatories and antioxidants from vegetables and fruits, and, incidentally, only 10% of calories coming from fat.

Ornish had a drop-out rate of almost 50%, but of the 20 men who completed the 5-year study, there were fewer cardiac events and a significant reversal of atherosclerosis. But the public perception of this study—strongly reinforced by Ornish himself—was that his results were due to the low-fat component of the program. This *may* be true—but there is absolutely no way to know it from the study design. (Imagine that you gave patients a daily dose of a three-drug cocktail, changed their diet, fixed their sleep apnea, taught them to exercise, got them meditating, and then found out—after 5 years—that their incidence of asthma was greatly reduced compared to a control group. Could you reasonably claim with a straight face that your asthma-eradicating results were due to *one* of the drugs? Or, for that matter, due to the mediation? No beginning statistics student would ever make a mistake like that, yet that is exactly what Ornish did.)

There is absolutely no way to know whether the results of Ornish's reversing heart disease study were due to the high fiber, the whole foods, the lack of sugar, or some combination of the interventions. It is entirely possible that Ornish would have gotten the same or better results with a program of exercise, stress management, smoking cessation, group therapy, and whole foods—low-glycemic diet that included *plenty* of saturated fat and protein. Attributing his results to the low-fat diet is as silly as attributing the health benefits of the Mediterranean diet to a slightly lower amount of saturated fat.

Back to Keys, a perfect segue from the discussion of confirmation bias. There is much misinformation about Keys in the "cholesterol skeptic" community. It is widely believed that he deleted data from his famous Seven Countries study to make a stronger case for the fat–heart disease connection (not true), that he cherry picked evidence (true), and that when all the evidence he chose to ignore was put back into the equation, the association between fat and heart disease disappeared (partly true). Here is what actually happened.*

As we have seen, Keys proposed that saturated fat in the diet and cholesterol in the blood were the major variables responsible for the high rates of heart disease seen in industrialized countries such as the United States. He decided to demonstrate this by analyzing data on saturated fat consumption and heart disease in six different countries, producing an article that was known as the Six Countries Study. He presented that article—and his theory about fat and cholesterol—at a 1955 world Health Organization conference (its first Expert Committee on the Pathogenesis of Atherosclerosis), which met to discuss what was perceived as an "epidemic" of heart disease.

It did not go well.

"Ancel Keys, known for his sharp, blunt, and biting commentary, was reportedly true to form at the conference," writes Anthony Colpo.[26] "But when the outspoken Minnesotan confidently put forth his dietary theory of heart disease at this hallmark gathering, he was greeted with considerable skepticism. Henry Blackburn, a long time collaborator of Keys, recalls that the researcher was 'flabbergasted to find that his ideas were not accepted on the spot'."[26]

Apparently, when Keys prepared his "case" using the six countries where saturated fat and heart disease had a positive correlation, there was data available on 22 countries. Keys "selected" the countries he felt would make the strongest case for the association. When you factor in the other 22 countries, the association between saturated fat and heart disease all but disappears. (It is still there—but it is significantly weaker [and confounded by other seemingly contradictory associations like the *inverse* association between animal fat consumption and mortality[27]]). "Instead of a perfectly uniform pattern, the resultant graph looked more like the holes on an old dartboard—all over the place!," writes Colpo.[26] George Mann—a well-known researcher from the University of Vanderbilt who was an outspoken critic of the cholesterol hypothesis discovered that in many countries physical activity was the most accurate predictor of heart disease risk, and that Keys had conveniently deleted those countries from his presentation.[26]

Meanwhile, across the pond, another researcher was questioning Keys' views and offering a different hypothesis. John Yudkin, MD, from the University of London, believed that Keys was so focused on proving the connection between fat and heart disease that he was missing many other compelling connections between diet and heart disease. In an article published in *The Lancet* entitled "Diet and Coronary Thrombosis: Hypothesis and Fact"[28] he stated, "… one begins to have the uneasy feeling that both the proponents and opponents of a dietary hypothesis are quoting only those data which support their view."

---

* Much of this is known because of superb investigative health journalism by one Denise Minger. You can read her complete report on the chronology of events, complete with references, here: http://rawfoodsos.com/2011/12/22/the-truth-about-ancel-keys-weve-all-got-it-wrong/.

Yudkin's research showed there were countries that had similar intakes of fat but as much as a fourfold difference in coronary mortality. He also questioned the demonization of animal fat:

> It has been suggested that the amount of animal fats, from milk and from meat, is more important than the amount of total fat in causing coronary thrombosis. The figures do not support this, since the relationship is less direct than with total fats. Those who believe that the culprit is butter fat, from butter, milk, and cheese, receive even less support. Nor is there support for the view that vegetable fat is protective, for there is no relationship, either positive or negative between the intake of vegetable fat and coronary mortality.[28]

Yudkin's most important finding was there was indeed a dietary component that tracked well with heart disease, much better, in fact, than fat did. That dietary component was sugar. "There is a better relationship with intake of sugar than with any other nutrient we have examined," he writes.[28] "These international comparisons, then, do not support the view that total fat or animal fat is the direct and single cause of coronary thrombosis. Neither do they support the view that (saturated) fats are related at all to coronary thrombosis. The relationships which do emerge, especially that with sugar, suggest that coronary thrombosis is associated with higher living standards. This is supported by the relationship which exists between coronary mortality and national income per head."[28]

In fact, the very best correlations Yudkin's research uncovered was the highly significant correlation between coronary mortality and number of radio and television licenses, followed by the correlation between coronary mortality and the number of registered motor vehicles.[28] This is important to point out because it shows both the possibilities and the limits of correlational (association) studies. Although epidemiology can *suggest* hypotheses—saturated fat causes heart disease, television set ownership causes heart disease—it does not *test* these hypotheses, and that is the great limitation of epidemiology, and the great danger in making health policy based on epidemiological findings. On the other hand, the fact that so many things about modern life track with heart disease should open us to the possibility that stress is of far greater importance as a variable in disease than cholesterol ever was, a position suggested by the work of neurobiologist and McArthur Genius Grant recipient Professor Robert Sapolsky.[29,30]

Back once again, to Keys. Having been scorned and ridiculed at the World Health Organization meeting where he presented the Six Countries article, he decided, in Blackburn's words, to "show these guys."[26] In 1958, he designed the Seven Countries Study[31] that has formed the cornerstone of our dietary policy for the past four decades and which has informed our myopic focus on cholesterol since 1984. He handpicked seven countries the data from which he had good reason to think would support his theory. He concentrated on the variables he thought were important and ignored the rest. And—surprise, surprise—he got the expected results.

Denise Minger—whose research on this is both impeccable and wonderfully entertaining to read—puts it beautifully:

> I'm not going to pat Keys on the back for deliberately choosing countries to make his case look stronger, but in terms of historical accuracy, we can't say that he actually lied. His biggest error, in fact, had less to do with data-deletion and more to do with tunnel vision. Along with failing to explore reasons why fat might be linked to heart disease in a non-causal way, it seems Keys had his eyes locked so tightly on his lovely lipids that he didn't notice the role of other dietary factors.[32]

Preselecting the countries that "proved" this theory was only one of the many problems with the Seven Countries Study. There was also data in the study that did not add up. For example, there was significant variability in heart mortality *within* these seven countries, even though saturated fat consumption was identical. In Finland, for example, the intake of saturated fat was almost identical in two population groups (from Turku and North Karelia), but heart mortality was three times higher in North Karelia. Similarly, saturated fat intake was nearly identical on two Greek islands—Crete and Corfu. But heart mortality was a whopping 17 times higher on Corfu than it was on Crete![33]

How did Keys explain these facts, which were clearly present in his data?

Simple. He ignored them.

Keys was a member of the nutrition advisory committee of the American Heart Association, so despite the flaws in his study, he managed to get his theories officially incorporated into the 1961 American Heart Association dietary guidelines[34] where they have influenced government policy on heart disease, fat consumption, and cholesterol for decades.

These guidelines accomplished their goals, not least of all in the court of public opinion. A famous 1984 cover of *Time* magazine ("Cholesterol: And Now the Bad News....") showed a picture of two fried eggs and a piece of bacon arranged to look like a face making a frown. Both saturated fat and cholesterol had been successfully labeled as the primary bad actors in the development of heart disease, a perception that has not changed appreciably in the ensuing decades.

But does saturated fat *really* promote heart disease? And how much does lowering cholesterol really matter anyway?

In an excellent article published in the journal *Nutrition*, Robert Hoenselaar attempted to answer the first question.[35] He looked at the recommendations of leading U.S. and European advisory committees on saturated fat. He then compared their recommendations with the science they were based on. He argued that evidence-based dietary advice should be built on results from all studies available, according to a given methodology. So he examined what the science actually shows about the association between saturated fat intake and CVD and compared that with the results as they were presented by the advisory committees in their respective reports. He put the findings into perspective by examining studies that were not included in the advisory committee reports. For example, all three committee reports quoted research on the effect of saturated fat on LDL-C as evidence for the connection of saturated fat to CVD, but systematically ignored the effect of saturated fat on HDL. Hoenselaar also found that both U.S. reports failed to correctly describe the results from the prospective studies.

The advisory committees included three types of studies as support for their recommendations:

1. Controlled trials showing that saturated fat consumption increases (LDL) cholesterol levels.
2. Intervention studies showing that the decrease of saturated fat and the simultaneous increase of polyunsaturated fat in the diet decrease CVD risk.
3. Prospective cohort studies showing a positive association between saturated fat intake and coronary heart disease (CHD) risk.

But when Hoenselaar investigated the actual findings of the studies used to support the recommendations, a very different picture emerged than the one presented by the advisory committees. "Replacement of carbohydrates with tropical oils markedly raises total cholesterol, which is unfavorable, but the picture changes if effects on HDL and apolipoprotein B are taken into account," he writes.[35] Although the reports of the advisory committees included the effect of LDL-C on CVD in the evidence they cited, none of the reports considered the effect of HDL-C on CVD, even though, as Hoenselaar points out, a meta-analysis of 61 prospective studies published in *The Lancet*[36] showed that LDL-C and HDL-C were independent predictors of ischemic heart disease (IHD) mortality.[36] In fact, in that same *Lancet* study, the ratio of total to HDL-C was the strongest predictor of IHD mortality. None of the reports explained why they did not include the data on saturated fat and HDL.

In fact, the effect of saturated fat on cholesterol is more nuanced than was previously believed. Not only does saturated fat raise HDL-C but it has a profound effect on LDL particle size and distribution. Higher intake of saturated fat—in particular, myristic and palmitic acid—is inversely correlated with concentrations of small, dense LDL, and positively associated with increased concentrations of larger, cholesterol-enriched LDL.[37] If one looks only at total LDL numbers, this important (and positive) effect on LDL particle size and distribution is missed. "As long as information *directly linking* the consumption of certain fats and oils with CAD is lacking, we can never be sure what such fats and oils do to CAD risk," writes Hoenselaar.[35]

The danger of using cholesterol levels as a stand-in for heart disease has been demonstrated many times. There is no shortage of studies showing an association between saturated fat in the diet and cholesterol in the blood, but studies that investigated the direct result of saturated fat on hard end-points have been less frequently done. But at least three systemic reviews of prospective studies have been published examining the *direct* relationship between saturated fat and CVD.[6–8] They show a consistent lack of an association. One of these meta-analyses, done by Siri-Tarino et al., included the largest number of cohorts for the association between saturated fat and CHD and concluded that "there is no significant evidence for concluding that dietary saturated fat is associated with an increased risk of CHD or CVD."[8] Furthermore, the authors suggest that given the differential effects of dietary saturated fats and carbohydrates on concentrations of larger and smaller LDL particles, respectively, dietary efforts to improve the increasing burden of CVD risk associated with atherogenic dyslipidemia should primarily emphasize the limitation of refined carbohydrates.[8]

In fact, one study found that in postmenopausal women with relatively low total fat intake, a *greater* saturated fat intake was associated with *less* progression of coronary atherosclerosis, whereas carbohydrate intake was associated with a *greater* progression,[9] leading the *American Journal of Clinical Nutrition* to publish an editorial entitled, "Saturated fat prevents coronary artery disease? An American paradox."[38]

The second question—does LDL-C matter as much as previously believed—is another matter. In a recent article in the *Journal of Evaluation in Clinical Practice*, Petursson et al. asked the question, "Is the use of cholesterol in mortality risk algorithms in clinical guidelines valid?"[39] Using 10 years of prospective data from the Norwegian HUNT 2 study,[40] they assessed the association of total serum cholesterol with total mortality, as well as mortality from CVD and IHD, using Cox proportional hazard models. They found that among women, cholesterol had an *inverse* association with all-cause mortality (hazard ratio 0.94) as well as CVD mortality (hazard ratio 0.97). IHD mortality was not linear, but followed a U-shaped curve, as did the association of cholesterol with mortality from CVD and with all-cause mortality in men. The authors conclude, "If our findings are generalizable, clinical and public health recommendations regarding the 'dangers' of cholesterol should be revised. This is especially true for women, for whom moderately elevated cholesterol (by current standards) may prove to be not only harmless but even beneficial"[39]

Though research starting with the Framingham study has shown a strong positive association between high-plasma HDL and reduced risk of MI, it is not entirely clear if this association is causal. Voight et al.[41] used a Mendelian randomization model to test the hypothesis that the association of a plasma biomarker with disease is causal. They found that people who inherit genes (the *LIPG* 396*Ser* allele) that naturally give them higher HDL levels have no less heart disease than those who inherit genes that produce slightly lower levels. Though in observational epidemiological studies, a 1 SD increase in HDL cholesterol is associated with reduced risk of MI, the same 1 SD increase due to genetic score was not. The increase in HDL cholesterol associated with the *LIPG* 396*Ser* allele would have been expected to produce a 13% decreased risk of MI but in fact was not associated with any reduction in risk. Their data "challenge the concept that raising of plasma HDL cholesterol will uniformly translate into reductions in risk of myocardial infarction."[41]

Research article published in *The FASEB Journal* also suggests a rethinking of the HDL hypothesis. Scanu and Edelstein[42] found that the HDL from patients with chronic diseases (kidney disease, diabetes, and rheumatoid arthritis) is different from the HDL in healthy individuals, even when blood levels are comparable. In an interview with *Science Daily*,[43] Angelo Scanu, MD, a pioneer in blood lipid chemistry from the University of Chicago and the first author of the study, said: "For many years, HDL has been viewed as good cholesterol and has generated a false perception that the more HDL in the blood, the better. It is now apparent that subjects with high HDL are not necessarily protected from heart problems and should ask their doctor to find out whether their HDL is good or bad."

Other research also calls into question the idea that raising HDL-C always translates to a clinical benefit. In the AIM-HIGH trial,[44] patients with established CVD, who had achieved target LDL levels with statin therapy, were randomized to one of two treatments:

1. Simvastatin (40–80 mg/day) ± ezetimibe (10 mg/day) as necessary to maintain LDL-C below 70 mg/dL + placebo (a tiny dose of crystalline niacin to cause flushing)
2. As in point 1, with 1500–2000 mg/day of extended release niacin instead of placebo

After 2 years, the niacin group experienced a significant increase in plasma HDL-C but no improvement in patient survival. (The safety board halted the trial.) The dal-OUTCOMES study[45] randomized patients to either standard of care plus placebo or standard of care plus dalcetrapib, a CETP (cholesterylester transfer protein) inhibitor. (Inhibition of the CETP pathway, which facilitates transfer of triglyceride (TG) and cholesterol ester between lipoproteins, can increase concentrations of HDL-C.) Over the course of the trial, HDL-C levels increased from baseline by 4%–11% in the placebo group and by 31%–40% in the dalcetrapib group. At a prespecified interim analysis, the independent data and safety monitoring board recommended termination of the trial for futility. As compared with placebo, dalcetrapib did not alter the risk of the primary end point and did not have a significant effect on any component of the primary end point or on total mortality.

All of this begs another question, which may be even more relevant: are we measuring cholesterol in the most useful and accurate way?

Early on in this chapter, we expressed our opinion that the standard cholesterol test—given as part of a standard CBC—is out of date. Here's why. We have known for some time that there are different subtypes of HDL (e.g., HDL-2 and HDL-3) as well as different subtypes of LDL (LDL-a and LDL-b).

These behave quite differently in the body, yet these differences are obscured when we measure only HDL and LDL.

Although most HDL is indeed protective, all subtypes may not be equally so. HDL-2, for example, seems to be more protective, whereas the role of HDL-3 remains equivocal.[46] The differences in subtypes of LDL are even more dramatic.

LDL-a is a large molecule, which is less atherogenic than LDL-b, which is a small, dense, oxidized particle that can easily penetrate the endothelium. Particle tests that determine what kind of LDL one has (pattern "A" or the far less desirable pattern "B") are more sophisticated than standard cholesterol tests that simply divide cholesterol into "good" and "bad." But even more predictive than particle size is the actual number of particles.

Cromwell et al.[47] followed a Framingham offspring cohort of 3066 middle-aged white participants without CVD to compare the ability of alternative measures of LDL to provide CVD risk discrimination at relatively low levels consistent with current therapeutic targets. Specifically, they looked at particle number (LDL-P), and placed subjects into one of four possible groups:

1. High LDL-C, high LDL-P
2. High LDL-C, low LDL-P
3. Low LDL-C, high LDL-P
4. Low LDL-C, low LDL-P

They found that LDL-C is only a good predictor of adverse cardiac events when it is concordant with LDL-P (meaning both variables move in the same direction). When the two variables are discordant, LDL-C was found to be a poor predictor of risk. Those with the worst survival had low (below median) LDL-C but high LDL-P. They were also most likely to have either small LDL particles or TG-rich/cholesterol poor LDL particles, or both (e.g., those with insulin resistance, metabolic syndrome, or type II diabetes).

"Discordance between LDL-C and LDL-P is even greater in populations with metabolic syndrome, including patients with diabetes," writes Peter Attia, MD.[48] "Given the ubiquity of these conditions in the U.S. population, and the special risk such patients carry for cardiovascular disease, it is difficult to justify use of LDL-C, HDL-C, and TG alone for risk stratification in all but the most select patients." Attia points out that in patients without metabolic syndrome, LDL-C under-predicts cardiac risk 22% of the time. But in patients with metabolic syndrome, LDL-C under-predicts 63% of the time.[48]

In an article published in the *American Journal of Cardiology* in 2012, Malave et al.[49] assessed variations in lipoprotein particle concentrations in patients with diabetes with "very low" LDL-C and non-HDL-C levels to elucidate the drivers of cardiovascular risk. They concluded that patients with diabetes exhibited significant variation in LDL particle level, despite attainment of target LDL-C, "suggesting the persistence of potential residual coronary heart disease risk."

We began this chapter by discussing how what we see is affected by what we believe (confirmation bias). We can think of no better example than a study published in the *American Heart Journal*,[50] which tracked 231,986 hospitalizations from 541 hospitals. In this study, it was found that almost half the patients hospitalized with CAD had admission LDL levels <100 mg/dL, with less than 10% having HDL levels ≥60 mg/dL. Rather than concluding that LDL-C has outworn its usefulness as a predictor, the researchers suggest that their study provides "further support for recent guideline revisions with even lower LDL goals and for developing effective treatments to raise HDL."

The single-minded focus on cholesterol—particularly on LDL-C—has outlived its usefulness. Cholesterol is cargo on lipoprotein boats—we need to turn our attention to the boats themselves. The deterioration of lipoproteins, the oxidation of their membranes, the time they spend in the bloodstream, and the functionality of the LDL receptors all deserve careful attention. Heart disease is multifactorial and our preventive efforts should at least include a recognition that there are more sophisticated and useful measures than LDL-C, and that inflammation, oxidative damage, and stress play major—and largely unappreciated—roles in its development. The demonization of saturated fat has turned out to be not just wrong, but counterproductive. It has fostered the widespread belief that the wholesale replacement of saturated fat by (proinflammatory, omega-6-rich) vegetable oils is desirable. This has resulted in an unhealthy ratio of 16:1 omega-6 to omega-3 in the diet, and has contributed mightily to the inflammation, which underlines the atherosclerotic progression.[51]

"Empiricists are those of us who believe what we see, and rationalists are those who see what we believe," wrote the legendary teacher Sidney Baker, MD.[52] "It seems to me that the belief system of modern medicine has become something of a handicap in permitting us to see well."

REFERENCES

1. Chowdhury R, Warnakula S, Kunutsor S et al. Association of dietary, circulating, and supplement fatty acids with coronary risk: A systematic review and meta-analysis. *Ann Intern Med* 2014;160(6):398–406.
2. de Lorgeril M, Renaud S, Mamelle N et al. Mediterranean alpha-linolenic acid-rich diet in secondary prevention of coronary heart disease. *Lancet* 1994;143:1454–1459.
3. Krumholz HM, Seeman TE, Merrill SS et al. Lack of association between cholesterol and coronary heart disease mortality and morbidity and all-cause mortality in persons older than 70 years. *JAMA* 1995;272(17):1335–1340.
4. Castelli WP, Garrison RJ, Wilson PW, Abbott RD, Kalousdian S, Kannel WB. Incidence of coronary heart disease and lipoprotein cholesterol levels. The Framingham Study. *JAMA* 1986;256(20):2835–2838.
5. Castelli WP. Concerning the possibility of a nut. *JAMA* 1992;152(7):1371–1372.
6. Skeaff CM, Miller J. Dietary fat and coronary heart disease: Summary of evidence from prospective cohort and randomised controlled trials. *Ann Nutr Metab* 2009;55:173–201.
7. Mente A. A systematic review of the evidence supporting a causal link between dietary factors and coronary heart disease. Arch Intern Med 2009;169:659–669.
8. Siri-Tarino PW, Sun Q, Hu FB, Krauss RM. Meta-analysis of prospective cohort studies evaluating the association of saturated fat with cardiovascular disease. Am J Clin Nutr 2010;91:535–546.

9. Mozaffarian D, Rimm EB, Herrington DM. Dietary fats, carbohydrate, and progression of coronary atherosclerosis in postmenopausal women. *Am J Clin Nutr* 2004;80:1175–1184.

10. Jakobsen MU, Dethlefsen C, Joensen AM et al. Intake of carbohydrates compared with intake of saturated fatty acids and risk of myocardial infarction: Importance of the glycemic index. *Am J Clin Nutr* 2010;91:1764–1748.

11. Hu F. Are refined carbohydrates worse than saturated fat? *Am J Clin Nutr* 2010;91(6):1541–1542.

12. Kuhn T. *The Structure of Scientific Revolutions*, 4th Ed. Chicago, IL: University of Chicago Press; 2012.

13. Corr LA, Oliver MF. The low fat/low cholesterol diet is ineffective. *Eur Heart J* 1997;18:18–22.

14. Konstantinov I, Mejevoi N, Anichkov N, Nikolai N. Anichkov and his theory of atherosclerosis. *Tex Heart Inst J* 2006;33(4):417–423.

15. Dock W. Research in arteriosclerosis; the first fifty years. *Ann Intern Med* 1958;49:699–705.

16. Libby P. The molecular mechanisms of the thrombotic complications of atherosclerosis. *J Internal Med* 2008;264(5):517–527.

17. Spencer A, Saul AW. Vitamin C and Cardiovascular Disease: A Personal Viewpoint. Orthomolecular Medicine News Service, June 22, 2010 http://orthomolecular.org/resources/omns/v06n20.shtml (accessed March 22, 2014).

18. Simon JA. Vitamin C and cardiovascular disease: A review. *J Am Coll Nutr* 1992;11(2):107–125.

19. Pfister R, Sharp SJ, Luben R, Wareham NJ, Khaw KT. Plasma vitamin C predicts incident heart failure in men and women in European Prospective Investigation into Cancer and Nutrition–Norfolk prospective study. *Am Heart J* 2011;162(2):246–253.

20. Fleming P. *A Short History of Cardiology*. Atlanta, GA: Rodopi B. V. Editions, 1997.

21. Kalm L, Semba R. They starved so that others be better fed: Remembering Ancel Keys and the Minnesota experiment. *J Nutr* 2005;135(6):1347–1352.

22. Keys A (editor). *Seven Countries: A Multivariate Analysis of Death and Coronary Heart Disease*. Cambridge, MA: Harvard University Press; 1980.

23. Tapper R, Zubaida S. *A Taste of Thyme: Culinary Cultures of the Middle East*. London, UK: Tauris Parke Paperbacks; 2001, p. 43.

24. Willett W. *Eat, Drink and Be Healthy: The Harvard Medical School Guide to Healthy Eating*. New York: Fireside.

25. Ornish D. Intensive lifestyle changes for reversal of coronary heart disease. *JAMA* 1998;280(23):2001–2007.

26. Colpo A. The Great Cholesterol Con. Lulu.com, 2006 (republished by www.lulu.com, February 2012).

27. Yerushalmy J, Hilleboe HE. Fat in the diet and mortality from heart disease: A methodologic note. *NY State J Med* 1957;57(14):2343–2354.

28. Yudkin J. Diet and coronary thrombosis. *Lancet* 1957;270(6987):144–152.

29. Sapolsky R. *Why Zebras Don't Get Ulcers*, 2nd Ed. New York: W. H. Freeman, 1998.

30. Sapolsky R. *Stress and Your Body: 24 Lectures*. The Great Courses, The Teaching Company.

31. Keys A. Coronary heart disease in seven countries. *Circulation* 1970;41(1):1–211.

32. Minger D. The truth about Ancel Keys: We've all got it wrong. http://rawfoodsos.com/2011/12/22/the-truth-about-ancel-keys-weve-all-got-it-wrong/ (accessed March 22, 2014).

33. Ravnskov U. *Ignore the Awkward*. Seattle, WA: CreateSpace, 2010.

34. Page IH, Allen EV, Chamberlain FL, Keys A, Stamler J, Stare FL. Dietary fat and its relation to heart attacks and strokes. *Circulation* 1961;23:133–136.

35. Hoenselaar R. Saturated fat and cardiovascular disease: The discrepancy between the scientific literature and dietary advice. *Nutrition* 2012;28(2):118–123.

36. Prospective Studies Collaboration. Blood cholesterol and vascular mortality by age, sex, and blood pressure: A meta-analysis of individual data from 61 prospective studies with 55,000 vascular deaths. *Lancet* 2007;370(9602):1829–1839.

37. Dreon D, Fernstrom HA, Campos H, Blanche P, Williams PT, Krauss RM. Change in dietary saturated fat intake is correlated with change in mass of large low-density-lipoprotein particles in men. *Am J Clin Nutr* 1998;67(5):828–836.

38. Knopp R, Retzlaff B. Saturated fat prevents coronary artery disease? An American paradox. *Am J Clin Nutr* 2004;80(5):1102–1103.

39. Petursson H, Sigurdsson JA, Bengtsson C, Nilsen TI, Getz L. Is the use of cholesterol in mortality risk algorithms in clinical guidelines valid? Ten years prospective data from the Norwegian HUNT 2 study. *J Eval Clin Pract* 2012;18(1):159–168.

40. Holmen J, Midthjell K, Krüger O et al. The Nord-Trondelag Health Study 1995–97 (HUNT 2): Objectives, contents, methods and participation. *Norsk Epidemiologi* 2003;13:19–32.

41. Voight BF, Peloso GM, Orho-Melander M et al. Plasma HDL cholesterol and risk of myocardial infarction: A mendelian randomization study. *Lancet* 2012;380(9841):572–580.
42. Scanu A, Edelstein C. HDL: Bridging past and present with a look at the future. *FASEB* 2008;22(12):4044–4054.
43. Angelo Scanu MD. Interview with *Science Daily*. Some Good Cholesterol Is Actually Bad, Study Shows, December 3, 2008 http://www.sciencedaily.com/releases/2008/12/081201081713.htm (accessed March 22, 2014).
44. The AIM-HIGH investigators. Niacin in patients with low HDL cholesterol levels receiving intensive statin therapy. *N Eng J Med* 2011;365:2255–2267.
45. Schwartz GG, Olsson AG, Abt M et al. Effects of dalcetrapib in patients with a recent acute coronary syndrome. *N Engl J Med* 2012;367:2089–2099.
46. Salonen JT, Salonen R, Seppanen K, Rauramaa R, Tuomilehto J. HDL, HDL2, and HDL3 subfractions, and the risk of acute myocardial infarction. A prospective population study in eastern Finnish men. *Circulation* 1991;85(1):129–139.
47. Cromwell WC, Otvos JD, Keyes MJ et al. LDL particle number and risk of future cardiovascular disease in the Framingham Offspring Study: Implications for LDL management. *J Clin Lipidology* 2007;1(6):583–592.
48. Peter Attia MD. The straight dope on cholesterol—Part VI. http://eatingacademy.com/nutrition/the-straight-dope-on-cholesterol-part-vi (accessed March 22, 2014).
49. Malave H, Castro M, Burkle J et al. Evaluation of low-density lipoprotein particle number distribution in patients with type 2 diabetes mellitus with low-density lipoprotein cholesterol >50 mg/dl and non-high-density lipoprotein cholesterol <80 mg/dl. *Am J of Cardiology* 2012;110(5):662–665.
50. Sachdeva A, Cannon CP, Deedwania PC et al. Lipid levels in patients hospitalized with coronary artery disease: An analysis of 136,905 hospitalizations in Get With The Guidelines. *Am Heart J* 2009;147(1):111–117.
51. Simopoulos AP. Evolutionary aspects of the dietary omega-6:omega-3 fatty acid ratio: Medical implications. *World Review of Nutrition and Dietetics* 2009;100:1–21.
52. Baker S. *Detoxification and Healing*. New Canaan, CT: Keats Publishing; 1997.

2 Fats and Cardiovascular Disease

The Good, the Bad, and the Ugly

Beverly B. Teter

CONTENTS

The heart is one organ in the body that never gets to rest. It must work efficiently every day and all day—or within a few moments we are dead. However, it has to depend on other organs of the body to supply its needs for energy, oxygen, waste disposal, and sometimes exercise. In a sense every organ supports the heart and the heart supports every other organ by delivering the blood supply. The brain has to figure out how to find food, of course, and the eyes and ears also play a roll. The skeleton is essential for protection and support for internal organs and to support movement in the search for food. The intestinal tract has to process the food into a suitable form for efficient use along with the help of the liver. The liver is involved in processing toxins for disposal, making urea from ammonia, making and packaging lipids for transport throughout the body as lipoproteins (LDL, HDL, chylomicrons, etc.) and producing bile acids to aide digestion. The liver also processes fatty acids (FAs) to 3-oxybutyrates and ketone bodies, which can be used by the brain, muscles, kidneys, and the heart to produce more energy in the form of ATP and use less oxygen than if these tissues burned the FAs directly.[1] The lungs have to supply oxygen essential for producing the energy necessary to fuel the heart and all other organs and also for disposing carbon dioxide produced in the process. The kidneys need to clear toxic waste material and maintain appropriate electrolyte and urea levels as well as reabsorb water as needed. It is important to understand the energy needs of the heart to maintain its continuous function from the beginning of life to the end. The beta oxidation of fats in mitochondrial myocytes provides 60%–70% of energy in the heart. Thus, it is essential to have a clear understanding of the nature and basics of FAs as a nutritional strategy in cardiovascular disease.

TYPES OF DIETARY FATS

FATTY ACID-CONTAINING FATS

FAs are usually part of triglycerides (TGs) or phospholipids (PLs) and can be liberated from TGs, diglycerides (DGs), or monoglycerides (MGs) as well as PLs by lipase enzymes. FAs may be saturated (SFAs), monounsaturated (MFAs), or polyunsaturated (PUFAs). The degree of saturation depends on the number of double bonds in the FA carbon chain. The naturally occurring double bonds are in the *cis* confirmation due to the enzymes involved in desaturation. They may have *trans* double bonds from partial hydrogenation by either chemical (industrial) or bacterial (rumen) modification, in which case they may possess unique metabolic activity.

TGs are three FAs per molecule esterified to a glycerol backbone. These are found in animal depot fat and mammalian milks, lipoproteins in animal bodies (HDL, LDL, etc.), sea animals, as well as plant oils. They can be made by most animals and humans from either ingesting fatty acid-containing foods or synthesized from acetate. One of the functions of TG is that of an energy store. When needed, the depot fat can mobilize and provide FAs for energy.

PLs contain two FAs per molecule at the 1 and 2 positions and are found mostly in cell membranes of animals and plants. The third position on the glycerol of a PL molecule is occupied by phosphate. Often, the phosphate is bonded to another compound such as choline. PLs are the major lipids in cell membranes and intercellular membranes. Lung surfactant is di-palmitoyl phosphatidyl choline and is essential for proper lung function. PLs in the membranes of animal foods such as salmon, beef, or liver can provide an appreciable amount of our fatty acid intake and are rich in essential fatty acids (EFAs). EFAs need to be consumed in the diet as our body cannot make them. They can be modified once consumed, but the initial structure must be consumed as either omega-6 or omega-3 FAs usually attached to PLs.

Cholesterol esters (CEs) are a combination of one cholesterol molecule with one fatty acid. Cholesterol and other sterols from plants are usually present as an FA ester, often with PUFA as the FA. Cholesterol and its esters play a major role in maintaining the proper membrane fluidity for both cell membranes and the intercellular organelles such as mitochondria, endoplasmic reticulum (ER), and so on. Cholesterol is a precursor for CEs, bile salts, testosterone, β-estradiol, and 1,25-dihydroxyvitamin D_3.

To utilize the energy from the above lipid classes, the FAs need to be separated from the lipid molecule by various lipases. They are then converted to ketone bodies, mostly by the liver, and either used in situ or transported to tissues via the circulatory system.

TYPES OF FATTY ACIDS

FAs can be classified in several ways—by degree of saturation, by chain length, by position of the double bonds, and by metabolic functions. The SFAs have no double bonds. Their chain length is usually 4- to 18-carbon long but some of the waxes are much longer. The MFAs have one double bond, often at the Δ9 position of the carbon chain. The PUFAs have multiple double bonds mostly depending on their chain length. The most prevalent PUFA pattern of unsaturation is -C=C-C-C=C-, which is called methylene-interrupted double bonds.

Another class of FAs is the conjugated fatty acids (CLA). They have double bonds with a different pattern of unsaturation. Most are 18 or perhaps more carbons with two double bonds in the -C-C=C-C=C- configuration. Because of the preponderance of 18 carbon chain lengths, these FAs are called conjugated linoleic acid. They have unique properties depending on the carbon positions of the double bonds. The 9c, 11t—CLA has a *cis* bond at the 9th position and a *trans* bond at the 11th position of the chain. This isomer is very anticarcinogenic[2] and found in adequate quantities in full-fat cow's milk. It is enzymatically made in the rumen from the linoleic acid in the feed fed the cows. However, a CLA with the double bonds in the t10 and c-12 position, known as t-10, c-12-CLA, is pro-tumorogenic[3] and causes fatty liver in animals, and body weight loss just by shifting the position of the bonds and geometric configuration.

POLYUNSATURATED FATTY ACIDS

Omega-3 Fatty Acids

One group of PUFA is called omega-3 FAs. They can occur in TGs, CEs or PLs as well as free fatty acids (FFAs). They have a double bond at the n-3-position in the fatty acid chain. This is three carbons from the methyl end of the long-chain FAs. Since FAs are elongated from the carboxyl end of the chain, once established the double bond does not move during elongation and further desaturation. The prostaglandins and leukotrienes formed from these FAs are generally thought to be anti-inflammatory as opposed to the omega-6 FAs found in abundance in vegetable oils. The most abundant source of the omega-3 FAs is in fish oil from cold-water fish. They act as "antifreeze" for the fish because the long-chain omega-3s have very low melting points in the −11°C to −50°C range depending on the number of double bonds. Some melting points have not been determined. This means that they are fluid even at extreme temperatures despite having 20–24 or more carbons in their carbon chains. This confers fluidity to the cell membranes and allows proteins (enzymes) to assume their "favored" shapes for optimal activity. It is especially helpful for the cold-water fish and mammals that exist in extremely cold waters.

There is abundant evidence that the omega-3s are protective for heart diseases. This work was first done with northern Eskimos who have very low rates of heart disease on their normal diets.[4,5] Since this early work, there have been numerous studies that confirm the beneficial effects of omega-3s. The blood levels in patients are easily measured by a finger-stick sample mailed to labs for analysis. The fish or algal sources of these FAs are better to raise blood levels as the omega-3 FAs from plant sources are generally only 18 carbons long, thus the body needs to elongate and further desaturate them to the useful 20 to 24+ chain lengths. Some people, especially infants and elderly, cannot do this effectively if their liver enzymes are compromised. This lack of ability to elongate and desaturate is the reason that cats are obligatory carnivores, they need the omega-3s from their prey.

A recent research report[6] indicates that EPA (eicosapentaenoic acid) compared to other omega-3 FAs has a dramatic effect on cell metabolism. They studied the effects in THP-1 cells (a human leukemia cell line) when different oils were provided to the cultures to study various aspects of an oil rich in EPA on gene expression and activation of nuclear receptors. The EPA oil altered the expression of several genes including stearoyl-CoA-desaturase (SCD) and FA desaturase-1 and FA desaturase-2 (FASDS-1 and FASDS-2). The other omega-3s also resulted in altered gene expression for subsets of genes involved in lipid metabolism and inflammation. The EPA activated human peroxisome-proliferator-activated-receptor α (PPARα) and also PPARβ had minimal effects on PPARγ, liver-X-receptor, retinoid-X-receptor, Farnesoid-X-receptor, and retinoid-acid-receptor γ (RARγ). When the cultured cells were "fed" with serum from humans fed diets supplemented with oils using olive oil as the control and DHA and two levels of EPA as test supplements, the expression of SCD and FADS-2 in the cells treated with serum from omega-3-supplemented individuals was decreased. The authors conclude that the regulation of gene expression in the individuals treated with EPA is consistent with treating aspects of dyslipidemia and inflammation. These two conditions are considered risk factors for coronary heart disease (CHD).

Omega-6 Fatty Acids

Another grouping of PUFAs is the omega-6 group. In this group, the first double bond from the methyl end of the FA is in the omega-6 position. They also have additional double bonds in other positions of the carbon chain. The longer the chain, the more unsaturated the molecule is. This type of FA is found in large amounts in most dietary vegetable oils except olive oil, which is very rich in oleic acid. This family of FA can lead to more inflammation than the omega-3 version. The downstream metabolites formed such as leukotrienes, prostaglandins, and so on are often involved with inflammation. In the mid-1970s, it was discovered that linoleic acid was able to suppress the stimulation of the immune system by antigens and even more suppression was observed with the prostaglandins that were produced from the omega-6 FAs.[7]

In 1944 and 1946, Miller studied the effects of different dietary fats on the development of hepatomas. Rats were fed one of the following fats, and DMB (*p*-dimethylaminoazo-benzene)-induced tumor incidence was reported. The following fats were fed at 5% of the diet: corn oil, hydrogenated coconut oil (HCO), coconut oil (CO), trilaurin, or corn oil–HCO [4:1]. Rats fed corn oil or corn oil–HCO [4:1] exhibited the highest level of hepatomas. For the second study, the rats were fed 5% corn or olive oil, and either 20% corn oil, lard, or Crisco. The effects on DAB-induced hepatomas were studied. The animals fed corn oil or corn oil–HCO exhibited the highest levels of hepatomas.[8] The second study provided 5% corn or olive oil and 20% corn oil, lard, or Crisco to DAB-induced rats. Hepatomas observed at the 5% level of fat after 4 months were 73% for corn and 13% for olive oil. At the 20% level, the incidence of hepatomas was corn oil 100%, lard 60%, and Crisco 47%. The animals on a fat-free diet had 8% hepatomas, but displayed EFA deficiency.[9]

High omega-6 dietary oils have been used to suppress the immune system after kidney transplants. Unfortunately, these FAs are also associated with promoting tumor growth, possibly by damping down the body's immune system. This may happen due to oxidation and formation of peroxides. Another effect could be that they provide the PUFAs necessary for rapid growth of tumor cells that have to make cell walls and intracellular organelles such as mitochondria to provide energy for rapid growth. Cancer cells cannot live on fat or ketones. They have an absolute requirement for glucose to produce energy.

The omega-6 FAs are EFAs but are needed only in small amounts. The U.S. diet is overloaded with omega-6 FAs and undernourished with omega-3 FAs.

MONOUNSATURATED FATTY ACIDS

The monounsaturated fatty acids (MFAs) have intermediate properties between the PUFAs and SFAs. For the same chain length, i.e., 18 carbons, they have an intermediate melting point—stearate (18:0), the saturated 18-carbon fatty acid melts at 69.6°C; oleate (18:1Δ9cis) melts at 10.5°C, linoleic (all cis 9,12–18:2) melts at −8.0°C; while α-linolenic (18:3 all, cis 9,12,15) melts at −11°C. The melting points for the comparable FAs with the double bonds in the *trans* configuration would be −18:1t = 45°C; 18:2tt = 26.5°C. The reason for differences in metabolic action of the *trans* and *cis* isomers of FAs has been elusive. Dietary trans fatty acids (tFAs) are generally a mixture of isomers, which makes identifying the effect of any single isomer difficult.

A recent work using cultured macrophages studied the individual effects of *trans*-9 18:1 (elaidic acid) and *cis*-9 18:1 (oleic acid) in tissue culture where the conditions are controlled.[10] They observed that the *trans* isomer, elaidic acid, stabilized the macrophage ABCA1 (ATP-binding cassette transporter A1) protein levels compared to the *cis* isomer. This transporter is the rate-limiting step initiating apolipoprotein A-1 lipidation. The mechanism responsible for the different effects of oleic and elaidic acids on ABCA1 levels was due to protein degradation in cells treated with oleic acid. Thus, these two isomers, which differed only by the configuration of the double bond, caused different metabolic effects.

The most popular oleic-MFA is olive oil, which is considered the most representative food of the traditional Mediterranean diet. Observational studies from Mediterranean cohorts have suggested that dietary MFA are protective against not only cardiovascular disease but also age-related cognitive decline and Alzheimer's disease.[11] Although high-oleic safflower oil and sunflower oil have a predominance of monounsaturated fats, the most popular culinary and medicinal oil is olive oil, as the Mediterranean diet utilizing olive oil has been shown to improve cardiovascular risk, blood pressure, endothelial dysfunction, oxidative stress, and lipid profiles.[11]

Saturated Fatty Acids: A Controversial Subject

Saturated fatty acids (SFAs) are the end product of the synthesis of fat by human and animal bodies. FA synthesis takes place in the cytosol of the cells. Any food consumed that is not used immediately for energy is converted to fat to be stored until needed. The excess food is converted to acetyl-CoA in the mitochondria and sent to the cytosol where the FAs are made by the endoplasmic reticulum. The storage form is as TGs and the depot is adipose tissue. Saturated fat is only oxidized by appropriate enzymes used in the process of making ATP from the carbon chain of the FA or by being converted to ketone bodies that are the major energy source for most of the essential organs in the body, i.e., liver, kidney (except the medulla), and heart. The SFAs do not form ROS (reactive oxygen species) as do the unsaturated fatty acids. The more double bonds, the more ROSs can be formed. The liver makes ketones to send out to the rest of the body. Many organs can make them if necessary. During times of stress or low blood sugar, all the tissues of the body can convert to a ketone metabolism. Ketones are the most efficient substrate with which the body makes energy (see "Ketone Bodies").

After World War II, laws were passed that margarine could be colored to look like butter. During the war, butter was being shipped to the troops, and margarine for stateside consumption was white like shortening with a "color bubble" inside the plastic bag that could be broken and mixed to give it color. The dairy industry had lost its edge as the only table spread! To increase sales of margarine, it was packaged as "sticks of butter" and advertising campaigns were launched. The hydrogenation process had been developed to the point that margarine could be made to be soft and sold as a spread or to be made "hard" to be used as butter, or made in-between to be used as shortening. About the same time, the Diet/Heart Hypothesis was developed. This hypothesis was that saturated fat was unhealthy and the unsaturated fats were good for your health. The background for this is described in a book by Gary Taubes.[12] Consequently, consumption of all fats deemed to be saturated were discouraged and the newly available hydrogenated *trans* FA products (which were not saturated) were encouraged to be consumed. Vegetable oils replaced lard and tallow in many foods and especially in the fast-food market because of the low price. No one paid attention to the fact that lard and olive oil have very similar FA compositions! Thus, vegetable oils became good and animal fat (butter, lard, tallow, meat fat) became "bad." The historical fats had not changed but their perception had certainly changed.

Dr. Van Itallie in 1957[13] stated "Now, it is no longer possible to ignore the fact that under certain dietary conditions the serum cholesterol can be strikingly lowered by increasing the proportion of fat in the diet. Accordingly, the postulate relating quantity of fat intake to serum cholesterol level has had to be drastically revised."

The discussion of the roles of dietary saturated fat is still ongoing. Yamagishi et al.[14] report that increasing the saturated fat in the diets of two cohorts in Japan yielded mixed results. Cohort I was 45–64 years old in 1995 and followed until 2009. Cohort II was aged 45–74 in 1998 and followed until 2007. The total number of subjects was 38,084 men and 43,847 women. They found "inverse" associations between SFAs and total stroke ($p = .002$); intraparenchymal hemorrhage (p for trend = .005); ischemic stroke ($p = .08$); deep intraparenchymal hemorrhage (p for trend = .04); lacunar infarction ($p = .02$). They found a positive association between SFA intake and myocardial infarction (MI) ($p = .046$) but no association between SFA intake and incidence of subarachnoid hemorrhage or sudden cardiac death. Two other meta-analyses suggest that greater dietary SFA intake may not be associated with increased risk of coronary disease.[15,16] An article from the Harvard School of Public health[17] concludes the TC:HDL-C (total cholesterol to high density lipoprotein-cholesterol) ratio is nonsignificantly changed by consumption of myristic or palmitic acid and nonsignificantly decreased by stearic acid but significantly decreased by lauric acid (found in CO). In addition, replacing SFAs with carbohydrate has no effect and replacing it with monounsaturated fat has uncertain effects. An additional meta-analysis which concentrated on dairy foods, long thought to be a "bad" source of saturated fat, and the incidence of vascular disease and type 2 diabetes[18] concluded that "there appears to be an enormous mismatch between the evidence from long-term prospective studies and perceptions of harm from the consumption of dairy food items. This was based on the results of their meta-analysis that showed a reduction in risk in the subjects with the highest dairy intake compared to the lowest intake of 0.87 in all-cause deaths; 0.92 for ischemic heart disease; 0.79 for stroke; and 0.85 for incident diabetes. Thus we are back to Van Itallie's 1957 conclusion, now 57 years old.

ENERGY SUBSTRATES

FATTY ACIDS

Normally, all body cells can convert fatty acids into energy for their own use. However, some tissues prefer ketone bodies for energy (see "Energy Preferences of Tissues"). When one molecule of a 16-carbon saturated fatty acid (palmitic acid) is converted to energy, 106 ATPs are created—as 2 ATPs are used to form the palmitoyl CoA. However, when one molecule of glucose is converted to CO_2 and water, only 32 ATPs are produced. If these calculations are corrected for the number of glucose carbons involved, then the total for 16 carbons is 85 ATP which is less than 80% of the ATP yield of the 16-carbon FA. This difference derives from the fact that glucose is already partially oxidized. As an additional bonus, 123 water molecules are formed for every molecule of palmitoyl CoA oxidized. When a PUFA such as linoleate is converted to energy, two additional enzymes are needed and even more ATPs are lost. Thus, the more unsaturated a fat is, the less energy can be produced relative to the chain length. In case of severe exercise or in early starvation, the muscle cells can make their own energy but at an expense. The longer the chain length of the FA, the more ATP can be made; however, it will cost the cell more oxygen and enzymes. SFAs yield the highest energy for the length of the carbon chain. The yield of high-energy phosphate (ATP) from fatty acid oxidation is more from SFAs than from unsaturated fatty acids.

Hummingbirds are a prime example of the use of fat for energy. The ruby-throated hummingbird summers and breeds along the east coast from New England south and winters in the West Indies. They fly nonstop over water for a distance of about 2400 km at a velocity of about 40 km/hour for 60 hours or so. No protein is degraded during the flight so that their fat conversion to ketones must be rapid. They have very large fat stores that fuel such long flights. Oxidation of the fat provides water (123 water molecules for every molecule of palmitoyl CoA that is oxidized while they fly over salty ocean water on their flight). The nonmigrating birds do not have such large body fat stores. Another animal benefitting from a large fat store is the camel; the hump(s) provides energy and water for long desert trips.

An additional benefit of saturated fatty acids as an energy source is that they are, by nature, anhydrous. This allows them to be stored as "pure" energy and not be associated with water as are sugars and other carbohydrates. Ronald Amundsen, the Antarctic explorer, preferred a fat energy source over a carbohydrate one as they had to carry all their calories for the 1500-mile-round trip to the South Pole. As mentioned above it also provided them with fresh (warm) water.

TISSUE DIFFERENCES FOR PREFERRED SUBSTRATES FOR ENERGY

Kidney, liver, and heart use ketones as their preferred fuel even with high blood glucose levels. FAs can be utilized to make ketones on site in normal cells, but the liver generally makes ketones for the heart and other tissues. The liver is a large organ and has a good oxygenated blood supply.

When consuming a ketogenic diet, the liver makes ketones from the dietary fats consumed and sends them out to all other tissues of the body. This process has several beneficial effects. Liver has large blood supply that carries oxygenated blood. The oxygen required for making ketones is readily available in the liver and spares other tissues with a less oxygenated blood supply. Thus, when the ketones arrive at the peripheral tissues, they are ready to use and can pass through the cell membrane and into the mitochondria without carriers, insulin, oxygen, or any need to be modified for use by the mitochondria to be converted to energy. Furthermore, there are no waste products to be disposed of by the cells. All body tissues are capable of converting to a "ketone economy" within a few days of becoming ketonic. The brain can change in a few days but takes a little longer to completely adapt. Because ketones "burn" to carbon dioxide and water, the body actually produces metabolic water when using ketones for energy. The hump on a camel is fat to provide metabolic water when on long trips in the dessert. Marathon runners maintaining a ketogenic diet find that they do not "hit the wall" as severely as runners practicing carbohydrate loading (personal communication).

Historically, about 40%–45% cal of the U.S. diet came from fats. Recently, the low-fat diets recommended less than 30% from fat. Thus, since protein stays the same, the carbohydrate proportion increased to over 40% cal. It is questionable how effective these diets are since from 30% to 50% of the carbohydrates consumed at each meal is converted to TGs for energy.[19]

All body organs can convert to a ketone economy. Most are converted in about 3 days after starting a high-fat, ketogenic diet. The brain takes a few days longer to totally convert, but within 3 days is functioning well. The marathon runners maintaining a ketogenic diet claim that they do not have the problems of confusion, etc. during a long run, even the 100-mile runs. They also claim that their recovery time is shorter than when they were on a high-carbohydrate intake. The body cannot store excess sugars or other carbohydrates. Carbohydrates are converted to TGs to prevent damage from high glucose levels. High blood sugar levels are the cause of most of the diabetic side effects that cause disabilities in diabetes type 2 (DM2) patients, many of which are caused by inflammation induced by the sugars.

ENERGY PREFERENCES OF TISSUES

The myocardium preferentially uses FAs for energy under normal physiological conditions. However, it can efficiently use ketones as the energy substrate under ketotic conditions.[20] Under conditions of starvation or a chronic ketogenic diet, ketone bodies, lactate, amino acids, or acetate can be utilized to produce ATP in the heart mitochondria. Multiple energy sources ensure the continued functioning of this vital organ.

As discussed above, the preferred energy substrates and metabolic patterns of the brain, skeletal muscle, cardiac muscle, adipose tissues, and liver are all different and organ specific. Glucose is the preferred fuel for the brain in normal, well-fed people in today's U.S. population on high carbohydrate diets. However, it requires insulin to be able to cross the blood–brain barrier. Recently, there has been a report of diabetes—Type 3—diabetes of the brain. If brain insulin is low, the sugars cannot enter and conditions like Alzheimer's may develop. Many normal people who have switched to a ketogenic diet (one high in fat) report that they feel much better and seem to be thinking more clearly. During starvation or low blood sugar states, ketone bodies, especially, acetoacetate and 3-hydroxybutyrate become the main fuel for the brain. It has been estimated that after 3 days of low blood sugar, the brain gets 25% of its energy from ketone bodies and after 40 days about 70%.[21] At the beginning of starvation, the brain does not burn ketones as they are an important substrate for lipid synthesis in the brain. Other tissues can use fatty acids, protein, etc. Skeletal muscle can use glucose, fatty acids, and ketone bodies as fuel depending on the need at the time. At the beginning of exercise, and for short "spurts" of energy, the preferred fuel is glucose. Muscle is able to make glycogen as a fuel reserve for its own needs. However, a limited amount of glycogen can be stored within the muscle. The glucose in skeletal muscle is converted to pyruvate with the production of 2 ATPs made available for energy. The pyruvate is then converted to lactate and sent back to the liver where the lactate is converted back to pyruvate and with the addition of six phosphates converted back to glucose to go back to the peripheral muscles. These transformations are called the Cori cycle. This cycle shifts part of the metabolic energy burden back to the liver. After the first few minutes of heavy exercise, the ketones and fatty acids become the main energy source as they can be stored near the muscle cells and are more efficiently utilized. Marathon runners perform better on a ketogenic diet and recover quicker than on a high carbohydrate diet. The heart muscle generally runs on ketones provided by the liver because it needs a constant energy supply every day. The adipose tissue makes and stores TG from glucose delivered to it when insulin is high and releases the TG fatty acids when insulin drops. The liver is multifunctional to support other organs. It can make and mobilize glycogen to provide other organs. It also can perform gluconeogenesis to provide glucose to other organs. It can synthesize very low-density lipoproteins (VLDL) to send TGs to the adipose for storage. In the fasting state, these stored TGs are sent back to the liver to be converted to ketones. All these varied functions are integrated by hormones and metabolic signals in a ballet of sorts.

KETONE BODIES

What Are Ketone Bodies?

Ketone bodies are fuel molecules formed from fatty acids. They are molecules containing carbon, oxygen, and hydrogen. They are not particles, as the name suggests, but just small molecules. The shorter-chain FAs (butyric, capric, caprylic, decanoic, and lauric) are more easily converted to ketone bodies. However, the longer chain ones (palmitic16:0 to ~ 20:0) can also be converted. Coconut oil which has about 50% shorter-chain FAs is a good source for ketone production. The longer-chain unsaturated and polyunsaturated FAs do not yield as much energy per carbon as the saturated FAs. The ketones are carried dissolved in the blood plasma and pass directly into the cells through the cell membrane and into the mitochondria where they are converted to ATP—the energy currency of the cells.

The three main ketones produced in the mitochondria are acetone, acetoacetic acid, and β-hydroxybutyric acid. (Figure 2.1) Acetone is a three-carbon ketone derived from sequential oxidation of longer chain FAs. Acetic acid is metabolized to acetone, but in very small amounts. Sometimes, it can be detected from the breath of people doing a very long fast. Acetoacetic acid is a true ketone but beta-hydroxybutyric acid is actually a small carboxylic acid but acts like a ketone for combustion. Kidneys usually make their own ketones as they require them for energy. The liver provides most of the other ketones for itself and the heart. The heart can process fatty acids to make its own energy, but when necessary, the liver will provide ketones for the heart and the rest of the body.[20]

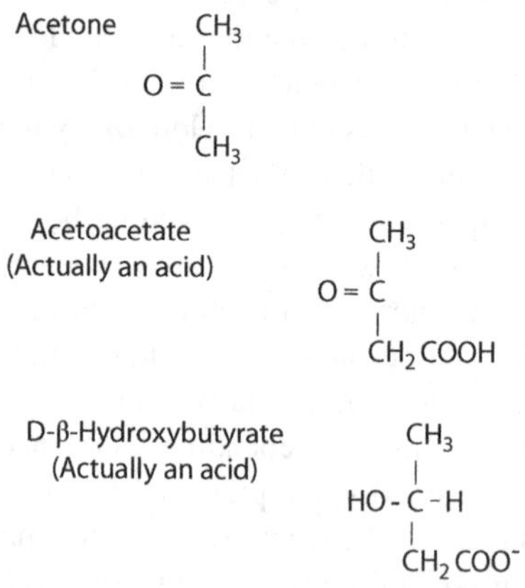

FIGURE 2.1   Ketone bodies.

When needed, the liver can supply the water-soluble ketones through the blood to other tissues that use the acetoacetate and beta-hydroxybutyrate, which can be converted quickly to acetyl-CoA to produce energy, using the citric acid cycle. Individual tissues have the capacity to produce ketones but it takes a few days of a ketogenic diet for the other tissues to convert to a ketone metabolic currency. The brain takes a few days and up to 2 or 3 weeks to completely adjust to ketosis. Prehistorically, the brain may have always used ketones but with the present-day diets being consumed it usually runs on glucose. A condition commonly called "diabetes type 3" has been identified in which the brain insulin is too low to process adequate glucose for the needed energy of the brain.[22] In diseases such as Alzheimer's, ALS, and Parkinson's, a ketogenic diet may be useful. It is interesting to note that the three major organs necessary to maintain life—kidney, liver, and heart all use ketone as their main energy source. Glucose levels can change rapidly during the day but ketones are more constant and do not depend on regular meals for substrate, because depot fat is constantly available.

Ketone bodies are formed when the glucose levels in the body become low. This can happen when the blood sugar becomes low due to low food intake, starvation, heavy exercise, or ingestion of a ketogenic diet (a diet with more fat than glucose). Ketosis, due to the ingestion of a ketogenic diet, is not to be confused with ketoacidosis, which is the result of uncontrolled diabetes and a dangerous medical emergency. Ketoacidosis is caused by excessive blood glucose and insufficient insulin to lower it, which tends to dehydrate the tissues. In the presence of low insulin, the adipose tissue can release FAs to the liver to form ketones for energy production. As ketone bodies accumulate, the pH of the blood drops and causes an acidic condition in the presence of ketones—ketoacidosis. The presence of high ketones and high blood sugar overwhelms the system and coma and often death occur. This is a medical emergency.

The ketotic state is a natural event when the diet is low in carbohydrates, including sugar. It occurs when the body runs out of glucose reserves and is forced to make ketone molecules from the fat reserves to use as fuel. Some people think that *ketosis* was the normal state for humans historically. Until grain crops were farmed, grazing was the normal way to obtain food, not gorging as we do now. Depending on the area of the world, most people would find a few seeds, nuts, and fruits as they traveled rather large distances. If hunting was good, they may share a "kill" with the tribe but then go back to grazing. There was likely very little obesity.

Some researchers refer to ketones as "high-octane fuel" compared to carbohydrates. They provide more energy to the cells because they have a higher energy of combustion, so each molecule can provide more energy. Second, they burn "clean" to carbon dioxide and water with no nitrogenous or other waste. Third, they require less oxygen per unit of energy (ATP). The ketone currency for energy also modifies the well-being of the cells by decreasing the generation of free radicals in the cells and increasing the concentration of glutathione in normal cells, which adds to their ability to neutralize free radicals from endogenous sources, chemotherapy, radiation, AGEs, and so on.

In addition, mutated cancer cells have an absolute requirement for glucose for energy, and a ketotic state denies them of their energy source.

AMINO ACIDS AND PROTEINS

Proteins and amino acids are not generally used for energy. In late stages of starvation, proteins begin to be used for energy. All known enzymes are proteins. They enhance reaction rates by as much as a million fold or more compared to simple chemical transformations. This is probably the reason they are not sacrificed to make energy, which also requires several enzymes to convert from CHO or fat to energy. There are also carrier proteins that help transport compounds around in the blood and aide in transporting molecules across cell membranes. Some of the compounds transported are oxygen (transported by hemoglobin in blood and myoglobin in muscle). Iron is transported by transferrin. Immune antibodies are proteins produced to defend against specific viruses and bacteria as well as other foreign substances. Proteins are involved in the generation and transport of nerve impulses, and control of growth and differentiation of cells. The metabolic adaptations during starvation are made to minimize protein degradation. Ketone bodies are formed from fat, and glucose is decreased as body stores are used up. After about 30 days of starvation, the body begins to use its own protein for energy, but it is near the end since protein in the diaphragm and other essential muscles are used up, and this causes death.

SHORT HISTORY LESSON

Beginning in the 1950s, the public was taught that dietary fat is responsible for the "epidemic" of heart disease. This became known as the "Diet-Heart Hypothesis." It was never proven and significantly altered the U.S. diet by promoting reduced intake of all dietary fat and decreased saturated fat with an increase in polyunsaturated vegetable oils. Despite all the advice and with many people adhering to such a diet, the "epidemic" was not significantly slowed. In the 1980s, there was a large campaign to severely decrease the total fat and especially the saturated fat in the diet. This advice led to the "obesity epidemic" after 1980 (Figure 2.2). By 1980, the *trans* fatty acid content of the U.S. diet had just about peaked and natural fats such as animal, dairy, and so on were greatly decreased compared to the 1930s and 1940s. The "healthy" vegetable oils were greatly increased due to the decrease in butter and meat fat consumption. The CHD deaths were not decreased, however. The so-called "epidemic" of CHD may not ever have been an epidemic because the ability to identify CHD early and definitively was greatly increased during these same years. Diagnostic techniques and treatments were better and more available. However, the incidence continued to be elevated and there was no evidence of abatement despite improved treatments and surgeries.

During the period from 1980 to about 2012, the recommended diets were very high in carbohydrates and low in fat, especially natural fats. The U.S. protein consumption has not changed since 1900 and remains at about 20% of the calories. Thus, if fat intake is lowered, the carbohydrate intake will increase. The diets recommended very low fat intake (20%–30% of calories), which left 50% to 60% cal of carbohydrate (CHO). The form of the CHO determines the speed with which it is converted to sugar not the end product. Sugars are the end product of the digestion of sugar, flours, grains, whole grains, fiber, and so on. When CHOs are digested, the body sees a sugar—usually glucose. But with fruit ingestion, it may see fructose, especially with sweetened soft drinks and other products where fructose is used instead of glucose. The glucose signals the pancreas to secrete insulin, which stimulates the body to store glucose. The liver and adipose cannot store too

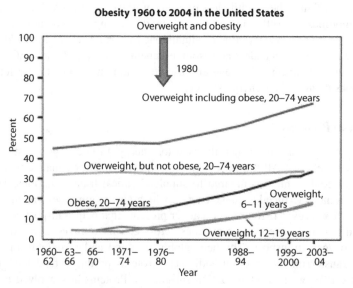

FIGURE 2.2 Obesity data from the CDC.

much sugar or glycogen, so the liver makes TGs out of the sugars. It also cannot store too much TG because it causes non-alcoholic fatty liver disease (NAFL). Therefore, it makes low-density lipoprotein (LDL) to ship the TG out to the body to use as energy. To make the LDL, it needs not only TG but also cholesterol, so it makes cholesterol to be able to assemble the LDL to ship the components to the rest of the body. Meanwhile, the adipose tissue is making fat from glucose that goes directly to the adipose tissue where it is stored as TG for future use. However, with the high-CHO diet, the blood sugar seldom gets low enough to allow the insulin levels to decrease to the point that the TG can leave the depot fat to supply energy to the rest of the body. Thus we are seeing the "obesity" epidemic (Figure 2.2).

Fructose has been linked to cardiovascular and DM2 risk factors in teens. A study in teenagers found that the ones who consumed higher levels of fructose had a higher risk of cardiovascular problems than their peers that consumed less. In addition. they had increased visceral adiposity, an additional risk factor for CVD as well as diabetes.[23] Fructose is the major sweetener used in processed foods and drinks. The adolescents consuming higher levels of fructose displayed higher levels of risk factors associated with CVD and DM2 including increased systolic blood pressure, TG, LDL-cholesterol, inflammatory markers, and glucose intolerance. The authors cite a relationship between abdominal fat and fructose consumption. This fat pad is metabolically different than the subcutaneous adipose tissue in thighs and legs. When the measure of visceral adiposity was added to the statistical equation, the relationships strengthened, indicating a strong relationship with the adiposity. Because of this relationship, the author suggests that fructose may promote visceral fat accumulation. This fat pad surrounds the abdominal organs and can release factors associated with CVD as well as insulin resistance and inflammatory disease. The relationship was evident in subjects as young as 14–18 years old. This observation is consistent with the "obesity" epidemic in young children since the 1980s (Figure 2.2).

To compound the heart disease problem, the levels of tFAs were at their highest during this time (~1980+) until the labeling laws took effect and partially hydrogenated oils were decreased in the diet. The combination of the industrially produced tFAs and the obesity epidemic compounded the problems for heart disease. The isomers of tFAs formed naturally in the rumen of cattle, cows, sheep, and goats are very different from the industrially formed ones. The shapes of the molecules, their melting points, and metabolic effects are very different. The industrially formed isomers are randomly formed based on the temperature and pressure of the reaction used to introduce the hydrogen into the double bonds of the FA. However, the tFAs formed by the rumen organisms of the animals are directed by enzymes that have specific requirements for where they will introduce the *trans* double bond. The main tFAs formed is *trans*-vaccenic acid, which has the *trans* bond at the number 11 position of the 18-carbon FA. This isomer does not depress milk fat production and can be formed in our bodies into the 9c,11t- CLA (conjugated linoleic acid), which is a powerful anticarcinogen.[2] The other isomers present are in much smaller amounts and their effects are not known yet. However, the industrially formed CLA isomers are rich in 10t, 12c-CLA, which is toxic to the liver and some reproductive processes as well as pro-carcinogenic for mammary cancer by accelerating mammary tumorigenesis and stimulating lung metastasis in a mouse model.[3] Also the *trans*-10 monene is the major one produced when the hydrogenation proceeds longer. The *trans*-10 isomer, significantly ($p < .003$), depresses milk fat in lactating mice as does trans-9 ($p < .01$) and vegetable shortening ($p < .002$) which is a mixture of isomers (unpublished data by this author). Another problem with the TFAs is that during the hydrogenation process, most of the EFAs are destroyed by being totally hydrogenated or modified by creating *trans* double bonds that are not effective EFAs.

Chemically made trans FAs (tFAi) have been shown to be related to heart disease. Mensik and Katan published one of the first studies in 1990. They demonstrated that increased consumption of tFAi increased the occurrence of heart disease in their study group.[24] The USDA[25,26] studies that followed confirmed many of the changes noted by Katan et al. More recently, Mozaffarian et al.[27] reported that tFAi consumption adversely affects CHD risk factors as well as increased the risk of

CHD. Deleterious effects of tFA consumption include increased LDL-C levels, decreased HDL-C levels, impairment of insulin sensitivity in the presence of insulin resistance, pro-inflammatory effects, endothelial dysfunction, aberrant PPARg responses, and decreased synthesis of milk fat in nursing mothers.

An article published in JAMA[28] cites evidence that the CVD rates as well as the risk factors have decreased because of the effect of trans fat labeling. This is consistent with the original article published by Mensik and Katan[24] that the commercial tFAs in the U.S. and European food supply were not beneficial for heart disease. A study conducted by the USDA has reported that their saturated fat test diet significantly lowered Lp(a)[25] (lipoprotein(a), a highly inflammatory small-particle LDL with a disulfide bridge). But a subset, with initially high levels of Lp(a) (>30 mg/dL), when consuming chemically produced tFAs, responded to the high *trans* diet with a 5% increase in Lp(a). In a later study,[26] they found that C-reactive protein (CRP) concentrations were higher after consuming a *trans* fat-containing diet than after a carbohydrate rich diet. The E-selectin concentrations were higher after the TFA diet than after the CHO or SFA diets.

The FDA estimated the average U.S. consumption of tFAi has decreased from about 4.6 g/person/ day in the late 1990s to 1.3 g/person/d in 2010. This amount is about 28% of the earlier intake. Vesper et al.[29] measured a 50% decrease in tFAi. Part of this discrepancy could be that if a product has 0.49 g/serving of tFAs, it can be labeled as "trans" is zero. Combined with the reduction in serving sizes to allow "zero trans" labeling, a person could eat nearly a gram of tFA by eating two servings and not be aware that they ate any tFA. Blood levels probably are a better estimate as they reflect actual consumption.

NUCLEAR RECEPTOR TRANSCRIPTION FACTORS AND CO-ACTIVATORS

Peroxisome Proliferator-Activated Receptors

To understand the impact of certain fatty acids on the metabolism and effects of different types of fatty acids, it is necessary to have a basic understanding of the peroxisome proliferator-activated receptors (PPARs) and their functions. The *PPARs are nuclear messengers responsible for the translation of nutritional, pharmacological, and metabolic stimuli into changes in the expression of genes involved in lipid metabolism.* PPARs are members of the nuclear hormone receptor superfamily that are activated by natural FAs and some xenobiotics and drug ligands. They are primarily involved in lipid metabolism by regulating the genes involved but also are involved in adipocyte differentiation. Their name is derived from the first member of the family now called PPARα, which responds to various compounds that induce peroxisome proliferation. Dietary tFAs are one of these compounds. The other PPARs do not do this. There are three PPARs (α, Δ, and γ), which have specific expression patterns in different tissues and cell types.

The PPARα increases fatty acid oxidation; the PPARγ decreases fatty acid oxidation and leads to storage; and PPARβ has poorly defined roles.

EPIDEMIOLOGY

Most commonly used animal models tend to have high HDL-C compared to humans and very low LDL-C. Hamsters are an exception to this generalization and carry most of the dietary fat in the LDL-C fraction of lipoproteins.[30] In the case of rabbits and other herbivores, they have never eaten cholesterol, so probably do not have the metabolic systems to effectively deal with it. In addition, it is very likely that the cholesterol added to the experimental diets is oxidized in the process of formulating the diets, and in storage, because it is unprotected while on the reagent shelf. The cholesterol consumed by humans is integral to the tissue cells or milk of the animals consumed, which conveys a certain degree of protection from oxidation. There seems to be a general consensus among researchers that the pig is the best model for human coronary and circulatory studies, but they are more expensive and difficult to use. Consequently, most research has been done with laboratory animals. In light of the above considerations, several large-scale human studies have been and are being conducted. The Framingham Study is probably the oldest and is still yielding multigenerational data collected from human subjects. There are numerous others that have looked at specific questions about diet, exercise, dietary fats, lifestyles, and genetic makeup as well as ethnic comparisons.

SUMMARY: THE ROLE OF INFLAMMATION AND CARDIOVASCULAR DISEASE

There is increasing evidence that dietary cholesterol is not the "cause" of CHD. It is most likely present in the atheroma plaque as a natural response to inflammation of the artery walls. Because cholesterol was easy to measure as early as the 1930s, it was likely detected and blamed for the plaque because the other components were not known yet or could not be identified and measured. Dietary cholesterol is a very, very, small portion of the amount made by the liver. It is estimated that the liver makes about 5 g per day of cholesterol. Dietary intake is ~0.3–0.5 g/d, which is 10% or less of what the liver makes and even less than what the enterohepatic reabsorption recovers from the intestine. The enterohepatic pathway is designed to actually conserve cholesterol by reabsorbing bile acids and dietary cholesterol from the gut. Cholesterol is an "expensive" molecule for the body to synthesize (30 carbons and many enzyme reactions) and also a critical one for the proper functioning of cell membranes, wound healing, brain synapse function, nutrient absorption, steroid hormones, and so on.

The omega-6 FAs are known to be more proinflammatory than the omega-3 FAs. As discussed above, they are at very high levels in the U.S. diets and the ratio of omega-6 to omega-3 fatty acids is way out of line with the omega-6s being excessively high.

A recent article in the *Canadian Journal of Cardiology*[31] commented that "Atherosclerosis is a complex inflammatory disease that results from lipid accumulation and oxidation in the arterial wall combined with an active inflammatory reaction involving transmigration of monocytes and other inflammatory cells from the blood stream into the vessel wall."

The Men's Health Study[32] reported that the level of CRP, an inflammatory marker that was measured at the beginning of the study, was significantly related to the risk of future MI by the end of the study. Their conclusions were that (1) baseline levels of inflammation, as measured by CRP, predicts the risk of first MI; (2) CRP is not associated with venous thrombosis; (3) CRP is not a short-term indicator of risk; and (4) The benefits of aspirin may be modified by underlying inflammation involving both anti-inflammatory and antiplatelet effects.

Statins, even at low doses, have anti-inflammatory effects. This may be the real value of statin treatment, not the lowering of cholesterol. Coenzyme Q10 (CoQ_{10}) is also lowered by statins. CoQ_{10} is necessary for the electron transport system in mitochondria. Coenzyme Q10 is a compound made by all the cells in our bodies. All the body cells can make it and it is used to produce energy for all the necessary functions of the cells. It is essential for the cells ability to make ATP (adenosine triphosphate), the main energy currency of all the cells. The ATP is found in all cells and usually is in the mitochondria associated with the electron transport system that converts the food we eat to usable energy for growth and maintenance. It also acts as an antioxidant to protect the body from oxidative damage. Statins inhibit the production of CoQ10 and may be the main cause of the bad side effects people often experience when taking statin drugs.

Because the heart is a muscle that has to work continuously, it does not make much sense to treat with high doses of a drug that decreases the efficiency of that muscle, as well as others, to work properly. This statin-induced decrease in CoQ_{10} may be related to the muscle pain experienced by many patients on statin therapy as well as cognitive side effects. Other important downstream compounds after the HMG-reductase step, which are partially blocked by statins, are also decreased. These include steroids, bile salts, diolcols, squalene, and so on. There is increasing evidence that blood lipids are not the sole determinants of CVD risk, if at all. About half of the people dying of heart attacks have normal blood lipids.

Low-grade inflammation is a common feature in patients with DM2. Heart disease, metabolic syndrome, and DM2 are often comorbidities displayed together and all have increased concentrations of circulatory cytokines, indicating the presence of inflammation.[33] Also, atherosclerosis, obesity, and insulin resistance (IR) all are associated with increased cytokines. These conditions often appear together in DM2 patients.

Another possible source of inflammation is the presence of latent viruses or bacteria such as herpes simplex, cytomegalovirus (CMV), *Helicobacter pylori*, or *Chlamydia pneumonia* could be the initiators of inflammation. There is some evidence in the literature that they have been identified with atheroma in the body of patients. The same species identified in the atheroma were also found in dental infections for some organisms, especially spirochetes. CMV infection has been shown to be associated with CVD. CMV infection has been shown to cause an increase in arterial blood pressure in infected mice. In addition, it has been shown that CMV along with a high cholesterol diet in mice causes an even higher blood pressure and classic atherosclerotic plaque formation. Much research is needed to follow-up on these observations.

In a recently published Commentary in the *Journal of the American College of Nutrition*,[34] we discussed the saturated fat and cholesterol controversy as well as statin use. There is a growing literature that inflammation, not serum cholesterol, is associated with CVD. High carbohydrate diets lead to higher levels of inflammation. Malhotra[35] argues in a recent article that saturated fat is not the issue. He reports that the LDL-C that increases with saturated fat consumption is the large buoyant (type A) LDL and not the small dense LDL (type B) that is more inflammatory and associated with CVD. This type B-LDL is associated with and responsive to carbohydrate intake and not with the saturated fat intake.

CONCLUSIONS

We have not made a lot of progress in preventing CHD. Treatment options such as surgery, stents, and diagnoses have improved but dietary advice has not contained or even improved the incidence of CVD to any extent. Perhaps, it is time to step back and look at the big picture. It is obvious that the Diet/Heart Hypothesis is just that—a hypothesis.

A recent study by Chowdhury et al.[36] of a meta-analysis of studies totaling 659,298 subjects through 2013, concluded that "Current evidence does not clearly support cardiovascular guidelines that encourage high consumption of polyunsaturated fatty acids and low consumption of total saturated fats." The only obvious fatty acid group that appeared to increase risk was the *t*FAs that produced a relative risk of 1.16 (1.05 − 1.27). Total long-chain omega-3 FAs decreased the relative risk to 0.93. The other groupings had a relative risk of 0.99 to −1.0.

Perhaps, it is time that we step back and look at the big picture and begin to consider some of the less popular theories about CVD and test them. Inflammation is one factor that has quite a bit of evidence in its favor. Likewise, omega-3 FA intake has good scientific evidence not only for alleviating CVD but also for improved mental function. The consumption of omega-3 FAs in the United States is much less than the omega-6s. There is quite a bit of evidence that SFAs are not causing CHD. In fact, the level of fat in the diet is probably not the problem either. Since the dietary recommendations in 1980, the obesity epidemic has increased due to the high carbohydrate consumption. Why not blame carbohydrates or fructose drinks?

Although the overconsumption of industrial trans fats and omega-6s will bolster inflammatory responses, the saturated, monounsaturated, and the omega-3 fats offer protection in cardiovascular disease. Saturated fats should no longer be vilified as they are the most resistant to oxidation. Making smart choices will include utilizing fats that are the most productive and omitting fats that are the most destructive. Thus, the discernment of fats is crucial. We must strongly utilize omega-3s and olive oil/MUFA (the good) and use less of the omega-6 (the bad) and avoid at all costs the industrial trans fats (the ugly) as a nutritional strategy in the prevention of cardiovascular disease.

REFERENCES

1. McGilvery RW, Goldstein G. *Biochemistry: A Functional Approach*, 2nd Ed. Philadelphia, PA: W.B. Saunders; 1979.
2. Ip MM, Masso-Welch PA, Ip C. Prevention of mammary cancer with conjugated linoleic acid: Role of the stroma and the epithelium. *Can Res* 2002;62:4383–4389.
3. Ip MM, McGee, Masso-Welch PA, Ip C, Meng X, Ou L, Shoemaker SF. The t10, c12 isomer of conjugated linoleic acid stimulates mammary tumorigenesis in transgenic mice over-expressing erbB2 in the mammary epithelium. *Carcinogenesis* 2007;28:1269–1272.
4. Burr GO, Burr MM. A new deficiency disease produced by the rigid exclusion of fat from the diet. *J Biol Chem* 1929;82:345–367.
5. Burr GO, Burr MM. On the nature and role of the fatty acids essential in nutrition. *J Biol Chem* 1930;86:587–621.
6. Gillies, PJ., Bhatia SK, Belcher LA, Hannon DB, Thompson JT, Vanden Heuvel JP. Regulation of inflammatory and lipid metabolism by eicosapentaenoic acid-rich oil. *J Lipid Res* 2012;53:1679–1689.
7. Gurr MI, James RT. *Lipid Biochemistry, an Introduction*, 3rd Ed. London, UK: Chapman and Hall; 1980, pp 229F.
8. Miller JA, Kline BE, Rusch HP, Baumann CA. The effect of certain lipids on the carcinogenicity of p-dimethylaminoazobenzene. *Cancer Res* 1944;4:756–761.
9. Kline BE, Miller JA, Rusch HP, Baumann CA. The carcinogenicity of p-dimethylaminoazobenzene in diets containing the fatty acids of hydrogenated coconut oil or of corn oil. *Cancer Res* 1946;6:5–7.
10. Shao F, Ford DA. Differential regulation of ABCA1 and macrophage cholesterol efflux by elaidic and oleic acids. *Lipids* 2013;48:757–767.
11. Miranda JL, Jimenez FP. Olive oil and health: Summary of the II international conference on olive oil and health consensus report. *Nutrition, Metabolism and Cardiovascular Dis* 2010;20:284–294.
12. Taubes G. *Good Calories, Bad Calories*. New York: Random House; 2008.
13. Van Itallie TB. Experimental and clinical evidence relating to the effect of dietary fat upon health in man. *Am J of Public Health* 1957;1530.
14. Yamagishi KH, Iso Y, Kokubo et al. Dietary intake of saturated fatty acids and incident stroke and coronary heart disease in Japanese communities: the JPHC Study. *Eur Heart J* 2013;34(16):1225–1232.
15. Mente A, de Koning L, Shannon H, Anand S. A systematic review of the evidence supporting a causal link between dietary factors and coronary heart disease. *Arch Intern Med* 2009;169:659–669.
16. Siri-Tarino P, Sun Q, Krauss R. Meta-analysis of prospective cohort studies evaluating the association of saturated fat with cardiovascular disease. *Am J Clin Nutr* 2010;91:535–546.
17. Micha R, Mozaffarian D. Saturated fat and cardiometabolic risk factors, coronary heart disease, stroke, and diabetes: A fresh look at the evidence. *Lipids* 2010;45:893–905.
18. Elwood PC, Pickering JE, Givens DI, Gallacher JE. The consumption of milk and dairy foods and the incidence of vascular disease and diabetes: An overview of the evidence. *Lipids* 2010;45:925–939.
19. Guyton AC, *Basic Human Physiology*. Philadelphia, PA: W.B. Saunders; 1977.
20. Kodde IF, van der Stok J, Smolenski RT, de Jong JW. Metabolic and genetic regulation of cardiac energy substrate preference. *Comp Biochem Physiol Part a Mol Integra Physiol* 2007;146(1):26–39.
21. Hasselbalch SG, Knudsen GM, Jakobsen J et al. Brain metabolism during short-term starvation in humans. *J cerebral blood flow and metabolism* 1994;14(1):125–131.
22. Kodde IF, van der Stok J, Smolenski RT, de Jong JW. Metabolic and genetic regulation of cardiac energy substrate preference. *Cop Biochem Physiol Part A Mol Integr Physiol* 2007;14691:26–39.
23. Steen E, Terry BM, Rivera EJ et al. Impaired insulin and insulin-like growth factor expression and signaling mechanisms in Alzheimer's disease—is this type 3 diabetes? *J Alzheimer's Disease* 2005;7:63–80.
24. Bundy, V. Fructose linked to cardiovascular risk in teens. *Academic Sourceguide*, April 2012, P.21.
25. Menisnk R, Katan M. Effect of dietary trans fatty acids on high-density and low-density lipoprotein cholesterol in healthy subjects. *N Engl J Med* 1990;23:439–445.
26. Clevidence BA, Judd J, Schaefer E et al. Plasma lipoprotein (a) levels in man and women consuming diets enriched in saturated, *cis-* or *trans*-monounsaturated fatty acids. *Arterioscler Thromb Vasc Biol* 1997;17:1657–1661.
27. Baer DJ, Judd JT, Clevidence BA, Tracy RP. Dietary fatty acids affect plasma markers of inflammation in healthy men fed controlled diets: a randomized crossover study. *Am J Clin Nutr* 2004;79:969–973.
28. Mozaffarian D, Aro A, Willett WC. Health effects of trans-fatty acids: experimental and observational evidence. *Eur J Clin Nutr* 2009;63(suppl 2):S5–521.

29. Vesper HW, Kuiper HC, Mirel LB, Johnson CL, Pirkle JL. Levels of plasma trans-fatty acids in non-Hispanic white adults in the United States in 2000 and 2009. *JAMA* 212;307(6) Feb. 6, 2012.
30. Vesper HW, Kuiper HC, Mirel LB, Johnson CL, Pinkle JL. Levels of plasma trans-fatty acids in non-Hispanic white adults in the United States in 2000 and 2009. *JAMA* 2012;306(6):562–563.
31. Tyburczy C, Major C, Lock AL et al. Individual trans octadecnoic acids and partially hydrogenated vegetable oil differentially affect hepatic lipid and lipoprotein metabolism in golden Syrian hamsters. *J Nutr* 2009;139:257–263.
32. Duchatelle V, Kritikou E, Tardif JC. Clinical value of drugs targeting inflammation for the management of coronary artery disease. *Can J Cardiol* 2012;28:678–686.
33. Ridker P, Cushman M, Stampfer M et al. Inflammation, Aspirin, and the Risk of Cardiovascular Disease in Apparently Healthy Men. *NEJM* 1997;336:973–979.
34. Calle M, Fernandez M. *Diabetes & Metabolism* 2012;38:183–191.
35. Sinatra S, Teter BB, Bowden J, Houston MC, Martinez-Gonzalez MA. The saturated fat, cholesterol and statin controversy: A commentary. *J Am Coll Nutr* 2014;33(1):79–88.
36. Malhotra A. Saturated fat is not the major issue. *Brit Med J* 2013;22:347:f6340.
37. Cowdhury R, Warnakula S, Kunutsor S et al. Association of dietary, circulating, and supplement fatty acids with coronary risk. *Ann Inter Med* 2014;160:398–406.

3 Has Statin Therapy Been Oversold?

A Call for a Reevaluation of the Standards for Treatment*

Stephen T. Sinatra and Jonny Bowden

CONTENTS

In Chapter 1, we discussed what we have colloquially referred to as "The Great Cholesterol Myth," defined as a belief system based on a collection of deeply intertwined hypotheses about cholesterol, saturated fat, heart disease, and treatment. The origins of this belief system can be found in the "Lipid Hypothesis," which holds that high cholesterol in the blood leads to heart disease, and the "Diet-Heart Hypothesis," which further postulates that saturated fat in the diet is the major cause of elevated serum cholesterol and, therefore, by definition, a causal actor in the development of heart disease. Accepting these notions about fat and cholesterol invariably leads to two conclusions: (1) saturated fat has little place in a healthy diet and (2) high cholesterol needs to be treated.

The Diet-Heart Hypothesis holds that saturated fat in the diet and, in some versions of the hypothesis, dietary cholesterol are major contributors to heart disease. And though there have always been naysayers who felt that the decision to blame heart disease on saturated fat and cholesterol was both premature and unwarranted, their warnings went largely unheeded.[1] The Diet-Heart Hypothesis was largely accepted by major health organizations. Saturated fat became the demon in our diet. Even today, the American Heart Association recommends getting no more than 7% of calories from saturated fat[2] and the USDA's Dietary Guidelines for Americans (2010) recommends no more than 10%.[3] Meanwhile, cholesterol-lowering drugs became a cash cow for their makers—particularly Pfizer, whose Lipitor was the best-selling drug of all time, generating, according to Forbes magazine, global sales of $141 billion, nearly double that of its closest competitor on their list of best-selling drugs.[4]

The demonization of saturated fat was accompanied by an even more virulent war on cholesterol in general. The National Cholesterol Expert Panel, Adult Treatment Panel III treatment recommendations targeting low-density lipoprotein cholesterol (LDL-C) as an entity to be treated aggressively by the use of hydroxymethylglutaryl coenzyme A (HMG-CoA) reductase inhibitors (statins) was launched in 2001. One in six American adults could potentially be advised to take these drugs, at a cost of approximately 30 billion a year.[5] In 2004, the therapeutic guidelines emphasized reaching a more targeted LDL level. The U.S. National Education Cholesterol Program Guidelines suggested that the objective in high-risk patients should generally be to reduce LDL cholesterol to

---

* Some of this material was adapted from a previous commentary in the *Journal of the American College of Nutrition*: Sinatra ST, Teter BB, Bowden J, Houston MC, Martinez-Gonzalez MA. The saturated fat, cholesterol, and statin controversy: A commentary. *J Am Coll Nutr* 2014;33(1):79–88.

below 100 mg/dL or optimally, for very high risk patients, to below 70 mg/dL.[6] For more than a decade, the doctrine and established medical dogma were to get lower and lower LDL levels.

The demonization of saturated fat was made complete with a *Time* magazine cover showing two eggs and a strip of bacon making the shape of a frowning face with the headline "And now the bad news: Cholesterol." Food companies started switching to hydrogenated vegetable oils (because anything was "better" than saturated fats); no-fat foods became all the rage; and a multibillion-dollar pharmaceutical industry developed around lowering the molecule said to be at the heart of the problem—cholesterol, which was widely believed to be raised by saturated fat. This perception, and the idea that "saturated fat and cholesterol clog your arteries," became what would now be called a cultural "meme," and we are still living with it today, despite the fact that it is wildly past its expiration date and simply not supported by the evidence.

Again in Chapter 1, we discussed the first of these, and what we believe to be serious flaws in the argument against saturated fat. We discussed the paucity of evidence for the "dangers" of saturated fat, and the emerging research that absolves dietary saturated fat of a causal role in heart disease.[7,8] And we discussed our deepening understanding of the relationship between "high cholesterol" and heart disease, a relationship far more nuanced and variable than is widely believed.

In this chapter, we will turn our attention toward statin therapy, which is widely considered first-line therapy for high cholesterol. But before we can even have a productive discussion about treatment options for dyslipidemia—treatment options that should most certainly include statin drugs, albeit perhaps in a much more circumscribed way—we should first clarify how we are quantifying dyslipidemia in the first place. What exactly does "high cholesterol" mean, and what is its significance? Though it may seem like those questions have been long settled, the truth is that they are not. In this chapter, we will make the case for a fresh evaluation of the accepted criteria for statin therapy and for a fresh evaluation of the efficacy (and potential dangers) of the therapy itself.

One of the many "great cholesterol myths" we have called attention to concerns the very nature of the measurements on which most physicians base their recommendations for statin therapy. High-density lipoproteins (HDL) and LDL are not two distinct classes of homogeneous molecules, rendering obsolete the commonly used division of cholesterol into "good" (HDL) and "bad" (LDL). A more sophisticated and complete assessment of cholesterol subclasses has been available for some time, and in our opinion, should always be used preferentially to the cruder measurement (high cholesterol), which may not, and frequently *does* not, correlate with risk.

For example, while most HDL is, in fact, beneficial, it is suggested that HDL2 is more protective than HDL3.[9] The importance of LDL subtypes is even more significant. LDLs have two distinct subtypes, LDL-a and LDL-b, both of which look and behave quite differently in the body. LDL-a is a large, fluffy molecule with less potential for atherogenic mischief, whereas LDL-b is quite the opposite—a small, dense, molecule that brings with it the potential for significant inflammation and ultimate vascular injury. Those with a preponderance of LDL-a particles (i.e., Pattern A) have a significantly different risk profile than those with a preponderance of LDL-b particles (Pattern B).[10] Particle size distribution should certainly be taken into account when determining whether a patient's cholesterol levels are of concern or not.

Furthermore, growing evidence suggests that overall particle number is a far better predictor of coronary events than LDL alone.[11] Yet, most prescriptions for statin drugs have been written on the basis of overall LDL numbers, the crudest and least revealing of the available cholesterol tests. As we will see in this chapter, these drugs are very far from universally benign. Every effort should be made to ensure that they are prescribed only to people who are most likely to benefit from them. The current tests for cholesterol do not allow us to make that distinction effectively. In Chapter 4, Dr. Richard Delany meticulously takes cholesterol and lipid subfraction testing to the next level , offering opinions that may seem a bit contrary to this chapter. Although the cholesterol theory of heart disease remains controversial and poorly understood by many health professionals, we will attempt to sort out this confusion by giving the reader the opportunity to see multiple sides of the cholesterol dilemma.

Although we are often accused of being antistatin, the truth is far more nuanced. To paraphrase Shakespeare, we come *not* to bury statins—but neither do we come to praise them, nor to misrepresent their benefits. We believe statins have a place in treatment. But emerging evidence suggests that the side-effect profile of statins is considerably more serious than statin advocates would have us believe, while their benefits have been wildly oversold.[12,13]

This has happened for three reasons:

1. The relatively modest beneficial effect of statin drugs for middle-aged males with existing cardiovascular disease (CVD) has been exaggerated.[14]
2. The assumption that because benefits have been observed in high-risk middle-aged men on statin medication for secondary prevention, those benefits would accrue to the general population.
3. The underreporting by physicians of the considerable side-effect profile of statin medication.[13]

We are deeply concerned that these drugs are now being enthusiastically recommended for populations in which they have shown no appreciable benefit (women, primary prevention, the elderly) and in which they may reasonably be expected to do quite a bit of potential harm (children).

Does this mean statins should never be used? Of course, not. Any good physician will use a drug—even one with potential side effects—if the risk of *not* using the drug is greater than the risk of using it. But she *will not* do so if the benefit is likely to be minimal, whereas the potential for danger is moderate to substantial. All of us would take a drug that would reduce our risk of cancer by 25% if the only side effect were a small chance of getting the temporary sniffles. But would we take a drug that *might* reduce the risk of a cold, but would likely cause a significant increase in the risk for bladder cancer? Most of us would consider this a bad bargain—a lot of risk for very little reward. If a given drug was the only thing standing between any of us and a life-threatening disease, and if the benefit of that particular drug were significant and demonstrable, we might be willing to take a chance. Yet, if the benefits of that drug had been oversold to us, while the risks had been largely underpublicized—or, worse, hidden in plain sight—we (both patients and doctors) would be unable to make an informed decision based on an accurate analysis of the "risk/benefit" ratio.

And that is precisely the situation we find ourselves in today vis-à-vis statin drugs. Although there have certainly been drugs with a far worse side-effect profile than statins (thalidomide, for one), the fact exists that statins have a number of potential and serious side effects, including muscle pain, fatigue, loss of libido, and everything from mild memory loss to transient global amnesia. Some statin studies have also shown a disturbing elevation in the risk for diabetes[15] and, in some research, cancer.[16,17] In one study, statin use was actually associated with an increased risk of death.[18] In that study, in a population of 300 adults diagnosed with heart failure and followed for an average of 3.7 years, those who were taking statins and had the lowest levels of LDL were found to have the highest rates of mortality. (Conversely, those with the highest levels of cholesterol had a lower risk of death.) And, as we will see shortly, few, if any, studies show a benefit to statin users in all-cause mortality, meaning the notion of taking a statin drug to extend your life is simply unsupported by any real evidence.

Would not it, therefore, make good sense to know precisely who will benefit the most from these drugs (and who is *unlikely* to benefit) before prescribing them willy-nilly to virtually every person over 40 on the assumptions that (1) they are completely benign substances that will never harm anyone and (2) that they actually save lives?

Furthermore, although statins do, as mentioned, have a modest beneficial effect for secondary prevention in middle-aged men, it is widely assumed (and unquestioned in the mainstream media) that they accomplish this modest benefit primarily by lowering cholesterol levels. But what if this were not true? What if, in fact, statins produced any positive effect that they produced *despite* the fact that they lowered cholesterol, not because of it?

Here is an example: cherries are widely known to have compounds in them (anthocyanadins) that reduce inflammation, and are effective at reducing pain, particularly from gout. Imagine a primitive society that discovered this relationship, but then wrongly concluded that "red foods cure gout." Their observation that cherries have demonstrable healing properties might be spot on, but they would be guilty of making a *false attribution*, by ascribing the healing properties of cherries to their "redness." The *observation* would be correct but the *explanation* would be wrong, and following the "red foods cure gout" theory would be expected to produce some miserable failures (except, of course, when the red food in question happens to be cherries!).

What if the same situation existed with statin drugs? The observed benefit (modest though it is) with statin drugs is *attributed* to their ability to lower cholesterol, just as cherries' ability to lower inflammation might be wrongly attributed to their red color. But what if the *real* reason for statin benefit lies elsewhere, just as the *real* benefit of cherries has little to do with their color? Would not it be important to know that?

We believe that the benefit of statin drugs in middle-aged men with existing heart disease may come from the well-known ability of statins to lower inflammation and to thin the blood.[19] If this is so, and if the negative side effects of statins are in fact related *only* to their cholesterol-lowering activity, this information would be extremely valuable. It would let the drug manufacturers develop a much safer statin-*like* drug that simply attacked inflammation and platelet aggregation and left cholesterol lowering and the side effects that come with it alone.

But that is not going to happen as long as we continue to fervently believe the cultural meme that cholesterol causes or is in some *direct* way responsible for heart disease, and that statins "work" because they lower cholesterol.

The argument that the "value" of statins comes from something *other* than their cholesterol-lowering activity is given quite a bit of weight by an analysis of the cholesterol-lowering studies that took place prestatin drugs. If cholesterol lowering reduces the risk of heart disease, then you would expect to see that effect regardless of the method used to lower cholesterol, provided, of course, that the method did not involve some diabolical, unsafe, and medically unsound procedure.

Well, as it turns out, there were a good 16 studies on lowering cholesterol well before statins became the front runner as a first-order treatment for the "medical" condition of high cholesterol. These 16 studies were brilliantly analyzed by two researchers: Russell Smith, PhD, an American experimental psychologist with a strong background in physiology, math, and engineering, and Edward Pinckney, MD, the editor of four medical journals and former coeditor of the *Journal of the American Medical Association*.[20]

Smith and Pinckney reviewed all the cholesterol-lowering trials that had been done before 1991. The studies found that using drugs to lower cholesterol was quite effective. The problem was that they were not much good for anything else. If cholesterol lowering was an effective way to reduce the risk of heart disease and death, then we would expect the research to show a reduction in heart attacks, strokes, and deaths when cholesterol was effectively lowered. However, this is not what happened. Smith and Pinckney: "Drugs were used to lower blood cholesterol levels in twelve trials. Eight of these trials were both randomized and blinded. Of the eight that met this standard, total deaths in six trials were the same or greater in the treatment group than in the control group. For the remaining four trials (either nonrandomized or unblinded), there were no differences between the treatment group and the control group."[20]

So, if lowering cholesterol does not make a big difference, as the overwhelming majority of these 16 studies showed, but statin drugs, which also lower cholesterol, *are* making a big difference (as the manufacturers and marketing departments of these drugs love to keep telling us), then logically, the benefit of statin drugs *cannot* be due to their cholesterol lowering ability, and *has* to be due to something else.

We believe the number one candidate for that "something else" is the ability of statins to lower inflammation. Which might lead to the reasonable question, "so what?" If statins lower inflammation and are essentially safe drugs with little downside, what is the problem? (Indeed, some doctors with big media platforms and best-selling popular books are going on talk shows waxing eloquently about statins, stopping just short of suggesting that they be added to the water supply.)[21]

There are two main problems with using statins as a first-line therapy against inflammation and, ironic and counterintuitive as it may seem, the first of those problems is that statins actually lower cholesterol. And that may turn out to be a very dangerous situation for the brain.

"When cholesterol levels are low," writes neurologist David Perlmutter, MD, "the brain simply doesn't work well, and individuals are at a significantly increased risk for neurological problems as a consequence."[22] One of the fundamental roles of the much-maligned LDL molecule, which, of course, is not cholesterol per se, but a lipoprotein, is to transport cholesterol to the neuron where it performs important functions. But, when free radicals or sugar damage the LDL molecule, its ability to deliver cholesterol to the brain is compromised. Oxidized LDL, as opposed to native, unoxidized LDL, is emerging as a significant risk factor for atherosclerosis. Hence, as Perlmutter points out, we should put our efforts into reducing the risk of LDL *oxidation,* not necessarily reducing levels of LDL itself.

That there could be collateral damage resulting from indiscriminate cholesterol lowering is an emerging concern. Depression runs much higher in people with low cholesterol.[23] Elderly men with low cholesterol have a 300% higher risk of depression than their cohorts with high cholesterol,[24] whereas in a sample of 300 healthy women, depression was also significantly higher among those in the lowest cholesterol group.[25] Lower cholesterol (under 160) is associated with a significantly greater likelihood of suicide,[26] with a significantly greater likelihood of external-cause mortality,[27] and with a 350% increase in the risk for Parkinson's.[28]

The second problem with using statins as a first-line therapy against inflammation is that it is simply inefficient. There are far more benevolent ways to accomplish the same goal, with far less potential for mischief. It is certainly worth exploring whether a greater anti-inflammatory effect can be had at considerably less economic cost and with none of the potential side effects of statins from pharmaceutical-grade fish oil, either as a stand-alone intervention or as part of a decidedly nontoxic cocktail of known anti-inflammatories such as curcumin and resveratrol. If lowering inflammation is the real benefit of statins, and that benefit could be had with less risk for less money, would not it be important to know that? And if the main benefit from statins is in fact their ability to lower systemic inflammation, why continue to use a potentially dangerous medicine to accomplish that which can be accomplished with a few weekly servings of salmon or a daily supplement of omega-3 fatty acids?

A careful examination of the research suggests that statins do whatever good they do independently of their ability to lower cholesterol. The Heart Protection Study (HPS)[29] evaluated women, the elderly, diabetics, people with low baseline cholesterol levels, and those with prior occlusive non-coronary vascular disease. Results demonstrated the positive impact of Simvastatin therapy across all patient groups, *independent* of cholesterol levels. Even in subjects with acceptable LDL-C levels (<100 mg/dL), there was a clear reduction in the incidence of major cardiovascular events, suggesting that risk reduction for CVD is not the result of the ability of HMG-CoA to reduce LDL-C level.

In other words, cholesterol is found at the scene of the crime but is it the perpetrator? Statins lower circulating lipoproteins, but they have multiple pleotropic and antiatherogenic effects as well.[30] The researchers in the WOSCOPS Study[19] indicated that the positive impact of statins had more to do with their favorable properties on blood rheology and blood viscosity. In the Jupiter Study,[31] there was a 53% reduction in venous thromboembolism and the abrupt withdrawal of statins in the setting of unstable angina or acute coronary syndrome could be hazardous and even fatal. We have learned that statins should be strictly avoided in any situation of a central nervous system bleed as demonstrated by the Massachusetts General Hospital researchers.[32] Clearly, statins at some level are thinning the blood and will be especially protective in the setting of acute ischemia or in very high-risk men as demonstrated in the WOSCOPS Study.[19]

Perhaps the ENHANCE[33] trial put the major nail in the coffin of the cholesterol theory of heart disease. The ENHANCE Study became a highly controversial issue given the fact that the study concluded in early 2006, but the release of its results was delayed until early 2008. This delay caused considerable angst in the medical community. The ENHANCE Study enrolled 720 patients with familial hypercholesterolemia who were randomized to receive either a statin drug Zocor (Simvastatin) or the anticholesterol drug Vytorin (which consists of Zocor plus ezetimbe—a drug that blocks cholesterol absorption from the gut). The trial was expected to demonstrate that patients on Vytorin would have less plaque expansion than patients taking Zocor alone. For those who believed that cholesterol is the main cause of coronary heart disease (CHD), ENHANCE was constructed not to fail. The administration of two drugs with different mechanisms of action in the same patient resulted in a drastic reduction of cholesterol levels but significant reductions in LDL levels achieved with both Zocor (41%) and Vytorin (58%), artherosclerosis progressed as the measurement in carotid intima-media thickness (IMT) increased in both groups.

These surprising and very disappointing data might be the reason why the results of ENHANCE were hidden from the medical community for nearly 2 years. How important is lowering cholesterol when a drastic reduction resulted in an increase in plaque of the carotid vessels?

After multiple cholesterol-lowering drug trials, the emergence of new data has raised new and provocative questions. Dr. Michel de Lorgeril, the architect of the Mediterranean Diet for secondary prevention, has called for a full reappraisal of the cholesterol theory.[34] He points out that major trials published after the enforcement of clinical trial regulations put in place by the FDA in 2008/2009 following the Vioxx affair were either negative or disappointing.

In 1994–2004, there were highly positive trials with statins that were used to issue guidelines for medical practitioners. de Lorgeril is asking for a reappraisal of these studies by experts independent from the pharmaceutical industry. In other words, will these earlier trials hold up to scientific scrutiny following a reexamination of the data?[34]

Debates over the cholesterol theory of heart disease and the merits of statin therapy in primary prevention will continue to go on indefinitely.[35] Both opponents and proponents will cite cherry-picked studies to support their arguments. But if the studies are exaggerated, flawed, not credible, or unethical, how are we to arrive at reasonable conclusions? What about the unpublished negative studies that do not support the pharmaceutical agenda? And when the rules are being made by those with conflicts of interest, the guidelines may be tarnished.

The recent newly developed guidelines by the American College of Cardiology and the American Heart Association has now created a policy that could double the number of patients taking statins in the United States. These organizations are suggesting that statins should be taken by both men and women with coronary artery disease (CAD), all subjects with type 1 and type-2 diabetes, as well as all individuals with LDL cholesterol levels greater than 190 and in those having a heart attack risk of greater than 7.5% over a 10-year period.[36] These guidelines appear to be a gross oversimplification and puts patients into jeopardy by creating standard of care algorithms for doctors placing patients on statin drugs. Most troubling of all is the fact that the risk calculator used to calculate the target figure of 7.5% risk over a 10-year period was found to overpredict risk by 75%–150%![37]—which led to a critical editorial in *The Lancet*[38] suggesting that the risk prediction algorithm used in the guidelines "systematically overestimated" cardiovascular risks could therefore lead to overtreatment of a substantial fraction of the 33 million Americans potentially affected by the guideline. *The Lancet* called for careful reanalysis before the new guideline goes into effect.[39]

Those of us who have used statins in clinical situations can all agree that statins are powerful drugs and can be a blessing or a curse. It makes good sense to use a statin in any male under the age of 75 with CAD. Ridker and Wilson[40] clearly state: "In 2013, the continued use of absolute risk assessment to guide prescription will most likely over treat many who do not benefit and undertreat many for whom efficacy is certain." And, we believe, that is a male with documented coronary disease regardless of his cholesterol level as the benefits clearly surpass the risks! However, women will need to be treated on an individual basis as the efficacy of statins in women is not as certain as in men and the risk profile is more significant and substantial in women.[41]

Recently, a trial in women 55–75 years of age on a 10-year or more statin treatment had more than double risk of lobular and ductal breast carcinoma.[17] And the recent data on increased cataracts with statins is also alarming suggesting a caution in low-risk populations.[42,43] Although it can seem reasonable to treat an LDL over 190 in a patient with familial hypercholesterolemia, autosomal dominant (1 in 500 cases), it is not smart medicine to prescribe statins to every patient with an LDL greater than 190 or is it reasonable to treat all diabetics and especially those without CAD. For example, statins in diabetic males may accelerate coronary artery calcification[44] and statins can increase cataracts that are more prevalent in diabetics as well. And the Women's Health Initiative showing an age-adjusted increase of 48% risk of diabetes in postmenopausal females receiving statins is disconcerting.[45] Previously, another meta-analysis of statin trials[46] showed new onset diabetes occurring frequently in the statin group. There are safer lifestyle, dietary and nutraceutical supports that can be used in the insulin-resistant or type-2 diabetic patient.

For example, the modification of lifestyle changes was particularly effective in preventing type-2 diabetes as the incidence of diabetes was reduced by 58% with lifestyle interventions and 31% with the pharmaceutical drug metformin as compared to placebo in a study of 3234 patients.[47] The superiority of a 7% loss of weight with a 150-minute brisk walking program per week showed almost twice the efficacy over pharmaceutical therapy.[47] Other nutraceutical supports that have recently been popular in treating blood sugar include pycnogenol[48] and benfotiamine for advanced glycation end products[49,50] as well as diabetic retinopathy.[51] In addition, a Mediterranean dietary pattern rich in extra-virgin olive oil has been recently proved to significantly reduce the incidence of new-onset cases of type-2 diabetes in the primary prevention PREDIMED randomized trial. This finding represents first-level evidence to support the beneficial effects of a high-quality dietary pattern on insulin resistance.[52]

Clearly in any diabetic patient, it makes sense to use pharmaceutical therapies only when necessary and certainly choose safer options as statins in the diabetic, as we have seen, can create significant adverse effects. Unfortunately, statin side effects are grossly underreported and may cause serious harm[41]; and in some instances, statins caused multiple deaths when cerivastatin was abruptly removed from the world market.[53]

Patient complaints about possible side effects must be listened to as statins have the power to literally form or deform a person's life. How do we protect low-risk populations of people, especially women, the elderly, and children from the unnecessary use of statins? There is little justification for subjecting any very low-risk population to the strong possibility of adverse effects if the evidence does not justify the expectation of benefits outweighing the risks.[41] Physicians must be more compassionate and listen carefully when the patient is voicing side effects however subtle they may be.

There are going to be gray areas where the physician may be confused about choosing a statin, particularly in primary prevention. The assessment of risk is a subjective situation involving dietary habits, emotional stress, overweight status, hypertension, family history, diabetes, smoking, metabolic syndrome traits, and so on. Although there will be high-risk patients treated with lifestyle factors, anti-inflammatory diets, hypertensive control, cessation of smoking, healing emotional stress, detoxification, and taking targeted nutritional supplements, some patients, and especially those with low HDL, with higher risk profiles, should be treated with low-dose statins in combination with lifestyle improvements. The most recent meta-analyses showing a reduction of cardiovascular events in individuals at lower cardiovascular risk requires more scrutiny when considering statin therapy.[54,55] However, treating low-risk patients for primary prevention will cause us to pause because the hazards of type-2 diabetes,[15,46] adverse quality of life,[41,56] and hemorrhagic stroke[57] will need to be considered in the strategic care of the patient.[55] Patients who cannot tolerate statins because of intolerable side effects can use other options.

Important scientific information and clinical studies have defined the present role of natural agents in the management of inflammation and dyslipidemia. There are multiple nutraceuticals that can have a positive impact on inflammatory cytokines and lipid markers, which can help to ease carotid intimal medial thickness and obstruction, plaque progression, coronary artery calcium score by electron beam tomography (EBT), generalized atherosclerosis, and endothelial function. Niacin, omega-3 essential fatty acids, and *Citrus bergamia*, to mention a few, may have favorable effects on HDL, triglycerides (TGs), blood sugar, and LDL particle size and particle number.[58–62]

Niacin has a dose-related effect (1–3 g/day) in reducing total cholesterol (TC), LDL, apolipoprotein B (APO-B), LDL particle number, TGs, very-low-density lipoprotein (VLDL), increasing LDL size from small type B to large type A, and increasing HDL, especially the protective and larger HDL 2b particle and apolipoprotein (APO-A1).[59,63]

Niacin inhibits LDL oxidation; increases TG lipolysis in adipose tissue; increases APO-B degradation; reduces the fractional catabolic rate of HDL-APOA-1; inhibits platelet function; induces fibrinolysis; decreases cytokines, cell adhesion molecules (CAMs); lowers Lp(a), increases adiponectin; and is a potent antioxidant.[58,61,62] The niacin dose should be gradually increased, administered at meal time, pretreated with an 81-mg aspirin and taken with apple pectin to reduce flushing.[58] The effective dosing range is 500–3000 mg/day. Only vitamin B3 niacin is effective in dyslipidemia. The non-flush niacin (inositol hexanicotinate—IHN) does not improve lipid profiles and is not recommended.[58] The side effects of niacin include hyperuricemia, gout, hepatitis, flushing, rash, pruritis, hyperpigmentation, hyperhomocysteinemia, gastritis, ulcers, bruising, tachycardia, palpitations, and hyperglycemia. Niacin is not recommended in the diabetic population. Although the side effects can be unpleasant, the flushing and pruritis can cause discontinuation of the supplement. However, if the doses are slowly and gradually increased without missing doses and taken on a regular basis, the flushing is minimized.

Observational, epidemiologic and controlled clinical trials for omega-3 essential fatty acids have shown significant reductions in serum TG, VLDL decreased LDL particle number and increased LDL and HDL particle size as well as major reductions in all CVD events.[58,64–71]) The DART trial[65] demonstrated a decrease in mortality of 29% in men after MI and the GISSI prevention trial found a decrease in total mortality of 20%, CV deaths of 30%, and sudden death of 45%.[66] The Kuppio Heart Study demonstrated a 44% reduction in fatal and nonfatal CHD in subjects in the highest quintile of omega-3 intake compared to the lowest quintile.[67] Omega-3 fatty acids reduce CHD progression, stabilize plaque, reduce coronary artery stent restenosis, and CABG occlusion.[58]

Omega-3 fatty acids are anti-inflammatory and antithrombotic; lower BP, heart rate; and improve heart rate variability.[58,64] There is a decrease in fatty acid synthesis and an increase in fatty acid oxidation with consistent weight loss.[58] Insulin resistance is improved and there are no significant changes in fasting glucose or hemoglobin A1C with long-term treatment.[72]

Citrus bergamia is an active flavanone polyphenol extract that originates from the coast of southern Italy. It has been evaluated in several clinical prospective trials in humans. In doses of 1000 mg/day, this compound lowers LDL up to 36% and TG up to 39%, increases HDL 40% by inhibiting HMG CoA reductase, increases cholesterol and bile acid excretion, and reduces reactive oxygen species (ROS), blood sugar, and oxLDL.[73,74] The active ingredients include naringin, neroeriocitrin, neohesperidin, poncerin, rutin, neodesmin, rhoifolin, melitidine, and brutelidine.[73,74] This very small sample of nutritional and nutraceutical supplements could be a valid alternative for patients that are statin intolerant, cannot take other drugs for the treatment of dyslipidemia, or in those who prefer alternative treatments.

To summarize, the saturated fat–cholesterol–statin paradigm will continue to raise more questions than answers. Unfortunately, the focus on cholesterol as the cardinal factor in atherosclerosis will detract from other inflammatory etiologies resulting from excessive sugar/insulin relationships, trans fatty acids, and overzealous use of omega-6 oils. Oxidized LDL-C, particle size and number, and especially Lp(a) are also potent factors causing inflammation at the endothelial level.

Statins are potent pleotropic agents and work in several mechanisms in reducing cardiac risk including antioxidant status, plaque stabilization, reduction in CRP levels, reduction in inflammation, as well as having a favorable impact on blood and plasma viscosity.[19,75] We need to ask ourselves the question: How much benefit seen from statins is actually due to cholesterol lowering and how much benefit is due to some of these other mechanisms? We know, for example, that in patients with established CAD, statin prescription reduces subsequent risk even if baseline cholesterol levels are not substantially elevated. Although reducing LDL particle size and number may indeed be significant, much of the available evidence is consistent with the theory that it is the statins themselves that reduce cardiac risk rather than the reduction in cholesterol levels achieved by statins. Although it will require significant time to sort this out, should we use the precautionary principle in low-risk populations? Physicians will need to be more creative in identifying patients with cardiovascular risk, making lifestyle changes when necessary while trying to temporize the probability of a cardiac event. Certainly, some physicians will be more skilled and thus comfortable than others in the assessment of such a probability.

In this modern pharmaceutical age, the practice of medicine is becoming less and less of a science. Physicians need to bring back the art of medicine. Empowering the patient with the right knowledge is a key element in healing. Although the use of statins in men and some women with proven CAD is good medicine, standards, guidelines, and algorithms, will only cause a rush to judgment and overtreat many low-risk people who will not benefit from statins and be vulnerable to side effects at the same time. Choosing statin pharmaceutical drug therapy must be employed with caution and specifically tailored to complement the patient's needs. Physicians should not make their decisions on dogmatic policies but rather see the guidelines as only a guide and definitely not use statin drugs to treat cholesterol numbers alone.[76,77] We must treat the patient thoughtfully and choose statin drugs carefully with extreme diligence to avoid side effects. To use Francis Peabody's 1927 eloquent[78] statement in JAMA—"The most important aspect in the care of the patient, is the care of the patient."

As all drugs carry some risk, good medicine asks the question, "who has the most to gain from this drug, and who has the least to gain from it?" Without knowing the answer to that question, it is impossible to make a wise decision about whether or not the potential benefit of a medication outweighs the risk in a given patient.

To summarize, we believe statin therapy is best utilized in any male under the age of 75 with proven and established CAD.

REFERENCES

1. Mann GV. Coronary Heart Disease—"Doing the Wrong Things." *Nutrition Today* 1985;20(4):12–14.
2. American Heart Association Website, The American Heart Association's Diet and Lifestyle Recommendations   https://www.heart.org/HEARTORG/GettingHealthy/NutritionCenter/HealthyDietGoals/The-American-Heart-Associations-Diet-and-Lifestyle-Recommendations_UCM_305855_Article.jsp (accessed March 17, 2014).
3. Dietary Saturated Fat and Cardiovascular Health, Nutrition Insight 44, USDA Center for Nutrition Policy and Promotion, July 2011 http://www.cnpp.usda.gov/Publications/NutritionInsights/Insight44.pdf (accessed march 17, 2014).
4. Simon K. The Best Selling Drugs Since 1996—Why AbbVie's Humira Is Set to Eclipse Pfizer's Lipitor, Forbes, July 15, 2013 http://www.forbes.com/sites/simonking/2013/07/15/the-best-selling-drugs-since-1996-why-abbvies-humira-is-set-to-eclipse-pfizers-lipitor/ (accessed March 17, 2014).
5. Expert Panel on Detection, Evaluation and Treatment of High Blood Cholesterol in Adults. Executive summary of the third report of the National Cholesterol Education Program (NCEP) expert panel on detection, evaluation and treatment of high blood cholesterol in adults. *JAMA* 2001;285:2486–2497.
6. Grundy SM, Cleeman JI, Merz CNB. Implications of recent trials for the National Cholesterol Education Program Adult Treatment Panel III Guidelines. *J Am Coll Cardiol* 2004;44:720–732.
7. Chowdhury R, Warnakula S, Kunustor S et al. Association of dietary, circulating, and supplement fatty acids with coronary risk: A systematic review and meta-analysis. *Ann Intern Med* 2014;160(6):398–406.
8. Siri-Tarino PW, Sun Q, Hu FB, Krauss RM. Meta-analysis of prospective cohort studies evaluating the association of saturated fat with cardiovascular disease. *Am J Clin Nutr* 2010;91(3):535–546.
9. Salonen JT, Salonen R, Seppanen K, Rauramaa R, Tuomilehto J. HDL, HDL2, and HDL3 subfractions, and the risk of acute myocardial infarction. A prospective population study in eastern Finnish men. *Circulation* 1991;85(1):129–39.
10. Arsenault BJ, Lemieux I, Despres JP et al. Cholesterol levels in small LDL particles predict the risk of coronary heart disease in the EPIC-Norfolk prospective population study. *Eur Heart J* 2007;28:2770–2777.

11. Cromwell WC, Otvos JD, Keyes MJ et al. LDL particle number and risk of future cardiovascular disease in the Framingham Offspring Study: Implications for LDL management. *J Clin Lipidol* 2007;(6):583–592.
12. Golomb BA, Evans MA. Statin adverse effects: A review of the literature and evidence for a mitochondrial mechanism. *Am J Cardiovasc Drugs* 2008;8(6):373–418.
13. Golomb, BA, McGraw JJ, Evans MA, Dimsdale JE. Physician response to patient reports of averse drug effects: Implications for patient-targeted adverse effect surveillance. *Drug Saf* 2007;30(8):669–675.
14. An Interview with John Abramson, MD: The Overselling of Statins, Townsend Letter, June 2008.
15. Culver AL, Ockene IS, Balasubramanian R et al. Statin use and risk of diabetes mellitus in postmenopausal women in the women's health initiative. *Arch Intern Med* 2012;172(2):144–152.
16. Chang CC, Ho SC, Chiu HF, Yang CY. Statins increase the risk of prostate cancer: A population-based case-control study. *Prostate* 2011;71(16):1818–1824.
17. McDougall JA, Malone KE, Daling JR, Cushing-Haugen KL, Porter PL, Li CI. Long-term statin use and risk of ductal and lobular breast cancer among women 55 to 74 years of age. *Cancer Epidemiol Biomarkers Prev* 2013;22(9):1529–1537.
18. Charach G, George J, Roth A et al. Baseline low-density lipoprotein cholesterol levels and outcome in patients with heart failure. *Am J Cardiol* 2010;105(1):100–104.
19. Lowe G, Rumley A, Norrie J et al. Blood rheology, cardiovascular risk factors and cardiovascular disease: The West of Scotland Coronary Prevention Study. *Thromb Haemost* 2000;84:553–558.
20. Smith RL, Pinckney ER. *The Cholesterol Conspiracy*. St. Louis, MO: Warren Green; 1991.
21. Dr. Agus' Alternative Health Guide, The Dr. Oz Show website, http://www.doctoroz.com/videos /dr-agus-alternative-health-guide (accessed March 22, 2014).
22. Perlmutter D. *Grain Brain*. New York: Little, Brown & Co., 2013.
23. Shin JY, Suls J, Martin R. Are cholesterol and depression inversely related? A meta-analysis of the association between two cardiac risk factors. *Ann Behav Med* 2008;36(1):33–43.
24. Morgan RE, Palinkas LA, Barrett-Connor EL, Wingard DL. Plasma cholesterol and depressive symptoms in older men. *Lancet* 1993;341(8837):75–79.
25. Horsten M, Wamala SP, Vingerhoets A, Orth-Gomer K. Depressive symptoms, social support, and lipid profile in healthy middle-aged women. *Psychosom Med* 1997;59(5):521–528.
26. Neaton JD, Blackburn H, Jacobs D et al. Serum cholesterol level and mortality findings for men screened in the Multiple Risk Factor Intervention Trial. *Arch Intern Med* 1992;152(7):1490–1500.
27. Boscarino JA, Erlich PM, Hoffman SN. Low serum cholesterol and external-cause mortality: Potential implications for research and surveillance. *J Psychiatr Res* 2009;43(9):848–854.
28. Huang X, Abbott RD, Petrovitch H, Mailman RB, Ross GW. Low LDL cholesterol and increased risks of Parkinson's disease: Prospective results from Honolulu-Asia Aging Study. *Mov Disord* 2008;23(7):1013–1018.
29. Collins R, Peto R, Armitage J. The MRC/BHF heart protection study: Preliminary results. *Int J Clin Pract* 2002;56:53–56.
30. Davignon J. Beneficial cardiovascular pleiotropic effects on statins. *Circulation* 2004;109:III39–III43.
31. Ridker PM, Pradhan A, MacFadyen JG et al. Cardiovascular benefits and diabetes risk of statin therapy in primary prevention: An analysis from the JUPITER trial. *Lancet* 2012;380:565–571.
32. Westover MB, Bianchi MT, Eckman MH, Greenberg SM. Statin use following intracerebral hemorrhage: A decision analysis. *Arch Neurol* 2011;68(5):573–579.
33. Kastelein JJ, Akdim F, Stroes ES, ENHANCE investigators. Simvastatin with or without ezetimibe in familial hypercholesterolemia. *N Engl J Med* 2008;358:1431–1443.
34. De Lorgeril M, Salen P. Recent cholesterol-lowering drug trials: New data, new questions. *J Lipid Nutr* 2010;19(1):65–92.
35. Joshi PH, Chaudhari S, Blaha MJ et al. A point by point response to recent arguments against the use of statins in primary prevention. *Clin Cardiol* 2012;35(7):404–409.
36. Stone NJ, Robinson J, Lichenstein AH et al. 2013 ACC/AHA guideline on the treatment of blood cholesterol to reduce atherosclerotic cardiovascular risk in adults: A report of the American College of Cardiology/American Heart Association Task Force on practice guidelines. *J Am Coll Cardiol 2014*; 63(25_PA):2889–2934.
37. Kolata G. Risk Calculator for Cholesterol Appears Flawed, *New York Times*, November 17, 2013.
38. Ridker PM, Cook NR. Statins: New American Guidelines for prevention of cardiovascular disease. *Lancet* 2013;382(9907):1762–1765.
39. Statins: New US guidelines sparks controversy. *Lancet* 2013;382(9906):1680.

40. Ridker PM, Wilson PW. A trial-based approach to statin guidelines. *JAMA* 2013;310(11):1123–1124.

41. Golomb B. The importance of monitoring adverse events in statin, and other, clinical trials. *Clin Invest* 2013;3(10):913–916.

42. Machan CM, Hrynchak PK, Irving EL. Age-related cataract is associated with type 2 diabetes and statin use. *Optom Vis Sci* 2012;89(8):1165–1171.

43. Leuschen J, Mortensen EM, Frei CR, Mansi EA, Panday V, Mansi I. Association of statin use with cataracts: A propensity score-matched analysis. *JAMA Ophthalmol* 2013;131(11):1427–1434.

44. Saremi A, Bahn G, Reaven PD, VAT Investigators. Progression of vascular calcification is increased with statin use in the Veterans Affairs Diabetes Trial (VADT). *Diabetes Care* 2012;35(11):2390–2392.

45. Culver AL, Ockene IS, Balasubramanian R et al. Statin use and risk of diabetes mellitus in postmenopausal women in the Women's Health Initiative. *Arch Intern Med* 2012;172:144–152.

46. Sattar N, Preiss D, Murray HM et al. Statins and risk of incident diabetes: A collaborative meta-analysis of randomized statin trials. *Lancet* 2010;375(9716):735–742.

47. Diabetes Prevention Program Research Group. Reduction in the incidence of type 2 diabetes with lifestyle intervention or metformin. *N Engl J Med* 2002;346(6):393–403.

48. Schafer A, Hogger P. Oligomeric procyanidins of French maritime pink bark extract (Pycnogenol) effectively inhibit a-glucosidase. *Diabetes Res Clin Pract* 2007;77(1):41–46.

49. Lin J, Alt A, Liersch J, Bretzel RG, Brownlee MA, Hammes HP. Benfotiamin inhibits formation of advanced glycation endproducts in vivo. *Diabetes* 2000;49(Suppl 1):A143(P 583).

50. Hammes HP, Du X, Edelstein D et al. Benfotiamine blocks three major pathways of hyperglycemic damage and prevents experimental diabetic retinopathy. *Nat Med* 2003;9(3):294–299.

51. Haupt E, Ledermann H, Kopcke W. Benfotiamine in the treatment of diabetic polyneuropathy—a three-week randomized, controlled pilot study (BEDIP Study). *Int J Clin Pharmacol Ther* 2005;43(2):71–77.

52. Salas-Salvado J, Bullo M, Estruch R et al. Prevention of diabetes with Mediterranean diets. *Ann Intern Med* 2014;160(1):1–10.

53. Furbert CD, Pitt B. Withdrawal of cerivastatin from the world market. *Curr Control Trials Cardiovasc Med* 2001;2:205–207.

54. Cholesterol Treatment Trialists' (CTT) Collaborators, Mihaylova B, Emberson J et al. The effects of lowering LDL cholesterol with statin therapy in people at low risk of vascular disease: Meta-analysis of individual data from 27 randomised trials. *Lancet* 2012;380(9841):581–590.

55. Taylor F, Huffman M, Ebrahim S. Statin therapy for primary prevention of cardiovascular disease. *JAMA* 2013;310(22):2451–2452.

56. Golomb BA, Evans MA, Dimsdale JE, White HL. Effects of statins on energy and fatigue with exertion. *Arch Intern Med* 2012;172(15):1180–1182.

57. Westover MB, Bianchi MT, Eckman MH, Greenberg SM. Statin use following intracerebral hemorrhage: A decision analysis. *Arch Neurol* 2011;68(5):573–579.

58. Houston MC, Fazio S, Chilton FH et al. Non-pharmacologic treatment of dyslipidemia. *Prog Cardiovasc Dis* 2009;52(2):61–94.

59. Nijjar PS, Burke FM, Bioesch A, Rader DJ. Role of dietary supplements in lowering low-density lipoprotein cholesterol: A review. *J Clin Lipidol* 2010;4(4):248–258.

60. Houston MC, Cooil B, Olafsson BJ, Raggi P. Juice powder concentrate and systemic blood pressure, progression of coronary artery calcium and antioxidant status in hypertensive subjects: A pilot study. *Evid Based Complement Alternat Med* 2007;4(4):455–462.

61. Budoff MJ, Ahmadi N, Gul KM et al. Aged garlic extract supplemented with B vitamins, folic acid and L-arginine retards progression of subclinical atherosclerosis: A randomized clinical trial. *Prev Med* 2009;49(2–3):101–107.

62. Ruparelia N, Digby JE, Choudhury RP. Effects of niacin on atherosclerosis and vascular function. *Curr Opin Cardiol* 2010;26(1):66–70.

63. Al-Mohissen MA, Pun SC, Frohlich JJ. Niacin: From mechanisms of action to therapeutic uses. *Mini Rev Med Chem* 2010;10(3):204–217.

64. Saremi A, Arora R. The utility of omega-3 fatty acids in cardiovascular disease. *Am J Ther* 2009;16(5):421–436.

65. Burr ML, Fehily AM, Gilbert JF et al. Effects of changes in fat, fish, and fibre intakes on death and myocardial reinfarction: Diet and reinfarction trial (DART). *Lancet* 1989;2:757–761.

66. GISSI-Prevenzione Investigators. Dietary supplementation with n-3 polyunsaturated fatty acids and vitamin E after myocardial infarction: Results of the GISSI-Prevenzione trial. *Lancet* 1999;354:447–455.

67. Rissanen T, Voutilainen S, Nyyssonen K, Lakka TA, Salonen JT. Fish oil-derived fatty acids, docosa-hexaenoic acid and docosapentaenoic acid and the risk of acute coronary events: The Kuopio ischaemic heart disease risk factor study. *Circ* 2000;102(22):2677–2679.
68. Davis W, Rockway S, Kwasny M. Effect of a combined therapeutic approach of intensive lipid management, omega 3 fatty acid supplementation, and increased serum 25(OH) D on coronary calcium scores in asymptomatic adults. *Am J Ther* 2009;16(4):326–332.
69. Yokoyama M, Origasa H, Matsuzaki M et al. Japan EPA lipid intervention study (JELIS) Investigators. *Lancet* 2007;369(9567):1090–1098.
70. Ryan AS, Keske MA, Hoffman JP, Nelson EB. Clinical overview of algal-docosahexaenoic acid: Effects on triglyceride levels and other cardiovascular risk factors. *Am J Ther* 2009;16(2):183–192.
71. Kelley DS, Siegal D, Vemuri M, Chung GH, Mackey BE. Docosahexaenoic acid supplementation decreases remnant-like particle cholesterol and increases the (n-3) index in hypertriglyceridemic men. *J Nutr* 2008;138(1):30–35.
72. Mori TA, Burke V, Puddey IB et al. Purified eicosapentaenoic and docosahexaenoic acids have differential effects on serum lipids and lipoproteins, LDL particle size, glucose, and insulin in mildly hyperlipidemic men. *Am J Clin Nutr* 2000;71(5):1085–1094.
73. DiDonna L, DeLuca G, Mazzotti F et al. Statin-like principles of bergamot fruit (*Citrus bergamia*): Isolation of 3 hydroxymethylglutaryl flavonoid glycosides. *J Nat Prod* 2009;72(7):1352–1354.
74. Mollace V, Sacco I, Janda E et al. Hypolipidemic and hypoglycaemic activity of bergamot polyphenols: From animal models to human studies. *Fitoterapia* 2011;82(3):309–316.
75. Davignon J. Beneficial cardiovascular pleiotropic effects on statins. *Circulation* 2004;109:III39–III43.
76. Sinatra ST. Is cholesterol lowering with statins the gold standard for treating patients with cardiovascular risk and disease? *South Med J* 2003;96:220–222.
77. Hayward RA, Krumholz HM. Three reasons to abandon low-density lipoprotein targets: An open letter to the adult treatment panel IV of the National Institutes of Health. *Circ Cardiovasc Qual Outcomes* 2012;5(1):2–5.
78. Peabody F. The care of the patient. *JAMA* 1927;88:877–882.

4 Lipid Subfraction Testing

Richard Delany

CONTENTS

Why is lipid subfraction testing information included in a book entitled *Nutritional Strategies for Cardiovascular Disease?* How might this information be of help? When and how could it be helpful in the discussion of nutritional strategies for cardiovascular disease (CVD)?

Lipid subfraction testing helps to identify an individual's "residual risk" of atherosclerosis by determining the presence of high-risk lipoproteins. Patients who are at risk of or who already have evidence of atherosclerosis benefit from the development and implementation of personalized strategies. To be successful in the personal reduction of cardiovascular risk, physicians and health-care providers need to possess a keen knowledge of the pathophysiological basis behind a patient's specific cardiovascular risk factors. A working knowledge of the well-accepted risk reduction studies is also important. Such an understanding helps guide the physician to move from the knowledge acquired from studies of "groups" of patients to decide what to do for the unique "individual" patient that is seen in the personal encounter in an examination or consultation room.

Nutritional strategies are very important and can be successful but are often difficult to implement and maintain successfully. However, effective individual implementation should translate into individual clinical benefit. Risk factors linked to the causation of CVD can improve with successful nutritional and lifestyle strategies. Monitoring the improvement of an individual's underlying atherogenic lipoprotein levels is one way to assess the short-term benefits of a nutritional/lifestyle strategy. If successful, one would predict a future risk reduction or decreased progression of CVD.

One example of the effect of nutritional strategies in cardiovascular risk reduction is the improvement in lipid subfraction values when patients successfully eradicate metabolic syndrome. Complex lipid abnormalities often normalize with the loss of total weight, abdominal fat, and insulin resistance. A case study will be presented later that is an example of that type of result. Improvement in lipid measurements and other risk factors without pharmacological intervention illustrates the power of successful nutritional strategy.

In summary, lipid subfraction testing can both serve as a way to identify an individual's "residual risk" of atherosclerosis and as a measurement of nutritional success.

ATHEROSCLEROSIS

Atherosclerotic cardiovascular disease (ASCVD) is a leading cause of mortality and morbidity and is a major health problem in the United States and in many countries, accounting for 16.7 million deaths each year.[1] Coronary artery disease (CAD) and cerebrovascular disease are the most common forms of ASCVD. The lifetime risk of ASCVD is substantial and the condition is often silent, often striking without warning.

Historically, the primary view of the cause of atherosclerosis was believed to be due to the passive accumulation of cholesterol into the walls of medium-sized to large blood vessels. Currently, atherosclerosis is now also felt to be linked to the presence of three main bodily imbalances: (1) abnormal atherogenic lipoproteins, (2) chronic "sterile" inflammation, and (3) an enhanced tendency toward forming blood clots. Of these three predisposing factors, the cause(s) of the complex and chronic "sterile" inflammation linked to ASCVD remains unknown.

The specific events linked to the occurrence of an atherosclerotic plaque have been well described. The initial event is felt to be a qualitative change in the endothelial cells that cover the inner surface of arteries. Especially, small dense and/or oxidized LDL lipoproteins are allowed to enter and remain within the arterial wall. The usual protective HDL molecules that are present, are either too few in number and/or are dysfunctional in their reverse transport process. Triglyceride-rich lipoproteins (VLDL [very low density lipoprotein] and remnant particles) add to the mix becoming pro-inflammatory contributing to a pro-atherosclerotic state. Smooth muscle cells, already present in the intima or arriving from the media portion of the blood vessel wall, are thought to play a sustaining role in the developing plaque. Impaired clearance of dead cells from the intimal wall also contributes to the development of an atherosclerotic plaque. Monocytes become pro-inflammatory macrophages, changing from a more healthy M1 type to a less healthy M2 type. In addition, different types of T cells also become active pro-inflammatory participants. The innate immune system via pattern recognition receptors (PRRs) and the adaptive immune system are now understood to play important sustaining roles to the existence of chronic "sterile inflammation."[2,3]

The development of an atherosclerotic plaque is a complex chronic biological event with lipid, inflammatory, and thrombotic elements. Modern medicine has begun to understand in great detail what is happening but still does not clearly understand why it is happening!

ASSESSING YOUR PERSONAL RISK OF ATHEROSCLEROSIS

USE OF A CALCULATOR AND USE OF A GLOBAL RISK FACTOR ASSESSMENT

Blood lipid testing results, whether obtained by traditional or specialized subfraction lipid testing, are used as a way to help assess an individual's risk of developing future coronary heart disease (CHD) or stroke.

If an individual already has evidence of atherosclerosis, it becomes more urgent to discover and treat any modifiable risk factors (and possible causes) that make up the often hidden-from-view residual risk of another atherosclerotic event.

In asymptomatic individuals, the identification of underlying lipid abnormalities with no history or clinical evidence of atherosclerosis is helpful to identify the future risk of atherosclerotic events. Once a patient has been identified as having an increased risk of atherosclerosis, this should trigger the institution of a personalized strategy with some combination of changes in lifestyle and diet and the possible addition of nutritional supplements and/or drugs—all designed to safely reduce the risk of ASCVD. Such a strategy is crucial to prevent or delay the future occurrence of heart attacks, peripheral vascular disease, or strokes.

Using an accurate automatic calculator is an easy way to determine an individual's future risk of ASCVD. Three helpful scoring systems: (1) The Reynolds Risk Score, (2) The Canadian Framingham Risk Score Modification and (3) the Framingham CHD Risk Score.

The calculations from these scoring systems provide an estimate of individual's risk of developing a cardiovascular event over the next 10-year period as either low, moderate, or high. If an individual's risk is in the moderate or high category, ideally, there should be a focused implementation of a personalized combination of changes in lifestyle, diet, and the careful consideration of key nutritional supplements and/or drugs. It is important to stress that drugs need not be automatically added especially in an asymptomatic individual with no prior history of any CVD. However, if based on a personalized global risk factor assessment and the use of an accurate calculator, a person is at high risk of future clinical ASCVD over the next 10 years, the use of a statin should be strongly considered as an important part of the preventive strategy. Choose your calculator. I like the Reynolds the best.

The Reynolds Risk Score: An Easy Automatic Calculation: http://www.reynoldsriskscore.org
Canadian Framingham Risk Score Modification: An Easy Automatic Calculation; http://www.palmedpage.com/Framingham/CCSFramingham.html
The Framingham Risk Score: A Point System (-1 to 17 Points) http://www.nhlbi.nih.gov/guidelines/cholesterol/risk_tbl.htm

GLOBAL RISK FACTOR ASSESSMENT

CLINICAL DECISIONS REQUIRE AN ASSESSMENT OF INDIVIDUAL RISK

A global risk factor approach is an approach that involves the identification of the disease-specific risk factors associated with the chronic disease in question. Atherosclerosis is an example of a chronic disease that responds partially to the identification and treatment of underlying risk factors.[4] Once an individual's risk factors are identified, a treatment plan can be created directed at modifiable risk factors. Such a risk factor approach promotes a personalized integrative approach toward the prevention and treatment of atherosclerosis.

When a modifiable risk factor linked to atherosclerosis is identified, the hardest task is often the ability to achieve the desired target in an individual patient. This is especially true when it involves lifestyle changes but is also true in "getting to goal" of various metabolic blood tests and bodily measurements such as LDL particle number (LDL-P), high-sensitivity C-reactive protein (hsCRP), hemoglobin A1c, fasting blood sugar (FBS), body weight, blood pressure levels, and body mass index.

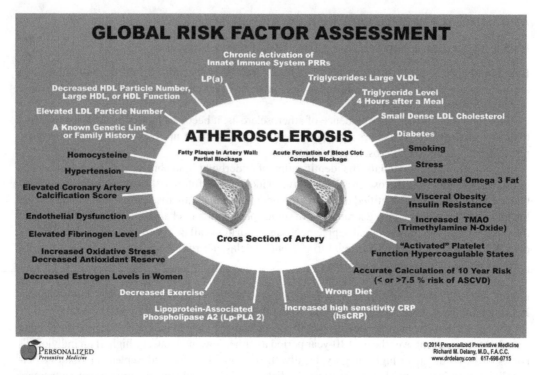

FIGURE 4.1   Disease causes, disease promoters, and disease risk identifiers.

Successful achievement of specific endpoints in risk factor modification clearly requires focus and commitment by both the patient and the physician.

My list of atherosclerotic risk factors (Figure 4.1) contains both officially accepted risk factors and also members that have not been universally accepted as "group-associated" risk factors. However, these "unofficial" risk factors possess biological plausibility and may contribute to the development of atherosclerosis in individual patients. In 2011, the National Lipid Association summarized their recommendations regarding lipid subfraction testing and other markers that are on my list below.[5]

Lipid subfraction testing is becoming increasingly accepted as an important part of a global risk factor assessment in patients at risk of atherosclerosis. Most importantly, the results of lipid subfraction testing often lead to modifications in the specific treatment plan addressing dyslipidemia risk in individual patients.

ATHEROSCLEROTIC RISK FACTORS

1. Presence of unknown immune-mediated inflammatory disease (IMID) or "sterile" inflammation[6,7]
2. Hyperlipidemia/dyslipidemia
3. Lp(a)—a special apoB lipoprotein
4. Decreased exercise
5. Wrong diet
6. Known genetic causation or strong family history
7. Inflammatory markers
   a. Increased hsCRP
   b. Increased lipoprotein-associated phospholipase A2 (Lp-PLA 2)
   c. Increased myeloperoxidase[8–11]
8. Diabetes mellitus

9. Hypertension
10. Insulin resistance with/without visceral obesity
11. Elevated coronary artery calcium score
12. Hypercoagulability
13. Endothelial dysfunction
14. Increased homocysteine
15. Decreased omega-3 fat (intake and/or absorption)
16. Increased TMAO (trimethylamine *N*-oxide) linked to the human microbiome[12–21]
17. Chronic stress

ATHEROSCLEROSIS

How Do Statins Work to Reduce ASCVD Risk?

Lipid lowering and inflammation reducing—These are the two mechanisms of how statin drugs reduce an individual's risk of a heart attack or stroke. Statins block a key enzyme in the mevalonate pathway (Figure 4.2). This leads to a reduction in downstream compounds with an important branch point seen at farnesyl pyrophosphate. From that point, cholesterol production occurs on one side and prenylated protein production occurs on the other. A reduction in cholesterol production stimulates a liver receptor to take more cholesterol out of the bloodstream. A reduction in prenylated proteins causes inflammation associated with arteries in the body to diminish. Most of the side effects seen with statins appear to occur due to a reduction in prenylated proteins.

When a patient takes a statin drug, both parts of the downstream mevalonate pathway are affected. Two of the main effects are beneficial: specifically a reduction in the blood level of LDL cholesterol and a reduction in inflammation.[22,23]

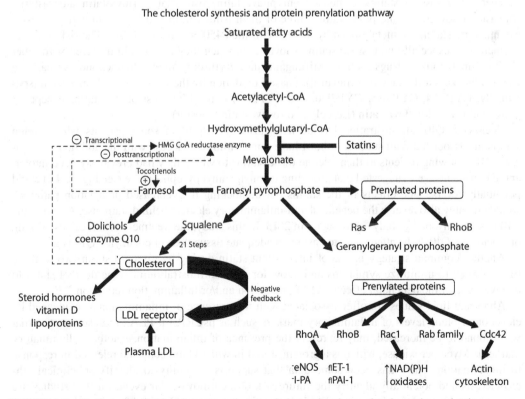

FIGURE 4.2 Statins work by blocking two pathways: cholesterol and prenylated protein production.

However, some of the effects of statins can be associated with mild symptoms or are actually clinically harmful, e.g., muscle aches, fatigue, memory loss, and mental status changes. Many of these symptoms (both the mild and the harmful) typically can come on slowly and insidiously and can be unappreciated by both the patient and the physician. As such, physicians need to be keenly aware of these symptoms and remain vigilant to the discovery of unsuspected clinically relevant statin toxicity.

I consider five issues before starting a patient on a statin who is starting the statin in an outpatient setting. (1) I try to normalize an individual's vitamin D levels before starting a statin, (2) I try to start at a low dose of the statin (so as not to assault their enzyme systems abruptly) and I then titrate upward at different speeds monitoring for side effects, (3) I spend time educating the patient about potential side effects and remain vigilant in monitoring the patient for symptoms and at times the use of blood tests measuring liver function tests and muscle enzymes (CPK and Aldolase levels), (4) I carefully consider the choice of water-soluble statins (pravastatin (Pravachol), rosuvastatin (Crestor), pitavastatin (Lialdo), and fluvastatin (Lescol) if the patient or family members have had a history of statin intolerance, and (5) in selected patients who have already shown intolerance, I use a water-soluble statin once or twice a week following the patient's lipid levels and symptoms or muscle enzyme levels. There are a number of genetic risk factors that have been identified that can identify patients at increased risk of statin toxicity.

The SLCO1B1 gene encodes for a protein in liver cells that is responsible for the transport of statins into the liver cells. Some common variations in the SLCO1B1 gene are associated with a reduced ability to process some of the statins resulting in higher blood concentration and higher muscle tissue exposure. One statin, fluvastatin, does not require this pathway for entry and would be an alternate choice of a statin for a patient who has symptomatic muscular complaints with the presence of the genetic variation. The statins that use this pathway are atorvastatin, simvastatin, rosuvastatin, and pravastatin. Boston Heart Diagnostics Laboratory includes gene testing for variants of SLCO1B1.[24]

There are 7 possible statins to choose from: pitavastatin, rosuvastatin , fluvastatin, atorvastatin, simvastatin, lovastatin, and pravastatin. Three of them (simvastatin and lovastatin and to a lesser extent, atorvastatin) are metabolized by the cytochrome P450 enzyme CYP3A4. The risk of toxicity increases, especially with simvastatin or lovastatin, when they are co-administered with other CYP3A4 metabolized drugs such as antifungal drugs, erythromycin, colchicine, and two calcium channel blockers (diltiazem or verapamil). Phase I oxidation by the cytochrome P450 system (specifically: CYP3A4, CYP3A5, CYP2D6, and CYP2C9) is used by most of the statins except for pitavastatin (Lialdo), fluvastatin (Lescol), and rosuvastatin (Crestor).

Coenzyme Q10 administration has been historically helpful in some patients who develop symptoms associated with statin use, but I have found minimal success with the addition of coenzyme Q10 allowing patients to then tolerate those statins to which they had previously been intolerant. Experiments have suggested that providing geranylgeranyl pyrophosphate (see Figure 4.2) could potentially reverse side effects of the statins but unblocking the decreased prenylation pathways would probably also reverse the beneficial anti-inflammatory element behind statin use. A coenzyme Q10 in statin myopathy study[25] was begun in 2013. In this study, the treatment arm receives 600 mg of Coenzyme Q10 daily, attempting to ensure an adequate tissue dose of coenzyme Q10 is given.

Another common strategy is one of intermittent statin dosing by giving a statin two to three times a week to minimize symptoms and allow for safe administration of some dose of statin to receive some of the beneficial effects of LDL reduction and/or inflammation reduction.[26,27]

Abnormal lipid values are often associated with the presence of inflammation as evidenced by elevation of blood levels of inflammatory markers such as hsCRP. Lp-PLA2 represents a test that when found to be increased, may represent the presence of inflammation. Another inflammatory marker is Myeloperoxidase, which is a protein stored in white blood cells and released in response to inflammation. There has been some data that supports its ability to identify subclinical atherosclerosis and potentially identify the future risk of a cardiovascular event. Further studies are needed to understand the clear clinical and prognostic usefulness of Lp-PLA2 and myeloperoxidase measurements. At this time, successful reduction of high-risk lipid values along with the reduction of hsCRP has been shown in multiple studies to reduce CHD risk on an average of 36% (up to 46% in diabetic patients).

Even with successful administration of a statin and its ability to lower both the LDL cholesterol and hsCRP of patients, there still remains a significant residual risk of CHD. "The decrease in cardiovascular mortality due to statin therapy still allows two thirds of cardiovascular events to occur."[28] I believe that while the primary cause(s) of the chronic inflammation are still not understood, the use of lipid subfraction testing to help identify and correct an individual's abnormal lipid subfractions can reduce residual CHD risk.

LIPID TESTING AND ATHEROSCLEROSIS

Lipoproteins are a group of particles that are responsible for transporting lipids throughout the body. Each type of lipoprotein contains a combination of protein, cholesterol, triglyceride, and phospholipid molecules.[29] There are a number of factors that affect an individual's concentration and function of the various lipoproteins. A dynamic, primarily bloodstream-based process results in daily modifications of the various lipoproteins as they are able to drop off or pick up different components in the blood, liver, or other tissues. Large triglyceride lipoproteins (VLDL) formed by the liver in response to dietary fat intake are typically modified once they arrive in the bloodstream. The specific activity of different enzymes within an individual's bloodstream and tissues (e.g., lipoprotein lipase [LPL] and cholesterol ester transfer protein [CETP]) help shape the amount and type of lipoproteins. Additional modifications of the lipoproteins also occur throughout the day in response to one's diet, level of exercise, the presence of insulin resistance, the nature and the degree of any underlying chronic inflammatory states, and lastly, the individual genetic expression of the individual patient.

A traditional lipid panel testing measures the amount of cholesterol and triglyceride within the various types of lipoproteins providing a snapshot view of a complex array of lipoproteins that vary from each other in size, composition and function (Figure 4.3). The complexity of the various lipoproteins are better understood by realizing that they are made up of a number of different elements: chylomicrons, chylomicron remnants, VLDL (triglyceride) particles (total, large, and small), LDL particles (total, large, intermediate, and small), Lp(a), and HDL particles (total, large, medium and small, or HDL2 and HDL3).[30]

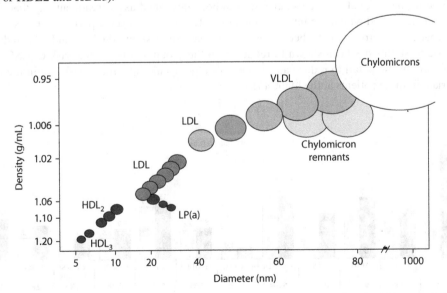

FIGURE 4.3 A view of the lipoprotein subclasses. (From Otvos JD, *Handbook of Lipoprotein Testing*, AACC Press, Washington, DC, 2000.)

All the high-risk atherogenic lipoproteins (VLDL, IDL [intermediate-density lipoprotein], LDL, and Lp(a)) have in common the presence of one molecule of apolipoprotein B. Apolipoprotein B levels (apoB) and the LDL particle number (LDL-P) currently represent two available tests that accurately provide a direct measurement of atherogenic particles[31] and are superior to the traditionally measured LDL cholesterol level (LDL-C).

Although a non-HDL cholesterol level (non-HDL-C) is better at determining the presence of residual atherogenic particles missed by a traditionally measured LDL-C, it does not accurately measure the total level of atherogenic particles[32,33] that measurements of apoB and LDL-P both provide. As such, some residual risk of CHD can be missed by relying solely on a non-HDL-C measurement.

ApoB levels are readily available in many commercial laboratories and medical centers using a number of different methodologies. Nuclear magnetic resonance (NMR) measurement of LDL-P may actually be more precise than apoB, but the real advantages of NMR over apoB is the ability of the NMR LipoProfile to provide more information about the other major lipoprotein classes,[32] especially the level of small dense LDL, the total HDL-P, the large HDL, and the large VLDL.

WHY LIPID SUBFRACTION TESTING?

- To obtain an accurate measurement of an individual's atherogenic lipoproteins
- To better assess potential clinical risk
- To assess successful improvement of high risk lipoproteins after treatment

A significant degree of "residual risk"[28] exists in many patients after being treated with statins as evidenced in the major stain trials (Figure 4.4).[34] Residual risk is found particularly in patients with insulin resistance and/or type 2 diabetes mellitus. In 2008,[35] a "residual risk reduction initiative" was formed to focus specifically on a plan to treat the common atherogenic lipid abnormalities found in obese patients with metabolic syndrome and type II diabetes. Initially, in the earlier studies such as the Scandinavian Simvastatin Survival Study (4S), a 20% cardiovascular (CV) event rate was found in statin-treated patients. However, recent statin studies using high-dose statin therapy to achieve intensive LDL-C lowering have shown a further reduction in the risk of CHD. Nevertheless, there still exists an approximately 9% residual risk despite intensive LDL-C lowering.[36] A persistent presence of atherogenic lipoproteins unrecognized by the traditional lipid panel is now felt to play a role in the residual risk. This situation has been described as "a treatment gap that can be recognized and closed with more intensive therapy only if the atherogenic particle is measured."[31]

Atherogenic lipoproteins have been shown to increase the risk of ASCVD, and their reduction by the use of statins has been shown to reduce both the group and individual risk of ASCVD. If lifestyle modifications fail to reduce an individual's atherogenic lipoprotein risk, statin therapy is appropriate in those patients at the highest risk.

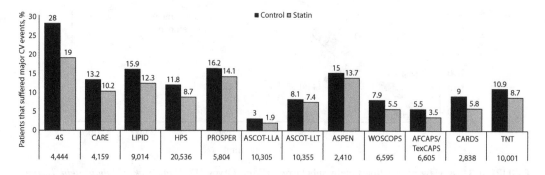

FIGURE 4.4 Presence of residual cardiovascular risk in large prospective studies of optimal statin therapy.

Until December 2013, the major assessment of success of an individual's risk reduction has been by the results of a specific target LDL-C value obtained by traditional lipid testing. Using this measurement, "clinical studies indicate that treatment with statins reduces the risk of major CV events by 21% for every 39 mg/dL decrease in LDL-C and that when LDL-C is lowered below 70 mg/dL, further reduction in CV risk is accomplished."[36] Overall, the amount of risk reduction by the use of statin therapy is approximately 30% when given moderately intensive statin therapy and up to a risk reduction of 45% for more intensive therapy when LDL-C is reduced by up to 50%.[37]

The focus of the late 2013 ACC/AHA Guidelines was away from the use of statin therapy based on goals to achieve specific LDL-C and non-HDL-C targets. Instead, the new recommended focus was on the use of statin therapy for "all individuals at increased ASCVD risk who are likely to benefit from risk reduction." While lifestyle modification is recognized as a cornerstone of therapy before and during therapy, the new guidelines identified 4 statin benefit groups while at the same time reinforcing the need for either "moderate-intensity or high-intensity statin therapy" to lower LDL-C by 30%–50%.[38] The 2013 ACC/AHA Guidelines produce evidence from multiple studies supporting statin therapy as an important tool to achieve documented risk reduction.

I feel that the approach should be more individual-based relying on a working knowledge of the key studies of risk reduction with and without statin use and a keen awareness and ability to follow a patient carefully who is prescribed a statin. There are clearly some clinically identifiable high-risk patients whose underlying abnormal lipid subfraction values result in further treatment leading to further risk reduction. Such treatment requires analysis of the individual's persistent high-risk lipid subfractions to guide individualized therapy.

I determine an estimate of an individual's risk of future atherosclerotic events after obtaining a lifestyle history, a family history, stress test results, lab data analysis, a physical examination, and a global risk factor assessment, which may include a lipid subfraction analysis. If there is a high future risk or atherosclerosis is already present, I do not hesitate to add in a statin with clear goals to obtain safe lipid-lowering and inflammation-lowering results. In such high-risk patients, I want to know the lipid subfraction data to both guide and judge my therapy. The goal is the maximal risk reduction for the individual patient.

Tables 4.1 and 4.2 summarize and compare the current components of the traditional lipid profile panel and the NMR LipoProfile lipid subfraction panel. Table 4.3 summarizes the benefits and the drawback associated with the traditional lipid profile.

TABLE 4.1
Traditional Lipid Profile

- Total cholesterol
- LDL cholesterol [TC − (HDL + TG/5)]
- non-HDL cholesterol (TC − HDL)
- HDL cholesterol
- Triglyceride

TABLE 4.2
NMR LipoProfile

- LDL particle concentration: LDL–P
- LDL-small dense LDL subclass
- HDL particle concentration: HDL–P
- HDL large HDL subclass
- Triglyceride subclass: large VLDL–P

The traditional lipid panel testing measures the amount of cholesterol and triglyceride within various types of lipoproteins providing an LDL-C level. The NMR lipoprofile measures directly the amount of lipoprotein molecules providing an LDL particle number (LDL-P). The NMR method quantifies the signals broadcast by lipoproteins of different size to accurately measure the concentration of each subclass of lipoproteins.[39] Although the traditional lipid panel uses the cholesterol content as surrogate markers for the levels of the lipoproteins, the NMR LipoProfile measures directly the amount of atherogenic lipoproteins avoiding the likelihood of a "treatment gap" due to hidden atherogenic lipoproteins.

Figures 4.5 and 4.6[40] illustrate how the NMR LipoProfile obtains the specific measurements of the various lipoproteins. The particle concentration of different-sized lipoprotein subclasses are derived from the NMR measured amplitudes of the terminal methyl groups of the specific lipoproteins. The concentrations used are nmol/L for LDL and VLDL particles and μmol/L for HDL particles compared to concentrations of mg/dL for the traditionally measured lipoproteins.

Lipoprotein subclasses do not have all the same associations with CHD. In Figure 4.7,[39] the breakdown of the various NMR-derived lipoproteins are displayed. There are 3 subtypes of VLDL with the large VLDL felt to be of higher risk. There are 4 subtypes of LDL-all of which make up the LDL-P. The small, dense LDL lipoproteins are of higher risk in many subgroups of patients but especially those with insulin resistance and/or metabolic syndrome. There are three subtypes of HDL and the large HDL may be more protective than the small HDL in most (but possibly not all) subgroups of

---

TABLE 4.3
Traditional Lipid Profile: Benefits and Drawbacks

Benefits	Drawbacks
• Availability	• The presence of a treatment gap:
• Historical data	• An underestimation of true risk by LDL-C
	• TG elevation can hide the true LDL level
	• Small dense LDL – not measured
	• Total HDL-P & HDL subclasses – not measured
	• Higher risk TG subclass – not measured

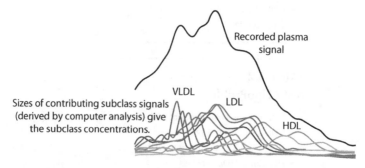

Each lipoprotein subclass broadcasts a unique NMR "sound."

V6 V5 V4 V3 V2 V1   IDL L3 L2   L1 H5 H4 H3 H2 H1

Simultaneous "ringing" of the plasma lipoproteins produces a recorded signal.

Recorded plasma signal

Sizes of contributing subclass signals (derived by computer analysis) give the subclass concentrations.

VLDL

LDL

HDL

FIGURE 4.5 Lipoprotein subclasses broadcast unique signals allowing for individual identification and quantification.

Each different-size lipoprotein particle broadcasts a distinguishable NMR signal. The signal amplitudes give the concentrations of the particles.

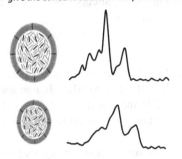

FIGURE 4.6 Different shaped signals and different amplitudes allow for accurate identification and quantification.

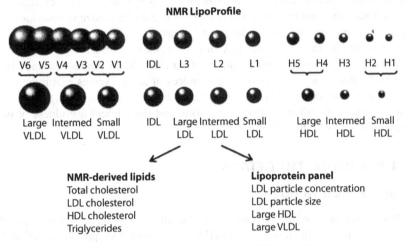

FIGURE 4.7 A summary view of the spectrum of NMR-derived lipoproteins.

patients. It would not be surprising to find that the large HDL subfractions may be beneficial and predictive of lower risk in some subgroups of patients such as metabolic syndrome and yet not helpful in other genetically acquired dyslipidemias. I expect that the use of some lipid subfractions will be found to be specifically helpful in the assessment and treatment for a specific clinical subtype of patient.

Detecting and diminishing atherogenic subfractions have the potential to reduce the risk of ASCVD. Nevertheless, controversy exists as to whether (1) any lipid subfractions should be tested and (2) which patients (based on either clinical/family history issues or preliminary laboratory data) should have this additional testing performed.[5,37,41–43]

The most widely agreed on helpful measurement is the LDL-P, which provides a better assessment of ASCVD risk in many high-risk patients than the traditionally measured LDL-C. The LDL-P represents the sum total of all the LDL lipoproteins measured by NMR. This value is very comparable to an apoB level because it, like an apoB level, represents an accurate level of an individual's atherogenic lipoproteins.

Comparative clinical studies have shown that the levels of the various lipoproteins themselves, rather than the cholesterol content, in many (but not all) patients, better determine the risks of atherosclerosis.[44] The cholesterol content of the lipoproteins as measured by the traditional lipid panel testing are best viewed as surrogate markers[39] for the underlying level of lipoproteins. The main issue is that while the traditional lipid panel is accurate for many patients, it often fails to identify the higher risk that some patients possess.

This summary of the possible role and benefits of lipid subfraction testing derives from a 13-year clinical use of the NMR LipoProfile.[45] I use NMR LipoProfile testing as part of a global risk factor assessment (Figure 4.1) in evaluating those patients who possess an increased risk of ASCVD or who already have evidence of atherosclerosis.

OTHER TESTING COMPANIES

Berkley Heart Lab, now a part of Quest Laboratory,[46] utilizes ion mobility analysis to directly measure LDL-P and subfractions of LDL, VLDL, and HDL. In one study,[47] LDL subfractions obtained by this technology found evidence of an increased risk of ASCVD associated with the presence of small to medium dense LDL particles and a decreased risk of atherosclerosis associated with higher values of large HDL particles.

Atherotech[48] currently offers lipid subfraction testing that includes measurements of LDL-particle and subclasses, total HDL and subclasses, and remnant lipoproteins.

Boston Heart Diagnostics[49] offers lipid subfraction testing along with an extensive array of biologically plausible risk factors. Boston Heart Diagnostics is the only laboratory that provides the HDL map, which identifies and quantifies the amount of five different-size subfractions of maturing HDL molecules. The measurement of the largest HDL using The HDL map methodology has been shown to be predictive of cardiovascular risk in both women and men.[50–55] Additionally, Boston Heart Diagnostic provides unique measurements of an individual's production and absorption of cholesterol, which allows for more personalized choices of statins versus ezetimibe or the use of both together. The methodology of small dense LDL testing by Boston Heart Diagnostic differs from the small dense LDL NMR Liposcience testing and the clinical usefulness of one method versus the other has yet to be directly studied.

THE NMR LIPOPROFILE: THE DETAILS

LDL LIPOPROTEIN PARTICLE NUMBER

Traditional lipid panel lipid testing fails to always identify the presence of high-risk atherogenic lipoproteins. Although the calculation of non-HDL cholesterol does provide additional information about "hidden" triglyceride-rich" atherogenic lipoproteins, it reflects the cholesterol content of atherogenic particles, but not the accurate number of atherogenic particles as does the NMR LipoProfile and apoB levels.[56]

The NMR LipoProfile provides 5 potentially important lipid subfractions that can help assess risk and guide therapy in the individual patient. The most commonly accepted helpful marker is the LDL particle number (LDL-P) (Table 4.4).

Because the LDL-C relies on the cholesterol content of lipoproteins and the NMR LipoProfile measures the number of particles by themselves, there can exist "discordance" between the results when tested simultaneously. Discordance is defined as a situation when the traditionally measured LDL-C level and the LDL particle number (LDL-P) differ significantly from each while testing the

---

TABLE 4.4

Details of NMR LipoProfile

- LDL particle concentration: LDL-P
- LDL-small dense LDL subclass
- HDL particle concentration: HDL-P
- HDL large HDL subclass
- Triglyceride subclass: large VLDL-P

---

same specimen at the same time. This can result in one LDL measurement being reported as normal while the other LDL measurement would be reported as abnormal. Hence a discordance exists.

When discordance exists between these two tests of LDL concentration, the LDL-C is often found to either underestimate or overestimate the true level of underlying atherogenic lipoproteins compared to the LDL-P measurement.

The more common directional type of discordance occurs with an underestimation of the risk. When this occurs, the more accurate predictive risk lies with the LDL-P measurement rather than the LDL-C measurement. In this scenario, if the LDL-C was found to be normal and the LDL-P was found to still be elevated, more treatment might be added because of the higher risk predicted by an elevated LDL-P.

Conversely, there can be discordance in the opposite direction. In this instance, the LDL-C reports out a measurement that is normal while the simultaneous LDL-P reports out a low measurement. Similar to the other directional discordance, the LDL-P measurement has been found to be the more correct value as it relates to a reduced predictive risk compared to a higher, LDL-C measurement.

An example of this dual type of directional discordance between LDL-P and LDL-C is seen in the analysis Figure 4.8. In this study, 516 patients on the high end of risk are more accurately defined by LDL-P; and 553 patients on the low end of risk are more accurately defined by LDL-P.[44]

In Figure 4.9 from the Framingham Offspring Study,[57] the risk of future CV events over 15 years was higher in 282 patients who were found to simultaneously have high LDL-P values and yet lower LDL-C values. This again demonstrates the discordance that can exist between LDL-P and LDL-C. In both these studies, a significant number of patients were determined to have a residual ASCVD risk uncovered by LDL-P testing.

A recent analysis of data from the HealthCore Integrated Research Database from 16 Wellpoint/Anthem plans of commercially insured patients supported the importance of measuring LDL-P over LDL-C. Those high-risk adult patients who ended up receiving more intensive treatment based on attempts to successfully achieve an LDL-P goal of <1000 µg/dL compared to patients who successfully achieved an LDL-C goal of <100 mg/dL had a clear reduction in cardiovascular event rates over the subsequent 12–36 months.[58]

Two 2013 summary reviews[59,60] of the benefits of LDL-P testing over LDL-C testing reinforced this issue of hidden discordance. The final assessment was that the use of LDL-P for monitoring lipid-lowering therapy, especially for those patients on statins, can provide a more accurate assessment of residual cardiovascular risk.

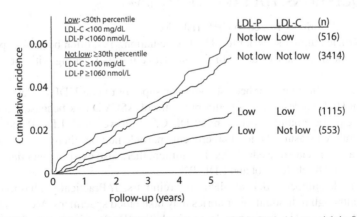

FIGURE 4.8 MESA study. Higher risk in 516 patients based on LDL-P; and lower risk in 553 patients based on LDL-P.

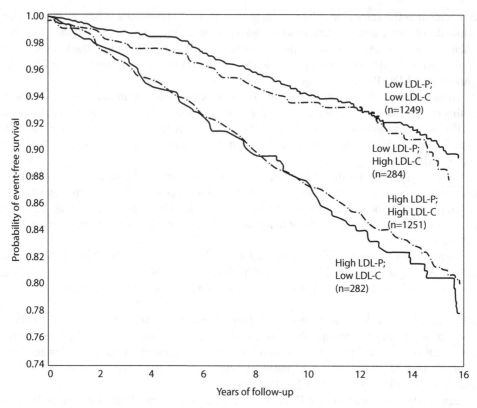

FIGURE 4.9   Framingham offspring study: Higher risk in 282 patients with a high LDL-P and a low LDL-C; Lower risk in 284 patients with a low LDL-P and a high LDL-C.

In summary, benefits that result from the use of Lipid Subfraction Testing to assess LDL-P are

1. To better assess the presence of a residual risk due to an underestimated presence of residual atherogenic lipoproteins, i.e., the identification of a "Treatment Gap"
2. To guide and judge the success of treatment plans designed to eradicate residual atherogenic lipoproteins

SUMMARY QUESTIONS: LDL PARTICLE NUMBER

1. Is LDL particle number linked to CHD risk? Yes.
2. Is LDL particle number superior to LDL-C calculation? Yes, often because typically there is a 25%–33% discordance rate with the predictive results tracking with the LDL-P over the LDL-C.
3. Has the LDL particle number been shown to be superior to non-HDL cholesterol measurement? Non-HDL cholesterol is a better predictor of ASCVD risk because it measures the atherogenic particle number better than LDL-C.[60] However, both LDL-P and apoB levels more accurately measure the total atherogenic particle number thereby more successfully capturing any associated residual risk. In addition, there also exists a potential discordance between non-HDL cholesterol and LDL-P.[61]
4. Is LDL particle number widely available and reimbursed? Practically it has to be drawn in the office although individual laboratories may take blood specimens. Medicare covers the test; $99 if uncovered by insurance. Increasingly the NMR derived LDL-P is also becoming available as one element of testing within specialized lipid panels (Figure 4.10).

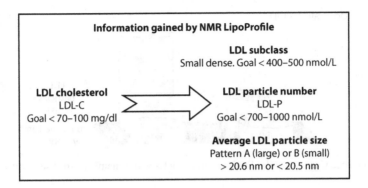

FIGURE 4.10   NMR derived LDL lipoprotein information versus LDL-C.

5. Has the LDL particle number been shown to better predict the presence of treatable residual risk reduction when the non-HDL is calculated? It remains to be studied fully but there
is published evidence of clear discordance between the risk defined by non-HDL measurements and LDL-P.[61,62]

6. Current National Lipid Association recommendations[5] for LDL particle number testing: reasonable for many patients who have intermediate risk score, family history, recurrent events;
it is fine to consider for selected patients with CHD or CHD equivalent.[5] I strongly agree,
especially with patients who have metabolic syndrome, elevated triglycerides, or who develop
cardiovascular events despite being on "successful" therapy based on traditional lipid testing.

THE SMALL DENSE LDL PARTICLES

The LDL particles measured by the NMR LipoProfile can be separated into small dense or larger
sizes. A number of clinical studies have shown higher CHD risk associated with increased levels of
small dense LDL.[63–66] In the 1997 Quebec Cardiovascular Study[67] (Figure 4.11), men were stratified
by apoB level and LDL particle size. High apoB was associated with CHD. The presence of both
high apoB and small dense LDL was associated with a marked increase in CHD risk. Treatment
options would include (1) lowering apoB levels and LDL levels with a statin, and (2) attempting to
change any significant number of residual small dense LDL particles to a larger size via the use of
Niacin, omega-3 fat, fibrates, or a statin itself.

A 13-year follow-up data analysis of the Quebec Cardiovascular Study was published in 2005.[68]
It reaffirmed the importance of small dense LDL particles in risk of CHD especially in the first
7 years of follow-up. The analysis also revealed that the larger LDL particles were not associated
with an increase in CHD over the 13-year follow-up. However, there are other studies that have suggested that larger LDL particles may be associated with a higher risk.[69–71]

The MESA study published in 2007[72] utilized NMR LipoProfile testing in analyzing LDL particle subclasses, LDL size, and the incidence of carotid atherosclerosis. The MESA study found that
small and large LDL particles were both significantly associated with subclinical atherosclerosis
and felt strongly there was no higher risk with small dense LDL. However, in a recent January 2014
study[73] of the same MESA group of patients, a new automated homogeneous assay[74] of small dense
LDL identified a higher risk of CHD in patients with small dense LDL but only in normoglycemic
individuals while simultaneous NMR-derived small dense LDL data did not discover a higher risk.

There are now at least 5 available techniques that are able to determine LDL particle size and
thus are able to give some measurement of the level of small dense LDL particles. These include (1)
segmented gradient gel electrophoresis (SGGe), (2) ultracentrifugation vertical auto profile (VAP),
(3) nuclear magnetic resonance (NMR), (4) ion mobility (IM),[75] and (5) a simple heparin-magnesium
precipitation method (direct homogenous LDL assay).[74,76,77]

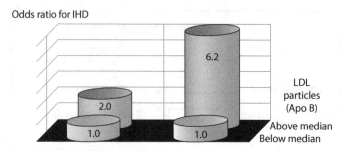

FIGURE 4.11   Quebec Cardiovascular Study: LDL particles and ischemic heart disease risk.

While one study[75] compared the first four methods of LDL particle size and found substantial agreement between them, the more recently published and utilized simple precipitation method of the small dense LDL[74,76,77] may be more sensitive and/or more specific. This possibility is based on a comparison of the data from the Multi-Ethnic Study of Atherosclerosis (MESA) lipoprotein sub-fraction analysis published in 2007 utilizing the NMR small dense testing method versus testing the same blood samples from the MESA lipoprotein subfraction analysis published in 2014 utilizing the simple precipitation, direct homogeneous assay method.

There are subgroups of patients both with and without obvious clinical insulin resistance who have atherosclerosis and possess measurable levels of small dense LDL that identify increased ASCVD risk. It is important to consider lowering the levels of all LDL particles into an optimal range but especially in those patients who have a significant proportion of their LDL particles made up of the small dense pattern.

Additionally I have found similar discordant results in some patients whom I have simultaneously tested for the level of small dense LDL by NMR and the simple precipitation-homogeneous assay. My preliminary results have found a number of patients who had low levels of small dense LDL-P by NMR and yet elevated levels by the simple precipitation-homogeneous assay. The accuracy of this observation and the percentage of patients who exhibit this discordance between the various small dense LDL testing modalities and the clinical relevance is unclear at this time. It requires further study in order to both confirm and to understand the clinical relevance.

The simple precipitation method of small dense LDL testing has had a number of publications[77–86] that attest to its ability to predict atherosclerotic risk.

I believe that the presence of elevated levels of predominantly small dense LDL particles represent, in some patients, a much higher risk than if the LDL particles were mostly large. An accurate and risk predictive measurement of small dense LDL particles is an important tool in guiding the development of treatment strategies. Such strategies should be designed to reduce the risk of cardio-vascular events in both groups of patients and in individual patients who are found to be at risk of or who already possess atherosclerosis.

In addition, it should be recognized that patients who cannot tolerate statins are often left with persistent elevated total level of LDL particles. Non-statin therapy such as Niaspan, omega-3 fat, or possibly fibrates, should be used to shift the size of the small dense higher risk LDL to a lower risk larger size LDL. I believe that patients who cannot tolerate statins should not be left with high levels of small dense LDL lipoproteins if a shift can be accomplished toward the larger size.

In my experience, it is not uncommon to find elderly women with no evidence of atherosclerosis but with elevated levels of total cholesterol and LDL-P particles of which almost all are in the large size. These women also typically possess elevated levels of HDL-P and large HDL levels, and are thin without any abdominal fat. In this subgroup, the presence of elevated large LDL particles do not appear to be associated with an increased risk of ASCVD and I typically do not treat them with a statin if there are no other risk factors placing the patient at increased risk.

Individuals with familial hypercholesterolemia[87,88] have both increased large LDL particle numbers along with very high total LDL-C levels and this group of patients possess a clear risk of early onset of heart disease. However, when familial hypercholesterolemia patients were given Simvastatin alone versus Simvastatin and Ezetimibe (Zetia) for 2 years in the AIM-HIGH Study,[89] the group given Simvastatin and Ezetimibe reached significantly lower total LDL-C levels and yet surprisingly did not do as well as the group given Simvastatin alone. This finding may be explained, in part, by possibility of an unrecognized shift of LDL particles from the possibly lower risk large LDL subfraction toward the higher risk small dense LDL subfraction that appears to occur in an as yet undetermined percentage of patients when Ezetimibe (Zetia) is added to a patient already taking a statin. Lipid subfraction data were not performed in this study. This hidden shift may occur in 30%–40% of patients but it needs to be studied using the most sensitive and specific assay of small dense LDL.

Ezetimibe (Zetia)[90] has been shown to shift the proportion of large LDL-C particles toward the small dense particles, which might explain the lack of carotid artery benefit from the additional cholesterol lowering in the group receiving both Ezetimibe and a statin (Richard M. Delany, Unpublished observations, 2008). If this potentially harmful essentially hidden-from-view "ezetimibe LDL shift" is shown to occur in a significant percentage of patients when combined with a statin, it would give more credence to the potential higher risk of small LDL particles over large LDL particles.

Further studies, utilizing the most sensitive and specific small dense LDL particle assay, should be performed in statin naïve patients, defining both their unique baseline cholesterol absorption and production status along with their lipid subfractions. Repeat studies should then be performed on a statin alone, on ezetimibe alone, and when ezetimibe is added to patient already on a statin. I believe it is important to confirm or exclude whether or not an essentially hidden "ezetimibe shift" might be occurring in a significant percentage of patients or in specific subtype of patient.

Patients with familial combined hyperlipidemia have predominantly small dense LDL lipoproteins and these particles appear to be directly related to cardiovascular events, independent of metabolic syndrome, total cholesterol, and apoB.[91]

The risk of small dense LDL particles may primarily be related to the fact that patients with small dense LDL have more particles than those with same level of cholesterol that are large LDL (Figure 4.12)[40] In some patients, a greater ASCVD risk reduction can be achieved by lowering elevated levels of small dense LDL particles. This is especially important in patients with metabolic syndrome.

It should be noted that overweight individuals who are able to achieve a weight reduction of 20–30 pounds accompanied by a loss of their truncal obesity often normalize their NMR LipoProfile without the need for a statin (to be discussed in a following first case study). In this type of clinical scenario of resolution of metabolic syndrome with diet alone, the total LDL-P becomes markedly decreased along with a significant lowering of small dense LDL-P and an actual rise in the large LDL-P and a moderate increase in the large HDL. I believe this type of abnormal NMR LipoProfile reversal with or without lipid-lowering drugs is associated with a decreased risk of CHD.

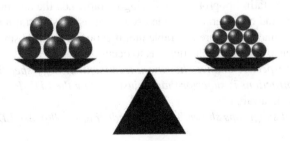

FIGURE 4.12 Large buoyant LDL particles versus small dense LDL particles; at the same level of LDL cholesterol, the small dense group of patients have 25% more particles.

In summary, it appears that the size of the LDL and the associated risk can be different for different subgroups of patients. Patients with familial hypercholesteremia do appear to have elevated levels of large LDL that promote atherosclerosis. However, for most other groups, I believe that elevated small dense LDL particles, do in fact, point to a higher risk.

The fact that small dense LDL-P is not as a high a risk for one group of patients as it is for another does not mean that it should not be viewed as a potential modifiable risk factor in many patients at risk of or already with atherosclerosis. Individualizing patient assessment and treatment is a common everyday event in the offices of health-care practitioners. The use of lipid subfraction testing as it relates to the assessment of individual patients at risk is especially helpful in patients with clinical features of metabolic syndrome or who possess lipid patterns revealing high triglycerides and low HDL and a discordance between LDL-C and LDL-P. In many patients, the discovery of elevated small dense LDL levels identify higher risk and often provide an opportunity to further reduce an individual's risk.

SUMMARY QUESTIONS: LDL SUBFRACTIONS: SMALL DENSE VERSUS LARGE BUOYANT

1. *Is small dense LDL a strong risk marker of CHD risk?*

    Probably yes, especially in patients with insulin resistance and/or metabolic syndrome. However, in the 2007 MESA study, the risk linked more to the LDL-P concentration rather than to either large and small LDL subclasses. Yet, a recent retesting of MESA study serum using a new automated small dense LDL technique found higher risk in normoglycemic men with elevated small dense LDL particles.

    A persistently elevated small dense LDL-P should be carefully assessed and treatment should be considered to lower it and/or to promote its shift into a larger LDL-P subtype. Both statin and non-statin therapies can be used, especially if the patient cannot successfully lower his LDL-P < 1000 nmol/L.

2. *What reduces the small dense LDL while increasing the large buoyant LDL?*

    Weight loss in patients with metabolic syndrome, control of diabetes, lowering of triglycerides, niacin, omega-3, fibrates, and possible withdrawal of ezetimibe (via cessation of a possible ezetimibe shift of large LDL toward small dense LDL).

3. *What can move the large LDL toward a small dense LDL?*

    Weight gain, especially truncal obesity; addition of ezetimide to a patient already on a statin; excess carbohydrate intake; poorly controlled diabetes; and increased trans fat/saturated fat intake.

    A patient with risk factors for atherosclerosis who also is found to have an elevated small dense LDL particle number increases the importance of instituting a global risk factor approach to the individual patient. Typically, this leads to monitoring the lipid values more carefully, aggressively attempting to eradicate insulin resistance by exercise, diet, and the use of non-statin lipoprotein-modifying therapy, i.e., the addition of omega-3 fat, niacin or fibrates, and consideration of the use of statins. Rosuvastatin (Crestor), a potent statin medication, may have more favorable modification of existing small dense LDL-P,[92] but more experience and data collection has to occur.

4. *Are there any prospective studies showing a treatment strategy specifically designed to change LDL subfractions is superior than to just treating the LDL-P or LDL-C?*

    No, not that I am aware of.

5. *Have any clinical subgroups shown benefit by reducing small dense LDL and increasing large LDL?*

    Yes, but it often occurs by lowering total LDL-P and correcting other modifiable risk factors making it difficult to know the specific benefit attained specifically by the lowering small dense LDL particles and the raising of the large LDL particle numbers.

I approach the issue of the possibility of less of a risk of increased large LDL particles versus increased small dense LDL particles by separating patients into clinical and lipid subfraction subgroups: (1) Patients with predominantly all large LDL: If they have familial hypercholesterolemiia, I recommend aggressive treatment. (2) A second group are very healthy with no other worrisome lipid subfractions and no clinical risk factors. With these group of patients, I don't routinely start them on a statin and I focus primarily on non-pharmacologic therapy. I used the LDL-P measurement as a guideline seeking ideally to have it < 1000 nmol/L and I use a water soluble statin when I do give them a statin. (3) A third, more common subgroup are those who have elevated large LDL-P and large LDL, having typically shifted or in the process of shifting from small dense to large LDL particles. These patients have usually typically been placed on a therapy or life style change that has caused a beneficial shift away from small dense to the large buoyant LDL particles. It's more important to keep the LDL in the large subgroup than in the small but I would also try to lower their LDL-P to below 1000 nmol/L. I would not want to lower the Large LDL at the expense of raising the amount of small dense LDL particles. This can occur with the addition of ezteimibe to an unknown percentage of patients already on a statin.

6. *Are there any current (11/2013) National Lipid Association recommendations[93] for LDL particle subclasses?*

"Don't test for them" was the recommendation in November 2013. I currently believe in testing for small dense LDL in patients who have evidence of residual risk (patients who have gone on to develop more atherosclerosis while on therapy) and patients in those clinical subgroups who are likely to have elevated levels of small dense LDL—those with metabolic syndrome, elevated triglycerides or diabetes.

LARGE VLDL PARTICLE NUMBER

The large VLDL particle level (VLDL-P) is another reported NMR-derived lipoprotein (Figure 4.13). This is best viewed as a potentially high risk triglyceride subgroup. The large VLDL or triglyceride may represent a higher risk than other smaller VLDL lipoproteins.[94] The response of this lipid subfraction to the implementation of broad-based treatment plans encompassing lifestyle issues such as diet, weight loss, better control of diabetes, and regular weekly exercise along with omega-3 fat intake and niacin, can be very rewarding for the patient and physician alike.

The triglyceride value is often regarded as not a "statistically significant risk factor" when analyzed via group analysis. However, I feel the triglyceride is another example of matching the relevance of the lipoprotein abnormality to the individual. This individual-focused concept has been best stated by Dr. Allan Sniderman:

> The actual hazard that a factor poses to an individual depends on the actual level of that factor within the individual not on the average hazard of the factor for the group....Clinical decisions should be based on the risk in the individual not on risk in the group.[95]

Individuals with elevated triglyceride (VLDL) values often have associated truncal obesity, insulin resistance, and glucose intolerance. Triglyceride elevation may not be a formally recognized

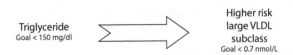

FIGURE 4.13 Information gained by the NMR LipoProfile, specifically the large VLDL subclass.

risk factor, but it is clearly associated with these other atherogenic clinical elements that promote atherosclerosis. Effective treatment of elevated triglycerides have effects on small dense LDL, HDL, and blood sugar control—all of which translate into reduced risk for the individual.

SUMMARY KEY QUESTIONS: LARGE VLDL

1. *Has large VLDL particle number been linked to CHD risk?*

    Variable and difficult to evaluate in isolation. However, in the HATS trial, where patients received simvastatin and niacin, decreased coronary artery stenosis was seen in patients whose large VLDL became lower along with lowering of small dense LDL and an increase in large HDL.[94]

2. *Is the large VLDL particle number associated with more CV risk?*

    Possibly because it remodels to become small dense LDL particles, and when large triglyceride-rich VLDL particles are not remodeled to LDL, they become more pro-atherogenic.[96]

3. *What reduces the large VLDL level?*

    Fish oil, low carbohydrate diet, loss of abdominal obesity, improvement in the control of diabetes, Niaspan, fibrates, and some statins (Atorvastatin) may be better than others.

4. *Are there clinical subgroups who have no increased risk from the presence of increased large VLDL?*

    Unknown; it is difficult to study in isolation from LDL-P and HDL.

5. *National Lipid Association recommendations for VLDL testing?*

    Do not test for it! Because it is a routine part of the NMR LipoProfile, we can realize its limitations and we can individually assess its potential relevance in the individual patient. Seeing it improve with a life style change is a nice conversation to have with a patient.

HDL CHOLESTEROL: THE "GOOD" CHOLESTEROL

HDL has multiple beneficial functions, but the most well-recognized function is the reverse transport function whereby cholesterol from cells in the peripheral sites in the body (including from atherosclerotic plaques) are delivered to the liver for breakdown (Figure 4.14). Other functions are anti-inflammatory, antioxidant, antiapoptotic, anti-infective, and the capacity to modulate insulin secretion.

Thus, HDL is not just a single molecule but possesses a high level of complexity linked to its protein and lipid components, which vary from one group of HDL molecules to another.[97] Viewing the HDL subfractions as the large HDL as being good and the small HDL as being bad is probably an oversimplification. We have to wait for greater understanding of the functional aspects of different HDL molecules and how to test for them and promote their antiatherogenic functionality.

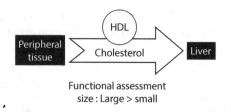

FIGURE 4.14   Reverse cholesterol transport pathway.

HDL PARTICLE NUMBER

The NMR LipoProfile provides the total HDL particle number (HDL-P) that measures accurately the total number of HDL particles. The traditional HDL cholesterol (HDL-C) measures the cholesterol content as opposed to the particle number themselves similar to the limitations of LDL-C versus LDL-P.

From an epidemiologic standpoint, low serum levels of HDL-C have been found to be one of the best predictors of CHD risk. It is still accepted and agreed upon that individuals who naturally possess higher levels of HDL-C are statistically (as a group) at a lower risk of CHD, and those who naturally possess lower values are at a higher risk of CHD. Also raising HDL levels in animals have been shown to reduce future atherosclerosis.

However, problems have occurred when it has been tried to extend those facts to the belief in the "HDL Hypothesis." This is defined as a belief that "actively raising HDL levels in humans would reduce clinical CHD events."

The Familial Atherosclerosis Treatment Study (FATS)[98] and the HDL Atherosclerosis Treatment Study (HATS)[99] studies revealed that powerful LDL-C lowering by a statin and HDL-C raising with Niacin could substantially reduce cardiovascular morbidity and mortality. However, these two studies did not address whether Niacin and/or HDL-raising added any benefit to the LDL-lowering effect of a statin. Four additional studies (ARBITER 2, ARBITER 3, ARBITER 6, and the Oxford Niaspan Study) also showed positive results when Niaspan was added to a statin, but they still did not answer the question if Niacin and/or HDL raising by themselves contributed to the positive results.

Four subsequent studies (The AIM-HIGH,[89,100] HPS2-THRIVE,[101] ILLUMINATE,[102] and dal-OUTCOMES[103]) placed the HDL cholesterol hypothesis at risk because of no benefit or the actual risk of harm. However, these four studies had a number of flaws that suggests that the HDL Hypothesis should not yet be discarded. One of the flaws possibly was the use of Ezetimibe (Zetia) in the AIM-HIGH trial because of its hidden effect of possibly increasing small dense LDL particles at the expense of large LDL being lowered.[90] Nevertheless, these events have led to a current consensus that HDL-C-targeted therapies, in general, and Niacin, specifically, may not be helpful.

In the Jupiter Trial, HDL-P was found to be a better marker of residual risk than chemically measured HDL-C or apoA-1.[104] Additionally, two studies that included testing of HDL-P and HDL size have supported the fact that HDL size and HDL-P are individually associated with decreased risk of CAD[105] and that increasing HDL-P with a fibrate alone produced clinical benefit out of proportion to the modest increase in HDL-C, and that this may have occurred because HDL-P increased more.[106,107] This data, while limited in scope, mirrors somewhat the LDL-C versus LDL-P data in that HDL-C is a poor test to follow as you treat a patient to raise the HDL but possibly HDL-P has some predictive benefit. Future studies will probably clarify these issues more completely (see Figure 4.15).

At this time, there is an active search for tests of HDL function that could lead to effective treatment linked to reduction of ASCVD risk. Meanwhile, testing of the HDL-P and the large HDL level are best viewed with more questions than answers as to their role in the individual patient.

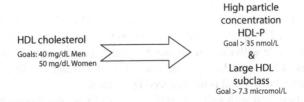

FIGURE 4.15 HDL cholesterol information gained by the NMR LipoProfile.

Practically speaking, an NMR LipoProfile provides the HDL information along with the beneficial data of an individual's LDL-P and small dense LDL. Reviewing the HDL data of an individual while realizing its limitations seems potentially helpful if such an analysis might answer the question: Does HDL-P and /or the large HDL concentration increase as healthy lifestyle and global risk modifications are successfully implemented? I have commonly seen the large HDL increase and the small HDL decrease as patients' lifestyle improves. Reviewing HDL data while realizing its limitations seems reasonable especially if such an analysis might answer the question: does HDL-P and large HDL increase as healthy lifestyles and global risk factor modifications are implemented? I typically see the large HDL and the small HDL decrease as patient's lifestyle changes improve their overall health.

Boston Heart Diagnostics has developed a unique HDL Map that has very supportive published data [57-63] confirming its ability to predict risk

SUMMARY QUESTIONS: TOTAL HDL PARTICLE NUMBER AND HDL LARGE OR SMALL

1. *Is HDL-P linked to CHD risk?*

Unknown but probably lower values (possibly < 34 mg/dl) supports the possibility of higher risk and raising the HDL-P with a fibrate may reduce risk (i.e., VA-HIT Study). HDL-P was a better marker of residual risk in the Jupiter Trial, and an editorial discussing HDL-P's strong inverse relationship with cardiovascular events suggested it might be time to "move from a cholesterol-based to a particle-based world."[108]

2. *Is the small HDL less protective than large HDL?*

Unknown but possibly. Based on some studies, the small HDL appears to be associated with increased risk in some clinical subgroups, whereas the larger HDL appears to reduce risk. But we really just do not yet know for sure. HDL functional assessment may well be the future.

3. *What treatment options tend to promote a shift from the small HDL toward the large HDL?*

Niacin, triglyceride reduction, possibly consumption of predominant docosahexaenoic acid (DHA) (from fish oil), correction of metabolic syndrome with loss of abdominal obesity.

4. *Have any clinical subgroups shown benefit from having elevated small HDL levels?*

Unknown. There are a few scattered reports of small HDL being beneficial but we do not know if any size is truly helpful. As noted, most studies suggest that large HDL might be more protective. Clearly, when patients lose weight, exercise, and eat well, the large HDL goes up and the small HDL goes down.

5. *Current National Lipid Association recommendations HDL subfractions?*

No proven benefit, do not test for it.

The value of the HDL-P particle concentration is unknown but it may be helpful in predicting risk in some subjects. Additionally I often seen the large HDL go up in patients who have lost weight, have changed their eating habits and exercise regularly.

LIPOPROTEIN(A)

Lipoprotein(a) (Lp[a]) consists of an LDL particle containing "little" protein that is attached to the apoB component of LDL. The apoA is a liver-derived protein that belongs to the plasminogen family suggesting a possible role with thrombosis but it actually has, as yet, no known function.

Even though it is like LDL and VLDL, because it has apoB and an LDL-like lipoprotein features, Lp(a) has a different metabolism and is not reduced by a statin.

Lp(a) is typically associated with a strong family history of vascular disease because it possesses a strong hereditary component.[109] An elevated value is associated with CHD,[110,111] stroke, venous thromboembolism,[112] and an increased incidence of restenosis after angioplasty.

The cardiovascular risk starts at an Lp(a) > 25 mg/dL. Lp(a) values greater than 25–39 mg/dL are present in 30% of Caucasians and 60%–70% of blacks.

Who should be treated?[113–115] A value of Lp(a) > 50 mg/dl is associated with a 20% s risk. Patients who have elevated values of Lp(a) in the 30-50 mg/dl range ma have a higher risk if they possess other risk factors (i.e., elevated small dense LDL elevated LDL-P, low HDL)

The discovery of a patient's elevated Lp(a) value represents an opportunity to reduce an individual's cardiovascular risk. The independent residual risk of Lp(a) is substantial.[116]

Treatment primarily with Niacin (1–3 g daily) and estrogens lower Lp(a) values and reduce major coronary events by 25%, stroke by 26%, and any cardiovascular event by 27%.[117]

EZETIMIBE (ZETIA) STORY: A HIDDEN RISK UNCOVERED BY LIPID SUBFRACTION TESTING

The discovery of unknown harm that may be occurring can be another advantage of testing lipid subfractions. Ezetimibe (brand name: Zetia) is a drug that is used as a LDL-C-lowering agent that accomplishes the LDL-lowering effect by blocking the absorption of cholesterol. It is almost always used in conjunction with a statin drug and together they lower the measured LDL-C more completely than either agent used alone.

In 2008, a study was published in the *New England Journal of Medicine*[118] titled the ENHANCE Trial, that tested the use of a statin drug (Simvastatin: brand name Zocor) alone or with use of Ezetimibe. The goal was to lower cholesterol in two groups of patients with a genetic disorder (familial hypercholesterolemia) causing high LDL-C values with the study lasting for 2 years. One group received simvastatin alone and the other group received both drugs. A measure of the rate of expected progressive increased thickness of the lining of the carotid arteries over the 2 years served as the differentiating test. The expectation was that the expected lowering of the LDL in the group of patients who took both drugs would achieve a much lower cholesterol (which occurred) and a lower rate of progressive thickening (which surprisingly did not occur).

After the 2008 publication of the ENHANCE Trial, I chose a few of my patients who were on Ezetimibe and a statin, obtained baseline lipid subfraction levels and stopped the Ezetimibe and repeated the lipid subfraction values 4–6 weeks later. I found that while the total LDL-C went up off Ezetimibe, high levels of small dense LDL that had been present while on the dual therapy of a statin and ezetimibe, went markedly down. in some, but not all, of the patients. The number of patients were too small to accurately gauge the percentage of patients who exhibit an apparent shift of LDL particles from large to small when ezetimibe (Zetia) is added to a statin and the reverse occurring when it is stopped. This tendency of ezetimibe to enhance the production of small dense LDL at the expense of large LDL has been noted and published by Berneis et al. in 2010.[89]

It appears that Ezetimibe, when combined with a statin, appears to promote the conversion of large LDL lipoproteins into small dense lipoproteins. It is unclear what percentage of patients exhibit this change from large to small dense lipoprotein. These small dense LDL particles are essentially hidden from view unless they are specifically tested for through the use of lipid subfraction testing. As noted, small dense LDL lipoproteins have been shown in a number of studies to be more proatherogenic than the larger LDL cholesterol, but opinions still differ. Also it is now appreciated that the various Lipid subfraction small dense LDL testing techniques may differ in their ability to accurate measure the level of small dense LDL. The latest measurement[74] may be the most sensitive and specific small dense LDL assay.

I discovered the "ezetimibe shift" using nuclear magnetic resonance in 2008. Berneis[90] used gradient gel electrophoresis and found the same shift toward the small dense LDL, offsetting the favorable effect of a statin alone in reducing the level of small dense LDL.

Because of the Simple Precipitation-Homogeneous Assay's[74] ability to possibly discover the presence of small dense more accurately than the other available measures, I believe this assay should be used along with NMR to clarify the presence of an ezetimibe shift when added to a statin and, if present, the percentage of patients who experience this potentially harmful shift. If this shift is confirmed to be present, understanding to whom it occurs and why would be important.

I sent a letter to the editor of the *New England Journal of Medicine* weeks after the study was published summarizing these findings, but the letter was not published. Since then, a study has been published in the *European Heart Journal*[90] in 2010 supporting the same findings. This 2010 study also found that small dense LDL particles appear to frequently increase when ezetimibe is combined with a statin.

It should be noted that one of the studies[89] (AIM-HIGH TRIAL) with Niacin that showed no benefit in reducing risk when raising HDL also had patients taking Ezetimibe to try to keep the LDL-C levels at the same level during the trial. Lipid subfractions were not obtained. A hidden-from-view shift from large LDL to the small dense LDL may have occurred during the AIM-HIGH-Trial possibly explaining the negative effects of Niacin on HDL raising and CHD risk reduction. (See Tables 4.5 and 4.6 Figures 4.16 and 4.17.)

In November 2014, the results of the IMPROVE IT Trial of ezetemibe(Zetia) plus simvastatin (Zocor) 40 mg was presented at the American Heart Association 2014 Scientific Sessions.[119] The study lasted 7 years and included more than 18,000 patients from 39 countries who were stable (< 10 days) after a recent acute coronary syndrome.

Patients were randomized to one of two treatment arms: simvastatin (Zocor) 40 mg alone and simvastatin (Zocor) 40 mg plus ezetimibe 10 mg (Zetia). They were followed for a minimum of

---

TABLE 4.5
Lipid Goals

Traditional Lipid Profile

- Total cholesterol < 200 mg/dl
- LDL cholesterol < 70–100 mg/dl
- HDL cholesterol > 40 mg/dl (Men); > 50 mg/dl (Women)
- Triglycerides < 150 mg/dl

NMR LipoProfile

- LDL particle concentration: LDL-P < 700–1000 nmol/L
- LDL particle size: more large & buoyant > 20.6 nm
- LDL small dense subclass: less small dense LDL ≤ 400–500 nmol/L
- HDL particle concentration: HDL-P > 35 nmol/L
- HDL subclass: more large HDL > 7.3 micromol/L
- VLDL(TG) subclasses: less large VLDL-P <0.7 nmol/L

Boston Heart Diagnostics

- Direct LDL: < 100 mg/dl
- ApoB: < 80 mg/dl
- LDL-P < 1000 nmol/L
- Small dense LDL: < 20 mg/dl
- Triglycerides < 150 mg/dl
- VLDL-C/TG < 0.2

HDL Map

- Apo A-1 (mg/dl) levels in HDL particles
- alpha-1: > 20 mg.dl
- alpha-2: > 55 mg/dl
- alpha-3: < 25 mg/dl
- VLDL-C < 30 mg/dl

Source: Courtesy of Richard M. Delany, MD, FACC.

TABLE 4.6

Treatment Order of Importance

Traditional Lipid Profile

1. Elevated LDL
2. Depressed HDL
3. Elevated triglyceride

NMR LipoProfile

1. Elevated LDL particle number
2. Elevated small LDL subclass→Large LDL
3. Elevated large VLDL
4. Low total HDL-P
5. Low large HDL subclass

Boston Heart Diagnostics

1. Elevated LDL particle number
2. Elevated apo B
3. Elevated small dense LDL
4. Abnormal HDL map
5. Elevated VLDL-C

Source: Courtesy of Richard M. Delany, MD, FACC.

2.5 years or until 5250 events occurred in the study participants. The LDL-C with simvastatin alone at 1 year was 69.9 mg/dl; the LDL-C with simvastatin and ezetimibe at 1 year was 53.2 mg/dl.

The end points of cardiovascular death, heart attack, unstable angina requiring hospitalization, coronary artery bypass grating, or stroke was reduced 6.4% in patients on the combination of simvastatin and ezetimibe versus simvastatin alone. The absolute reduction over 7 years was 2.0% with 32.7% of patients in the simvastain /Zetia arm experiencing a primary end point versus 34.7 % in the simvastatin alone arm experiencing an event. The major event reduction occurred in the occurrence of a heart attack or stroke but the all-cause mortality was not affected by the treatment.

This is one of the first trials where Zetia combined with a statin showed improvement over a statin alone. While the results were modest, the risk of cardiovascular events were clearly slightly less within the ezetimibe/simvastatin arm. There was no lipid subfraction data obtained before or during this study.

How does this study affect my concern about combining ezetimibe with a statin to achieve a reduced risk of cardiovascular events? I believe we still need to find the answers to some questions:

- Is there a tendency of Zetia to shift the absolute number of small dense LDL particles to a higher level (typically unseen by traditional lipid testing level)?
- If present, how frequently does it occur and does it persist over the long term?
- Is small dense LDL not as atherogenic when the LDL-C is brought to levels < 70 mg/dl? (and LDL-P levels below 800 nmol/L?)
- Does the knowledge of a patient's level of cholesterol absorption and production at baseline and over time affect the occurrence and duration of an ezetimibe shift?
- Is there a subgroup patients who should not take ezetimibe because of this shift and if so, how can we identify them clinically or by laboratory testing?
- Does an ezetimibe shift only occur with some statins and not with others, and if so, why?
- Does starting the statin and ezetimibe at the same time have a different effect than when Zetia is added to a statin to the same patient?

Lipoprotein effects of lipid modifying therapy

	Statins	Niaspan	Delta Tocotrienol	Fibrates	EPA	Diet	Exercise
↓LDL	+++	+	+	+	0	+/++	0/+
↑HDL	−/+/++	+++	0	++	0	0/+	+/++
↓TG	+/++	++/+++	0	+++	++	+/++	+/++

FIGURE 4.16   Summarizes the effects of lipid modifying therapy on the parameters measured by the traditional lipid profile. (Courtesy of Richard M. Delany, MD, FACC.)

Lipoprotein effects of lipid modifying therapy

	Statins	Niaspan	Fibrates	EPA	Diet	Exercise
↓LDL particle #	+++	+	+	0	+/++	0/+
↑LDL size	+	+++	++	++	+/++	+/++
↑HDL	−/+/++	+++	++	0	0/+	+/++
↑Large HDL	?	+++	+/++	+/++	?	?
↓Small HDL	?	+/++	+	+/++	?	?
↓Large VLDL	+/++	++/+++	+++	++	?	?

FIGURE 4.17   Summarizes the effects of lipid modifying therapy on the parameters measured by the NMR LipoProfile. (Courtesy of Richard M. Delany, MD, FACC.)

While we wait for the literature to answer these questions, I still recommend remaining cautious about adding ezetimibe to a statin without obtaining baseline level of LDL-P and small dense LDL.

Ideally obtaining baseline levels of LDL-P and small dense LDL before Zetia is added to a statin and then rechecking the same testing 4-6 weeks later would no longer allow any shifts to be hidden from the view of the prescribing physician.

If a patient is already on a statin/ezetimibe combination, stopping ezetimibe alone for 4–6 weeks and repeating the testing would also provide the information about the presence of a hidden small dense LDL shift in the individual patient.

WHY LIPID SUBFRACTION TESTING?

Lipid subfraction testing is performed to obtain additional information about a patient's often hidden-from-view potential atherogenic lipoproteins. Lipid subfraction testing provides some answers to important questions: (1) Does the patient possess high risk lipoprotein levels that place him/her at risk? (2) Does the patient, therefore, need additional therapy to reduce any potential residual risk that still exists? (3) Has the patient's total treatment strategy (drugs, diet, lifestyle, exercise, nutritional supplements) been successful in correcting parameters that have been shown to be linked to increased risk? (4) Has a specific treatment helped, hurt and has been neutral with regard to the lipoprotein abnormality of interest? I believe that by obtaining a lipid subfraction test (NMR from Liposcience or from other lipid subfraction testing laboratories), a hidden persistent risk of ASCVD can be uncovered in a significant number of patients. Once identified, a treatment plan can then be implemented in an attempt to correct the specific imbalances.

The treatment plan does not have to be a drug but could very well be a lifestyle change or a change in diet. However, if the test result and clinical assessment identifies the patient to be in a high-risk subgroup that has shown (by well-documented meta-analysis)[120] to significantly benefit from the LDL lowering and hsCRP anti-inflammatory effects of statins, then a statin should be seriously considered. As Sniderman et al. commented in his discussion about choosing to use a statin in primary prevention: "Not acting, not using statins in primary prevention is as real an act as using them."[121]

The key point is that when any test is found to discover the presence of hidden atherosclerotic risk, a treatment plan should be implemented that realistically, safely, and with the full understanding of the patient proceeds to achieve specific goals. Any or all treatment plans can always be reviewed and changed as needed based on clinical results, side effects, new medical conditions, or new knowledge.

The results of a lipid subfraction test often leads to a goal to achieve a greater reduction in the LDL Particle number, the most widely accepted value that helps guide treatment. However, the existence of other hidden-from-view lipid subfractions also often leads to therapies to potentially improve an individual's risk. I believe this includes too many small dense LDL particles (accurately obtained) in the setting of insulin resistance or metabolic syndrome with type II diabetes. This might include too many small dense LDL particles in the setting of insulin resistance or metabolic syndrome with type 2 diabetes. Another example of a hidden-from-view lipid abnormality is the presence of a normal fasting traditional triglyceride value but with the finding of an elevated large VLDL subfraction. In this instance, an emphasis might now focus on the need for a lower carbohydrate diet and possible further testing of his lipid panel 1–2 hours after a meal. Some patients have elevated triglyceride-rich lipoproteins 1–2 hours after eating, placing them at a higher risk.

SUMMARY COMMENTS

1. Lipid subfraction testing: An opportunity to obtain important information in patients with an increased risk of CHD. A hidden-from-view group of atherogenic lipoproteins are often discovered that leads to specific adjustments designed to reduce an individual's risk.

2. Teaching moments with patients: Once on a treatment plan, the discovery of improvement or lack of improvement in a patient's lipid subfraction testing data allows for "teaching moments" with patients. These conversations can enhance the patient's understanding leading to improved compliance and success with the various components of the individualized treatment plan. These components include diet, exercise, other lifestyle choices, nutritional supplement choices and dosages, and drug choices and dosages.

3. Top eight lipid subfractions
   a. LDL-P ideally <1000 nmol/L
   b. ApoB: ideally <80 mg/dL
   c. Small dense LDL level, ideally <400 nmol/L
   d. Boston Heart Diagnostics HDL Map: alpha-1: > 20 mg.dl, alpha-2: > 55 mg/dl, alpha-3: < 25 mg/dl
   e. Total HDL-P > 35.0 µmol/L
   f. Large HDL > 7.0 µmol/L
   g. Large VLDL, ideally <0.7 nmol/L
   h. Lp(a) < 50 mg/dL

4. Other important parameters
   a. hsCRP
   b. FBS and hemoglobin A1C
   c. Family history
   d. Physical examination
5. Patients need physicians to choose carefully and wisely for their patients. The decision to start a drug, specifically a statin, should be based on a patient's risk and the ability of the physician to monitor and reduce that risk safely. Not to start a patient on a statin who has a high risk of CHD with the presence of high-risk atherogenic proteins is a missed opportunity at future cardiovascular risk reduction; not to monitor the patient carefully is a failed responsibility.

REFERENCES

1. Hansson GK, Hermanasson A. The immune system in atherosclerosis. *Nat Immunol* 2011;12:204–212.
2. Lundberg AM, Hansson GK. Innate immune signals in atherosclerosis. *Clin Immunol* 2010;134:5–24.
3. Libby P, Ridker P, Hansson GK. Progress and challenges in translating the biology of atherosclerosis. *Nature* 2011;473:317–324.
4. Ford ES, Ajani UA, Croft JB et al. Explaining the decrease in US deaths from coronary disease, 1980–2000. *N Engl J Med* 2007;356:2388–2398.
5. Davidon MH, Ballantyne CM, Jacobson TA et al. Clinical utility of inflammatory markers and advanced lipoprotein testing: Advice from an expert panel of lipid specialists. *J Clin Lipidol* 2011;5:338–367.
6. Kuek A, Hazleman BL, Ostör AJ. Immune Mediated Inflammatory Diseases (IMIDs) and biologic therapy. *PostGrad Med J* 2007;83:251–260.
7. Baeton D, van Hagen PM. Use of TNF blockers and other targeted therapies in rare refractory immune-mediated inflammatory diseases: Evidence-based or rational? *Ann Rhem Dis* 2010;69:2067–2073.
8. Apple F, Smith SW, Pearce LA et al. Myeloperoxidae improves risk stratification in patients with ischemia and normal cardiac troponin I concentrations. *Clin Chem* 2011;57(4):603–608.
9. Meuwese MC, Stroes ESG, Hazen SL et al. Serum myleoperoxidase levels are associated with the future risk of coronary artery disease in apparently healthy individuals. *J AM Coll Cardiol* 2007;50:159–165.
10. Schindhelm RK, van der Zwan LP, Terlink, T, Scheffer, PG. Myeloperoxidase: A useful biomarker for cardiovascular disease risk stratification? *Clin Chem* 2009;55(8):1462–1470.
11. Wong ND, Gransar H, Narula J et al. Myeloperoxidase, subclinical atherosclerosis, and cardiovascular events. *JACC Cardiovascular Imaging* 2009;2:1093–1099.
12. Rak K, Rader D J. The diet-microbe morbid union. *Nature* 2011;472:40–41.
13. Wang Z, Klipfell E, Bennett BJ et al. Gut flora metabolism of phosphatidylcholine promotes cardiovascular disease. *Nature* 2011;472:57–63.
14. Howitt MR, Garrettet WS. Gut microbiota and cardiovascular connectivity. *Nature Medicine* 2012;18(8)1188–1189.
15. Koeth RA, Wang Z, Levison BS et al. Intestinal microbiota metabolism of L-carnitine, a nutrient in red meat, promotes atherosclerosis. *Nature Medicine* 2013;576–585.
16. Tang WHW, Wang Z, Levison BS et al. Intestinal microbial metabolism of phosphatidylcholine and cardiovascular risk. *NEJM* 2013;368:1575–1584.
17. Wang Z, Tang WHW, Buffa JA et al. Prognostic value of choline and betaine depends on intestinal microbiota-generated metabolite trimethylamine-N-oxide. *Eur Heart J* 2014;35:904–910.
18. Tang WHW, Hazen SL. The contributory role of gut microbiota in cardiovascular disease. *J Clin Invest* 2014;124:4204–4211.
19. Tang WH Wilson, Wang Z et al. Prognostic value of elevated levels of intestinal microbe-generated metabolite trimethylamine-N-oxide in patients with heart failure. *J Am Coll Cardiol* 2014;64:1908–1914.
20. Claus SP. Mammalian-microbial cometabolism of L-carnitine in the context of atherosclerosis. *Cell Metabolism* 2014;20:699–700.
21. Koeth RA, Levison BS, Culley MK et al. Gamma butyrobetaine is a proatherogenic intermediate in gut microbial metabolism of L-carnitine to TMAO. *Cell Metabolism* 2014;20:799–812.
22. Abeles AM, Pillinger MH. Statins as antiinflammatory and immunomodulatory agents: A future in rheumatologic therapy? *Arthritis Rheum* 2006;54:393–407.
23. Liao, JK. Isoprenoids as mediators of the biological effects of statins. *J Clin Invest* 2002;110:285–288.

24. Mombelli G, Pavanello C. Statin muscle toxicity and genetic risk factors. *Int J Genomic Med* 2013;1:(2)1–5.
25. Parker BA, Gregory SM, Lorson L, Polk D, White CM, Thompson PD. A randomized trial of coenzyme Q10 in patients with statin myopathy: Rationale and study design. *J Clinical Lipidology* 2013;7:187–193.
26. Sorrentino M. An Update on Statin Alternatives and Adjuncts. *Clin Lipidology* 2012;7(6):721–730.
27. Kennedy SP, Barnas GP, Schmidt MJ et al. Efficacy and tolerability of once-weekly rosuvastain in patients with previous statin intolerance. *J Clin Lipidol* 2011;5(4):308–315.
28. Libby P. The Forgotten majority. Unfinished business in cardiovascular risk reduction. *J Am Coll Cardiol* 2005;46:1225–1228.
29. Lusis AJ, Pajukanta P. A treasure trove for lipoprotein biology. Nat. Genet. 2008; 40: 129–130. Figure One.
30. Otvos JD. *Handbook of Lipoprotein Testing.* Washington, DC: AACC Press, 2000.
31. Sniderman AD. Differential response of cholesterol and particle measures of atherogenic lipoproteins to LDL-lowering therapy: Implications for clinical practice. *J Clin Lipidol* 2008;2:36–42.
32. AACC Lipoproteins and Vascular Diseases Division Working Group on Best Practices, Cole TG, Contois JH et al. Association of apolipoprotein B and nuclear magnetic resonance spectroscopy-derived LDL particle number with outcomes in 25 clinical studies: Assessment by the AACC lipoprotein and vascular disease division working group best practices. *Clin Chem* 2013;59(5):753–770.
33. Sniderman AD et al. A meta-analysis of low density lipoprotein cholesterol, non-high density lipoprotein cholesterol, and apolipoprotein B as markers of cardiovascular risk. *Circ Cardiovasc Qual Outcomes* 2011;4:337–345.
34. Sampson UK, Fazio S, Linton, M. Residual cardiovascular risk despite optimal LDL reduction with statins: The evidence, etiology, and therapeutic challenges. *Curr Atheroscler Rep* 2012;14:1–10.
35. Fruchart JC, Sacks F, Hermans MP et al. The residual risk initiative: A call to action to reduce residual vascular risk in patients with dyslipidemia. *Am J Card* 2008;102(10 suppl):1K–34K.
36. Sampson UK, Fazio S, Linton M. Residual cardiovascular risk despite optimal LDL reduction with Statins: The evidence, etiology, and therapeutic challenges. *Curr Atheroscler Rep* 2012;14:1–10.
37. Robinson J. What is the role of advanced lipoprotein analysis in practice? *J Am Coll Cardiol* 2012;60:2607–2615.
38. Stone NJ, Robinson J, Lichtenstein AH et al. 2013 ACC/AHA guideline on the treatment of blood cholesterol to reduce atherosclerotic cardiovascular disease risk in adults. *J Am Coll Cardiol* 2013;63(25 Pt B):2889–934.
39. Otvos JD, Jeyarajah EJ, Cromwell CC. Measurement issues related to lipoprotein heterogeneity. *Am J Cardiol* 2002;90(8A):22i–29i.
40. Otvos JD. Measurement of lipoprotein subclass profiles by nuclear magnetic resonance spectroscopy. *Clin Lab* 2002;48:171–180.
41. Ip, S, Lichtenstein AH, Chung M, Lau J, Balk EM. Systematic review: Association of low-density lipoprotein subfractions with cardiovascular outcomes. *Ann Intern Med* 2009;150:474–484.
42. Mora S. Advanced lipoprotein testing and subfractionation are not (yet) ready for routine clinical use. *Circulation* 2009;119:2396–2404.
43. Superko HR. Advanced lipoprotein testing and subfractionation are clinically useful. *Circulation* 2009;119:2383–2395.
44. Otvos JD, Mora S, ShaLaurova I, Greenland P, Mackey RH, Goff DC Jr. Clinical implication of discordance between low-density lipoprotein cholesterol and particle number. *J Clin Lipidol* 2011;5:105–113.
45. LipoScience. 2500 Sumner Blvd, Raleigh, NC 27616: 919-212-1954. www.liposcience.com
46. Quest Diagnostics Laboratory. Ion mobility: Advance lipid analysis for management of cardiovascular risk. www.questdiagnostics.com
47. Musuburu K, Orho-Melander M, Caulfield MP et al. Ion Mobility analysis of lipoprotein subfractions identifies three independent areas of cardiovascular risk. *Arterioscler Thromb Vasc Biol* 2009;29:1375–1380.
48. Atherotech Diagnostic Lab. 201 London Parkway, Birmingham, Alabama 35211: 877-901-8510. www.Atherotech.com
49. Boston Heart Diagnostics 175 Crossing Boulevard, Suite 100 Framingham, MA 01702. www.boston-heartdiagnostics.com
50. Asztalos BF, Swarbrick MM, Schaefer EJ et al. Effects of weight loss, induced by gastric bypass surgery, on HDL remodeling in obese women. *J Lipid Res* 2010;51(8):2405–2412.
51. Asztalos BF, Batista M, Horvath KV et al. Change in alpha 1 HDL concentration predicts progression in coronary artery stenosis. *Arterioscler Thromb Vasc Biol* 2003;23:847–852.

52. Asztalos BF, Cupples LA, Demissie S et al. High-density lipoprotein subpopulation profile and coronary heart disease prevalence in male participants of the Framingham offspring study. *Arterioscler Thromb Vasc Biol* 2004;24:2181–2187.

53. Asztalos BF, Collins D, Cupples LA et al. Value of high-density lipoprotein (HDL) subpopulations in predicting recurrent cardiovascular events in the veterans affairs HDL intervention trial. *Arterioscler Thromb Vasc Biol* 2005;25:2185–2191.

54. Lamon-Fava S, Herrington DM, Reboussin DM et al. Plasma levels of HDL subpopulations and remnant lipoproteins predict the extent of angiographically-defined coronary artery disease in postmenopausal women. *Arterioscler Thromb Vasc Biol* 2008;28:575–579.

55. Asztalos BF, de la Llera-Moya M, Dallal GE, Horvath KV, Schaefer EJ, Rothblat GH. Differential effects of HDL subpopulations on cellular ABCA1- and SR-B1-mediated cholesterol efflux. *J Lipid Res* 2005;46:2246–2253.

56. Rosenson RS, Davidson MH, Pourfarzib,R. Underappreciated opportunities for low-density lipoprotein management in patients with cardiometabolic residual risk. *Atherosclerosis* 2010;213:1–7.

57. Cromwell WC, Otvos JD, Keyes MJ et al. LDL Particle number and risk for future cardiovascular disease in the Framingham Offspring Study: Implications for LDL management. *J Clin Lipidol* 2007;1:583–592.

58. Jacobson T, Peter P. Toth. Comparison of Cardiovascular Events Between Patients Achieving Low-Density Lipoprotein Particle Targets and Patients Achieving Low-Density Lipoprotein Cholesterol Targets. American College of Cardiology Poster Presentation: ACC Convention, Washington, DC, March 31, 2014.

59. Rosenson SR, Underberg JA. Systematic review: Evaluating the effect of lipid-lowering therapy on lipoprotein and lipid values. *Cardiovasc Drugs Ther* 2013;27:465–479.

60. AACC Lipoproteins and Vascular Diseases Division Working Group on Best Practices, Cole TG, Contois JH et al. Association of apolipoprotein b and nuclear magnetic resonance spectroscopy—derived LDL particle number with outcomes in 25 clinical studies: Assessment by the AACC lipoprotein and vascular diseases division working group on best practices. *Clin Chem* 2013;59(5):752–770.

61. deGoma EM, Davis MD, Dunbar RL, Mohler ER 3rd, Greenland P, French B et al. Discordance between non-HDL cholesterol and LDL-particle measurements: Results from the multi-ethnic study of atherosclerosis. *Atherosclerosis* 2013;229:517–523.

62. Malave H, Castro M, Burkle J et al. Evaluation of low-density lipoprotein particle number distribution in patients with type 2 diabetes mellitus with low-density lipoprotein cholesterol <50 mg/dl and non-high-density lipoprotein cholesterol <80 mg/dl. *Am J Cardiol* 2012;110:662–665.

63. El Harchaoui K, van der Steeg WA, Stroes ES et al. Value of low-density lipoprotein particle number and size as predictors of coronary artery disease in apparently healthy men and women: The EPIC-Norfolk prospective population study. *J Am Coll Cardiol* 2007;49:547–553.

64. Kamigaki AS, Siscovick DS, Schwartz SM et al. Low density lipoprotein particle size and risk of early-onset myocardial infarction in women. *Am J Epidemiol* 2001;153:939–945.

65. Zeljkovic A, Vekic J, Spasojevic-Kalimanovska V et al. LDL and HDL subclasses in acute ischemic stroke: Prediction of risk and short term mortality. *Atherosclerosis* 2010;210:548–554.

66. Blake GJ, Otvos JD, Rifai N et al. Low density lipoprotein particle concentration and size as determined by nuclear magnetic resonance spectroscopy as predictors of cardiovascular disease in women. *Circulation* 2002;106:1930–1937.

67. Lamarche B, Tchernof A, Moorjani S et al. Small Dense Low-density lipoprotein particles as a predictor of ischemic heart disease in men. *Circulation* 1997;95:69–75.

68. St-Pierre AC, Cantin B, Dagenais GR et al. Low-density lipoprotein subfractions and the long-term risk of ischemic heart disease in men. 13-year follow-up data from the Quebec cardiovascular study. *Arterioscler Thromb Vasc Biol* 2005;25(3):553–559.

69. Campos H, Roederer GO, Lussier-Cacan S, Davignon J, Krauss RM. Predominance of large LDL and reduced HDL 2 cholesterol in normolilidemic men with coronary artery disease. *Arterioscler Thromb Vasc Biol* 1995;15:1043–1048.

70. Ruotolo G, Tettamanti C, Garancini MP et al. Smaller denser LDL particles are not a risk factor for cardiovascular disease in healthy nonagenarian women of the Cremona Population Study. *Atherosclerosis* 1998;140:65–70.

71. Campos H, Moye LA, Glasser SP, Stampfer MJ, Sacks FM. Low density lipoprotein size, pravastatin treatment, and coronary events. *JAMA* 2001;286:1468–1474.

72. Mora S, Szklo M, Otvose JD et al. LDL particle subclasses, LDL particle size, and carotid atherosclerosis in the Multi-Ethnic Study of Atherosclerosis (MESA). *Atherosclerosis* 2007;192:211–217.

73. Tsai MY, Steffen BT, Guan W, McClelland RI et al. New automated assay of small dense lipoprotein cholesterol identifies risk of coronary heart disease: The multi-ethnic study of atherosclerosis. *Arterioscler Thromb Vasc Biol* 2014;34:196–201.

74. Ito Y, Fujimura M, Ohta M et al. Development of a homogeneous assay for measurement of small dense LDL cholesterol. *Clinical Chemistry* 2011;57:57–65.

75. Sninsk JJ, Powland MS, Baca AM et al. Classification of LDL phenotypes by 4 methods of determining lipoprotein particle size. *J Investig Med* 2013;61:942–949.

76. Hirano T, Ito Y, Saegusa H, Yoshino G. A novel and simple method for quantification of small dense LDL. *J Lipid Research* 2003;44:2193–2201.

77. Hirano T, Ito Y, Yoshino G. Measurement of small dense low-density lipoprotein particles *J Atheroscler Thromb* 2005;12:67–72.

78. Koba S, Hirano T, Ito Y, et al. Significance of small dense low-density lipoprotein cholesterol concentrations in relation to the severity of coronary heart diseases. *Atherosclerosis* 2006;189:206–214.

79. Tokuno A, Hirano T, Hayashi T et al. The effects of statin and fibrate on lowering small dense LDL-cholesterol in hyperlipidemic patients with type 2 diabetes. *J Atheroscler Thromb* 2007;14:128–132.

80. Nozue N, Michishita I, Ishibashi Y et al. Small dense low-density lipoprotein cholesterol is a useful marker of metabolic syndrome in patients with coronary disease. *J Atheroscler Thromb* 2007;14:202–207.

81. Nozue T, Michishita I, Ito Y et al. Effects of statin on small dense low-density lipoprotein cholesterol and remnant-like particle cholesterol in heterozygous familial hypercholesterolemia. *J Atheroscler Thromb* 2008;15:146–153.

82. Koba S, Yokota Y, Hirano T et al. Small LDL cholesterol is superior to LDL cholesterol for determining severe coronary atherosclerosis. *J Atheroscler Thromb* 2008;15:250–260.

83. Masumi A, Otokozawa S, Asztalos BF et al. Small dense LDL cholesterol and coronary heart disease: Results from the Framingham Offspring Study. *Clinical Chemistry* 2010;56:967–976.

84. Ito Y, Fujimura M, Ohta M, Hirano T. Development of a homogeneous assay for measurement of small dense LDL cholesterol. *Clinical Chemistry* 2011;57:57–65.

85. Tsai M, Steffen B, Guan W et al. New automated assay of small dense low-density lipoprotein cholesterol identifies risk of coronary heart disease: The multi-ethnic study of atherosclerosis. *Arterioscler Thromb Vasc Biol* 2014;34:196–201.

86. Hoogeveen R, Gaubatz JW, Sun W et al. Small dense low-density lipoprotein cholesterol concentrations predict risk for coronary heart disease: The Atherosclerosis Risk in Communities (ARIC) study. *Arterioscler Thromb Vasc Biol* 2014; 34: 1069–1077.

87. Brunzell JD. Increased ApoB in small dense LDL particles predicts premature coronary artery disease. *Arterioscler Thromb Vasc Biol* 2005;25:474–475.

88. Ayyobi A, McGladdery SH, McNeely M, Austin MA, Motulsky AG, Brunzell JD. Small dense LDL and elevated apolipoprotein B are the common characteristics for the three major lipid phenotypes of familial combined hyperlipidemia. *Arterioscler Thromb Vasc Biol* 2003;23:1289–1294.

89. AIM-HIGH Investigators, Boden WE, Probstfield JL et al. Niacin in patients with low HDL cholesterol levels receiving intensive statin therapy. *N Engl J Med* 2011;365:2255–2267.

90. Berneis K, Rizzo M, Berthold HK, Spinas GA, Krone W, Gouni-Berthold I. Ezetimibe alone or in combination with simvastatin increases small dense low-density lipoproteins in healthy men: A randomized trial. *European Heart J* 2010;31:1633–1639.

91. Pauciullo P, Gentile M, Marotta G et al. Small dense low-density lipoprotein in familial combined hyperlipidemia: Independent of metabolic syndrome and related to history of cardiovascular events. *Atherosclerosis* 2009;203:320–324.

92. Ai M, Otokozawa S, Asztalos BF et al. Effects of maximal doses of atorvastatin versus rosuvastain on small dense low-density lipoprotein cholesterol levels. *Am J Cardiol* 2008;101:315–318.

93. Davidon MH, Ballantyne CM, Jacobson TA et al. Clinical utility of inflammatory markers and advanced lipoprotein testing: Advice from an expert panel of lipid specialists. *J Clin Lipidol* 2011;5:338–367.

94. Dobiasova M, Frohlich J, Sedová M, Cheung MC, Brown BG. Cholesterol esterification and atherogenic index of plasma correlate with lipoprotein size and findings on coronary angiography. *J Lipid Res* 2011;52:566–571.

95. Sniderman AD, Williams K, McQueen MJ, Furberg CD. When is equal not equal? *J Clin Lipidol* 2010;4(2):83–88.

96. McEneny J, McMaster C, Trimble ER, Young IS. Rapid Isolation of VLDL subfractions: Assessment of composition and susceptibility to copper-mediated oxidation. *J Lipid Research* 2002;43(5):824–831.

97. Toth PP, Barter PJ, Rosenson RS et al. High-density lipoproteins: A consensus statement from the National Lipid Association. *J Clin Lipidol* 2013;7:484–525.
98. Brown BG, Brockenbrough A, Zhao XQ et al. Very intensive lipid therapy with lovastatin, niacin, colestipol for prevention of death and myocardial infarction: A 10 year familial atherosclerosis treatment study(FATS) follow up. *Circulation* 1998;98(suppl 1):1–635.
99. Brown BG, Zhao X, Chait A et al. Simvastatin, and niacin, antioxidant vitamins or the combination for the prevention of coronary disease. *N Engl J Med* 2001;345:1583–1592.
100. AIM-HIGH Investigators. The role of niacin in raising high density lipoprotein cholesterol to reduce cardiovascular events in patients with atherosclerotic cardiovascular disease and optimally treated low density lipoprotein cholesterol. Rationale and study design. The atherothrombosis intervention in metabolic syndrome with low HDL/high triglycerides: Impact on global health outcomes. (AIM-HIGH). *AM Heart J* 2011;161:471–444.
101. HPS2-THRIVE Collaborative Group. HPS2-THRIVE randomized placebo-controlled trial in 25,673 high-risk patients of ER niacin/laropiprant: Trial design, pre-specified muscle and liver outcomes, and reasons for stopping study treatment. *Eur Heart J* 2013;34:1279–1291.
102. Barter PJ,Caulfield M, Eriksson M et al. Effects of torcetrapib in patients with low HDL cholesterol levels receiving intensive statin therapy. *N Engl J Med* 2011;365:2255–2267.
103. Schwartz GG, Olsson AG, Abt M et al. Effects of dalcetrapib in patents with an acute coronary syndrome. *N Engl J Med* 2012;367:2089–2099.
104. Mora S, Glynn RJ, Ridker PM. High density lipoprotein cholesterol, size, particle number, and residual vascular risk after potent statin therapy. *Circulation* 2013;128:1189–1197.
105. Harchaoui K El, Arsenault BJ, Franssen R et al. High–density lipoprotein particle size and concentration and coronary risk. *Ann Intern Med* 2009;150:84–93.
106. Otvos JD, Collins D, Freedman DS et al. Low-density lipoprotein and high-dense lipoprotein particle subclasses predict coronary events and are favorably changed by gemfibrozil therapy in the veterans affairs high density lipoprotein intervention trial. *Circulation* 2006;113:1556–1563.
107. Brown WV, Mackey RH, Rosenson RS, Underberg JA, Wright R. Managing atherosclerotic risk with a particle focus. A Roundtable Discussion IMNG Medical Media, 2011.
108. Nicholls SJ, Puri R. Is it time for HDL to Change its Tune? *Circulation* 2013;128:1175–1176.
109. Tsimikas S, Hall JL. Lipoprotein(a) as a potential causal genetic risk factor of cardiovascular disease. *J Am Coll Cardiol* 2012;60:716–721.
110. Emerging Risk Factors Collaboration, Erqou S, Kaptoge S et al. Lipoprotein (a) concentration and the risk of coronary heart disease, stroke and nonvascular mortality. *JAMA* 2009;302:412–423.
111. Bennet A, Di Angelantonio E, Erqou S et al. Lipoprotein(a) levels and risk of future coronary heart disease: Large-scale prospective data. *Arch Intern Med* 2008;168:598–608.
112. Sofi F, Marcucci R, Abbate R, Gensini GF, Prisco D. Lipoprotin (a) and venousthromboembolism in adults: A meta-analysis. *Am J Med* 2007;120:728–733.
113. Nordestgaard BG, Chapman MJ, Ray K et al. Lipoprotein (a) as a cardiovascular risk factor: Current status. *Eur Heart J* 2010;31:2844–2853.
114. Rubenfire M, Vodnala D, Krishnan SM et al. Lipoprotein (a): Perspectives from a lipid referral program. *J Clin Lipidol* 2012;6:66–73.
115. Brown WV, Ballantyne CM, Jones PH, Marcovina S. Management of Lp(a). *J Clin Lipidol* 2010; 4:240–247.
116. Helgadottir A, Gretarsdottir S, Thorleifsson G et al. Apolipoprotein (a) genetic sequence variants associated with systemic atherosclerosis and coronary atherosclerosis burden but not with venous thromboembolism. *J Am Coll Cardiol* 2012;60:722–729.
117. Bruckert E, Labreuche J, Amarenco P. Meta-analysis of the effect of nicotinic acid alone or in combination on cardiovascular events and atherosclerosis. *Atherosclerosis* 2010:210;353–361.
118. Kastelein JI, Akdim F, Stroes ES et al. Simvastatin with or without ezetimibe in familial hypercholesterolemia. *N Engl J Med* 2008;358:1431–1443.
119. Cannon CP. IMPROVE -IT Trial: A comparison of ezetimibe/simvastatin versus simvastatin monotherapy on cardiovascular outcomes after coronary syndomes. American Heart Association Sessions November 17, 2014, Chicago, Ill. http://www.medscape.com/viewarticle/835030_print (accessed December 6, 2014).
120. Cholesterol Treatment Trialists' (CTT) Collaboration, Baigent C, Blackwell L et al. Efficacy and safety of more intensive lowering of LDL cholesterol: A meta-analysis of data from 170,000 participants in 26 randomised cv trials. *Lancet* 2010;376:1670–1681.
121. Sniderman AD, Thanassoulis G, Couture P et al. Counterpoint: Statins do reduce fatal events. *J Clin Lipidology* 2013;7:225–227.

5 The Role of Nutrition and Nutritional Supplements in the Treatment of Dyslipidemia

Mark Houston

CONTENTS

INTRODUCTION, NEW CONCEPTS, AND PERSPECTIVES

Dyslipidemia is considered one the of top five risk factors for cardiovascular disease (CVD), along with hypertension, diabetes mellitus (DM), smoking, and obesity.[1] There are an infinite number of vascular insults but only three finite responses of vascular endothelium, and vascular and cardiac smooth muscles. The mechanisms by which certain lipids induce vascular damage are complex, but from a pathophysiologic and functional medicine viewpoint, the three finite responses are inflammation, oxidative stress, and autoimmune dysfunction.[2–4] These pathophysiologic mechanisms lead to endothelial dysfunction and vascular smooth muscle and cardiac dysfunction. The vascular consequences are CVD, coronary heart disease (CHD), myocardial infarction (MI), and cerebrovascular accidents (CVA).[4]

Genetics, chronic inflammatory micro and macronutrient intake, obesity (visceral obesity), chronic infections, toxins and some specific pharmacological agents such as selective beta blockers and diuretics, tobacco products, DM, and lack of exercise contribute to dyslipidemia.[5] For example, several genetic phenotypes, such as apolipoprotein E (APO-E), result in variable serum lipid responses to diet, as well as CHD and MI risk.[6,7] In addition, high-density lipoprotein (HDL) proteomics that affect PON-1 (paroxonase-1) and SR-BI (scavenger receptor B-1) increase CVD.[8] The Sortilin I allele variants on Chromosome 1p13 increases low-density lipoprotein (LDL) and CHD risk by 29%.[9]

Recent studies suggest that increasing dietary cholesterol intake will not alter serum total cholesterol (TC) or LDL cholesterol (LDL-C) levels or CHD significantly. Some saturated fats depending on their carbon chain length have a minimal influence on serum lipids and CHD risk, whereas monounsaturated and omega-3 polyunsaturated fats have a favorable influence on serum lipids and CHD risk. Increased refined carbohydrate intake, may be more important in changing serum lipids and lipid subfractions than saturated fats and cholesterol. Refined carbohydrates have more adverse effects on insulin resistance, atherogenic LDL, small dense LDL, LDL particle number (LDL-P), VLDL, triglycerides (TGs), total HDL, HDL subfractions, and HDL particle number (HDL-P), thus contributing to CHD risk more than saturated fats.[5,10–16] Postprandial hyperglycemia, hypertriglyceridemia, and endotoxemia coupled with inflammation, oxidative stress, and immune vascular dysfunction is highly associated with atherosclerosis.[17–20] Activation of chylomicron and cholecystokinin, GLP-1, low nitric oxide (NO), elevated asymmetric dimethylarginine (ADMA), increased lipid peroxidation, inflammatory cytokines, tumor necrosis factor alpha (TNF-alpha) and stimulation of nuclear factor kB (NFkB), pattern recognition receptors (PRR), toll-like receptors (TLR 2 and 4) and nucleotide-binding oligomerization domain (NOD)-like receptors (NLR), caveolae and lipid rafts increase the inflammatory pathways after meals inducing endothelial dysfunction.[17–20]

Increased dietary intake of sodium chloride, not balanced with potassium further increases the endothelial dysfunction (ED) and ADMA and reduces NO. Many phytoalexins, phytonutrients, and polyphenols may block the TLR and NLR inflammatory response.[21,22] In addition, a "metabolic memory" of cells and the blood vessel exists due to an innate immune response with increased inflammation. These responses are perpetuated long after the original insult and are heightened with smaller insults.[17]

The validity of the "Diet Heart Hypothesis" that implies that dietary saturated fats, dietary cholesterol, and eggs increase the risk of CHD has been questioned.[11–13] Trans fatty acids (trans FAs) have definite adverse effects and increase CVD and CHD risk, but omega-3 FAS and monounsaturated fats improve serum lipids and reduce CVD risk.[5,10,12,14–16] Trans fats suppress TGF-B responsiveness that increases the deposition of cholesterol into cellular plasma membranes in vascular tissue.[15]

Expanded lipid profiles that measure lipids, lipid subfractions, particle size and number, and APO-B and A are preferred to standard obsolete lipid profiles that measure only the TC, LDL, TG, or HDL. These expanded lipid profiles such as the LPP (lipoprotein particles; Spectracell labs), NMR (nuclear magnetic resonance) (LipoScience, Raleigh, North Carolina), Berkley Heart Labs and VAP (vertical auto profile) (Atherotec, Birmingham, Alabama) improve serum lipid analysis and CHD risk profiling.[23,24]

It is now proven that LDL-P value over 700 is the primary lipid parameter that drives the risk for CHD and MI as well as coronary artery calcification (CAC) as measured by computed tomography

(CT) angiogram.[25,26] Dense LDL type B or LDL type 3 or 4 have a secondary role in CHD only if the LDL–P is elevated over 700–900. Dysfunctional HDL[27–30] may become inflammatory, atherogenic and lose its atheroprotective effects especially in patients with DM, metabolic syndrome, and obesity due to the vascular inflammatory effects of cardiometabolic syndrome.[30] Oxidation and inflammation of APO-A1 often results in higher levels of HDL that are dysfunctional and not protective.[30] The ability to evaluate HDL functionality, either directly or indirectly, measuring reverse cholesterol transport[28] or myeloperoxidase (MPO)[29,30] will allow even better assessment of dyslipidemia-induced vascular disease, CHD risk, and treatment.

An understanding of the pathophysiological steps in dyslipidemia-induced vascular damage is mandatory for optimal and logical treatment (Figure 5.1). The ability to interrupt all of the various steps in this pathway will allow more specific functional and metabolic medicine treatments to reduce vascular injury, improve vascular repair systems, and to maintain or restore vascular health.

Native LDL, especially large type A LDL, is not usually atherogenic until modified. However, there exists an alternate pinocytosis mechanism that allows macrophage ingestion of native LDL, which accounts for up to 30% of foam cell formation in the subendothelium that occur during chronic inflammation or infections.[31,32]

For example, decreasing LDL modification, the atherogenic form of LDL-C, though decreases in oxidized (oxLDL), glycated (glyLDL), glyco-oxidized LDL (gly-oxLDL) and acetylated LDL (acLDL), decreasing the uptake of modified LDL into macrophages by the scavenger receptors (CD 36 SR), decreasing the inflammatory, oxidative stress and autoimmune responses will reduce vascular damage beyond just treating the LDL-C level.[33–38] There are at least 38 mechanistic pathways that can be treated to interrupt the dyslipidemia-induced vascular damage and disease (Table 5.1). Reduction in high-sensitivity C-reactive protein (HS-CRP), an inflammatory marker, reduces vascular events independent of reductions in LDL-C through numerous mechanisms.[39]

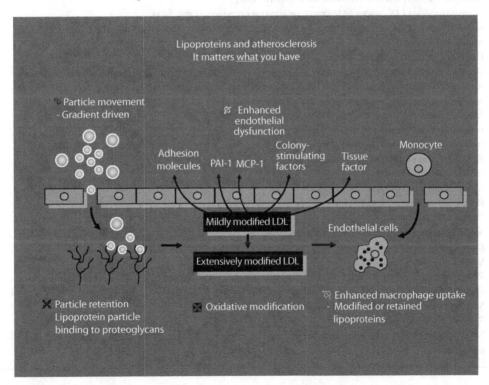

FIGURE 5.1   (See color insert.) The various steps in the uptake of LDL cholesterol, modification, macrophage ingestion with scavenger receptors, foam cell formation, oxidative stress, inflammation, and autoimmune cytokines and chemokine production.

TABLE 5.1

Thirty-Eight Mechanisms for Treatment of Dyslipidemia-Induced Vascular Disease

1. Decrease endothelial permeability, gap junctions, endothelial dysfunction, and improve endothelial repair. Aged garlic: increase NO; reduce A-II effects; increase EPCs; BP control; reduce inflammation, oxidative stress, and vascular immune dysfunction.
2. Modify caveolae, caveolin-1, lipid rafts, membrane microdomains, unesterified cholesterol, and cholesterol crystals. Lycopene, omega-3 FAs, and statins.
3. Increase eNOS and nitric oxide. Arginine/citrullene, resveratrol, flax seed, omega-3 FAs, co-enzyme Q10, R-lipoic acid, NAC, taurine, pycnogenol, grape seed extract, pomegranate, aged garlic.
4. Modify pattern recognition receptor (PRR) activation and toll like receptors. Niacin, EGCG, pantethine, resveratrol, MUFA, curcumin, pomegranate, aged garlic, sesame, gamma/delta tocotrienols, lycopene.
5. Decrease cholesterol crystals, LDL phospholipids, oxLDL, APO-B, and 7 ketosteroids that activate PRR. Omega-3 FAs and statins.
6. Decrease LDL burden (Table 5.4).
7. Reduce cholesterol absorption (Table 5.6).
8. Increase cholesterol bile excretion (Table 5.17).
9. Decrease LDL particle number (Table 5.13).
10. Decrease APO-B (Table 5.15).
11. Decrease LDL modification/oxidation (Table 5.2).
12. Inhibit LDL glycation (Table 5.3).
13. Increase LDL size (Table 5.5).
14. Modify LDL composition. Omega-3 FAs, MUFA, reduce inflammation, oxidative stress, and immune dysfunction.
15. Upregulate LDL receptor (Table 5.17).
16. Regulate sortilins and SORLA.
17. Deactivate the LOX-1 receptor. Reduce BP, reduce HS-CRP.
18. Decrease modified LDL macrophage uptake by scavenger receptors (Table 5.11).
19. Decrease native LDL macrophage uptake by pinocytosis. Decrease infections and inflammation, decrease modified LDL.
20. Decrease LDL signaling. Plant sterols.
21. Decrease CAMs, macrophage recruitment and migration. NAC, resveratrol, luteolin, glutathione, and curcumin.
22. Alter macrophage phenotype. Omega-3 FA, plant sterols, sterolins, and glycosides.
23. Modify signaling pathways. Plant sterols and phytosterolins.
24. Increase reverse cholesterol transport (Table 5.12).
25. Increase HDL and increase HDL size (Table 5.10).
26. Improve HDL function. Reduce inflammation, oxidative stress, and immune dysfunction. Quercetin, pomegranate, EGCG, resveratrol, glutathione, lycopene.
27. Increase APO-A1 (Table 5.16).
28. Increase PON 1 and PON 2 (Table 5.18).
29. Reduce inflammation (Table 5.14).
30. Reduce oxidative stress.
31. Modulate immune dysfunction. Plant sterols and sterolins.
32. Decrease VLDL and TG (Table 5.9).
33. Lower Lp(a) (Table 5.8).
34. Reduce foam cell and fatty streak formation. Resveratrol, NAC, phytosterolins.
35. Reduce trapping of foam cells in the subendothelium. Resveratrol, NAC.
36. Stabilize plaque. Omega-3 FAs, vitamin K2MK7, aged garlic.
37. Reduce LpPLA2 Omega-3 FAs, niacin.
38. Reduce plaque burden, progression, and increase regression. Omega-3 FAs, vitamin K2 MK 7, aged garlic, pomegranate.

Many patients cannot or will not use pharmacologic treatments such as statins, fibrates, bile acid resin binders, or ezetimibe to treat dyslipidemia.[5] Statin-induced or fibrate-induced muscle disease, abnormal liver function tests, neuropathy, memory loss, mental status changes, gastrointestinal disturbances, glucose intolerance, or DM are some of the reasons.[41–44] However, many patients have other clinical symptoms or lab abnormalities such as chronic fatigue, exercise-induced fatigue, myalgias, muscle weakness, memory loss, decrease lean muscle mass, reduced exercise tolerance, reductions on Coenzyme Q10 carnitine, vitamin E, vitamin D, omega-3 FAs, selenium and free T3 levels (hypothyroidism) with prolonged usage, or the administration of high-dose statins.[5,40,45–52] New treatment approaches that combine weight loss, reduction in visceral and total body fat, increase in lean muscle mass, optimal aerobic and resistance exercise, scientifically proven nutrition, and use of nutraceutical supplements offer not only improvement in serum lipids but also reductions in inflammation, oxidative stress, immune dysfunction, and endothelial and vascular smooth muscle dysfunction. In addition, surrogate markers for vascular disease or clinical vascular target organ damage such as CHD and carotid intimal medial thickness (IMT) are reduced in many clinical trials.[5]

NUTRACEUTICAL SUPPLEMENTS AND THE MANAGEMENT OF DYSLIPIDEMIA

Nutraceutical supplement management of dyslipidemia has been infrequently reviewed.[5,53,54] New important scientific information and clinical studies are required to understand the present role of these natural agents in the management of dyslipidemia.[5,53,54] Studies include clinical trials that show excellent reductions in serum lipids and CHD with niacin, omega-3 FAs, red yeast rice, fiber and alpha linolenic acid (ALA), and smaller studies using surrogate vascular markers such as carotid intimal medial thickness and obstruction, plaque progression, CAC score by electron beam tomography (EBT) and CT angiogram, generalized atherosclerosis, and endothelial function.[5,54–56] The proposed mechanisms of action of some of the nutraceutical supplements on the mammalian cholesterol pathway are shown in Figure 5.2.

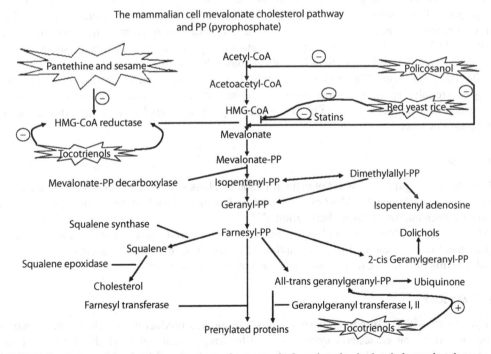

FIGURE 5.2 Proposed mechanisms of actions of nutraceuticals and statins in the cholesterol pathway.

NIACIN (VITAMIN B3)

Niacin has a dose-related effect (1–4 g/day) in reducing TC, LDL, APO-B, LDL-P, TGs, VLDL, increasing LDL size from small type B to large type A, increasing HDL especially the protective and larger HDL 2b particle and APO-A1).[5] However, niacin does not increase HDL-P (the predominant protective lipid parameter) much, if at all.[57,58] Niacin has a logarithmic dose–response on HDL with smaller doses having a large effect, but the effect on LDL reduction is a linear dose–response that requires higher doses.[57]

The changes are dose related and vary from about 10%–30% for each lipid, including HDL, LDL and triglycerides.[5,59,60] Niacin inhibits LDL oxidation, increases TG lipolysis in adipose tissue, increases APO-B degradation, reduces the fractional catabolic rate of HDL–APO-A1, inhibits platelet function, induces fibrinolysis, decreases cytokines, cell adhesion molecules (CAMs), lowers Lp(a), increases adiponectin—which provides antioxidant activity, inhibits cholesterol ester transfer protein (CETP), and increases reverse cholesterol transport.[5,57,59,60] However, despite an improved lipid profile and all other parameters, there is no improvement in endothelial or microvascular function.[61] Randomized clinical trials such as the Coronary Drug Project, HATS trial, ARBITOR 2, Oxford Niaspan Study, FATS, CLAS I and CLAS II, and AFRS have shown reduction in coronary events, decreases in coronary atheroma (plaque) and decreases in carotid IMT.[5,59,60,62–65] The recent negative findings in the AIMHIGH study[66,67] do not detract from these positive clinical trials, as this study has numerous methodological design flaws and was not powered to statistically determine CVD endpoints.

The recent THRIVE trial of 26,000 patients using 2 g of extended-release niacin plus the anti-flushing agent laropiprant daily or placebo on top of a background therapy of simvastatin with or without ezetimibe did not reduce CV events despite an increased HDL of 17% and decreased LDL of 20%.[68,69] Whether the inhibition of flushing by laropiprant or some other unknown effect of this agent interfered with the HDL function and the CV outcomes is not clear. However, the recommendation by some not to use niacin in face of other positive studies is clearly premature.

The effective dosing range is from 500 to 4000 mg/day. Only vitamin B3 (niacin) is effective in dyslipidemia. The nonflush niacin (inositol hexanicotinate-IHN) does not improve lipid profiles, and is not recommended.[5,70] The side effects of niacin include hyperglycemia, hyperuricemia, gout, hepatitis, flushing, rash, pruritus, hyperpigmentation, hyperhomocysteinemia, gastritis, ulcers, bruising, tachycardia, and palpitations.[5,59,60] Elevations in homocysteine should be treated with vitamin B6, B12, and folate. Niacin-induced flushing is minimized by increasing the dose gradually, taking on a regular basis without missing doses, taking with meals, avoiding alcohol within 4 hours of ingestion of niacin, consumption of 81 mg baby aspirin, and supplemental quercetin, apples or apple pectin or sauce.[5]

POLICOSANOL

Policosanol is a sugar cane extract of eight aliphatic alcohols that has undergone extensive clinical studies with variable results.[5] Most of the earlier studies that showed positive results performed in Cuba have been questioned as to their validity.[5,54,71,72]

The more recent double-blind placebo-controlled clinical trials have not shown any significant improvement in any measured lipids including TC, LDL, TG, or HDL. Policosanol is not recommended at this time for the treatment of any form of dyslipidemia.[5,54,71,72]

RED YEAST RICE

Red yeast rice—RYR (*Monascus purpureus*) is a fermented product of rice that contains monocolins, which inhibit cholesterol synthesis via 3-hydroxy-3-methyl-glutaryl (HMG) CoA reductase and thus has "statin-like" properties (13 natural statins).[5,54,73–75] RYR also contains ergosterol, amino acids, flavonoids, trace elements, alkaloids, sterols, isoflavones, and monounsaturated FAs.

RYR administered orally to adults subjects with dyslipidemia at 2400 mg/day reduced LDL-C by 22% ($p < .001$), TG by 12% with little change in HDL.[5,54,73] RYR reduces the risk of abdominal aortic aneurysms (AAA) by suppressing angiotensin II levels.[74] In a recent placebo-controlled Chinese study of 5000 subjects over 4.5 years, an extract of RYR reduced LDL 17.6% ($p < .001$) and increased HDL 4.2% ($p < .001$).[75]

A highly purified and certified RYR must be used to avoid potential renal damage induced by mycotoxin and citrinin.[5,54,73]

The recommended dose is 2400–4800 mg of a standardized RYR. Although reductions in Coenzyme Q 10 may occur in predisposed patients and those on prolonged high-dose RYR due to its weaker "statin-like" effect. RYR is an excellent alternative to patients with statin-induced myopathy.[5,54,73]

PLANT STEROLS (PHYTOSTEROLS)

The plant sterols, which are similar to cholesterol molecules, are naturally occurring sterols of plant origin that include B-sitosterol (the most abundant), campesterol, stigmasterol (4-desmethyl sterols of the cholestane series), and the stanols, which are saturated.[5,54,76–78] The plant sterols are much better absorbed than the plant stanols. The daily intake of plant sterols in the United States is about 150–400 mg/day mostly from soybean oil, various nuts, and tall pine tree oil.[54] These have a dose-dependent reduction in serum lipids.[77] TC is decreased 8%, LDL is decreased 10% (range 6%–15%) with no change in TG and HDL on doses of 2–3 g/day in divided doses with meals.[5,54,76,77] A recent meta-analysis of 84 trials showed that an average intake of 2.15 g/day reduced LDL by 8.8% with no improvement with higher doses.[77] The mechanism of action is primarily to decrease the incorporation of dietary and biliary cholesterol into micelles due to lower micellar solubility of cholesterol, which reduces cholesterol absorption and increases bile acid secretion. In addition, there is an interaction with enterocyte ATP-binding cassette transport proteins (ABCG8 and ABCG5) that directs cholesterol back into the intestinal lumen.[5,54,76] The only difference between cholesterol and sitosterol consists of an additional ethyl group at position C-24 in sitosterol, which is responsible for its poor absorption. The plant sterols have a higher affinity than cholesterol for the micelles. Patients that have the rare homozygote mutations of the ATP-binding cassette are hyperabsorbers of sitosterol (absorb 15%–60% instead of the normal 5%) and will develop premature atherosclerosis.[54] This is a rare autosomal recessive disorder termed sitosterolemia. The plant sterols are also anti-inflammatory and decrease the levels of proinflammatory cytokines such as HS-CRP, IL-6, IL1b, TNF alpha, PLA 2, and fibrinogen, but these effects vary among the various phytosterols.[78,79] Other potential mechanisms include modulation of signaling pathways, activation of cellular stress responses, growth arrest, reduction of APO-B48 secretion from intestinal and hepatic cells, reduction of cholesterol synthesis with suppression of HMG COA reductase and CYP7A1, interference with sterol regulatory element-binding protein (SREBP), and promotion of reverse cholesterol transport via ATP-binding cassette transporter (ABCA1) and ATP-binding cassette sub-family G member 1 (ABCG1).[79] The biological activity of phytosterols is both cell-type and sterol specific.[79]

The plant sterols can interfere with absorption of lipid-soluble compounds such as fat soluble vitamins and carotenoids such as vitamins D, E, and K, and alpha carotene.[5,54] Some studies have shown reduction in atherosclerosis progression, reduced carotid IMT, and decreased plaque progression, but the results have been conflicting.[5,54] There are no studies on CHD or other CVD outcomes. The recommended dose is about 2–2.5 g/day (average 2.15 g/day).

SOY

Numerous studies have shown mild improvements in serum lipids with soy at doses of about 30–50 g/day.[5,54,80,81] TC decreased 2%–9.3%, LDL decreased 4%–12.9%, TG decreased 10.5%, and HDL increased up to 2.4%. However, the studies are conflicting due to differences in the type and dose of soy used in the studies, as well as nonstandardized methodology.[5,54,94,95] Soy decreases the micellar content and absorption of lipids through a combination of fiber, isoflavones (genistin, glycitin, and diadzin) and phytoestrogens.[5,54,80,81] Soy also reduces SREBP, HMG-COA reductase, increases LDL receptor density, and increases the antioxidant activity of SOD and catalase. Most reduction is seen with soy-enriched isoflavones with soy protein. Fermented soy is preferred.

GREEN TEA EXTRACT AND GREEN TEA

Catechins, especially epigallocatechin-3-gallate (EGCG), may improve the lipid profile by interfering with micellar solubilization of cholesterol in the GI tract and reduce absorption.[5] In addition, EGCG reduces the FA gene expression, inhibits HMG CoA reductase, increases mitochondrial energy expenditure, reduces oxLDL, increases PON-1, upregulates the LDL receptor, decreases APO-B lipoprotein secretion from cells, mimics the action of insulin, improves endothelial dysfunction, activates Nrf2, increases heme oxygenase-1 (HO-1) expression, decreases inflammation, displaces caveolin-1 from cell membranes, increases NO, reduces endothelial inflammation, and decreases body fat.[5,82–85]

A meta-analysis of human studies of 14 trials show that EGCG at 224–674 mg/day or 60 oz of green tea per day reduced TC 7.2 mg/dL and LDL 2.19 mg/dL ($p < .001$ for both). There was no significant change in HDL or TG levels.[86] The recommended dose is a standardized EGCG extract 500–1000 mg/day.

OMEGA-3 FATTY ACIDS

Observational, epidemiologic, and controlled clinical trials have shown significant reductions in serum TG, VLDL, decreased LDL-P, and increased LDL and HDL particle size as well as major reductions in all CVD events.[5,87–94] The DART trial demonstrated a decrease in mortality of 29% in men post MI and the Gruppo Italiano per lo Studio della Sopravvivenza nell'Infarto (GISSI) prevention trial found a decrease in total mortality of 20%, CV deaths of 30% and sudden death of 45%. The Kuppio Heart Study demonstrated a 44% reduction in fatal and nonfatal CHD in subjects in the highest quintile of omega-3 intake compared to the lowest quintile.[5,87,88] Omega-3 FA reduce CHD progression, stabilize plaque, reduce coronary artery stent restenosis, and coronary artery bypass graft eicosapentaenoic acid (CABG) occlusion.[5,89] In the JELIS study, the addition of 1.8 g of omega EPA to a statin resulted in an additional 19% relative risk reduction (RRR) in major coronary events and nonfatal MI and a 20% decrease in CVA.[5,90] There is a dose-related reduction in VLDL of up to 50%, TG of up to 50%, with little to no change or decrease in total TC, LDL, APO-B and no change to slight increase in HDL.[5,91–94] However, the number of LDL particles decrease and LDL particle size increases from small type B to large type A (increase of 25 nm). The antiatherogenic HDL 2b is also increases by up to 29%. The rate of entry of VLDL particles into the circulation is decreased and APO-CIII is reduced which allows lipoprotein lipase to be more active.[26] There is a decrease in remnant chylomicrons and remnant lipoproteins.[5,92] Patients with LDL over 100 mg% usually have reductions in total LDL and those that are below 80 mg% have mild increases.[93] However, in both cases, the LDL-P decreases, the dense LDL B increases in size to the less atherogenic LDL A particle and APO-B levels decrease. There is a net decrease in the concentration of cholesterol carried by all atherogenic particles and decreases in non-HDL-C. Omega-3 FA are anti-inflammatory, antithrombotic, lower BP and heart rate, improve heart rate variability,[5,87] decrease FA synthesis, increase FA oxidation, and reduce body fat and weight.[5] Omega-3 FAs are one of the only substances that lower lipoprotein-associated phospholipase A2 (Lp-LPA2).[26]

Insulin resistance is improved and there are no significant changes in fasting glucose or hemoglobin A1C with long-term treatment.[95] Doses of 3 g/day of combined EPA and DHA at a 3:2

ratio with GLA at 50% of the total EPA and DHA content and 700 mg of gamma/delta tocopherol at 80% and 20% alpha tocopherol per 3 g of DHA and EPA are recommended.[5] DHA and EPA may have variable but favorable effects on the various lipid levels.[5,91,92,95,96] EPA does not usually increase LDL, is less effective in lowering TG than DHA but does not alter the LDL and HDL particle size. However, DHA may increase total LDL, but increases LDL and HDL size and lowers TG more.[96] The combination of plant sterols and omega-3 FAs are synergistic in improving lipids and inflammation.[94] New free FA forms of omega-3 FAs have a fourfold greater area under the plasma n-3 PUFA curve than prescription Lovaza and thus a more potent reduction in TG levels.[96] The data of krill oil on dyslipidemia is limited to only one study in which a dose-related response to LDL-C reduction up to 39%, TG reduction of 27%, and HDL increase of 60% was found.[97] These findings with krill oil require confirmation with additional controlled trials.

FLAX

Flax seeds and flax lignan complex with SDG (secoisolariciresinol diglucoside) and increased intake of ALA from other sources such as walnuts have been shown in several meta-analyses to reduce TC and LDL by 5%–15%, Lp(a) by 14%, TG by up to 36% with either no change or a slight reduction in HDL.[5,98–100] These properties do not apply to flax seed oil. In the Seven Countries study, CHD was reduced with increased consumption of ALA. In the Lyon diet trial at the end of 4 years, intake of flax reduced CHD and total deaths by 50%–70%.[5] Flax seeds contain fiber and lignins and decrease the levels of 7 alpha hydroylase and acyl CoA cholesterol transferase.[5,98–100] Flax seeds and ALA are anti-inflammatory, reduce HS-CRP, decrease TG, increase HDL, decrease insulin resistance and risk of type 2 DM, reduce visceral obesity and systolic BP, increase eNOS, and improve endothelial dysfunction. Flax contains phytoestrogens, decreases vascular smooth muscle hypertrophy, reduces oxidative stress, increases cholesterol efflux in macrophage-derived foam cells by decreasing stearoyl CoA desaturase-1 expressions and farnesoid X receptor mechanism of action, and retard development of atherosclerosis.[5,98–102] The dose required for these effects is from 14 to 40 g of flax seeds per day.[5,98–100] Chia seeds (*Salvia hispanica*) are the richest botanical source of ALA at 60% wt/volume.[101] The dose of chia seeds is 25 g/day.

MONOUNSATURATED FATS

Monounsaturated fats (MUFAs) such as olives, olive oil, and nuts reduce LDL by 5%–10%, lower TG by 10%–15%, increase HDL by 5%, decrease oxLDL, reduce oxidation and inflammation, improve ED, lower BP, decrease thrombosis and reduce the incidence of CHD (Mediterranean diet).[5,103–107] MUFA reduces CD40L gene expression and its downstream products (IL23a, adrenergic B-2 receptor, oxLDL receptor 1, IL-8 receptor) and related genes involved in atherogenic and inflammatory process in vivo in humans.[107] MUFA are one of the most potent agents to reduce oxLDL in humans.

The equivalent of 3–4 tablespoons (40–50 g) per day of extra-virgin olive oil (EVOO) with MUFA content is recommended for the maximum effect in conjunction with omega-3 FAs. However, the caloric intake of this amount of MUFA must be balanced with the other beneficial effects.

SESAME

Sesame at 40 g/day reduces LDL by 9% through inhibition of intestinal absorption, increasing biliary secretion, decreasing HMG CoA reductase activity, upregulating the LDL receptor gene, upregulating 7 alpha hydroxylase gene expression, and upregulating the SREBP 2 genes.[108,109] A randomized placebo-controlled crossover study of 26 postmenopausal women who consumed 50 g of sesame powder daily for 5 weeks had a 5% decrease in TC and a 10% decrease in LDL-C.[108]

TOCOTRIENOLS

Tocotrienols are a family of unsaturated forms of vitamin E termed alpha, beta, gamma, and delta.[5] The gamma and delta tocotrienols lower TC up to 17%, LDL 24%, APO-B 15%, and Lp(a) 17% with minimal changes in HDL or APO-A1 in 50% of subjects at doses of 200 mg/day given at night with food.[5,110–112] The gamma/delta form of tocotrienols inhibits cholesterol synthesis by suppression of HMG-CoA reductase activity by two posttranscriptional actions.[5,110–112] These include increased controlled degradation of the reductase protein and decreased efficiency of translation of HMG CoA reductase mRNA. These effects are mediated by sterol binding of the reductase enzyme to the endoplasmic reticulum membrane proteins called INSIGS.[111] The tocotrienols have natural farnesylated analogues of tocopherols, which give them their effects on HMG CoA reductase.[111] In addition, the LDL receptor is augmented and they exhibit antioxidant activity.

The tocotrienol dose is very important as increased dosing will induce its own metabolism and reduce effectiveness, whereas lower doses are not as effective.[5] Also, concomitant intake (less than 12 hours) of alpha tocopherol reduces tocotrienol absorption. Increased intake of alpha tocopherol over 20% of total tocopherols may interfere with the lipid-lowering effect.[5,110]

Tocotrienols are metabolized by successive beta oxidation and then catalyzed by the CYP P450 enzymes 3A4 and CYP 4F2.[5] The combination of a statin with gamma/delta tocotrienols further reduces LDL-C by 10%.[110] The tocotrienols block the adaptive response of upregulation of HMG-CoA reductase secondary to competitive inhibition by the statins.[5,110] Carotid artery stenosis regression has been reported in about 30% of subjects given tocotrienols over 18 months. They also slow progression of generalized atherosclerosis.[5,112] The recommended dose is 200 mg of gamma delta tocotrienol at night with food.

PANTETHINE

Pantethine is the disulfide derivative of pantothenic acid and is metabolized to cystamine-SH, which is the active form in treating dyslipidemia.[5,113–117] Over 28 clinical trials have shown consistent and significant improvement in serum lipids. TC is decreased 15%, LDL by 20%, APO-B by 27.6%, and TG by 36.5% over 4–9 months. HDL and APO-A1 are increased 8%.[5,113–118] The effects on lipids are slow with peak effects at 4 months but may take up to 6–9 months.[5,113–118] In addition, pantethine reduces lipid peroxidation of LDL, decreases lipid deposition, intimal thickening and fatty streak formation in the aorta and coronary arteries.[5,113–117] Pantethine inhibits cholesterol synthesis and accelerates FA metabolism in the mitochondria by inhibiting hepatic acetyl-CoA carboxylase, increases CoA in the cytoplasm, which stimulates the oxidation of acetate at the expense of FA and cholesterol synthesis, and increases the Krebs cycle activity.[5,113–117] In addition, cholesterol esterase activity increases and HMG-CoA reductase activity is decreased.[5,113–117] There is 50% inhibition of FA synthesis and 80% inhibition of cholesterol synthesis.[5] Its lipid effects are additive to statins, niacin, and fibrates. The recommended effective dose is 300 mg three times per day or 450 mg twice per day with or without food.[5,113–118]

GUGGULIPIDS

Guggulipids are resins from the Mukul myrrh tree (*Commiphora wightii*) that contain active lipid-lowering compounds called guggulsterones.[5,119–121] These increase hepatic LDL receptors, bile acid secretion, and decrease cholesterol synthesis in animal experiments.[5,119] However, controlled human clinical trials have not shown these agents to be effective in improving serum lipids.[119–121] One study of 103 subjects on 50–75 mg of guggulsterones per day for 8 weeks actually had a 5% increase in LDL, no change in TC, TG, or HDL, and insignificant reductions in Lp(a) and HS-CRP.[119] Guggulipids are not recommended at this time.

GARLIC

Numerous placebo-controlled clinical trials in humans indicate reductions in TC and LDL of about 9%–12% at doses of 600–900 mg/day of a standardized extract of allicin and ajoene.[5,122,123] Many studies have been poorly controlled and use variable types and doses of garlic, which have given inconsistent results.[5,122,123] Aged garlic (AGE) has shown the best results related to improvement in serum lipids as well as lowering BP, improving endothelial function and arterial elasticity, decreasing CAC and plaque progression, and lowering HS-CRP.[5,56,122–126] Garlic reduces intestinal cholesterol absorption, inhibits enzymes involved in cholesterol synthesis, and deactivates HMG COA reductase.[5,122] In addition, AGE reduces vascular smooth muscle proliferation and transformation; decreases oxidative stress and inflammation; decreases oxLDL; prevents entry of lipids into the arterial wall and macrophages; increases eNOS and NO; increases glutathione, glutathione reductase, and superoxide dismutase; has fibrinolytic activity and antiplatelet activity.[5,56,122] AGE has been used in these studies alone or in conjunction with B vitamins, folate, arginine, and statins.[123–126]

RESVERATROL

Resveratrol reduces oxLDL; inhibits ACAT activity and cholesterol ester formation; increases bile acid excretion; reduces TC, TG, and LDL; increases PON-1 activity and HDL; inhibits NADPH oxidase in macrophages and blocks the uptake of modified LDL by CD36 SR (scavenger receptors).[127,128] N-Acetylcysteine (NAC) has this same effect on CD 36 DR and should be used in conjunction with resveratrol.[127] The dose of trans-resveratrol is 250 mg/day and NAC is 1000 mg twice per day.

CURCUMIN

Curcumin is a phenolic compound in turmeric.[5,129] It induces changes in the expression of genes involved in cholesterol synthesis such as the LDL receptor mRNA, HMG CoA reductase, SREBP, cholesterol 7 alpha hydrolyze, peroxisome proliferator-activated receptors (PPAR), liver X receptors (LXR), affects the expression of genes involved in leukocyte adhesion and transendothelial migration to inhibit atherosclerosis.[5,129,130] In one human study of 10 patients consuming 500 mg/day of curcumin, the HDL increased 29% and total cholesterol decreased 12%.[5,129] This needs confirmation in larger randomized clinical trials.

POMEGRANATE

Pomegranate increases PON 1 binding to HDL and increases PON 2 in macrophages, which improves the function of HDL cholesterol and increases reverse cholesterol transport. It is a potent antioxidant, increases total antioxidant status (TAS), lowers oxLDL, decreases antibodies to oxLDL, inhibits platelet function, reduces glycosylated LDL, decreases macrophage LDL uptake, reduces lipid deposition in the arterial wall, decreases progression of carotid artery IMT, and lowers blood pressure especially in subjects with the highest oxidative stress, known carotid artery plaque, and the greatest abnormalities in TG and HDL levels.[131–136] Consuming about 8 oz of pomegranate juice per day or 1–2 cups of pomegranate seeds is recommended.

CITRUS BERGAMIA

Citrus bergamia has been evaluated in several clinical prospective trials in humans. In doses of 1000 mg/day, this compound lowers LDL up to 36%, TG up to 39%, increases HDL up to 40% by inhibiting HMG CoA reductase, increases cholesterol and bile acid excretion, reduces ROS and oxLDL, improves glucose via AMPK and GLUT 4 receptor, reduces weight, and binds to the ACAT receptor.[137–139] The active ingredients include naringin, neroeriocitrin, neohesperidin, poncerin, rutin, neodesmin, rhoifolin, melitidine, and brutelidine.[137,139]

Vitamin C

Vitamin C supplementation lowers serum LDL-C and TGs.[140] A meta-analysis of 13 randomized controlled trials in subjects given at least 500 mg of vitamin C daily for 3–24 weeks found a reduction in LDL-C of 7.9 mg/dL ($p < .0001$) TG reduction of 20.1 mg/dL ($p < .003$). HDL did not change. The reductions in LDL and TG were greatest in those with the highest initial lipid levels and the lowest serum vitamin C levels.[141]

Lycopene

Lycopene is an acyclic carotenoid with a high concentration in tomatoes.

It has been shown in tissue culture to inhibit HMG CoA reductase; induce Rho inactivation; increase PPAR gamma, LXR receptor, and RXR activities; increase reverse cholesterol transport and efflux with ABCA1, APO-AI expression and caveolin-1 expression, increase HDL 2 and 3, improve HDL functionality, reduce SAA, decrease CETP, increase PON 1, and reduce inflammation in humans.[142–144] This reduces intracellular cholesterol and lowers cholesterol in lipid domains, which alters membrane-induced cellular signal transduction. The two unconjugated double bonds in the lycopene molecule have high activity against ROS. Higher serum lycopene levels are associated with reduction in carotid IMT and carotid atherosclerosis.[145]

Probiotics

Mixed high-dose probiotics at 60–100 billion organisms per day reduce TC by 9%, LDL-C by 8%, and TG by 10%.[146,147] Probiotics precipitate bile salts, deconjugate bile salts, and are incorporated into cell membranes and into the assimilation of cholesterol.

Berberine HCL

Berberine HCL is an alkaloid present in roots, rhizomes, and stem barks of selected plants.[148–150] In a study of 32 dyslipidemic patients, 500 mg/day of berberine HCL decreased TC by 29%, LDL-C by 25%, and TG by 35% in 3 months.[149] Berberine increases hepatic LDL-R and is additive to statins in its lipid-lowering effect.[148,149] The recommended dose is 500 mg/day to bid. Berberine has additive LDL-lowering effects with statins[148] and ezetimibe.[150] However, berberine is more effective and has fewer adverse effects compared to ezetimibe monotherapy.

Combinations

A recent prospective open-label human clinical trial of 30 patients for 2 months, which is not as rigorous as a placebo-controlled trial, showed significant improvement in serum lipids using a proprietary product with a combination of pantethine, plant sterols, EGCG, gamma/delta tocotrienols, and phytolens.[151] There was a reduction of TC by 14%, LDL by 14%, VLDL by 20%, and small dense LDL particles by 25% (type III and IV) (100). In another study using the same proprietary product with RYR 2400 mg/day and niacin 500 mg/day, the TC dropped by 34%, LDL decreased by 34%, LDL-P dropped by 35%, VLDL dropped by 27%, and HDL increased by 10% (Houston MC, Personal Communication, 2011). Studies indicate an RRR of CVD mortality with omega-3 FAs of .68, with resins of .70 and with statins of .78.[152] Combining statins with omega-3 FAs (EFA) decreases CHD 19% more.[90] The combination of gamma/delta tocotrienols and a statin reduces LDL-C by an additional 10%.[110] Plant sterols with omega-3 FAs have synergistic lipid-lowering and anti-inflammatory effects.[94] A combination of red yeast rice, bitter gourd, chlorella, soy protein, and licorice resulted in significant reductions in TC, TG, and LDL as well as BP in 228 subjects in a controlled clinical trial.[153] AGE alone or in combination with B vitamins, folate, arginine, Coenzyme Q10, or statins improves lipids and other markers of endothelial function, vascular elasticity, NO, inflammation, HS-CRP, CAC, and plaque regression.[5,56,122–126] Future studies are needed to evaluate various other combinations on serum lipids, surrogate vascular endpoints, and CHD and CVD morbidity and mortality.

NUTRITIONAL MANAGEMENT OF DYSLIPIDEMIA

Nutrition is an important treatment for dyslipidemia, CHD risk factors, and for the prevention and treatment of CVD. Numerous epidemiological studies and prospective clinical trials including the Framingham Heart Study,[154,155] Seven Countries Study,[156,157] Pritikin diet studies,[158–160] Ornish Lifestyle Heart Trial,[161–164] Omni Heart Trial,[155] Portfolio diet,[165–168] MD,[169–172] Lyon Diet Heart Study,[172] Indian Heart Study,[173] Predimed study,[174,175] and Paleolithic diet have clearly established the relationship between diet, serum lipids, inflammation, and CVD including CHD and stroke.

Three cohorts of the Framingham Heart Study with over 10,000 subjects have demonstrated improved CV risk on lipid lowering diets that decrease total and LDL-C, TG, and increase HDL.[154,155] The Seven Countries Study was an international study that investigated lifestyle and diet.[156,157] A high fat diet increased prevalence of CVD. The Pritikin Principle Diet, which included low-fat diet (10% of total calories) with primarily vegetables, grains, and fruits, combined with exercise, improved the lipid profile.[158–160]

Ornish evaluated an intensive therapeutic approach that combined a low fat (10% total calories, low cholesterol of 10 mg/day, complex carbohydrate, low refined carbohydrate vegetarian diet, exercise, and other lifestyle changes such as stress reduction, smoking cessation, and group psychosocial support).[161–164] The experimental group compared to the control group had statistically significant reductions in LDL-C, frequency of angina episodes, and regression in coronary artery stenosis at years 1 and 5.

The Optimal Macronutrient Intake for Heart Health Trial (OmniHeart Trial) was a randomized controlled intervention crossover study of 164 adults using a Mediterranean-style diet to evaluate plasma lipids and blood pressure.[155] Three diets were included—a carbohydrate-rich diet, a protein-rich diet with 50% from plant sources, and a diet rich in monounsaturated fat. The monounsaturated fat-rich diet increased HDL-C levels, lowered TG, with no change in LDL-C. The protein-rich diet decreased LDL-C, TG, and HDL-C compared to the carbohydrate diet. Substitution of the carbohydrates with either proteins or monounsaturated fat lowered blood pressure, improved serum lipid levels, and reduced CV risk.[168]

The Portfolio Diet Study was a randomized control trial of 14 dyslipidemic subjects[165] given a vegetarian diet, with additional soluble fiber, nuts, soy protein, and plant sterols. At 4 weeks, the LDL-C dropped by 29.6% and TG by 9.3% in the diet group versus 8.5% in the control group. There was a 33.3% decrease in LDL-C and 11% decrease in TG in those given a statin drug. In a follow-up study of the Portfolio diet in 66 dyslipidemic adults for 1 year, 31 participants had reductions in LDL-C > 20% related to compliance with the diet.[166] The most recent Portfolio diet of 351 subjects showed an LDL-C reduction of 13.8% vs. 3% in the control group.[167,168] Increasing the monounsaturated fat content increased serum HDL-C levels but maintained the reduction in LDL-C.[167,168]

The Mediterranean-style diet[169] consists of a high intake of vegetables and fruits, bread and other cereal grains, potatoes, legumes, nuts, seeds, monounsaturated fat as olive products (15%–20% of total calories), animal products (meat, poultry, fish, dairy, eggs) at a low-to-moderate level, and red wine. The Lyon Diet Heart Study was the first randomized single-blind secondary prevention trial 600 participants over 4 years with a prior MI to investigate the effect of a Mediterranean-style diet on CVD.[170–172] The primary outcome measurement of fatal or nonfatal MI was significantly reduced. For example, the total fat in the experimental diet was 30.5% but had only 12.5% MUFA and was enriched in ALA, an omega-3 polyunsaturated fat. The recent 4.8-year study of 7447 subjects given the MD in primary prevention of CVD found a 28%–30% reduction in major CV events in those on the MD with EVOO or nuts.[176]

The Indian Heart Study was a one year evaluation of a Mediterranean-style diet enriched in ALA administered to the treated group, while the control group was advised on smoking cessation, stress management, regular exercise, reduction of dietary fat and alcohol.[173] Compared to the control group, the treated group had a 38% reduction in nonfatal MI and a 32% reduction in fatal MI.

The Prevención con Dieta Mediterránea (PREDIMED)[174] was a 3 month randomized cross-sectional study of 772 asymptomatic Spanish adults at high risk for CVD treated with one of 3 diets. A control group and two experimental arms that used a Mediterranean-style diets, differing only in the primary fat source: EVOO at 1 L/week or mixed nuts at 30 g/day. The treated groups showed a reduction in the TC:HDL-C ratio, at −0.38 (95% CI, −0.55 to −0.22) for those on the Mediterranean/EVOO diet and of −0.26 (95% CI, −0.42 to −0.10) for those on the Mediterranean/nuts diet. In addition, four inflammatory markers were significantly reduced in the EVOO group including HS-CRP, interleukin-6 (IL-6), intracellular adhesion molecule-1 (ICAM-1), and vascular cell adhesion molecule-1 (VCAM-1). All but the HS-CRP were reduced in the nut consumption group.[174,175]

The hunter–gatherer diet or Paleolithic diet[177–178] is considered close to human ancestral diet and consisted of a diet high in foliage, leafy vegetables, fruits, seeds, nuts, plant sterols, vegetable protein, fiber, omega-3 FAs, and lean animal protein that improves lipids and CVD risk.

SUMMARY OF NUTRITION, DYSLIPIDEMIA, AND CVD

Although many questions still exist regarding the optimal intake of fats, the types of fats, types and quality of protein, and the dietary intake of complex and refined carbohydrates, most studies clearly indicate that trans FAs and refined carbohydrates have an adverse effect on serum lipids and CV outcomes.[181] Some saturated fats may be adverse, others neutral, and some potentially beneficial. The MUFA and omega-3 FAs are consistently beneficial for dyslipidemia and CVD. The vegetarian diet with increased complex carbohydrates and fiber with lower dietary cholesterol is also beneficial. Protein intake of lean, wild and organic types of protein, and cold-water fish improves lipids and CHD risk factors.

SUMMARY AND CONCLUSIONS

The combination of a lipid-lowering diet and selected scientifically proven nutraceutical supplements have the ability to reduce LDL-C by up to 50%, increase LDL particle size, decrease LDL-P, lower TG and VLDL, and increase total and type 2 b HDL. In addition, inflammation, oxidative stress, and immune responses are decreased. Many surrogates for vascular target organ damage are improved, such as carotid IMT and plaque, aortic fatty streaks, CAC, plaque regression and morphology changes, endothelial function, vascular smooth muscle hypertrophy and elasticity, CABG and stent occlusion, and heart rate variability. Hard CV endpoints are also improved such as atherosclerosis, CVA, CVD, CHD, MI, abdominal aortic aneurysms, sudden death, and total mortality.

In several prospective clinical trials, CHD and CVD have been reduced with many of the nutraceutical supplements such as omega-3 FAs, RYR, ALA, and niacin. This nutritional and nutraceutical supplement treatment is a valid alternative for patients that are statin intolerant, cannot take other drugs for the treatment of dyslipidemia, or in those who prefer alternative treatments. This new approach to lipid management to decrease vascular disease utilizes a more functional medicine approach with a broader treatment program that addresses the multitude of steps involved in dyslipidemia-induced vascular damage (Tables 5.1 through 5.20).

TABLE 5.2
Inhibition of LDL Oxidation

Niacin
EGCG and catechins
Quercetin
Pantethine
Resveratrol
Red wine
Grape seed extract
MUFA
Curcumin
Pomegranate
Garlic
Sesame
Gamma/delta tocotrienols
Lycopene
Polyphenols
Flavonoids
Oleic acid
Glutathione
Citrus bergamia
Tangerine extract
Policosanol
RBO (Ferulic acid gammaoryzanol)
Coenzyme Q10
Vitamin E
Polyphenols and flavonoids

TABLE 5.3
Inhibition of LDL Glycation

Carnosine
Histidine
Myricetin
Kaempferol
Rutin
Morin
Pomegranate
Organosulfur compounds

TABLE 5.4

Lower Low-Density Lipoprotein

Niacin
RYR
Plant sterols
Sesame
Tocotrienols (gamma/delta)
Pantethine
GLA
Citrus bergamia
EGCG
Omega-3 FAs
Flax seed
MUFA
Aged garlic
Resveratrol
Curcumin
Soluble fiber
Krill oil (?)
Soy
Lycopene
Fiber

TABLE 5.5

Convert Dense LDL B to Large LDL A

Niacin
Omega-3 FAs
Plant Sterols

TABLE 5.6

Reduce Intestinal Cholesterol Absorption

Plant sterols
Soy
EGCG
Flax seeds
Sesame
Garlic
Fiber

TABLE 5.7
HMG CoA Reductase Inhibition

RYR
Pantethine
Gamma-delta/tocotrienols
Sesame
EGCG
Omega-3 FAs
Citrus bergamia
Garlic
Curcumin
GLA
Plant sterols
Lycopene
Soy

TABLE 5.8
Lower Lp(a)

Niacin
NAC
Gamma delta tocotrienols
Omega-3 FAs
Flax seed
CoQ 10
Vitamin C
L Carnitine
L-Lysine
L-Arginine
Almonds

TABLE 5.9
Lower Triglycerides

Niacin
RYR
Omega-3 FAs
Pantethine
Citrus bergamia
Flax seed
MUFA
Resveratrol

TABLE 5.10
Increase Total HDL and HDL 2 b Levels and Convert HDL 3 to HDL 2 and 2 b

Niacin
Omega-3 FAs
Pantethine
Red yeast rice
MUFA
Resveratrol
Curcumin
Pomegranate
Citrus bergamia

TABLE 5.11
Alter Scavenger Receptor NADPH Oxidase and oxLDL Uptake into Macrophages

Resveratrol
NAC (N-Acetyl cysteine)
Aged garlic

TABLE 5.12
Increase Reverse Cholesterol Transport

Lycopene
Niacin
Plant sterols
Glutathione
Resveratrol
Various flavonoids and anthocyanins
Alpha linolenic acid

TABLE 5.13
Decrease LDL Particle Number

Niacin
Omega-3 FAs

TABLE 5.14

Reduce Inflammation

Niacin
Omega-3 FAs
Flax seed
MUFA
Plant sterols
Guggulipids
Resveratrol
Glutathione
Quercetin
Curcumin
Aged garlic

TABLE 5.15

Lower APO B Lipoprotein

Niacin
Omega-3 FAs
Plant sterols
EGCG

TABLE 5.16

Increase APO-A1 Lipoprotein

Niacin

TABLE 5.17

Upregulate the LDL Receptor

EGCG
Sesame
Tocotrienols
Curcumin
Policosanol
Plant sterols

TABLE 5.18

Increase PON 1 and PON 2

EGCG
Quercetin
Pomegranate
Resveratrol
Glutathione

TABLE 5.19

Increase Bile Acid Excretion

Resveratrol
Citrus bergamia
Fiber
Probiotics
Plant sterols
Sesame

TABLE 5.20

Summary of Nutraceutical Supplement Recommended Doses for the Treatment of Dyslipidemia

Supplement	Daily Dose
Niacin: Vitamin B3	500–4000 mg in divided doses
Phytosterols	2.15 g
Soy (fermented)	30–50 g
EGCG	500–1000 mg
Omega-3 FAs	3000–5000 mg
Flax seed	40 g
Monounsaturated fats	20–40 g
Sesame	40 g
Gamma/delta tocotrienols	200 mg
Pantethine	900 mg in divided doses
Resveratrol (trans form)	250 mg
N-Acetyl cysteine	2000 mg in divided doses
Curcumin	2000–5000 mg in divided doses
Pomegranate juice	8 oz
Pomegranate seeds	1 cup
Citrus bergamia	1000 mg
Vitamin C	500 mg
Quercetin	500–1000 mg

REFERENCES

1. Kannel WB, Castelli WD, Gordon T et al. Serum cholesterol, lipoproteins and risk of coronary artery disease. The Framingham Study. *Ann Intern Med* 1971;74:1–12.
2. Houston MC. Nutrition and nutraceutical supplements in the treatment of hypertension. *Expert Rev Cardiovasc Ther* 2010;8:821–833.
3. Tian N, Penman AD, Mawson AR, Manning RD Jr., Flessner MF. Association between circulating specific leukocyte types and blood pressure: The atherosclerosis risk in communities (ARIC) study. *J Am Soc Hypertension* 2010;4(6):272–483.
4. Ungvari Z, Kaley G, de Cabo R, Sonntag WE, Csiszar A. Mechanisms of vascular aging: New Perspectives. *J Gerontol A Biol Sci Med Sci* 2010;65(10):1028–1041.
5. Houston MC, Fazio S, Chilton FH et al. Non pharmacologic treatment of dyslipidemia. *Prog Cardiovasc Dis* 2009;52:61–94.
6. Plourde M, Vohl MC, Vandal M, Couture P, Lemieux S, Cunnane SC. Plasma n-3 fatty acid supplement is modulated by apoE epsilon 4 but not by the common PPAR-alpha L162 polymorphism in men. *Br J Nutr* 2009;102:1121–1124.

7. Neiminen T, Kahonen M, Viiri LE, Gronroos P, Lehtimaki T. Pharmacogenetics of apolipropro-tein E gene during lipid-lowering therapy: Lipid levels and prevention of coronary heart disease. *Pharmacogenomics* 2008;9(10):1475–1486.

8. Shih DM, Lusis AJ. The Roles of PON 1 and PON 2 in cardiovascular disease and innate immunity. *Curr Opin Lipidol* 2009;20(4):288–292.

9. Calkin AC, Tontonoz P. Genome-wide association studies identify new targets in cardiovascular disease. *Sci Transl Med* 2010;2(48):48.

10. Djousse L, Caziano JM. Dietary cholesterol and coronary artery disease: A systematic review. *Curr Atheroscler Rep* 2009;11(6):418–422.

11. Werko L. End of the road for the diet-heart theory? *Scand Cardiovasc J* 2008;42(4):250–255.

12. Erkkila A, de Mello VD, Riserus U, Laaksonen DE. Dietary fatty acids and cardiovascular disease: An epidemiological approach. *Prog Lipid Res* 2008;47(3):172–187.

13. Weinberg SL. The diet-heart hypothesis: A critique. *J Am Coll Cardiol* 2004;43(5):731–733.

14. Mozaffarian D, Willet WC. Trans fatty acids and cardiovascular risk: A unique cardiometabolic imprint. *Curr Atheroscler Rep* 2007;9(6):486–493.

15. Chen CL, Tetri LH, Neuschwander-Tetri BA, Huang SS, Huang JS. A mechanism by which dietary trans fats cause atherosclerosis. *J Nutr Biochem* 2011;22:649–655.

16. Siri-Tarino PW, Sun Q, Hu FB, Krauss RM. Saturated fat, carbohydrate and cardiovascular disease. *Am J Clin Nutr* 2010;91(3):502–509.

17. Youssef-Elabd EM, McGee KC, Tripathi G et al. Acute and chronic saturated fatty acid treatment as a key instigator of the TLR-mediated inflammatory response in human adipose tissue, in vitro. *J Nutr Biochem* 2012;23(1):39–50.

18. Lubbers T, de Haan JJ, Hadfoune M et al. Chylomicron formation and glucagon-like peptide 1 receptor are involved inactivation of the nutritional anti-inflammatory pathway. *J Nutr Biochem* 2011;22(12):1105–1111.

19. Bruno RS. Postprandial hyperglycemia on vascular endothelial function: Mechanisms and consequences. *Nutr Res* 2012;32(10):727–740.

20. Mah E, Noh SK, Ballard KD, Matos ME, Volek JS, Bruno RS. Postprandial hyperglycemia impairs vascular endothelial function in healthy men by inducing lipid peroxidation and increasing asymmetric dimethylarginine:arginine. *J Nutr* 2011;141(11):1961–1968.

21. Ghanim H, Sia CL, Upadhyay M et al. Orange juice neutralizes the proinflammatory effect of a high-fat, high-carbohydrate meal and prevents endotoxin increase and toll-like receptor expression. *Am J Clin Nutr* 2010;91(4):940–949.

22. Dickinson KM, Clifton PM, Keogh JB. Endothelial function is impaired after a high-salt meal in healthy subjects. *Am J Clin Nutr* 2011;93(3):500–505.

23. Otvos JD, Mora S, Shalaurova I, Greenland P, Mackey RH, Goff DC Jr. Clinical implications of discordance between low density lipoprotein cholesterols and particle number. *J Clin Lipidol* 2011;5(2):105–113.

24. Hodge AM, Jenkins AJ, English DR, O'Dea K, Giles GG. NMR determined lipoprotein subclass profile is associated with dietary composition and body size. *Nutr Metab Cardiovasc Dis* 2011;21(8):603–609.

25. Prado KB, Shugg S, Backstrand JR. Low-density lipoprotein particle number predicts coronary artery calcification in asymptomatic adults at intermediate risk of cardiovascular disease. *J Clin Lipidol* 2011;5:408–413.

26. Maki KC, Bay HE, Dicklin MR, Johnson SL, Shabbout M. Effects of prescription omega-3-acid ethyl esters, coadministered with atorvastatin in circulating levels of lipoprotein particles, apoprotein CIII and lipoprotein-assoicated phospholipase A2 mass in men and women with mixed dyslipidemia. *J Clin Lipidol* 2011;4:485–492.

27. Asztalos BF, Tani M, Schaefer E. Metabolic and functional relevance of HDL subspecies. *Curr Opin Lipidol* 2011;22:176–185.

28. Khera AV, Cuchel M, de la Llera-Moya M et al. Cholesterol efflux capacity, high-density lipoprotein function, and atherosclerosis. *N Engl J Med* 2011;364:127–135.

29. Karakas M, Koenig W, Zierer A et al. Myeloperoxidase is associated with incident coronary heart disease independently of traditional risk factors: Results from the MONICA/KORA Augsburg study. *J Intern Med* 2011;271:43–50.

30. Onat A, Hergenç G. Low-grade inflammation, and dysfunction of high-density lipoprotein and its apoli-poproteins as a major driver of cardiometabolic risk. *Metabolism.* 2011;60(4):499–512.

31. Lamarche B, Tchernof A, Mooriani S et al. Small, dense low-density lipoprotein particles as a predictor of the risk of ischemic heart disease in men. Prospective results from the Quebec Cardiovascular Study. *Circulation* 1997;95(1):69–75.

32. Kruth HS. Receptor-independent fluid-phase pinocytosis mechanisms for induction of foam cell formation with native low density lipoprotein particles. *Curr Opin Lipidol* 2011;22(5):386–393.

33. Zhao ZW, Zhu XL, Luo YK, Lin CG, Chen LL. Circulating soluble lectin-like oxidized low-density lipoprotein redeptor-1 levels are associated with angiographic coronary lesion complexity in patients with coronary artery disease. *Clin Cardiol* 2011;34(3):172–177.

34. Ehara S, Ueda M, Naruko T et al. Elevated levels of oxidized low density lipoprotein show a positive relationship with the severity of acute coronary syndromes. *Circulation* 2001;103(15):1955–1960.

35. Hansson GK. Inflammation, atherosclerosis, and coronary artery disease. *N Engl J Med* 2005;352(16):1685–1695.

36. Harper CR, Jacobson TA. Using apolipoprotein B to manage dyslipidemic patients: Time for a change? *Mayo Clin Proc* 2010;85(5):440–445.

37. Curtiss LK. Reversing atherosclerosis? *N Engl J Med* 2009;360(11):1144–1146.

38. Shen GX. Impact and mechanism for oxidized and glycated lipoproteins on generation of fibrinolytic regulators from vascular endothelial cells. *Mol Cell Biochem* 2003;246(1–2):69–74.

39. Ridker PM, Danielson E, Fonseca FA et al. Rosuvastatin to prevent vascular events in men and women with elevated C-reactive protein. *N Engl J Med* 2008;359(21):2195–2207.

40. Krishnan GM, Thompson PD. The effects of statins on skeletal muscle strength and exercise performance. *Curr Opin Lipidol* 2010;21(4):324–328.

41. Mills EJ, Wu P, Chong G et al. Efficacy and safety of statin treatment for cardiovascular disease: A network meta-analysis of 170,255 patients from 76 randomized trials. *QJM* 2011;104(2):109–124.

42. Mammen AL, Amato AA. Statin myopathy: A review of recent progress. *Curr Opin Rheumatol* 2010;22(6):544–550.

43. Russo MW, Scobev M, Bonkovsky HL. Drug-induced liver injury associated with statins. *Semin Liver Dis* 2009;29(4):412–422.

44. Preiss D, Sattar N. Statins and the risk of new-onset diabetes: A review of recent evidence. *Curr Opin Lipidol* 2011;22:460–468.

45. Moosmann B, Behl C. Selenoproteins, cholesterol-lowering durgs, and the consequences: Revisiting of the mevalonate pathway. *Trends cardiovasc Med* 2004;14(7):273–281.

46. Liu CS, Lii CK, Chang LL et al. Atorvastatin increases blood ratios of vitamin E/low-density lipoprotein cholesterol and coenzyme Q10/low-density lipoprotein cholesterol in hypercholesterolemic patients. *Nutr Res* 2010;30(2):118–124.

47. Wyman M, Leonard M, Morledge T. Coenzyme Q10: A therapy for hypertension and statin-induced myalgia? *Clev Clin J Med* 2010;77(7):435–442.

48. Mortensen SA. Low coenzyme Q levels and the outcome of statin Treatment in heart failure. *J Am Coll Cardiol* 2011;57(14):1569.

49. Shojaei M, Djalali M, Khatami M, Siassi F, Eshraghian M. Effects of carnitine and coenzyme Q10 on lipid profile and serum levels of lipoprotein (a) in maintenance hemodialysis patients on statin therapy. *Iran J Kidney Dis* 2011;5(20):114–118.

50. Gupta A, Thompson PD. The relationship of vitamin D deficiency to statin myopathy. *Atherosclerosis* 2011;215(1):23–29.

51. Avis HJ, Hargreaves IP, Ruiter JP, Land JM, Wanders RJ, Wijburg FA. Rosuvastatin lowers coenzyme Q10 levels, but not mitochondrial adenosine triphosphate synthesis, in children with familial hypercholesterolemia. *J Pediatr* 2011;158(3):458–462.

52. Kiernan TJ, Rochford M, McDermott JH. Simvastatin induced rhapdomyloysis and an important clinical link with hypothyroidism. *Int J Cardiol* 2007;119(3):374–376.

53. Houston M. The role of nutraceutical supplements in the treatment of dyslipidemia. *J Clin Hypertens* (Greenwich) 2012;14(2):121–132.

54. Nijjar PS, Burke FM, Bioesch A, Rader DJ. Role of dietary supplements in lowering low-density lipoprotein cholesterol: A review. *J Clin Lipidol* 2010;4:248–258.

55. Houston MC. Juice powder concentrate and systemic blood pressure, progression of coronary artery calcium and antioxidant status in hypertensive subjects: A Pilot Study. *Evid Based Complementary Alternat Med* 2007;4(4):455–462.

56. Budoff MJ, Ahmadi N, Gul KM et al. Aged garlic extract supplemented with B vitamins, folic acid and L-arginine retards progression of subclinical atherosclerosis: A randomized clinical trial. *Prev Med.* 2009;49(2–3):101–107.

57. Hcohholzer W, Berg DD, Giugliano RP. The facts behind niacin. *Ther Adv Cardiovasc Dis* 2011;5(5):227–2240.
58. Otvos JD. The surprising AIM-HIGH results are not surprising when viewed through a particle lens. *J Clin Lipidol* 2011;5(5):368–370.
59. Ruparelia N, Digby JE, Choudhury RP. Effects of niacin on atherosclerosis and vascular function. *Curr Opin Cardiol* 2011;26(1):66–70.
60. Al-Mohissen MA, Pun SC, Frohlich JJ. Niacin: From mechanisms of action to therapeutic uses. *Mini Rev Med Chem* 2010;10(3):204–217.
61. Philpott AC, Hubacek J, Sun YC, Hillard D, Anderson TJ. Niacin improves lipid profile but not endothelial function in patients with coronary artery disease on high dose statin therapy. *Atherosclerosis* 2013;226(2):453–458.
62. The Coronary Drug Project Group. Clofibrate and niacin in coronary heart disease. *JAMA* 1975;231:360–381.
63. Taylor AJ, Lee HJ, Sullenberger LE. The effect of 24 months of combination statin and extended release niacin on carotid intima-media thickness: ARBITER 3. *Curr Med Res Opin* 2006;22(11):2243–2250.
64. Lee JM, Robson MD, Yu LM et al. Effects of high dose modified release nicotinic acid on atherosclerosis and vascular function: A randomized, placebo controlled, magnetic resonance imaging study. *J Am Coll Cardiol* 2009;54(19):1787–1794.
65. Taylor AJ, Villines TC, Stanek EJ et al. Extended release niacin or ezetimibe and carotid intima media thickness. *N Engl J Med* 2009;361(22):2113–2122.
66. AIM HIGH Investigators. The role of niacin in raising high density lipoprotein cholesterols to reduce cardiovascular events in patients with atherosclerotic cardiovascular disease and optimally treated low density lipoprotein cholesterol: Baseline characteristics of study participants. The Atherothrombosis Intervention in Metabolic syndrome with low HDL/high triglycerides: Impact on global health outcomes (AIM-HIGH) trial. *Am Heart J* 2011;161(3):538–543.
67. The AIM–HIGH Investigators. Niacin in patients with low HDL cholesterol levels receiving intensive statin therapy. *N Engl J Med* 2011;365:2255–2267.
68. Gouni-Bertold I, Berthold HK. The role of niacin in lipid-lowering treatment: Are we aiming too high? *Curr Pharm Des* 2013;19(17):3094–3106.
69. Jancin B. Once a rising star of CV prevention, boosting HDL cholesterol falls to earth. *Internal Med News* 2013;46(2):1 and 33.
70. Keenan JM. Wax-matrix extended-release niacin vs inositol hexanicotinate: A comparison of wax-matrix, extended-release niacin to inositol hexanicotinate "no-flush" niacin in persons with mild to moderate dyslipidemia. *J Clin Lipidol* 2013;7(1):14–23.
71. Berthold HK, Unverdorben S, Degenhardt R, Bulitta M, Gourni Berthold I. Effect of policosanol on lipid levels among patients with hypercholesterolemia or combined hyperlipidemia: A randomized controlled trial. *JAMA* 2006;295(19):2262–2269.
72. Greyling A, De Witt C, Oosthuizen W, Jerling JC. Effects of a policosanol supplement on serum lipid concentrations in hypercholesterolemic and heterozygous familial hypercholesterolaemic subjects. *Br J Nutr* 2006;95(5):968–975.
73. Liu J, Zhang J, Shi Y, Grimsgaard S, Alraek T, Fonnebo V. Chinese red yeast rice (*Monascus purpureus*) for primary hyperlipidemia: A meta-analysis of randomized controlled trials. *Chin Med* 2006;1:4.
74. Wang JA, Xie X, Wang Y et al. Chinese red yeast rice attenuates the development of angiotensin II-induced abdominal aortic aneurysm and atherosclerosis. *Nutr Biochem* 2012;23(6):549–556.
75. Lu Z, Kou W, Du B et al. Effect of Xuezhikang, an extract from red yeast Chinese rice, on coronary events in a Chinese population with previous myocardial infarction. *Am J Cardiol* 2008;101(12):1689–1693.
76. Patch CS, Tapsell LC, Williams PG, Gordon M. Plant sterols as dietary adjuvants in the reduction of cardiovascular risk: Theory and evidence. *Vasc Health Risk Manag* 2006;2(2):157–162.
77. Demonty I, Ras RT, van der Knaap HC et al. Continuous dose response relationship of the LDL cholesterol lowering effect of phytosterol intake. *J Nutr* 2009;139(2):271–284.
78. Othman RA, Moghadasian MH. Beyond cholesterol lowering effects of plant sterols: Clinical and experimental evidence of anti-inflammatory properties. *Nutr Rev* 2011;69(7):371–382.
79. Sabeva NS, McPhaul CM, Li X, Cory TJ, Feola DJ, Graf GA. Phytosterols differently influence ABC transporter expression, cholesterol efflux and inflammatory cytokine Secretion in macrophage foam cells. *J Nutr Biochem* 2011;22:777–783.
80. Sacks FM, Lichtenstein A, Van Horn L et al. Soy protein, isoflavones, and cardiovascular health: An American Heart Association Science Advisory for professionals from the Nutrition Committee. *Circulation* 2006;113(7):1034–1044.

81. Harland JI, Haffner TA. Systemic review, meta-analysis and regression of randomized controlled tri-
    als reporting an association between an intake of circa 25g soya protein per day and blood cholesterol.
    Atherosclerosis 2008;200(1):13–27.
82. Singh DK, Banerjee S, Porter TD. Green and black tea extracts inhibit HMG-CoA reductase and activate
    AMP kinase to decrease cholesterol synthesis in hepatoma cells. *J Nutr Biochem* 2009;20(10):816–822.
83. Tinahones FJ, Rubio MA, Garrido-Sanchez L et al. Green tea reduces LDL oxidability and improves
    vascular function. *J Am Coll Nutr* 2008;27(2):209–213.
84. Brown AL, Lane J, Holyoak C, Nicol B, Mayes AE, Dadd T. Health effects of green tea catechins in
    overweight and obese men: A randomized controlled cross-over trial. *Br J Nut* 2011;7:1–10.
85. Zheng Y, Morris A, Sunkara M, Layne J, Toborek M, Hennig BJ. Epigallocatechin-gallate stimu-
    lates NF-E2-related factor and hemeoxygenase-1 viacaveolin-1 displacement. *Nutr Biochem* 2012;23
    (2):163–168.
86. Zheng XX, Xu YL, Li SH, Liu XX, Hui R, Huang XH. Green tea intake lowers fasting serum total
    and LDL cholesterol in adults: A meta-analysis of 14 randomized controlled trials. *Am J Clin Nutr*
    2011;94:601–610.
87. Saremi A, Arora R. The utility of omega-3 fatty acids in cardiovascular disease. *Am J Ther*
    2009;16(5):421–436.
88. Rissanen T, Voutilainen S, Nyyssonen K, Lakka TA, Salonen JT. Fish oil-derived fatty acids, docosa-
    hexaenoic acid and docosapentaenoic acid and the risk of acute coronary events: The Kuopio ischaemic
    heart disease risk factor study. *Circulation* 2000;102(22):2677–2679.
89. Davis W, Rockway S, Kwasny M. Effect of a combined therapeutic approach of intensive lipid manage-
    ment, omega 3 fatty acid supplementation, and increased serum 25(OH) D on coronary calcium scores in
    asymptomatic adults. *Am J Ther* 2009;16(4):326–332.
90. Yokoyama M, Origasa H, Matsuzaki M et al. Japan EPA lipid intervention study (JELIS) Investigators.
    Lancet 2007;369(9567):1090–1098.
91. Ryan AS, Keske MA, Hoffman JP, Nelson EB. Clinical overview of algal-docosahexaenoic acid: Effects
    on triglyceride levels and other cardiovascular risk factors. *Am J Ther* 2009;16(2):183–192.
92. Kelley DS, Siegal D, Vemuri M, Chung GH, Mackey BE. Docosahexaenoic acid supplementation
    decreases remnant-like particle cholesterol and increases the (n-3) index in hypertriglyceridemic men.
    J Nutr 2008;138(1):30–35.
93. Maki KC, Dicklin MR, Davidson MH, Doyle RT, Ballantyne CM. COMBination of prescription omega-3
    with Simvastatin (COMBOS) Investigators. *Am J Cardiol* 2010;105(10):1409–1412.
94. Micallef MA, Garg ML. The lipid-lowering effects of phytosterols and (n-3) polyunsatu-
    rated fatty acids are synergistic and complementary in hyperlipidemic men and women. *J Nutr*
    2008;138(6):1085–1090.
95. Mori TA, Burke V, Puddey IB et al. Purified eicosapentaenoic and docosahexaenoic acids have differen-
    tial effects on serum lipids and lipoproteins, LDL particle size, glucose and insulin in mildly hyperlipid-
    emic men. *Am J Clin Nutr* 2000;71(5):1085–1094.
96. Pauwels EK, Kostkiewicz M. Fatty acid facts, Part III: Cardiovascular disease, or, a fish diet is not fishy.
    Drug News Perspect 2008 Dec;21(10):552–61.
97. Bunea R, ElFarrah K, Deutsch L. Evaluation of the effects of Neptune Krill Oil on the clinical course of
    hyperlipidemia. *Altern Med Rev* 2004;9(4):420–428.
98. Prasad K. Flaxseed and cardiovascular health. *J Cardiovasc Pharmacol* 2009;54(5):369–377.
99. Bioedon LT, Balkai S, Chittams J et al. Flaxseed and cardiovascular risk factors: Results from a double-
    blind, randomized controlled clinical trial. *J Am Coll Nutr* 2008;27(1):65–74.
100. Mandasescu S, Mocanu V, Dascalita AM et al. Flaxseed supplementation in hyperlipidemic patients. *Rev
     Med Chir Soc Med Nat Iasi* 2005;109(3):502–506.
101. Poudyal H, Panchal SK, Waanders J, Ward L, Brown L. Lipid redistribution by α-linolenic acid-rich chia
     seed inhibits stearoyl-CoA desaturase-1 and induces cardiac and hepatic protection in diet-induced obese
     rats. *J Nutr Biochem* 2012;23(2):153–162.
102. Zhang J, Kris-Etherton PM, Thompson JT, Hannon DB, Gillies PJ, Heuvel JP. Alpha-linolenic acid
     increases cholesterol efflux in macrophage-derived foam cells by decreasing stearoyl CoA desatu-
     rase 1 expression: Evidence for a farnesoid-X-receptor mechanism of action. *J Nutr Biochem*
     2012;23(4):400–409.
103. Bester D, Esterhuyse AJ, Truter EJ, van Rooven J. Cardiovascular effects of edible oils: A comparison
     between four popular edible oils. *Nutr Res Rev* 2010;23(2):334–348.
104. Brown JM, Shelness GS, Rudel LL. Monounsaturated fatty acids and atherosclerosis: Opposing views
     from epidemiology and experimental animal models. *Curr Atherosclero Rep* 2007;9(6):494–500.

105. Bogani P, Gali C, Villa M, Visioli F. Postprandial anti-inflammatory and antioxidant effects of extra virgin olive oil. *Atherosclerosis* 2007;190(1):181–186.
106. Covas MI. Olive oil and the cardiovascular system. *Pharmacol Res* 2007;(55(3):175–186.
107. Castañer O, Covas MI, Khymenets O et al. Protection of LDL from oxidation by olive oil polyphenols is associated with a downregulation of CD40-ligand expression and its downstream products in vivo in humans. *Am J Clin Nutr* 2012;95(5):1238–1244.
108. Wu WH, Kang YP, Wang NH, Jou HJ, Want TA. Sesame ingestion affects sex hormones, antioxidant status and blood lipids in postmenopausal women. *J Nutr* 2006;136(5):1270–1275.
109. Namiki M. Nutraceutical functions of sesame: A review. *Crit Rev food Sci Nutr* 2007;47(7):651–73.
110. Qureshi AA, Sami SA, Salser WA, Khan FA. Synergistic effect of tocotrienol-rich fraction (TRF 25) of rice bran and lovastatin on lipid parameters in hypercholesterolemic humans. *J Nutr Biochem* 2001;12(6):318–329.
111. Song BL, DeBose-Boyd RA. Insig-dependent ubiquitination and degradation of 3-hydroxy-3 methylglutaryl coenzyme a reductase stimulated by delta-and gamma-tocotrienols. *J Biol Chem* 2006;281(35):54–61.
112. Prasad K. Tocotrienols and cardiovascular health. *Curr Pharm Des* 2011;17(21):2147–2154.
113. McRae MP. Treatment of hyperlipoproteinemia with pantethine: A review and analysis of efficacy and tolerability. *Nutr Res* 2005;25:319–333.
114. Kelly G. Pantethine: A review of its biochemistry and therapeutic applications. *Altern Med Rev* 1997;2:365–377.
115. Horvath Z, Vecsei L. Current medical aspects of pantethine. *Ideggyogy Sz* 2009;62(7–8):220–229.
116. Pins LL, Keenan JM. Dietary and nutraceutical options for managing the hypertriglyceridemic patient. *Prog Cardiovasc Nurs* 2006;21(2):89–93.
117. No Authors listed. Pantethine monograph. *Altern Med Rev* 2010;15(3):279–282.
118. Rumberger JA, Napolitano J, Azumano I, Kamiya T, Evans M. Pantethine, a derivative of vitamin B (5) used as a nutritional supplement, favorably alters low-density lipoprotein cholesterol metabolism in low- to moderate-cardiovascular risk North American subjects: A triple-blinded placebo and diet-controlled investigation. *Nutr Res* 2011;31(8):608–615.
119. Szapary PO, Wolfe ML, BLoedon LT et al. Guggulipid for the treatment of hypercholesterolemia: A randomized controlled trial. *JAMA* 2003;290(6):765–772.
120. Ulbricht C, Basch E, Szapary P et al. Guggul for hyperlipidemia: A review by the Natural Standard Research Collaboration. *Complement Ther Med* 2005;13(4):279–290.
121. Nohr LA, Rasmussen LB, Straand J. Resin from the Mukul Myrrh tree, guggul, can it be used for treating hypercholesterolemia: A randomized, controlled study. *Complement Ther Med* 2009;17(1):16–22.
122. Gardner CD, Lawson LD, Block E et al. Effect of raw garlic vs commercial garlic supplements on plasma lipid concentration in adults with moderate hypercholesterolemia: A randomized clinical trial. *Arch Intern Med* 2007;167(4):346–353.
123. Rai SK, Sharma M, Tiwari M. Inhibitory effect of novel diallyldisulfide analogs on HMG-CoA reductase expression in hypercholesterolemic rats: CREB as a potential upstream target. *LifeSci* 2009;85(5–6):211–219.
124. Ahmadi N, Tsimikas S, Hajsadeghi F et al. Relation of oxidative biomarkers, vascular dysfunction, and progression of coronary artery calcium. *Am J Cardiol* 2010;105(4):459–466.
125. Zeb I, Ahmadi N, Nasir K et al. Aged garlic extract and coenzyme Q10 have favorable effect on inflammatory markers and coronary atherosclerosis progression: A randomized clinical trial. *J Cardiovasc Dis Res*. 2012;3(3):185–190.
126. Larijani VN, Ahmadi N, Zeb I, Khan F, Flores F, Budoff M. Beneficial effects of aged garlic extract and coenzyme Q10 on vascular elasticity and endothelial function: The FAITH randomized clinical trial. *Nutrition* 2013;29(1):71–75.
127. Curtiss LK. Reversing atherosclerosis? *N Engl J Med* 2009;360(11):1144–1146.
128. Smoliga JM, Baur JA, Hausenblas HA. Resveratrol and health: A comprehensive review of human clinical trial. *Mol Nutr Food Res* 2011;55(8):1129–1141.
129. Soni KB, Kuttan R. Effect of oral curcumin administration on serum peroxides and cholesterol levels in human volunteers. *Indian J Physiol Pharmacol* 1992;36(4):273–275.
130. Coban D, Milenkovic D, Chanet A et al. Dietary curcumin inhibits atherosclerosis by affecting the expression of genes involved in leukocyte adhesion and transendothelial migration. *Mol Nutr Food Res* 2012;56(8):1270–1281.
131. Aviram M. Atherosclerosis: Cell biology and lipoproteins—oxidative stress and paraoxonases regulate atherogenesis. *Curr Opin Lipidol* 2010;21(2):163–164.

132. Fuhrman B, Volkova N, Aviram M. Pomegranate juice polyphenols increase recombinant paroxonase-1 binding to high density lipoprotein: Studies in vitro and in diabetic patients. *Nutrition* 2010;26(4): 359–366.

133. Avairam M, Rosenblat M, Gaitine D et al. Pomegranate juice consumption for 3 years by patients with carotid artery stenosis reduces common carotid intima-media thickness, blood pressure and LDL oxidation. *Clin Nutr* 2004;23(3):423–433.

134. Mattiello T, Trifiro E, Jotti GS, Pulcinelli FM. Effects of pomegranate juice and extract polypyenols on platelet function. *J Med Food* 2009;12(2):334–339.

135. Aviram M, Dornfeld L, Rosenblat M et al. Pomegranate juice consumption reduces oxidative stress, atherogenic modifications to LDL, and platelet aggregation: Studies in humans and in atherosclerotic apolipoprotein E-deficient mice. *Am J Clin Nutr* 2000;71(5):1062–1076.

136. Davidson MH, Maki KC, Dicklin MR et al. Effects of consumption of pomegranate juice on carotid intima-media thickness in men and women at moderate risk for coronary heart disease. *Am J Cardiol* 2009;104(7):936–942.

137. Di Donna L, De Luca G, Mazzotti F et al. Statin-like principles of bergamot fruit (Citrus bergamia): Isolation of 3 hydroxymethylglutaryl flavonoid glycosides. *J Nat Prod* 2009;72(7):1352–1354.

138. Leopoldini M, Malaj N, Toscano M, Sindona G, Russo N. On the inhibitor effects of bergamot juice flavonoids binding to the 3-hydroxy-3-methylglutaryl-CoA reductase (HMGR) enzyme. *J Agric Food Chem* 2010;58(19):10768–10773.

139. Mollace V, Sacco I, Janda E et al. Hypolipidemic and hypoglycaemic activity of bergamot polyphenols: from animal models to human studies. *Fitotherapia* 2011;82(3):309–316.

140. McRae MP. Vitamin C supplementation lowers serum low-density cholesterol and triglycerides: A meta-analysis of 13 randomized controlled trials. *J Chiropr Med* 2008;7(2):48–58.

141. McRae MP. The efficacy of vitamin C supplementation on reducing total serum cholesterol in human subjects: A review of 51 experimental trials. *J Chiropr Med* 2006;5(1):2–12.

142. Palozza P, Simone R, Gatalano A, Parrone N, Monego G, Ranelletti F. Lycopene regulation of cholesterol synthesis and efflux in human macrophages. *J Nutr Biochem* 2011;22:971–978.

143. Yang CM, Lu IH, Chen HY, Hu ML. Lycopene inhibits the proliferation of androgen-dependent human prostate tumor cells through activation of PPAR-gamma-LXR alpha and ABCA1 pathway. *J Nutr Biochem* 2012;23:8–17.

144. McEneny J, Wade L, Young IS et al. Lycopene intervention reduces inflammation and improves HDL functionality in moderately overweight middle-aged individuals. *J Nutr Biochem* 2013;24(1):163–168.

145. Riccioni G, Scotti L, DiIlio E et al. Lycopene and preclinical carotid atherosclerosis. *J Biol Regul Homeost Agents* 2011;25(3):435–441.

146. Lewis SJ, Burmeister S. A double-blind placebo-controlled study of the effects of *Lactobacillus acidophilus* on plasma lipids. *Eur J Clin Nutr* 2005 Jun;59(6):776–80.

147. Greany KA, Nettleton JA, Wangen KE, Thomas W, Kurzer MS. Probiotic consumption does not enhance the cholesterol-lowering effect of soy in postmenopausal women. *J Nutr* 2004;134(12):3277–3283.

148. Kong WJ, Wei J, Zuo ZY et al. Combination of simvastatin with berberine improves the lipid-lowering efficacy. *Metabolism* 2008;57(8):1029–1037.

149. Kong W, Wei J, Abidi P et al. Berberine is a novel cholesterol-lowering drug working through a unique mechanism distinct from statins. *Nat Med* 2004;10(12):1344–1351.

150. Pisciotta L, Bellocchio A, Bertolini S. Nutraceutical pill containing berberine versus ezetimibe on plasma lipid pattern in hypercholesterolemic subjects and its additive effect in patients with familial hypercholesterolemia on stable cholesterol-lowering treatment. *Lipids Health Dis* 2012;11:123.

151. Houston M, Sparks W. Effect of combination pantethine, plant sterols, green tea extract, delta-tocotrienol and phytolens on lipid profiles in patients with hyperlipidemia. *JANA* 2010;13(1):15–20.

152. Studer M, Briel M, Leimenstoll B, Glass TR, Bucher HC. Effect of different anti-lipidemic agents and diets on mortality: A systemic review. *Arch Int Med* 2005;165(7):725–730.

153. Lee IT, Lee WJ, Tsai CM, Su IJ, Yen HT, Sheu WH. Combined extractives of red yeast rice, bitter gourd, chorlella, soy protein and licorice improve total cholesterol, low-density lipoprotein cholesterol and triglyceride in subjects with metabolic syndrome. *Nutr Res* 2012;32:85–92.

154. Dawber TR, Meadors GF, Moore, FE. Epidemiological approaches to heart disease: the Framingham Study. *Am J Public Health* 1951;41:279–286.

155. Appel LJ, Sacks FM, Carey VJ et al. Effects of protein, monounsaturated fat, and carbohydrate intake on blood pressure and serum lipids: Results of the Omni Heart randomized trial. *JAMA* 2005;294:2455–64.

156. Keys A. Coronary heart disease in seven countries. *Circulation*. 1970;41(suppl 1):1–21.
157. Keys A, Menotti A, Karvonen MJ et al. The diet and 15-year death rate in the Seven Countries Study. *Am J Epidemiol* 1986;124:903–915.
158. Pritikin N. Dietary factors and hyperlipidemia. *Diabetes Care* 1982;5:647–648.
159. Pritikin N. The Pritikin diet. *JAMA*. 1984;251:1160–1161.
160. Barnard RJ, Lattimor eL, Holly RG, Cherny S, Pritikin N. Response of non-insulin-dependent diabetic patients to an intensive program of diet and exercise. *Diabetes Care* 1982;5:370–374.
161. Ornish D, Brown SE, Scherwitz LW et al. Can lifestyle changes reverse coronary heart disease? The Lifestyle Heart Trial. *Lancet* 1990;336:129–133.
162. Ornish D, Magbanua MJ, Weidner G et al. Changes in prostate gene expression in men undergoing an intensive nutrition and lifestyle intervention. *Proc Natl Acad Sci U S A* 2008;105:8369–8374.
163. Ornish D, Scherwitz LW, Billings JH et al. Intensive lifestyle changes for reversal of coronary heart disease. *JAMA* 1998;280:2001–2007. Erratum in: *JAMA* 1999;281:1380.
164. Ornish D, Scherwitz LW, Doody RS et al. Effects of stress management training and dietary changes in treating ischemic heart disease. *JAMA* 1983;249:54–59.
165. Jenkins DJ, Kendall CW, Marchie A et al. Effects of a dietary portfolio of cholesterol-lowering foods vs lovastatin on serum lipids and C-reactive protein. *JAMA*. 2003;290:502–510.
166. Jenkins DJ, Kendall CW, Faulkner DA et al. Assessment of the longer-term effects of a dietary portfolio of cholesterol-lowering foods in hypercholesterolemia. *Am J Clin Nutr* 2006;83:582–591.
167. Jenkins DJ, Chiavaroli L, Wong JM et al. Adding monounsaturated fatty acids to a dietary portfolio of cholesterol-lowering foods in hypercholesterolemia. *CMAJ* 2010;182:1961–1967.
168. Jenkins DJ, Jones PJ, Lamarche B et al. Effect of a dietary portfolio of cholesterol-lowering foods given at 2 levels of intensity of dietary advice on serum lipids in hyperlipidemia: A randomized controlled trial. *JAMA* 2011;306:831–839.
169. Kris-Etherton P, Eckel RH, Howard BV, St Jeor S, Bazzarre TL; Nutrition Committee Population Science Committee and Clinical Science Committee of the American Heart Association. AHA Science Advisory: Lyon Diet Heart Study. Benefits of a Mediterranean-style, National Cholesterol Education Program/American Heart Association Step I Dietary Pattern on Cardiovascular Disease. *Circulation* 2001;103:1823–1825.
170. de Lorgeril M, Renaud S, Mamelle N et al. Mediterranean alpha-linolenic acid-rich diet in secondary prevention of coronary heart disease. *Lancet* 1994;343:1454–1459. Erratum in: *Lancet* 1995;345:738.
171. de Lorgeril M, Salen P. The Mediterranean diet: Rationale and evidence for its benefit. *Curr Atheroscler Rep* 2008;10:518–522.
172. de Lorgeril M, Salen P, Martin JL, Monjaud I, Delaye J, Mamelle N. Mediterranean diet, traditional risk factors, and the rate of cardiovascular complications after myocardial infarction: Final report of the Lyon Diet Heart Study. *Circulation* 1999;99:779–785.
173. Rastogi T, Reddy KS, Vaz M et al. Diet and risk of ischemic heart disease in India. *Am J Clin Nutr* 2004;79:582–592.
174. Estruch R, Martínez-González MA, Corella D et al. Effects of a Mediterranean-style diet on cardiovascular risk factors: A randomized trial. *Ann Intern Med* 2006;145:1–11.
175. Salas-Salvadó J, Garcia-Arellano A, Estruch R et al. Components of the Mediterranean-type food pattern and serum inflammatory markers among patients at high risk for cardiovascular disease. *Eur J Clin Nutr* 2008;62:651–659.
176. Estruch R, Ros E, Salas-Salvadó J et al. Primary prevention of cardiovascular disease with a Mediterranean Diet. *N Engl J Med* 2013;368:1279–1290.
177. Konner M, Eaton SB. Paleolithic nutrition: Twenty-five years later. *Nutr Clin Pract* 2010;25:594–602.
178. Eaton SB, Konner MJ, Cordain L. Diet-dependent acid load, Paleolithic [corrected] nutrition, and evolutionary health promotion. *Am J Clin Nutr* 2010;91:295–297. Erratum in: *Am J Clin Nutr* 2010;91:1072.
179. O'Keefe JH Jr, Cordain L. Cardiovascular disease resulting from a diet and lifestyle at odds with our Paleolithic genome: How to become a 21st-century hunter-gatherer. *Mayo Clin Proc* 2004;79:101–108.
180. Jew S, AbuMweis SS, Jones PJ. Evolution of the human diet: linking our ancestral diet to modern functional foods as a means of chronic disease prevention. *J Med Food* 2009;12:925–934.
181. Van Horn L, McCoin M, Kris-Etherton PM et al. The evidence for dietary prevention and treatment of cardiovascular disease. *J Am Diet Assoc* 2008;108:287–331.

6 Healing the Heart with Whole Foods and Food Bioactives

Deanna Minich and Benjamin Brown

CONTENTS

INTRODUCTION: WHY FOODS FOR CARDIOVASCULAR HEALTH?

To our benefit, the well-recognized global health concern that is cardiovascular disease (CVD) seems to have an accessible, effective solution—food. The component nutrients of what we eat can be an effective strategy against the CVD morbidity and mortality that affects both men and women across a variety of ethnic groups. Over the past decades, increasing numbers of epidemiological studies have demonstrated an association between dietary patterns and the risk of CVD. Solidifying these population findings are prospective clinical trials that have investigated the influence of dietary interventions on cardiovascular endpoints, with the overall findings indicating beneficial effects on two major modifiable CVD risk factors, hypertension and elevated low-density lipoprotein (LDL) cholesterol, as well as reduced inflammatory markers. In addition, current research indicates the risk of developing CVD increases twofold with diabetes, a condition linked to obesity and commonly addressed through nutritional modifications. These findings have uncovered a more direct role of glucose dysregulation on vascular health.[1,2] As a result, dietary recommendations have been purported as a means to prevent and treat CVD by opinion leader organizations and cardiologists in clinical practice.

Although it is beneficial to have knowledge about healthful dietary patterns and the whole foods they are composed of from a cardiovascular perspective, it is imperative to apply these findings within the context of a personalized approach to the individual beyond the traditional nutritional recommendations established according to age, gender, ethnicity, and pregnancy. Indeed, the degree to which a person may respond to the influence of food on their cardiovascular risk factors is related to a large degree on their genetics and corresponding epigenetics. Studies over the past two decades have revealed associations between gene polymorphisms, foods/nutrients, and risk factors for chronic disease. More rigorous research is required to delineate how cohorts of patients with gene variants and subsequent propensity toward CVD respond to an intervention with select foods and food components. Preliminary discussion on personalized nutrition for CVD is establishing a foothold as the scientific literature continues to indicate the following examples of where this type of approach would be warranted: (1) only about 25% of individuals with hypercholesterolemia respond to dietary cholesterol limitation; (2) various degrees of salt sensitivity exist in individuals with hypertension; (3) apolipoprotein E (APOE) genotype heterogeneity may result in differential lipid responses to the long-chain omega-3 fatty acids, eicosapentaenoic acid (EPA) and docosahexaenoic acid (DHA)[3]; (4) genotypes at angiotensinogen, β_2-adrenergic receptor, and kallikrein single nucleotide polymorphisms (SNPs) directly impact the effects of blood pressure–lowering diets such as Dietary Approaches to Stop Hypertension (DASH).[4]

Furthermore, lifestyle and behaviors beyond nutrients need to be taken into account. As we know from the INTERHEART study,[5] there are nine potentially modifiable risk factors, including lifestyle aspects (e.g., exercise, fruit and vegetable intake, smoking, and alcohol) that account for over 90% of the risk of an initial acute myocardial infarction. Therefore, accounting for a comprehensive, individualized approach based on lifestyle medicine for the individual with CVD is consistent with where nutrition science is headed in the twenty-first century.

In this chapter, an overview of the recent science on whole foods, whole food patterns, and food constituents as they relate to CVD will be discussed, with a focus on nutrigenomic and epigenetic influences whenever available. Nutrigenomic and epigenetic influences relate to how nutrients can modify gene expression, either directly or through changes in the DNA conformation.

HEART-HEALTHY DIETARY PATTERNS

Individual food components have for a long time been the primary focus of nutritional science, policy and recommendations; however, it is becoming better appreciated that people eat food, not nutrients, and that these foods are eaten in complex dietary patterns.[6] Placing foods in the context of a dietary pattern has two major advantages. Firstly, food components work synergistically to influence health outcomes and foods, and their components may have additive or more than additive effects.[7] Thus, "food synergy" can act as an operational framework for understanding how complex dietary patterns may confer unique health effects beyond individual dietary components.[8] Secondly, a food-focused, as opposed to nutrient-focused, approach is far more practical in a clinical setting. For example, advising a patient to adopt healthful foods (e.g., olive oil), rather than the foods individual components (monounsaturated fatty acids) is far more pragmatic when facilitating dietary change.[9]

A number of dietary patterns and their relationship to cardiovascular health have been investigated including traditional diets such as those of Mediterranean and Japanese cultures, or even the combination of those two (MediterrAsian), as well as "prudent" or healthy dietary patterns and "western" or unhealthy dietary patterns. Although the characteristics and definitions of these dietary patterns vary, there are shared commonalities. In general, diets that feature plant-based foods (nuts, seeds, whole grains, legumes, fruits, vegetables, herbs, and spices), fish, seafood, and vegetables oils, in particular, olive oil, are associated with a low risk of chronic disease while western dietary patterns featuring high amounts of red and processed meats, refined carbohydrates such as sugars, sugar-sweetened beverages, desserts, sweets, refined cereals, and solid fats are associated with increased disease risk.[10]

The relationship between dietary patterns and biomarkers for CVD risk may be more meaningful than those of individual nutrients or foods, which can fail to capture the effects of food synergy.[11] Both prudent and western dietary patterns have been associated with several cardiovascular risk factors; body weight, fat mass, body mass index (BMI), waist circumference, systolic blood pressure, diastolic blood pressure, plasma insulin, homocysteine, total cholesterol, high-density lipoprotein (HDL) cholesterol, LDL cholesterol, and inflammatory markers such as C-reactive protein (CRP).[12–15]

There is also clear evidence to show that dietary patterns are associated with morbidity and mortality from CVD. Healthful dietary patterns have been associated with lower risk of myocardial infarction, stroke, atherosclerosis, and death from CVD.[16–19] In an illustrative prospective study, it was demonstrated that high adherence to a prudent dietary pattern was a strong predictor of cardiovascular death in women previously free of CVD.[20] Over an 18-year period, greater adherence to the prudent pattern was associated with a 28% lower risk of cardiovascular mortality while those with high adherence to a western dietary pattern had a 22% increase in fatal CVD.

Two dietary patterns that have been extensively studied in observational and prospective studies, as well as randomized controlled trials for associations with CVD, are the Mediterranean diet and the DASH diet.

MEDITERRANEAN DIET

The traditional Mediterranean diet first attracted interest when it was noticed that the dietary pattern of people living on the Greek island of Crete was associated with a greatly reduced risk of CVD.[21] Since this early observation, a vast body of literature has been accumulated and the traditional Mediterranean diet has emerged as the most likely dietary model for robust cardiovascular benefits.[22]

There is, of course, no standardized diet across the diverse cultures that surround the Mediterranean, and the traditional foods and eating practices of the poor and rural groups upon which the dietary pattern is based are being progressively replaced by the modernization and globalization of food production and culture. However, the essence and heritage of the traditional Mediterranean diet has been captured and the current definition of the traditional Mediterranean diet is broadly a dietary pattern that is "rich in plant foods (cereals, fruits, vegetables, legumes, tree nuts, seeds, and olives), with olive oil as the principal source of added fat, along with high to moderate intakes of fish and seafood; moderate consumption of eggs, poultry, and dairy products (cheese and yogurt); low consumption of red meat; and a moderate intake of alcohol (mainly wine during meals)."[23]

The Mediterranean diet pyramid was developed and published by Mediterranean Diet Foundation Expert Group to represent the diet and its wider lifestyle, social and environmental context (see Figure 6.1).[23]

Several observational studies have demonstrated striking cardiovascular benefits of the Mediterranean diet. A meta-analysis and review of prospective cohort studies found that each two-unit increment in the Mediterranean diet score was associated with a 10% lower incidence of non-fatal and fatal CVD.[24] In a more recent prospective cohort study in a multiethnic North American population, it was found that closer adherence to a Mediterranean dietary pattern was protective against ischemic stroke, myocardial infarction, and vascular death.[25] In a large Dutch cohort, higher adherence to a Mediterranean dietary pattern was associated with a 56% lower incidence of fatal CVD compared to lower adherence over a mean 11.8-year period.[26]

Controlled intervention trials have examined the effects of the Mediterranean diet on cardiovascular risk markers. A meta-analysis contrasting the impact of Mediterranean to low-fat diets found the former more effective for producing long-term, clinically relevant changes in body weight, BMI, systolic blood pressure, diastolic blood pressure, fasting plasma glucose, total cholesterol, and high-sensitivity C-reactive protein.[27] Intervention studies have demonstrated remarkable effects on disease

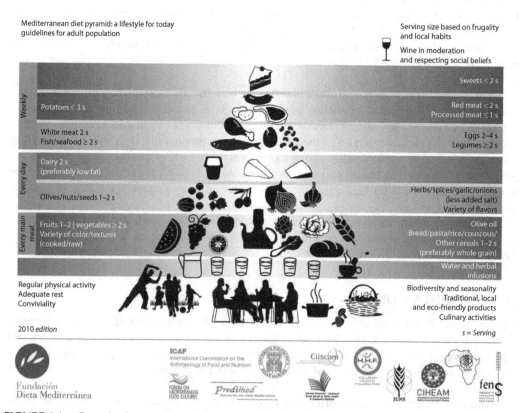

FIGURE 6.1　(**See color insert.**) The Mediterranean diet pyramid.

endpoints. A primary prevention study in a large, high-risk cohort found that a Mediterranean diet supplemented with walnuts or olive oil resulted in an approximately 30% reduction in major cardiovascular events, which was a combination of myocardial infarction, stroke, or death from cardiovascular causes, compared to a standard low-fat diet.[28] For the secondary prevention of CVD (after first myocardial infarction), the Lyon Diet Heart Study contrasted the effects of a Mediterranean style diet supplemented with α-linolenic acid against a prudent western diet. Compared to the control, the Mediterranean style diet was associated with a 76% lower risk of cardiac death and nonfatal myocardial infarction, and the protective effects were maintained for up to 4 years.[29,30]

DASH DIETARY PATTERN

While the Mediterranean diet had its origins in cultural history, the DASH dietary pattern was initially conceived in the early 1990s as a rational, evidence-based dietary prescription for reducing hypertension.[31] Taking into account that at the time of its development individual nutrients were primarily being studied, the DASH represented a tipping point in conventional nutritional wisdom. Rather than focusing on isolated foods or nutrients, the DASH was developed as complex, synergistic, dietary pattern.[32]

The DASH diet emphasizes fruit, vegetables, whole grains, beans, and low-fat dairy products while including poultry, fish, seeds and nuts, and limiting red meat, sweets, and sugar-containing beverages. Although the practical prescription focuses on foods, the diet was developed to minimize the intake of salt, added sugars, saturated fat, trans fat, and cholesterol while optimizing the intake of potassium, magnesium, and calcium; protein; and fiber.[33] Importantly, the first DASH diet (DASH 1) had a sodium content of about 3100 mg/day,[34] whereas the follow-up study diet (DASH 2) restricted sodium to 1500 mg daily and was able to demonstrate significantly greater reductions in blood pressure.[35]

Controlled clinical trials investigating the effects of the DASH diet for blood pressure reduction have found it to be at least as effective as antihypertensive medication.[34–36] Beyond blood pressure reduction, the DASH diet has been suggested to impact wider cardiovascular health. Using the Framingham risk equations to calculate 10-year risk of developing coronary heart disease (CHD) from the original DASH trial, it was estimated that the intervention would reduce disease risk by 11%.[37]

Prospective cohort studies have shown that closer adherence to a DASH dietary pattern may lower the incidence of CVD. In the Nurses Health Study, adherence to the DASH dietary pattern was associated with a lower risk of CHD and stroke. Incidence of CHD was 14% lower in those with the highest compared to the lowest adherence.[38] Similarly, in a large cohort of Swedish men, adherence to a DASH dietary pattern was associated with a 22% lower rate of heart failure events compared to low adherence.[39] In hypertensive adults in the Third National Health and Nutrition Examination Survey, adherence to a DASH diet was associated with lower all-cause mortality, including stroke.[40] These apparent benefits, however, have not been confirmed in all studies with some reports finding no or weak associations between the DASH diet and hypertension, CVD, or cardiovascular mortality.[41,42]

The DASH diet has been shown to favorably affect cardiovascular risk factors. In a dietary intervention study, the DASH resulted not only in blood pressure reduction but also in improvements in vascular and autonomic function (pulse wave velocity, baroreflex sensitivity) and reduction in left ventricular mass.[43] The diet has been shown to lower total cholesterol and LDL cholesterol; however, it also reduced HDL cholesterol and had no significant effects on triglycerides.[44] Reductions in homocysteine and inflammatory markers (CRP and interleukin-6) have been demonstrated.[38,45]

Gene–diet interactions may modify response to the DASH dietary intervention. Carriers of the A allele of the β_2-adrenergic receptor have a greater blood pressure–lowering response to the DASH diet, whereas those with the GG genotype had no significant effect.[4,46] Genotype of the β_2-adrenergic receptor has been shown to influence dietary sodium sensitivity.[47] Additionally, the low sodium DASH diet has been observed to lower oxidative stress in salt-sensitive individuals, but not in salt-resistant hypertensive patients suggesting further gene–diet interactions.[48]

EMERGING DIETARY CONCEPTS IN CARDIOVASCULAR NUTRITION

Promoting an individualized, complex diet and dietary behaviors that center on healthful foods is fundamental to clinical nutrition; however, our relationship with food is more complex and the construction of a heart-healthy diet may extend beyond simply eating the right food. A number of emerging concepts in clinical nutrition are proving to be very important for optimizing cardiovascular health, and these move beyond recommending a healthful dietary pattern. How much we eat (caloric restriction), how we prepare it (minimizing exposure to high-heat cooking by-products), and how alkaline it is (the influence on acid–alkaline balance) are examples of important areas that deserve clinical consideration.

CALORIC RESTRICTION

Caloric restriction in the context of human clinical nutrition refers to the reduction of energy intake to an individualized level that is sufficient to maintain a slightly low to normal body weight (i.e., BMI < 21 kg/m^2) without causing malnutrition (i.e., adequate intake of proteins and micronutrients).[49] In this context, long-term calorie restriction has been extensively studied in animal models and shown to be one of the most potent interventions for improving metabolic health, offsetting chronic disease and consequently extending life span.[50]

A number of cardiovascular benefits of caloric restriction have been identified in animal studies including reductions in oxidative stress and inflammation in the vasculature and heart, beneficial effects on endothelial function and arterial stiffness, protection against atherosclerosis, and attenuation of age-related changes in the heart (e.g., reduction in myocardial fibrosis and preservation or improvement in left ventricular diastolic function).[51] Although much of this research is limited to animal studies, there is telling evidence from human data that suggests some of these effects translate to human caloric restriction as well.[52]

An exemplary diet for caloric restriction is that of the people of the Japanese island of Okinawa, who are one of the few populations in the world who have experienced mild, long-term caloric restriction in a natural setting without malnutrition. The Okinawans are also unique in that they have an unusually low incidence of chronic diseases including CVD (18 deaths per 100,000 inhabitants per year compared to 100 in the United States) and are among the longest-lived people in the world (an average of 83.8 years compared to 78.9 years in the United States).[53] These differences in disease incidence and life span are thought to be at least in part due to diet.

Analysis of the traditional Okinawan diet has revealed that Okinawans were in a negative energy balance of approximately 11% until the 1960s (before progressive westernization of their diet).[54] Notably, the traditional Okinawan diet shares many general features of the Mediterranean and DASH diets, however, it also characteristically includes a high consumption of green leafy vegetables, sweet potato, soy foods, seaweeds, herbs and spices and low consumption of dairy products and daily green tea.[55]

Sustained calorie restriction has also been studied in a controlled clinical trial and in people practicing voluntary caloric restriction. These preliminary and observational human studies suggest that caloric restriction may improve a number of cardiovascular risk factors including body weight, visceral adipose tissue, inflammatory markers (e.g., CRP), blood pressure, fasting blood glucose and insulin, insulin sensitivity, cholesterol, and left ventricular diastolic function.[56]

Alternate-day fasting (ADF) or intermittent fasting is an approach that is gaining popularity and has experimental and clinical evidence to support its use. Typically, ADF involves consuming 25% of energy needs on the fast day and ad libitum food intake on the following day.[57] This regimen has been shown to significantly influence weight loss and cardiometabolic health with reductions in aortic vascular smooth muscle cell proliferation, CRP, adiponectin, leptin, total cholesterol, LDL cholesterol, triacylglycerol concentrations and systolic blood pressure, and increases in LDL particle size in a relatively short period.[58–60]

Caloric restriction could be practically achieved by constructing a personalized diet based on nutrient-dense, low-energy foods such as vegetables, fruits, whole grains, nuts, fish, low-fat dairy products, and lean meats and coaching in concepts such as volumetrics and low-glycemic index (GI) foods, as well as ensuring adequate protein and fiber at meals to improve satiety and adherence.[61]

ADVANCED GLYCATION END PRODUCTS (AGEs)

Modern dietary changes with importance for cardiovascular health include how we cook and pre-pare food. Advanced glycation end products (AGEs) are a group of oxidant, inflammatory com-pounds with significance in the pathogenesis of chronic diseases including CVD. AGEs are formed during a reaction between reducing sugars and free amino groups of proteins, lipids, or nucleic acids known as the Maillard reaction, which occurs during normal metabolism. In addition to AGEs produced during metabolism, diet is known to be a significant contributor to the endogenous AGE pool. Cooking methods associated with modern diets, including industrial heat processing, grilling, broiling, roasting, searing, and frying, significantly increase dietary AGE formation and exposure.[62]

Experimental research indicates that a low AGE diet may decrease circulating AGE levels, lower inflammatory mediators, and reduce atherosclerosis development.[63] In humans, a single high AGE meal has been shown to impair postprandial endothelial function.[64] Intervention with diet based on high AGE foods for 1 month was shown to influence a number of biomarkers relevant to car-diovascular risk (insulin sensitivity, plasma concentrations of omega-3 fatty acids, vitamins C and E, cholesterol, and triglycerides) in a group of healthy individuals.[65] A subsequent 6-week human intervention study with a low AGE diet in diabetic patients demonstrated a marked reduction in inflammation and oxidative stress compared to a standard diet.[66]

From a clinical perspective, dietary intake of AGEs can be reduced by two general means. First, avoiding foods that are known to be high in AGEs, including full-fat cheeses, meats, and highly processed foods, while increasing the consumption of fish, grains, low-fat milk products, fruits, and vegetables. Second, adopting traditional cooking methods such as boiling, poaching, and stewing, as well as steaming and slower cooking at a lower heat can markedly reduce dietary AGE exposure.[67]

DIETARY ACID LOAD

Diet-induced "low-grade" metabolic acidosis has been proposed to play an important role in the development of cardiovascular and other chronic diseases. An underlying basis for diet-induced low-grade metabolic acidosis is the notion that divergence from our ancestral diet, which would have featured predominantly in wild plant foods, toward cereal grains, dairy products, and a higher intake of meats with the agricultural revolution some 10,000 years ago, and more recently to a highly industrialized diet has resulted in a relative deficiency of potassium alkali salts and subse-quent increase in net systemic dietary acid load.[68]

In general, vegetables, fruits, and alkali-rich beverages (red wine and coffee) are alkaline, whereas fats and oils are neutral, and meats, dairy products, and cereal grains are acid producing.[69] Accordingly, a large population study showed that a diet higher in fruits and vegetables and lower in meats was strongly associated with a more alkaline physiological state.[70]

There is some evidence to suggest that a higher dietary acid load may be associated with CVD risk factors including systolic and diastolic blood pressure, total and LDL cholesterol, BMI, and waist circumference.[71] Dietary acid load has been associated with risk of hypertension in some, but not all studies.[72,73] Furthermore, diet-induced acidosis may contribute to insulin resistance and subsequent CVD risk.[74]

From a clinical standpoint, dietary acid load can be reduced by increasing the intake of fruits and vegetables and decreasing excessively high dietary protein intake.[75] Dietary intervention stud-ies are currently lacking, although one study found an alkaline diet effectively reduced urinary uric acid levels.[76] A short-term (10-day) intervention with a highly alkaline "paleolithic diet" resulted in a marked increase in potassium intake and improvements in vascular reactivity, blood pressure, glucose tolerance, insulin sensitivity, and lipid profiles.[77] Although the clinical effects of modification of dietary acid load on cardiovascular health are not yet clear, such dietary changes are in line with recommendations such as the Mediterranean style diet.

MACRONUTRIENTS

The difficulty in the discernment of the effect of specific macronutrients on cardiovascular function is that the overall dietary pattern consists of complex varieties of foods containing compounds other than macronutrients, which may impact the physiological effect of the food.[8] After all, macronutrients are not eaten in isolation, but are constituents as part of the larger whole pattern of eating. With this point taken under consideration, trends in foods that predominate in certain macronutrients and their relationship to CVD risk will be discussed.

PROTEIN

Proteins in the body serve a multitude of functions including acting as structural components, enzyme constituents, nutrient carriers, fluid balance regulators, and signaling molecules, to name a few. Thus, it would seem that dietary protein, and ensuring intake of the essential amino acids that cannot be made endogenously, is an important constituent to consider for cardiac structure and function. One example of a well-established role of dietary protein is the presence of key peptides, which serve as angiotensin-converting enzyme inhibitory (ACEI) compounds.

In some cases, the research may indicate that what the dietary protein may be replacing in the diet is more or less important than the mere inclusion of protein in the diet itself. Additionally, what has not been adequately explored in many studies investigating the impact of dietary protein on cardiovascular issues is the source, quality, and exact composition of the protein (e.g., Is the meat from a cow that has been grass-fed or corn-fed?) along with how individual subsets of the population and corresponding genotypes may respond differently to various types of protein. Therefore, with the best data currently available, this chapter will focus on the role of vegetable versus animal protein, soy, whey, and fish and their associations with CVD.

VEGETABLE VERSUS ANIMAL PROTEIN

CHD Risk Factors

Compelling research on the divergent effects of dietary animal versus vegetable protein on risk of CHD comes from the Nurses' Health Study data collection and subsequent lineage of publications. An early study by Hu et al.[78] on this large cohort of over 80,000 women for a duration of 14 years indicated that there was a positive association between the consumption of red meat and high-fat dairy products and the risk of CHD, whereas poultry, fish, and low-fat dairy intake were associated with a decreased risk. Further work on this same cohort was undertaken by Halton et al.[9] in which they indirectly investigated the association between dietary protein and CHD by primarily examining the effects of whether a low-carbohydrate diet influences CHD risk over 20 years of follow-up. Although they found that low-carbohydrate diets with compensatory increases in protein and fat were not associated with increased CHD, they did find that vegetable sources of protein (and fat) reduced the risk of CHD. Similar findings were observed in the prospective follow-up of the women in the Nurses' Health Study over a longer period of 26 years: higher intakes of red meat and high-fat dairy were significantly associated with greater risk of CHD, whereas consumption of poultry, fish, and nuts was associated with a lower risk. In comparison with one serving of red meat daily, 30%, 24%, 19%, and 13% lower risks of CHD were seen with one serving/day of nuts, fish, poultry, and low-fat dairy, respectively. A meta-analysis by Maki et al.[80] showed no significant differences in lipids (total cholesterol, HDL cholesterol, LDL cholesterol) in healthy individuals when comparing lean beef with either poultry or fish consumption. Thus, when it comes to CHD risk factors, the overall consensus from this large, prospective cohort of women over decades of observation is that vegetable protein appears to be somewhat more protective than animal protein; however, since the consumption of plant foods may be a marker of a healthy lifestyle, it is worthwhile to evaluate these findings in further trials.

HYPERTENSION

A number of observational studies have investigated the association between animal and plant protein and blood pressure, resulting in inconclusive results but indicating a general trend toward greater benefit with plant protein.[81–86] Further, in a meta-analysis to determine the effect of dietary protein consumption with blood pressure, Rebholz et al.[87] concluded from the 40 selected trials and over 3200 subjects that depending on the dietary variables being compared there were different findings on the role of protein. When compared to dietary carbohydrate, there was a statistically significant reduction in both mean systolic (−1.76 mmHg) and diastolic (−1.15 mmHg) blood pressure, and, in contrast to the data on CHD, there was no distinct difference between vegetable and animal protein and their blood pressure–lowering effects. In line with these findings relative to the difference between dietary carbohydrate and protein, He et al.[88] conducted a randomized, double-blind crossover trial to determine the effect of soy protein, milk protein, or carbohydrate (a mixture of sucrose, fructose, and maltodextrin with a GI of 98.9) supplementation on blood pressure in adults with prehypertension or stage 1 hypertension. Compared with the carbohydrate supplement, soy protein and milk protein both significantly lowered blood pressure, with no significant difference between the two. Thus, the overall clinical application of these collective findings may involve replacing dietary (high glycemic index) carbohydrate with protein when there are concerns about hypertension.

In a larger study with over 20,000 Dutch adults, proteins from a variety of different sources were investigated for their effects on blood pressure, including the intakes of total, plant, animal, dairy, meat, and grain protein.[89] Although the effects of total protein and meat protein appeared to be insignificant, there was a protective effect of plant protein, which was most pronounced in subjects with untreated hypertensive, quite possibly a more sensitive subset of the population and consistent with the OmniHeart study findings.[90] When the researchers looked more specifically at the types of plant protein that might be responsible for this effect, they found vegetable protein (and not protein intake from potatoes, legumes, and fruits) to have a small inverse relationship with blood pressure. Therefore, vegetables may be an indicator of a healthy lifestyle and have other attributes such as decreased net dietary acid load, which could further make them desirable dietary components for blood pressure reduction.

On the basis of the science available to suggest that there is an inverse relationship between dietary (vegetable) protein and hypertension, Altorf-van der Kuil et al.[91] examined whether certain amino acids, including glutamic acid, arginine, cysteine, lysine, or tyrosine, could be attributed to this association in a Dutch population over 6 years of follow-up. Although there was a statistically significant reduction in systolic blood pressure (−2.4 mmHg) with a higher intake of tyrosine (at ~0.3% of protein), the authors concluded that there was not a major role for any of these amino acids in the prediction of occurrence or risk of hypertension in this Dutch cohort. In another study investigating a smaller number of subjects who had prevalent CVD over a shorter duration of just 2 years, who were following one of two dietary patterns, it was noted that intakes of methionine and alanine were positively associated with higher blood pressure, whereas threonine and histidine had inverse associations.[92] An in vivo study conducted in 2007 measured the ACEI activity of peptides generated through milk fermentation using the lactic acid bacteria *Lactococcus lactic* and *Lactobacillus helveticus* and found foods containing ACEI peptides beneficial in lowering blood pressure.[93] In 2010, studies confirmed the potent hypotensive qualities of tripeptides valine, proline, proline and isoleucine, proline, proline extracted from *Lactobacillus helveticus* casein fermentations.[94] On the basis of these studies, it would seem that further delineation of specific amino acids and their effect on blood pressure in population groups is warranted.

STROKE

In a large, prospective study of 34,670 Swedish women without CVD over 10.4 years of follow-up, Larsson et al.[95] demonstrated a significant inverse association between total and animal protein and stroke events, especially for women with a history of hypertension. Similar findings were documented by Bernstein et al.[96] in a prospective study with 84,010 American women and 43,150 men without CVD after more than two decades of follow-up, respectively: greater consumption of red meat was associated with increased incidence of stroke, whereas poultry intake was associated with a lower risk. Substituting poultry, nuts, fish, and low-fat dairy for red meat led to 27%, 17%, 17%, and 11% reductions in risk for stroke, respectively, and there was no association with exchanging red meat for legumes or eggs. On the contrary, Preis et al.[97] did not find a statistically significant effect for increased risk of stroke for total and animal protein and decreased risk of stroke with vegetable protein in a large, prospective study with 43,960 Japanese men free of CVD followed over 18 years. The conflicting findings among the literature, may, in part, be due to the different protein sources and even genotypic responses to these proteins in the respective countries.

SOY PROTEIN

A meta-analysis by Anderson and Bush[98] assessed clinical trials related to soy protein intake and serum lipoprotein changes and found that soy protein intake at 15–30 g daily had favorable impacts on LDL cholesterol, HDL cholesterol, and triglycerides compared with non-soy controls. Furthermore, data exist to indicate that soy protein reduces LDL cholesterol and increases HDL cholesterol when specifically compared with milk protein.[99] Despite the number of studies indicating a positive effect of soy protein in the diet for cardiovascular markers, there has been debate about the inclusion of soy protein in the diet and whether the health claim on soy protein and heart health should be reconsidered.[100,101] One explanation for the variable effects of soy protein on cardiovascular parameters may be related to differences in population subgroups. For example, Hodis et al.[102] demonstrated that a soy protein/isoflavone supplement had no effect on atherosclerotic progression in postmenopausal women, but a favorable effect for healthy, premenopausal women. Furthermore, the variability in studies on soy may also be due to the heterogeneity of available soy products and their degree of processing, resulting in a variety of by-products formed. Tomatsu et al.[103] reported on novel ACEI peptides that could be derived from soy that are comparable with those peptides derived from other sources.

Finally, more recent studies have begun to explore the potential mechanisms for soy protein on cardiovascular markers. In a three-phase crossover trial in adults with 40 g of soy protein, 40 g of milk protein, and 40 g of complex carbohydrate, Rebholz et al.[104] found improvements in E-selectin compared with milk protein. Conversely, in individuals with prehypertension or stage 1 hypertension, no effect on cell adhesion molecules was found after 8 weeks of either a whole soy bean, soy protein isolate, or cow's milk beverage.[105]

WHEY PROTEIN

A number of studies demonstrate that chronic intake of several grams (typically 20 g) of whey protein has clinically significant blood pressure–lowering effects.[106–109] Additionally, whey protein reduces elevated triglycerides and cholesterol levels and even inflammation in patients with CVD and cerebrovascular disease.[107,110,111] There is some evidence that these benefits from whey protein may come from chronic consumption rather than an acute meal. Pal and Ellis[112] studied the acute meal effects of 45 g whey protein isolate compared with either the same amount of sodium caseinate or a glucose control in a randomized, three-way crossover design study with 20 overweight and obese postmenopausal women. They did not find any significant postprandial differences between the groups for vascular, inflammatory, or blood pressure changes.

The type of whey protein formulation may significantly impact results. For example, data from clinical trials indicate that whey protein must be hydrolyzed to ACEI peptides for it to have antihypertensive properties.[106–108,113,114] When proteins are broken down into individual peptides, some of these peptides can be used to act as inhibitors of angiotensin converting enzyme, a protein that is responsible for blood pressure regulation. Furthermore, it is worthwhile to note that certain whey protein preparations may result in a relatively higher insulin response relative to other protein sources, which may or may not be beneficial in some patient populations.[115,116]

Finally, there may also be food interactions that may enhance or potentiate the ACEI activity of peptides within whey protein. Murakami et al.[117] found that simultaneous consumption of tea with whey protein may reduce the blood pressure–lowering efficacy of the protein. Conversely, there may be particular whey formulations that lead to better results. A recent study by Petyaev et al.[118] demonstrated that when whey protein isolate was embedded into lycopene micelles and fed to patients with hypertension over 1 month, there were several favorable changes in cardiovascular function, plasma lipids, and inflammatory markers, compared with simple formulations of either the whey protein or the lycopene.

FISH

Overall, studies support fish consumption for cardiovascular health.[119] Mozaffarian and Rimm[120] found evidence to support that even modest consumption of fish at 1 to 2 servings weekly, especially higher omega-3 fatty acid-containing fish, reduces risk of coronary death by 36% and total mortality by 17%. They also advised consuming a variety of seafood with limited intake of high mercury-containing fish with greater fish consumption (≥5 servings/week). Two recent meta-analysis findings confirmed positive results for fish consumption: Li et al.[121] demonstrated that fish consumption is protective for heart failure with every increment of 20 g of daily fish intake associated with a 6% lower risk of this condition, whereas Chowdhury et al.[122] identified a similar, yet moderate, inverse association between fish consumption and cerebrovascular risk. Of note, there may be gender specific differences to the response of fish consumption. In a large prospective trial with 20,069 men and women followed over 8–13 years, de Goede et al.[123] found that increased fish intakes were associated with reduced stroke incidence in women while that same association could not be found in men. Moreover, there may be physiological differences from intakes of the different fish protein sources. Pilon et al.[124] compared metabolic effects of bonito, herring, mackerel, or salmon against casein in high-fat-, high-sucrose-fed rats and reported that all the fish proteins were superior to casein in reducing inflammatory markers; however, the salmon protein resulted in some differences in calcitonin levels compared with the other fish proteins.

There are actives within fish that add to its cardioprotective qualities. Studies have documented the presence of ACEI in fish such as bonito and sardines.[125–127] Oral consumption of sardine muscle protein, which contains valyl–tyrosine (Val–Tyr), by mildly hypertensive volunteers led to 9.7 and 5.3 mmHg reductions in systolic and diastolic blood pressure, respectively, within just 1 week.[128] The science to support the role of omega-3 fatty acids from fish in CVD will be addressed in the section "Fats and Oils."

In evaluating studies on fish consumption, it is important to consider that there could be confounding variables related to those who choose to eat fish such as other positive, healthful lifestyle factors as well as genetic factors.[129,130] In a study by Sofi et al.[130] in 647 Italian men, it was demonstrated that there was a significant gene–dietary interaction with one of the polymorphisms for the lipoprotein(a) [Lp(a)] gene (LPA 93C>T polymorphism) and fish intake, resulting in reduced Lp(a) concentrations with daily fish intake.

What is often not taken into consideration is the type of fish and its methylmercury levels, and further, the degree to which individuals can metabolize mercury based on polymorphisms they may have for the metallothionein protein[131] or glutathione-related genes.[132] Methylmercury has detrimental effects on cardiovascular health in certain populations, including increasing heart rate,[133] blood pressure,[134,135] and incidence of myocardial infarction[136]; however, ultimately, it has been suggested that the benefits of fish eating outweigh the risks from the potential toxins it contains.[120]

FATS AND OILS

Of all the macronutrients, dietary fats and oils have most likely received the most attention in the field of cardiovascular nutrition with the greatest degree of studies, including controlled feeding studies, randomized trials, and large cohort studies. As Willett[137] has suggested, the total fat amount may not be as important as the type of diet. If not oxidized for energy, dietary fatty acids may become cellular structural and functional components that may have far-reaching impacts on CVD processes such as inflammation. Essential fatty acids such as those from the omega-6 and omega-3 families must be consumed from food in proper quantities relative to other ingested fats to impact the regulation of inflammation through the production of eicosanoid-derived prostaglandins. Within this section, the individual fatty acid families will be discussed along with significant studies to demonstrate their role in CVD.

Trans Fats (TFAs)

TFAs can be found in nature and may be produced industrially. Vaccenic acid and the naturally occurring isomer of conjugated linoleic acid (CLA), cis-9, trans-11 CLA (c9, t11-CLA), are found in meat and milk products derived from ruminant animals.[138] Other TFAs may form in the industrial production of solid fats from liquid oils through the process of partial hydrogenation,[139] in addition to small amounts produced in the course of the deodorization and refinement of vegetable oils.[140] It is well established that the industrially produced TFAs (iTFAs), ubiquitous in the processed food supply, are detrimental to cardiovascular health due to their ability to impair endothelial function, elevate triglycerides and Lp(a) lipoprotein, increase thrombogenesis, reduce the particle size of LDL cholesterol, and increase LDL cholesterol while simultaneously decreasing HDL cholesterol.[141–144] Specifically, one meta-analysis found that a 2% increase in energy intake from TFAs was associated with a 23% increase in the incidence of CHD.[145] The presence of iTFAs in the systemic circulation favors inflammation, ultimately contributing to atherosclerosis, hypertension, and heart hypertrophy as well as other chronic diseases.[146,147] It has been proposed by Angelieri et al.[148] that TFA contributes to inflammation and metabolic disturbances by altering cell signaling via intracellular kinases and insulin receptor substrates.

From a nutrigenomic perspective, an animal study by Collison et al.[149] demonstrated that an iTFA-containing diet induced over twice as many cardiac differentially expressed genes (DEGs) in males compared to females, including downregulation of *Gata4*, *Mef2d*, and *Srebf2*. This type of nutrigenomic research needs to be evaluated in human clinical trials as this information would be invaluable for making dietary recommendations and improving patient compliance to eating regimens.

The limited studies that are available examining the effect of naturally occurring TFAs from ruminants indicate inconclusive results. Ganguly and Pierce[150] stated that there may be cardioprotective effects while a comprehensive review of studies by Gebauer et al.[151] led to the conclusion that more research is required to have a better understanding of the cardiovascular and generalized health effects of these ruminant TFAs, especially at levels normally found in the diet. Along similar lines, Smit et al.[152] demonstrated that when 61 healthy adults were fed diets containing 7% of energy from either oleic acid (18:1n-9, control diet), iTFAs, or CLA, inflammatory markers remained unaffected and urinary concentrations of 8-iso-PGF(2α) increased in the group fed CLA. Additional research is warranted to fully understand the effects of ruminant TFAs and their mechanisms of action.

Saturated Fats

From early work by Ancel Keys several decades ago, dietary saturated fats as a collective macronutrient category has been associated with increased incidence of cardiovascular events. This research had, in part, set the foundation for public health recommendations to restrict saturated fat consumption to reduce CVD risk due to its influence on increasing LDL cholesterol; however, it is well accepted that saturated fat also increases HDL cholesterol. Thus, it would seem that saturated fat would not significantly alter an important CVD risk marker, the total cholesterol to HDL cholesterol ratio.[153] This effect is differentially modulated by the individual saturated fatty acids when replacing dietary carbohydrate with stearic acid (18:0) having no effect on LDL or HDL cholesterol and with lauric acid (12:0) having the greatest effect on increasing both LDL and HDL cholesterol.[154] Therefore, the public health guidance to lower dietary saturated fat is under scrutiny and the aspect of the type of saturated fat is being more thoroughly investigated due to the lack of a strong association in prospective studies.

Newer studies continue to be contradictory and inconclusive.[155] Cooper et al.[156] reviewed several studies and found that reducing saturated fat by reducing and/or modifying dietary fat resulted in a 14% reduced risk in cardiovascular events. In contrast, Siri-Tarino et al.[157] assessed the evidence related to dietary saturated fat intake with risk of CHD, stroke, and CVD in 21 prospective epidemiologic studies which included 347,747 subjects over 5–23 years of follow-up. The findings revealed that there was no significant relationship between dietary saturated fat intake and increased risk of CHD or CVD. The authors suggested that more research is required to ascertain the effects of nutrients that are used to replace the saturated fat.

Along these lines, de Oliveira Otto et al.[158] investigated whether there was variability in the food source of saturated fat in relationship to CVD events and reported that a higher intake of dairy saturated fat was associated with a lower CVD risk, whereas a higher intake of meat saturated fat was associated with greater CVD risk. Substituting 2% of energy from meat saturated fat with energy from dairy saturated fat resulted in a 25% lower CVD risk. There was no association observed between plant or butter saturated fat, but the data were limited by the narrow range of intake. Furthermore, there are differential effects even within the dairy category of foods with cheeses having smaller effects on LDL cholesterol concentrations compared with butter and fermented dairy foods, such as yogurt and even certain probiotic microorganisms, being associated with reductions in LDL cholesterol. Hence, it may be that there are other constituents in foods that have effects on CVD risk, which are worthwhile to evaluate. It is important to assess the total food source of saturated fat when tailoring individual dietary recommendations.

Additionally, gene–diet interactions may be involved in an individual's response to dietary saturated fat.[154] An example of this nutrigenomic interaction was evident in a study[159] that investigated polymorphisms in the peroxisome proliferator–activated receptor (PPAR) gene and dietary intake. The researchers observed that a certain polymorphism (PPARα V162) was associated with smaller peak particle diameters of LDL cholesterol in subjects with higher saturated fat intakes compared with those with lower intakes. Another study[160] identified an association between endothelial nitric oxide synthase (eNOS) gene variations and effects of an acute, high saturated fat meal in young, healthy men. Finally, an interaction between the apoE-4 allele and a greater LDL response to saturated fat has been reported in some studies.[154]

Polyunsaturated Fats (PUFAs): Omega-3 and Omega-6 Fatty Acids

The beneficial effect of dietary inclusion of PUFAs has been demonstrated in a number of studies[161] with one of the meta-analyses[162] indicating that a 5% increase in energy from PUFAs led to a 10% reduction in risk for CVD. Other studies[163,164] have shown that substitution of saturated fat with PUFAs results in decreased total, LDL, and HDL cholesterol, with a greater reduction in LDL cholesterol compared with HDL cholesterol. Moreover, Willett[137] states that replacing saturated fat with PUFAs leads to the best result when compared with monounsaturated fats (MUFAs) and carbohydrate (depending on the type of carbohydrate).

The two main essential PUFA families are the omega-6 and omega-3 fatty acids, which are found in vegetable oils and nuts (omega-6 and the shorter chain omega-3) and fish (the longer chain omega-3). Although the ratio of these two important fatty acid families has been the focus of nutrition recommendations, with a focus on increasing omega-3 and limiting omega-6 fatty acids, especially linoleic acid (18:2n-6), due to their potential proinflammatory and prothrombotic effects. However, there is some controversy regarding this assumption about omega-6 fatty acids. A human clinical trial by Pischon et al.[165] demonstrated that the greatest degree of anti-inflammatory effects were observed with the combination of both omega-3 and omega-6 fatty acids in the diet. Further, Anton et al.[161] clarify that part of the controversy surrounding linoleic acid could come from a lack of studies distinguishing between naturally occurring linoleic acid such as from sunflower oil and chemically hydrogenated forms of this fatty acid, such as is seen with hydrogenated vegetable oil and TFAs overall.

It has been suggested that since both of the PUFA families are essential and important for CVD risk reduction, it would be better to not solely focus on the omega-6:omega-3 ratio but on the whole foods that will provide the desirable mixture of fatty acids and have been shown to be beneficial for reducing CVD incidence.[137] The American Heart Association supports the concept of ensuring healthy intakes of both omega-3 (about 500 mg/day from fish or fish oil supplements) and omega-6 fatty acids (12 g for women and 17 g for men per day) for the prevention and treatment of CVD.[166] According to Lavie et al.,[167] consumption of long-chain omega-3 PUFAs (EPA and DHA) should be at least 800–1000 mg/day for individuals with known CHD and heart failure. A large, prospective study[168] in 34,670 Swedish women over a mean of 10.4 years revealed an inverse relationship between dietary intake of long-chain omega-3 PUFAs and risk of stroke. However, there was no association between saturated fat, mononunsaturated fat, PUFA, α-linolenic acid, and omega-6 PUFAs and risk of stroke.

Select whole foods provide the essential fatty acids include nuts, seeds, nut and seed oils, leafy greens, algae and fish oils. Foods high in naturally occurring omega-6 PUFAs such as nuts, and in particular, walnuts, have been shown to be cardioprotective.[169,170] The different components of flaxseed, such as the α-linolenic acid-rich oil and the lignans, may each have cardioprotective effects. Fukumitsu et al.[171] found that 100 mg of the flaxseed lignan (secoisolariciresinol diglucoside) was effective at reducing blood cholesterol and hepatic enzymes in moderately hypercholesterolemic men. Both flaxseed oil and fish oil supplementation have been shown to increase longer chain omega-3 fatty acids in red blood cell membranes,[172] and flaxseed oil incorporation into the diet at 8 g/day for 12 weeks resulted in reduced blood pressure in dyslipidemic subjects compared to a high linoleic acid diet.[173] Omega-3 fatty acid supplementation may be useful for primary prevention of CVD[167]; however, a recent large meta-analysis[174] indicated that there was no demonstrable effect for secondary prevention, a finding which is quite opposed to conclusions from previous studies.[167]

A number of nutrigenomic studies have elucidated interactions between the omega-3 fatty acids and gene expression in relationship to molecular events at all stages of atherogenesis, specifically decreasing activation of the host of nuclear factor-kappa B transcription factors.[175] Schmidt et al.[176] investigated the effects of omega-3 PUFAs supplementation versus that of corn oil on genomic expression in healthy and dyslipidemic subjects after 4 hours, 1 week, and 12 weeks. Findings revealed that 12-week supplementation with omega-3 PUFAs led to downregulation in proinflammatory genes. In a separate publication, Schmidt et al.[177] identified that 1.56 g EPA and 1.14 g DHA for 12 weeks to healthy and dyslipidemic men resulted in increased expression of antioxidant enzymes and decreased expression of pro-oxidant enzymes, suggesting further protective effects of these long-chain PUFAs. Finally, Liang et al.[178] suggest that the variable results of long-chain omega-3 PUFAs on CVD biomarkers such as lipids may be due to interactions between the APOE genotype and the fatty acid. Personalized recommendations for dietary intake and supplementation may be warranted based on these preliminary findings. More research is required to examine the effects of omega-3 PUFA intake in different genotype groupings.

Monounsaturated Fats

The benefit of MUFAs in the diet, particularly oleic acid through consumption of olive oil, has been consistently touted as being cardioprotective. Data have shown that MUFAs tend to reduce LDL cholesterol without lowering HDL cholesterol[179]; however, there are inconclusive results for CVD, such as in the meta-analysis by Jakobsen et al.,[180] where there was a positive correlation between MUFA-containing diets and risk of coronary events, but not between MUFA-rich diets and risk of coronary deaths. It has been postulated that the differences in MUFA origin may account for these differences, with most of the MUFAs in the western diet from animal sources.

One of the main MUFA-containing foods in a healthful diet is olive oil. Previous studies on olive oil consumption indicate it has anti-inflammatory, antioxidant, and antithrombotic effects, particularly when high in phenol content.[181,182] Camargo et al.[183] explored whether the positive cardioprotective benefits of olive oil were due to the oil or the phenol content and reported 98 DEGs between phenol-rich and low-phenol olive oil, especially those related to inflammatory pathways. Along similar lines, individuals with a specific polymorphisms of the interleukin (IL)-6 gene (-174G/C), the minor allele frequency (C), had lower body weight gain when following the Mediterranean diet plus a high intake of virgin olive oil.

Despite the plethora of data accumulated to support the inclusion of olive oil and MUFAs into the diet for cardiovascular benefit, there are some studies that indicate questionable effects of MUFAs.[184] For example, a study in African green monkeys[185] fed MUFAs in place of saturated fat resulted in greater enrichment of LDL particles with cholesteryl oleate, an indicator of atherogenicity as shown in the Atherosclerosis Risk in Communities Study.[186,187] Further, Imamura et al.[188] proposes that long-chain MUFAs (22:1 and 24:1) found in a variety of food sources, including fish, poultry, meats, whole grains, and mustard, may be cardiotoxic due to their association with incident congestive heart failure (CHF) in two independent cohorts.

CARBOHYDRATE

Due to its implication in glucose and insulin balance, carbohydrate has been a significant focus in dietary recommendations for type 2 diabetes and CVD. Although, much like protein and fats, the overall quantity and quality of carbohydrate needs to be considered in dietary guidance for certain patient populations. Hyperglycemia is closely intertwined with cardiovascular issues such as hepatic lipid synthesis and endothelial function, thus, glycemic control is important to consider for CVD. Therefore, it has been suggested that low-glycemic carbohydrates or those food sources of carbohydrates that have negligible or moderate impact on postprandial blood glucose levels such as whole fruits, vegetables, legumes, and whole grains are most suitable for individuals with lifestyle-induced chronic disease such as CVD.

CARBOHYDRATE QUANTITY

A meta-analysis by Hu et al.[189] investigated the effect of low-carbohydrate and low-fat diets on metabolic risk factors in 23 trials with a total of 2788 participants. They found that low-carbohydrate diets led to better reductions in total cholesterol, LDL cholesterol, and triglycerides and an improvement in HDL cholesterol. This study's findings are in contrast to the meta-analysis from Nordmann et al.[190] in which they analyzed five trials of 447 overweight subjects and demonstrated favorable reductions in triglycerides and HDL cholesterol for the low-carbohydrate diet; however, the low-fat diet performed better on total cholesterol and LDL cholesterol. Finally, a review and meta-analysis by Santos et al.[191] in obese patients on a low-carbohydrate diet to assess cardiovascular risk factors found that this diet resulted in significant decreases in systolic and diastolic blood pressure, plasma triglycerides, an increase in HDL cholesterol, and no significant change in LDL cholesterol. The subtle discrepancies in the findings of these three meta-analyses may, in part, be due to the quality of carbohydrate consumed by the subjects.

LOW GI VERSUS HIGH GI

Although the role of GI has been well studied in the context of individuals with type 2 diabetes and metabolic syndrome, there has not been the same depth of exploration for cardiovascular conditions; however, due to the interrelationship between these two chronic diseases, it would seem that there would be some relevance of glycemic impact in association with cardiovascular risk factors. In a meta-analysis by Ma et al.,[192] 14 studies with 229,213 subjects were assessed to determine the role of GI and glycemic load (GL) on CVD risk. Both GI and GL were found to be associated with significant increased risk of CVD with a greater risk incurred for women compared with men. Another meta-analysis[193] that included 8 prospective studies and 220,050 subjects reported similar results with both high dietary GL and GI being associated with risk of CHD with the most striking correlation found in women (relative risk (RR): 1.69, 95% confidence interval [CI]: 1.32–2.16).

One of the mechanisms of how GI and GL may be associated with CVD may through modulation of inflammatory processes. Studies have indicated that a low-GI diet reduces markers of inflammation such as CRP.[194,195] In the FUNGENUT study, Kallio et al.[196] tested two types of carbohydrate meals varying in quality and GI, a low-GI rye pasta and a high-GI oat–wheat–potato combination in individuals with metabolic syndrome. They demonstrated a differential gene expression between the meals with the oat–wheat–potato diet causing upregulation of 62 genes related to stress, immunity, and inflammation after 12 weeks.

FIBER

High-fiber foods such as legumes, whole grains, vegetables, and fruits have beneficial effects on cardiovascular function. A number of studies have documented an inverse relationship between fiber intake and cardiovascular risk with a stronger association for cereal fiber than fruit or vegetable fiber, possibly due to multiple mechanistic effects such as reduction of lipids, body weight, glucose, blood pressure, and even inflammation.[197] According to Lee et al.,[198] a fiber increase of approximately 17 g/day can result in blood pressure decreases of 1.15 mmHg (systolic) and 1.65 mmHg (diastolic). Soluble fiber seems to lead to better results than insoluble fiber. Thus, tailoring the fiber source to the cardiovascular condition as a means of personalizing the approach may be indicated. Furthermore, the effects of high-fiber foods on CVD may be due to their role in inflammation. A significant inverse association between several cytokines (IL-1β, IL-4, IL-5, IL-6, IL-13, and tumor necrosis factor-α) and cereal fiber was noted in 88 cancer-free subjects.[199] At the end of 5 weeks of consumption of either high- or low-fiber intakes (48.0 and 30.2 g/day, respectively) from oat bran, rye bran, and sugar beet fiber, there was a significant reduction in CRP between the two fiber diets.[200]

Specific high-fiber foods have also been evaluated for their effects on cardiovascular biomarkers; however, it is not apparent whether their effects are due to their fiber content or other constituents such as the vast array of phytochemicals. In some cases, there may be synergy among the food components. For example, Lee et al.[198] commented that dietary protein combined with fiber may have additive effects on lowering blood pressure. Tighe et al.[201] determined that whole grain foods such as wheat and oats fed to middle-aged health individuals led to significant reductions in systolic blood pressure and pulse pressure (6 and 3 mmHg, respectively). Bazzano et al.[202] evaluated non-soy legume consumption on total cholesterol levels in 10 trials representing 268 subjects. The mean net change in total cholesterol on a non-soy legume diet was −11.8 mg/dL (95% CI: −16.1 to −7.5) and for LDL cholesterol, −8.0 mg/dL (95% CI: −11.4 to −4.6). Larsson et al.[203] followed 26,556 Finnish male smokers for 13.6 years and found that vegetable fiber intake, in addition to the consumption of fruit, vegetables, and cereals, was inversely associated with risk of stroke.

SWEETENERS

There is an overwhelming preponderance of added sugars such as sucrose and high-fructose corn syrup in the current diet, increasing the risk of obesity, metabolic syndrome, diabetes, and CVD due to consequences such as dyslipidemia, inflammation, and oxidative stress.[204,205] As a result, public health recommendations, such as those put forth by the American Heart Association, advocate reductions in added sugar intake from high-added sugar foods such as soft drinks, fruit drinks, desserts, sugars and jellies, candy, and ready-to-eat cereal, with no more than 100 and 150 cal for American women and men per day, respectively.[206]

Fructose is further implicated in cardiovascular concerns due to its ability to increase triglycerides and uric acid,[204] although there is discussion that low dietary amounts of fructose are beneficial while high excessive intake is associated with these metabolic impairments.[207,208] The work of Le et al.[209] suggests that there may even be intraindividual differences in the response to fructose linked with SNPs in genes involved in fructose transport, which can alter cardiometabolic risk.

Select risk factors for CVD have been shown to be impacted by dietary sugar intake. There are studies emerging to indicate a potential relationship between sugar-sweetened beverage consumption and hypertension.[210–213] In the Framingham Heart Study cohort, Dhingra et al.[213] noted that individuals who consumed as little as one or more soft drinks per day had increased incidence of high blood pressure, hypertriglyceridemia, and low HDL cholesterol. Similarly, fasting triglycerides appear to be elevated in the presence of high intakes (>20% of energy) of sugars (sucrose, glucose, and fructose) with more marked effects in specific populations such as (1) men compared with women, (2) those who are sedentary overweight or have metabolic syndrome, and (3) those individuals consuming low fiber,[214–217] thus warranting specific dietary recommendations for certain patient populations. Additionally, postprandial triglyceride elevations may be augmented by sucrose and fructose.[218,219]

Although artificial sweeteners have been the subject of concern for metabolic disturbances and obesity, there is limited information available with respect to their impact on CVD. In one study,[220] three different artificial sweeteners (aspartame, acesulfame K, and saccharin) were found to exhibit proatherogenic and senescence properties *in vitro*, with implications for impairment in structure and function of apoA-I and HDL cholesterol.

PHYTONUTRIENT-RICH FOODS

A number of the natural plant foods that comprise healthful dietary patterns have been shown to have particularly pronounced cardiovascular health benefits.[221] These phytonutrient-rich plant foods are referred to as functional foods, which by definition are "foods that, by virtue of physiologically active food components, provide health benefits beyond basic nutrition."[222] The construction of therapeutic diets based on combinations of functional foods has been shown to be an effective and practical approach to cardiovascular risk reduction.[223]

FRUITS AND VEGETABLES

A higher intake of fruits and vegetables has consistently been associated with a lower incidence of CVD in a dose-dependent fashion. A meta-analysis of nine observational cohort studies including 91,379 men and 129,701 women found fruit and vegetable consumption reduced CHD risk by 4% to 7% for each additional portion per day of vegetables or fruits, respectively.[224] A similar dose-dependent relationship was revealed in a meta-analysis examining the relationship between fruit and vegetable intake and risk of stroke.[225] An intervention with a higher fruit and vegetables diet in hypertensive patients was found to improve endothelial function, again in a dose-dependent relationship.[226]

Fruits and vegetables are rich in important nutrients such as fiber, vitamins, minerals, and phytochemicals, but they are low in energy, sodium, and TFAs and tend to displace unhealthy foods, making them a vital component of a dietary cardiovascular health plan.[227] The health benefits of fruits and vegetables appear to be in part due to their ability to reduce inflammation and oxidative stress.[228] Importantly, the anti-inflammatory effect of fruits and vegetables may be related more to a wider dietary variety of foods than the absolute amount, which from a practical standpoint emphasizes the importance of dietary diversity.[229]

LEGUMES

Consumption of legumes has been associated with a lower CVD risk, and clinical intervention studies have suggested cardiovascular-protective effects. A large epidemiological study in the U.S. population revealed an association between legume consumption and reduced risk of CHD. Soy foods in particular have attracted attention for cardiovascular health because of their favorable nutritional profile.[230] However, the available evidence suggests than non-soy legumes (e.g., beans such as pinto, kidney, and lima beans and peas such as split green peas or lentils) may be equally beneficial for heart health.[202]

WHOLE GRAINS

Whole grains are rich in dietary fiber, micronutrients, phytosterols, and other phytochemicals and may reduce oxidative stress, inflammation, and improve hyperlipidemia, blood pressure and vascular function.[231] A meta-analysis of clinical trials and prospective cohort studies estimated that people consuming three to five servings per day have an approximately 20% lower risk of CVD compared with rarely or never consumers of whole grains.[232]

Advise to consume whole grains may improve weight loss and CVD risk. Obese adults with metabolic syndrome, who were advised to consume whole grains in addition to a hypocaloric diet had a significantly greater reduction in CRP and percentage body fat in the abdominal region when compared to those eating their grain allowance as refined grains.[233]

NUTS

The benefits of nuts for cardiovascular health have been consistently demonstrated across a number of observational studies and clinical trials.[234] Mechanisms for the benefits of nut consumption include cholesterol-lowering effects, reductions in oxidative stress, inflammation, and improvements in vascular reactivity.[235]

Nuts are phytonutrient dense (including high-quality vegetable protein, fiber, minerals, tocopherols, phytosterols, and phenolic compounds) and rich in unsaturated fatty acids.[236] Despite being high in fat, regular nut consumption does not appear to induce weight gain.[237] In fact, a 12-month study of a Mediterranean diet supplemented with 30 g of nuts per day found a decrease in prevalence of metabolic syndrome, mainly due to reduced visceral adiposity.[238]

The effects of even modest nut consumption on CVD outcomes are striking. For example, in individuals with high cardiovascular risk a longitudinal cohort study found that subjects who consumed greater than three servings of nuts per week at baseline had a 55% lower risk of cardiovascular mortality.[239] Similarly, two large prospective cohort studies found a 20% reduction in total mortality, including CVD, with consumption of nuts seven or more times per week compared to those who ate no nuts.[240]

OLIVE OIL

Olive oil is the major source of calories in the traditional Mediterranean diet and beyond simply being rich in MUFAs is also an important source of phytochemicals naturally present in the oil.[241] There is an important distinction between "olive oil" and "extra virgin olive oil" with the former refined and virtually devoid of phytochemicals, whereas the latter contains up to 1 g/kg of these important substances.[242] Within the oily matrix of extra virgin olive oil (EVOO), there is a rich array of bioactive compounds including triterpenes, phytosterols, flavonoids, and lignans. These bioactive compounds are thought to be a major reason for the health benefits of virgin olive oil.[243]

The fatty acid composition of EVOO also account for its health effects. Oleic acid is the predominant MUFA in olive oil comprising 55%–83% of the total fatty acids and is thought to account for many of the unique effects of olive when compared to other vegetable oils. Oleic acid may play an important role in the beneficial effects of EVOO on postprandial metabolism including insulin release, nitric oxide bioavailability, vasodilation, blood pressure, inflammation, and blood coagulation.[244]

A large observational study in a Spanish cohort demonstrated a 26% lower risk of CVD and 44% reduction in overall mortality in the highest quartile of olive oil consumption.[245] Consumption of 30 mL of polyphenol-rich olive oil for 2 months in hypertensive women led to improvement in endothelial function, a significant decrease of 7.91 mmHg in systolic and 6.65 mmHg of diastolic blood pressure, and reductions in inflammation and oxidative stress.[246]

COCOA

Cocoa is a rich source of polyphenols, and cocoa and dark chocolate consumption has been associated with impressive cardiovascular health benefits in observational studies.[247] The combined data from seven large-scale population studies (with a combined total of 114,009 participants), for example, revealed that the highest levels of chocolate consumption was associated with a 37% reduction in heart disease, a 31% reduction in diabetes, and a 29% reduction in stroke compared with the lowest levels.[248]

A number of controlled clinical trials have also shown consistent acute and chronic benefits of cocoa on flow-mediated dilatation and insulin resistance, although it was concluded that more research is required to confirm the potential clinical benefits of cocoa as a cardiovascular medicine.[249]

TEA

Tea is a rich source of polyphenols, a class of phytonutrients with several important cardioprotective effects. Consumption of both green and black teas had been associated with a significant reduction in CHD and stroke risk in epidemiological studies with estimates ranging from a 10% to 20% reduction in disease risk.[250]

Robust support for the protective effects of teas comes from a meta-analysis of prospective cohort studies, which found a statistically significant inverse association between tea consumption and risk of stroke.[251] The analysis also revealed a dose-dependent relationship with each increase of three cups per day in tea consumption associated with a 13% reduction in stroke risk.

A relevant clinical trial demonstrated that black tea consumption (three cups per day) for 6 months significantly reduced 24-hour ambulatory systolic and diastolic blood pressure by between 2 and 3 mmHg, an effect that at a population level would be associated with a 10% reduction in the prevalence of hypertension and a 7%–10% reduction in the risk of CVD.[252]

An interaction between a slow allele of the CYP1A2 genotype, a caffeine-metabolizing enzyme, has been associated with increased risk for hypertension and nonfatal myocardial infarction in regular coffee drinkers.[253,254] However, it is unknown if tea, which contains a different group of bioactives and lower caffeine content than coffee, would have the same effect.

CAROTENOIDS

Carotenoids are natural pigments found in deeply colored yellow, orange, red, and dark green plants as well as in some animal source foods (e.g., salmon and egg yolks). Some of the best-studied carotenoids include beta-carotene, zeaxanthin, lycopene, and astaxanthin. A primary mechanism for the cardioprotective effects of carotenoids appears to be their ability to reduce oxidant stress and subsequently atherosclerosis progression. Indeed, there may be a relationship between carotenoid intake and reduced intima-media thickness of common carotid artery wall.[255]

A particularly prominent relationship has been found between dietary carotenoid intake and cardiovascular risk, although it may be that carotenoid intake is simply a surrogate marker of higher fruit and vegetable consumption.[256] In Finnish men, the highest quartile of serum lycopene concentration was associated with 59% and 55% lower risks of ischemic stroke and any stroke, compared with men in the lowest quartile. Similarly, men with the lowest quartile of serum β-carotene had an approximately threefold increased risk of CHF.[257]

Increasing consumption of foods that are rich in carotenoids may improve cardiovascular risk. A 7-day intervention with red orange juice (500 mL/day) significantly improved endothelial function and reduced inflammation in adults with increased cardiovascular risk.[258] Supplementation with 70 g of tomato paste over a period of 14 days improved endothelial function (measured with flow-mediated dilatation) and reduced serum oxidative stress.[259]

POLYPHENOLS/FLAVONOIDS

Flavonoids are the most common class of polyphenolic phytochemicals consumed in a plant-based diet. Although major food sources of flavonoids vary depending on dietary habits and culture, some of the richest and most frequently consumed dietary sources of flavonoids include soy foods, whole grains, tea, apples, onions, cocoa, wine, and citrus fruits.[260]

Flavonoids and flavonoid-rich foods have marked antioxidant and anti-inflammatory activity and may reduce blood cholesterol oxidation and improve endothelial function.[261] Intakes of various flavonoids has been inversely associated with lower serum CRP concentrations in U.S. adults, even after adjustment for fruit and vegetable consumption, suggesting an important role of flavonoid-rich foods in reducing cardiovascular risk.[262]

A large prospective cohort study of almost 100,000 U.S. men and women identified a lower risk of fatal CVD with greater intake of total flavonoids. Interestingly, most of the apparent benefits of dietary flavonoids appeared with modest intakes, suggesting beneficial effects occur even with relatively small amounts of flavonoid-rich foods.[263]

Currently, there is considerable supportive evidence to suggest that increasing dietary intake of flavonoid-rich foods (e.g., apples, cocoa, soy, and tea) and, to a lesser extent purified dietary supplements, may modify biomarkers of cardiovascular risk, in particular blood pressure and endothelial function.[264]

NITRATES

Dietary nitrate has received increasing interest as a major reason for the cardiovascular benefits of vegetables-rich diets. Dietary nitrate, which is predominately found in vegetables and some fruits, plays an important role in vascular homeostasis. Nitrate is utilized in the biosynthesis of nitric oxide and as a consequence plays an important role in endothelial function, vascular relaxation, and platelet aggregation. Subsequently, nitrate may be important for the treatment and prevention of CVD.[265]

Dietary nitrate (NO_3) is absorbed rapidly in the small intestine with 100% bioavailability, once in the blood stream about 25% of the nitrate concentrates in the salivary glands where it is secreted back into the mouth and metabolized and converted by commensal bacteria on the tongue into nitrite (NO_2). The nitrite is then swallowed and absorbed directly in the stomach. Nitrite can be reduced to form nitric oxide (NO), a molecule of crucial importance for cardiovascular health.[266] Of relevance, antiseptic mouthwash can almost completely impede oral nitrite production.[267]

Nitrate is also produced in your skin in response to ultraviolet light (UVA), much like vitamin D. In fact, one experiment found that exposure to UVA light resulted in a significant reduction in systolic and diastolic blood pressure of 11% within just 30 minutes and the effects persisted for at least an hour.[268] But it is dietary source that makes the vast contribution to your daily nitrate exposure, which has been estimated to be 81–106 mg/day in the typical Western diet.[269]

Supplementation with dietary nitrate or nitrate-rich vegetables may have important cardiovascular benefits. An acute meal of nitrate-rich spinach augmented nitric oxide status, enhanced endothelial function, and lowered blood pressure in healthy men and women.[270] Using beetroot juice as a source of nitrate it was found that daily beetroot juice was able to significantly reduce blood pressure in free-living healthy adults.[271] A 10-day study of a high nitrate traditional Japanese diet increased plasma nitrite and nitrate levels and lowered diastolic blood pressure by an average of 4.5 mmHg compared to Western style diet.[272]

Increasing dietary intake of nitrate via vegetable and vegetables juices may prove to be an important consideration when constructing a heart-healthy diet. Foods that are particularly high in dietary nitrate include celery, celeriac, chervil, Chinese cabbage, cress, endive, fennel, kohlrabi, leek, lettuce, parsley, red beetroot, spinach, and rocket.[273]

PROBIOTICS/PREBIOTICS

Probiotic bacteria are increasingly found in foods including cultured milks, yogurt, functional foods, and dietary supplements. There is some evidence to suggest that probiotic bacteria may have functional cardiovascular benefits, in particular, the ability to lower LDL cholesterol. A number of human clinical studies have suggested that certain probiotic supplements or fermented milk products may favorably influence serum LDL cholesterol.[274]

In one such study, hyperlipidemic patients who revived *Lactobacillus sporogenes* for 90 days showed a 35% and 32% decrease in their LDL and total cholesterol levels, respectively.[275] There may also be benefits beyond cholesterol lowering; administration of *Lactobacillus plantarum* 299v to smokers, for example. decreased blood pressure, fibrinogen, inflammation, and oxidative stress.[276] It is important to note, however, that each probiotic strain, independent of its genus and species, has unique properties and health effects. Thus, clinical applications cannot be generalized across all probiotics, and a therapeutic strain must be selected based on proven effects.[277]

Prebiotic plant fibers may also benefit cardiovascular health via their influence on the gastrointestinal microflora. A number of potential mechanisms of prebiotics have been proposed to account for their association with CVD including improvements in body weight, glucose homeostasis, plasma lipid profile, and reductions in inflammation.[278] A clinical trial in overweight adults found that supplementation with prebiotic galactooligosaccharides was able to improve composition of the gut microbiota and reduce plasma CRP, insulin, total cholesterol, and triglyceride concentrations within 12 weeks.[279]

Interestingly, pre- and probiotics may impact cardiometabolic health via reductions in circulating endotoxin. Western dietary patterns can result in alterations in the gut microbiota that favor production of gram-negative bacterial lipopolysaccharide (endotoxin) and increase circulating levels, a phenomena that has been termed low-grade metabolic endotoxemia.[280] Low-grade metabolic endotoxemia has been associated with cardiovascular risk in a linear fashion.[385] Modulation of the gut flora with pre- and probiotics may be an important approach to reducing low-grade metabolic endotoxemia and improving cardiometabolic health.[280]

SUMMARY

Overall, there is clearly strong evidence that food and food constituents impact CVD risk and even aspects of CVD such as hypertension, dyslipidemia, and metabolic disturbance. Dietary patterns such as the Mediterranean diet and DASH diet have sufficient evidence to warrant their use in the general population with CVD prevention concerns. There is general consensus that a healthy dietary portfolio of whole, unprocessed, mainly plant-based foods, including high proportions of fruits, vegetables, legumes, nuts, whole grains, olives, as well as limited amounts of cocoa, and tea, may be helpful for addressing mechanisms related to CVD such as cholesterol, blood pressure, endothelial function, inflammation, stress response, and insulin sensitivity (see Figure 6.2). Specific delineation of amounts of these foods and their bioactives can be found in Table 6.1.

As research continues to plug the existing knowledge gaps, there will be increasing scope to tailor a unique dietary prescription for CVD prevention to an individual's genomic information, including genes, polymorphisms, and even epigenetics. Personalization of nutrition along with relevant lifestyle factors for CVD, such as physical activity, will ultimately produce the most beneficial health outcomes.

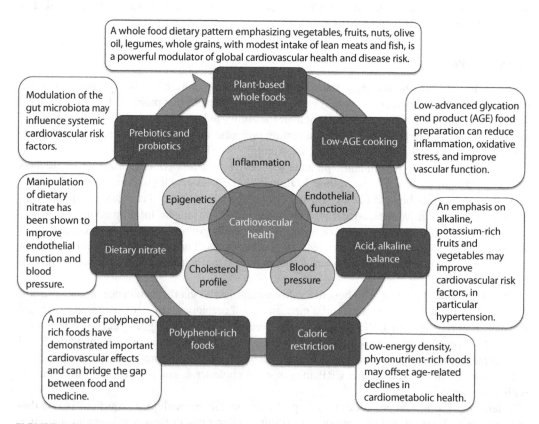

FIGURE 6.2 Healing the heart with whole foods and food bioactives. Each meal has potent acute and cumulative cardiovascular effects. A whole food, dietary pattern can influence global cardiovascular health and powerfully influence morbidity and mortality. Reduction in energy density appears to delay cardiovascular aging. Low-heat, slow-cooking methods (low-AGE cooking) may reduce the inflammatory and oxidative potential of food. And functional prebiotic-, polyphenol-, and nitrate-rich foods can be used to improve cardiometabolic health.

TABLE 6.1

Foods and Bioactives for Cardiovascular Health

Food category	Bioactive components	Effects on cardiovascular health	Guidance for consumption
Fruits and vegetables	Fruits and vegetables are abundant in fiber, vitamins, minerals, and phytochemicals, including carotenoids such as beta-carotene, zeaxanthin, lycopene, and astaxanthin. Dark leafy green vegetables contain short-chain omega-3 fatty acids and folic acid. Garlic contains allicin, the active ingredient thought to combat hypertension and high cholesterol.[281] Fruits and vegetables are also low in energy, sodium, saturated fatty acids, and TFAs. High K and Mg Increase K/Na ratio from 4 to 5:1.	Epidemiological data strongly associates fruit and vegetable intake with reduced risk for CVD.[282] Each additional portion of fruit and vegetables consumed reduces the risk of CHD by 4%, and each portion of fruit alone can reduce risk by up to 7%.[224] High carotenoid levels may also provide a two-third reduction in the risk of CHF.[257] Carotenoids are also associated with lower CRP levels,[262] reduced oxidative stress, atherosclerosis, and reduced thickening of the arterial wall.[264,228] For those with hypertension, fruits and vegetables improve endothelial function[226] and their naturally occurring nitrates reduce blood pressure.[264,265,270-272] Garlic also lowers blood pressure in those with hypertension.[283] In addition, for those with elevated total cholesterol levels, garlic consumption can lower total cholesterol and LDL cholesterol.[284]	Consume at least eight servings of a variety of fruits and vegetables per day.[229,282,285] Include plenty of dark green leafy vegetables, cruciferous vegetables, and vitamin C–rich fruits and vegetables, since higher consumption of these foods is associated with the lowest risk for heart disease.[286] To improve cholesterol levels, include garlic,[284] kiwifruit,[287] and strawberries.[288] To lower blood pressure, include vegetables with higher nitrite content such as celery, cress, chervil, lettuce, red beetroot, spinach, rocket (arugula), celeriac, Chinese cabbage, endive, fennel, kohlrabi, leek, and parsley.[273] The benefits of beetroot, orange, and garlic for lowering blood pressure, in particular, have been investigated specifically.[271,284,289] Daily consumption of antioxidant produce, including pomegranate grape, blueberry, tomato (including tomato paste), kiwi, and orange, will also enhance the vascular activity of nitric oxide, improve endothelial function, and protect against oxidative damage.[258,259,287,290,291] High levels of antioxidant carotenoids are found in yellow, orange, red, and dark green plants, and their bioavailability can be improved by cooking. Strawberries may help reduce the postmeal inflammatory response.[292]

(continued)

TABLE 6.1 (Continued)
Foods and Bioactives for Cardiovascular Health

Food category	Bioactive components	Effects on cardiovascular health	Guidance for consumption
Legumes	Legumes contain soluble dietary fiber, vegetable protein, oligosaccharides, isoflavones, phospholipids, MUFAs and PUFAs, saponins, and antioxidants.[293] Vitamins and minerals are also abundant, including folic acid, which promotes homocysteine metabolism.[293] Legumes provide high-quality vegetable protein, fiber, vitamins, and minerals in a low-GI, low-GL, and low-fat food.	Legume consumption is associated with lower overall CHD risk.[230] Isoflavones, found especially in soy beans, have antioxidant, antithrombotic, antiplatelet aggregation, and anti-inflammatory activity, as well as positive effects on blood cholesterol levels.[293] Although the benefits of soy have received much research attention,[98,99,230,282] non-soy legumes such as pinto, kidney, and lima beans, split peas, and lentils may be equally if not more beneficial.[202,293–295] For example, non-soy legumes, including pulses, have significantly favorable effects on serum lipids including total cholesterol, LDL cholesterol, triglycerides, and HDL cholesterol,[202,293] as well as blood pressure–lowering effects.[198] No less important, adequate protein and fiber, as provided by legumes and other heart-healthy whole foods, are important for satiety and adherence to a calorie-restricted diet.[61]	Consume legumes daily; at least 2/3 cup of cooked dried beans or 1/2 cup of canned beans per day.[98,293,294] Once again, variety is beneficial, including soy beans, pinto beans, kidney beans, lima beans, split peas, lentils, chickpeas (garbanzo beans), black-eyed peas, and navy beans. Legumes can be consumed instead of white potatoes and white rice, as well as served in chilis, stews, soups, and casseroles. Legume flours, such as chickpea or soy bean flour, can be included in breads and baked goods. Avoid soy-containing processed foods, however, including some processed meats, since these have been found to increase CVD risk.[282]
Fish	Fish contain long-chain omega-3 fatty acids (EPA and DHA). Some fish contain additional beneficial bioactives including ACEI,[126–128] carotenoids, and selenium.[119]	Regular fish consumption is strongly associated with cardiovascular and cerebrovascular health.[119,120–122,296] Long-chain omega-3 fatty acids appear to favorably alter lipoprotein profiles[299] and reduce inflammation markers, including as CRP[300] and Lp(a).[130] most reliably when consumed from dietary sources rather than supplements[298] and from oily fish rather than nonoily fish.[299] Other bioactive components found in fish may have cardioprotective effects, explaining some of the mixed results seen in trials using isolated supplements.[298] Fish oil intake is associated with lower incidence of hypertension,[300,301] which may be promoted by ACEI present in fish that work against the hypertension-promotion of ACEI.[120,125–128]	Consuming fish 1 to 2 times per week is associated with a 36% reduction in CVD risk,[120] and even greater protective effects are seen with intakes of 2–4 times or 5+ times per week.[121,122] Daily intake significantly lowers Lp(a) levels.[130] The highest concentrations of EPA and DHA can be found in salt water fish such as herring, salmon, sardines, and oysters.[302,303] Fish with ACEI include bonito,[125] tuna,[136] and sardines.[137] Choose a variety of fish with low mercury content, especially when consuming at higher frequency levels.[119,120] Avoid fish known to have high mercury content including shark, swordfish, king mackerel, tilefish, and albacore tuna (light tuna is a safer choice). Look for fresh sources where possible, since smoking or other preservation techniques can result in high levels of salt.[304]

Olive oil	Olive oil contains oleic acid, a MUFA, vitamin E, as well as phenols[241,182] such as oleuropein, hydroxytyrosol, and tyrosol.[305,306] One phenolic compound, secoiridoids, is unique to olives.[306]	As part of a Mediterranean diet, olive oil consumption is associated with decreased rates of CVD morbidity and mortality.[182,245] Although oleic acid was the first component investigated for heart health, other bioactives have since been recognized as beneficial. The phenolic antioxidant compounds and vitamin E found in olive oil have anti-inflammatory activity, reduce LDL oxidation,[181,182,305-308] improve HDL cholesterol,[181,313] and decrease prothrombotic effects. Olive oil has also been shown to improve endothelial function.[247,305,309] Not least, varieties rich in polyphenols appear to lower blood pressure,[246,310-312] even outshining the effects of MUFAs.[310,312]	10–30 mL (about 2–6 tbsp) of polyphenol-rich olive oil per day has been shown to exert positive effects on systolic and diastolic blood pressure, endothelial function, inflammation, and oxidative stress.[246,308,313] Interestingly, neither safflower oil nor sunflower oil, both rich in MUFAs have been found to have the same benefits.[314,315] The level of polyphenols appears to be important for enhancing the beneficial effects.[182,183,309,316,317] They are found at higher levels in unrefined, EVOOs[306] and give certain olive oils their characteristic bitter and astringent taste.
Nuts	Nuts are generally high in MUFAs and PUFAs, including omega-3 fatty acids, with a lower ratio of saturated fats. In addition, nuts contain important high-quality protein, vitamins, minerals, fiber, phytosterols, and phenolic compounds,[236] reservatrol and arginine.[282]	Strong evidence from large population studies and clinical trials supports nut consumption for cardiovascular health,[28,234,236,314,318-320] which may reduce risk by up to 35%.[282] Regular consumption also reduces the risk of sudden cardiac death,[235] which may be due to antiarrhythmic properties.[321] Various trials show that nuts can also reduce total cholesterol[117,314,322-325] and LDL cholesterol.[170,316,322,324-330] There is also some evidence that nuts can lower triglycerides[322] and apolipoprotein B.[314,325] Additional benefits include reduced inflammation and LDL oxidation,[235,236,329,330] as well as improved endothelial function, and vascular reactivity.[235,331] Although not all studies agree on the effects of nuts on blood pressure, there is some promising evidence,[295,332] which thought to be partly mediated by l-arginine present in nuts and a precursor to nitric oxide. Nitric oxide has important roles in maintaining endothelial function and reducing blood pressure via vasodilation.	The cardiovascular benefits of nut consumption increase in a dose-dependent manner,[318,323,333] with improvements seen even with consumption of 1 oz once a week.[319] However, the greatest benefits appearing when 1 oz nuts are consumed five or more times per week.[314,319] Among the varieties tested, the most potent cholesterol-lowering nuts appear to be walnuts, peanuts, and pistachios, followed closely by almonds, and then pecans and macadamia nuts.[327] Almonds and pecans have also been studied for their ability to reduce oxidized LDL,[327,329] and other nuts including Brazil nuts and hazelnuts (filberts) also confer cardiovascular benefits.[319] Nuts consumed in their unprocessed, whole form (including skins, but not shells) contain higher levels of antioxidants[236] and appear to counter the risks of weight gain[326] as well as protect against oxidation of their unsaturated fatty acids. Although uncooked nuts are preferable to maximize nutrient density,[334] roasting does preserve more antioxidants than blanching.[236,335] Avoid bleached pistachios since many of their antioxidants are destroyed by the bleaching process.[336]

(continued)

TABLE 6.1 (*Continued*)
Foods and Bioactives for Cardiovascular Health

Food category	Bioactive components	Effects on cardiovascular health	Guidance for consumption
Whole grains	Soluble and insoluble fiber, vitamins, minerals, antioxidants, phytosterols, and other phytochemicals.[231,337]	Whole grain consumption is associated with lower CVD mortality, an effect that is not found by consuming refined grains.[338–340] Cereal fiber found in whole grains may reduce CVD risk even more than fruit and vegetable fibers.[197] Consumption of whole grains is associated with lower levels of total cholesterol and LDL cholesterol,[201,282,341–343] as well as with the lowest BMI, weight, and waist circumference.[341,342] Whole grains can also reduce inflammation and oxidative stress[199,200,231,233] as well as lower blood pressure.[340,201]	At least three servings per day should be consumed to reduce the risk for CVD.[201,231,232] Aim to include grains with soluble fiber such as oats, since soluble fiber is found to have greater effects on reducing blood pressure.[198] Oats and barley also contain a specific form of fiber, β-glucan, which has cholesterol-lowering properties.[282,342–346]
Flaxseed	Short-chain omega-3 fatty acids (α-linolenic acid), lignans, as well as soluble and insoluble fibers.	Flaxseeds address dyslipidemia by lowering total cholesterol, LDL cholesterol,[347–350] and the LDL:HDL ratio.[171] This effect is thought to be imparted by their lignans and fiber content.[349,171] Flaxseeds may also reduce triglycerides and apolipoprotein B, although the evidence is less clear.[349,350] Some studies have also found a beneficial effect on blood pressure, including a large, ongoing prospective study.[173,332] Additional cardioprotective phytoestrogens are produced from the flaxseed lignans by bacteria in the human gut.[353,354] The anti-inflammatory effects of flaxseed[172,353] are thought to originate from short-chain omega-3 fatty acids, which can be partly converted in the body into long-chain omega-3 fatty acids, and then integrated into cellular membranes where their anti-inflammatory activity can be carried out.[172]	To reduce cholesterol levels, choose whole or ground flaxseed or lignans,[353] since flaxseed oil lacks the fiber and usually also the lignans that provide the desired effect.[348,354] Mixing the flax with liquid to dissolve the viscous fiber may be of additional benefit.[347] Flaxseed oil may still be useful, however, for its anti-inflammatory omega-3 content.[354] Although clinical trials have used varying amounts of flaxseed, it appears that 1–4 tbsp of ground flaxseed per day may be enough to generate positive effects on cholesterol, blood pressure, and other markers associated with cardiovascular disease.[350]

Cocoa	The benefits of cocoa consumption are thought to be derived from its flavonols.[247]	Multiple population studies have shown an inverse association between cocoa consumption and cardiovascular mortality and morbidity.[247,248,355] Clinical trials have also shown that cocoa can reduce total cholesterol and LDL cholesterol,[356] as well as improve flow-mediated dilation[357] and modestly reduce blood pressure.[247,357–360] Cocoa appears to increase nitric oxide levels, thereby improving endothelial function and flow-mediated dilation.[247] An inverse association between consumption of cocoa and dark chocolate, and hypertension has also been noted.[247] Potent antioxidant and antiplatelet aggregation activity may also contribute to the cardiovascular benefits.[247]	Small quantities of dark chocolate or cocoa consumed daily are the best choice due to its high caloric content.[282,357] The flavonol content of cocoa is reduced by processing, including fermentation and roasting.[247] Raw cocoa is, therefore, an option that maintains higher flavonol levels. Dark chocolate is also a better choice than milk or white chocolate, which have the lowest flavonol levels and have not been found to have the same benefits.[247,361]
Tea	Polyphenols, the most studied of which are the catechins, in particular epigallocatechin gallate, found especially in green tea.	Moderate tea consumption is associated with a lower risk of CVD in epidemiological studies.[362–365] Studies have shown that black tea and green tea can decrease blood pressure[252,366] and blood pressure variability.[367] A cholesterol-lowering effect has also been found for green tea[357,366,368,369] and possibly also black tea.[366] Green tea's hypocholesterolemic effects are thought to be achieved by increasing the excretion of cholesterol-rich bile acid.[370] In addition, the catechins found in teas have antioxidant activity, which may protect against LDL oxidation.[369] These components have also been found to improve endothelial function by increasing nitric oxide bioavailability and inhibiting reactive oxygen species.[369,370] They may also inhibit smooth muscle proliferation in the vascular walls.[370]	Up to 3 cups of tea per day have been found to deliver cardiovascular benefits.[252,367] More is not necessarily better.[273] In fact, consuming 5 cups/day of black or green tea may actually increase blood pressure.[372] Avoid adding bovine milk or soy milk, since this may counteract the vascular benefits.[373,374] Although black tea has been found to deliver benefits, green tea contains more antioxidant activity, since black tea catechins are lost during its more extensive processing.[375] In addition, there is evidence that green tea is more effective at improving lipid profiles and reducing CVD risk than black tea.[282,375] Other teas such as Redbush (rooibos) tea may also be considered. Redbush tea has been found to improve lipid profiles and antioxidant status[376] and may also inhibit angiotensin–converting enzyme, thereby favorably affecting blood pressure.[377]

Note: Diets that provide known cardioprotective and therapeutic effects are rich in plant foods, such as vegetables, fruits, whole grains, legumes, nuts, and seeds. Moderate consumption of fish, olive oil, cocoa, and tea has also shown benefits. These fundamental principles share many of the characteristics of the Mediterranean diet and the DASH recommendations, and traditional diets such as that of the Okinawans, who have unusually low rates of chronic disease, including cardiovascular conditions. In addition, calorie restriction, such as practiced by the Okinawans and food preparation techniques are increasingly realized as important potential influencers of cardiovascular health. This guide is intended to bridge the gap between typical recommended intakes of nutrients and calories, and practical advice for implementing dietary changes, recognizing that people eat food first, not nutrients.

ACKNOWLEDGMENT

Thanks to Romilly Hodges, who compiled the information found in Table 6.1.

BIBLIOGRAPHY

Bernstein AM, Pan A, Rexrode KM, et al. Dietary protein sources and the risk of stroke in men and women. *Stroke* 2012;43(3):637–644.

Bernstein AM, Sun Q, Hu FB, Stampfer MJ, Manson JE, Willett WC. Major dietary protein sources and risk of coronary heart disease in women. *Circulation* 2010;122(9):876–883.

Burdge GC, Hoilea SP, Lillycrop KA. Epigenetics: Are there implications for personalised nutrition? *Curr Opin Clin Nutr Metab Care* 2012;15:442–447.

de Oliveira Otto MC, Mozaffarian D, Kromhout D, et al. A high intake of industrial or ruminant trans fatty acids does not affect the plasma proteome in healthy men. *Proteomics* 2011;11(19):3928–3934.

German JB, Gibson RA, Krauss RM, et al. A reappraisal of the impact of dairy foods and milk fat on cardiovascular disease risk. *Eur J Nutr* 2009;48(4):191–203.

Görman U, Mathers JC, Grimaldi KA, Ahlgren J, Nordström K. Do we know enough? A scientific and ethical analysis of the basis for genetic-based personalized nutrition. *Genes Nutr* 2013;8(4):373–381.

Lenfant C. Prospects of personalized medicine in cardiovascular diseases. *Metabolism* 2013;62(Suppl 1):S6–S10.

Mann J. Dietary carbohydrate: Relationship to cardiovascular disease and disorders of carbohydrate metabolism. *Eur J Clin Nutr* 2007;61(suppl 1):S100–S111.

Miller MA, McTernan PG, Harte AL, et al. Ethnic and sex differences in circulating endotoxin levels: A novel marker of atherosclerotic and cardiovascular risk in a British multi-ethnic population. *Atherosclerosis* 2009;203(2):494–502.

Razquin C, Martinez JA, Martinez-Gonzalez MA, Fernández-Crehuet J, Santos JM, Marti A. A Mediterranean diet rich in virgin olive oil may reverse the effects of the -174G/C IL6 gene variant on 3-year body weight change. *Mol Nutr Food Res* 2010;54(suppl 1):S75–S82.

Robinson LE, Buchholz AC, Mazurak VC. Inflammation, obesity, and fatty acid metabolism: Influence of n-3 polyunsaturated fatty acids on factors contributing to metabolic syndrome. *Appl Physiol Nutr Metab* 2007;32(6):1008–1024.

Schwingshackl L, Hoffmann G. Monounsaturated fatty acids and risk of cardiovascular disease: Synopsis of the evidence available from systematic reviews and meta-analyses. *Nutrients* 2012;4(12):1989–2007.

REFERENCES

1. The Emerging Risk Factors Collaboration. Diabetes mellitus, fasting blood glucose concentration, and risk of vascular disease: A collaborative meta-analysis of 102 prospective studies. *Lancet* 2010;375(9733):2215–2222.

2. Badawi A, Klip A, Haddad P, et al. Type 2 diabetes mellitus and inflammation: Prospects for biomarkers of risk and nutritional intervention. *Diabetes Metab Syndr Obes* 2010;3:173–186.

3. Minich DM, Bland JS. Personalized lifestyle medicine: Relevance for nutrition and lifestyle recommendations. *Scientific World Journal* 2013;2013:129841.

4. Svetkey LP, Harris EL, Martin E, et al. Modulation of the BP response to diet by genes in the renin-angiotensin system and the adrenergic nervous system. *Am J Hypertens* 2011;24(2):209–217.

5. Yusuf S, Hawken S, Ounpuu S, et al. Effect of potentially modifiable risk factors associated with myocardial infarction in 52 countries (the INTERHEART study): Case-control study. *Lancet* 2004;364(9438):937–952.

6. Tucker KL. Dietary patterns, approaches, and multicultural perspective. *Appl Physiol Nutr Meta* 2010 Apr;35(2):211–8.

7. Jacobs DR Jr, Steffen LM. Nutrients, foods, and dietary patterns as exposures in research: A framework for food synergy. *Am J Clin Nutr* 2003 Sep;78(3 Suppl):508S–513S.

8. Jacobs DR, Tapsell LC. Food synergy: The key to a healthy diet. *Proc Nutr Soc* 2013;14:1–7.

9. Mozaffarian D, Ludwig DS. Dietary guidelines in the 21st century—A time for food. *JAMA* 2010 Aug 11;304(6):681–2.

10. Wirfält E, Drake I, Wallström P. What do review papers conclude about food and dietary patterns? *Food Nutr Res* 2013;57.

11. Jacques PF, Tucker KL. Are dietary patterns useful for understanding the role of diet in chronic disease? *Am J Clin Nutr* 2001 Jan;73(1):1–2.

12. Olinto MT, Gigante DP, Horta B, Silveira V, Oliveira I, Willett W. Major dietary patterns and cardiovascular risk factors among young Brazilian adults. *Eur J Nutr* 2012 Apr;51(3):281–91. doi: 10.1007/s00394-011-0213-4.

13. Sadakane A, Tsutsumi A, Gotoh T, Ishikawa S, Ojima T, Kario K, Nakamura Y, Kayaba K. Dietary patterns and levels of blood pressure and serum lipids in a Japanese population. *J Epidemiol* 2008;18(2):58–67.

14. Paradis AM, Godin G, Pérusse L, Vohl MC. Associations between dietary patterns and obesity phenotypes. *Int J Obes* (Lond.) 2009 Dec;33(12):1419–26.

15. Fung TT, Rimm EB, Spiegelman D, Rifai N, Tofler GH, Willett WC, Hu FB. Association between dietary patterns and plasma biomarkers of obesity and cardiovascular disease risk. *Am J Clin Nutr* 2001 Jan;73(1):61–7.

16. Lockheart MS, Steffen LM, Rebnord HM, Fimreite RL, Ringstad J, Thelle DS, Pedersen JI, Jacobs DR Jr. Dietary patterns, food groups and myocardial infarction: A case-control study. *Br J Nutr* 2007 Aug;98(2):380–7.

17. Sherzai A, Heim LT, Boothby C, Sherzai AD. Stroke, food groups, and dietary patterns: A systematic review. *Nutr Rev* 2012 Aug;70(8):423–35.

18. Millen BE, Quatromoni PA, Nam BH, O'Horo CE, Polak JF, D'Agostino RB. Dietary patterns and the odds of carotid atherosclerosis in women: The Framingham Nutrition Studies. *Prev Med* 2002 Dec;35(6):540–7.

19. Brunner EJ, Mosdøl A, Witte DR, Martikainen P, Stafford M, Shipley MJ, Marmot MG. Dietary patterns and 15-y risks of major coronary events, diabetes, and mortality. *Am J Clin Nutr* 2008 May;87(5):1414–21.

20. Heidemann C, Schulze MB, Franco OH, van Dam RM, Mantzoros CS, Hu FB. Dietary patterns and risk of mortality from cardiovascular disease, cancer, and all causes in a prospective cohort of women. *Circulation* 2008 Jul 15;118(3):230–7.

21. Simopoulos AP. The Mediterranean diets: What is so special about the diet of Greece? The scientific evidence. *J Nutr* 2001 Nov;131(11 Suppl):3065S–73S.

22. Mente A, de Koning L, Shannon HS, Anand SS. A systematic review of the evidence supporting a causal link between dietary factors and coronary heart disease. *Arch Intern Med* 2009 Apr 13;169(7):659–69.

23. Bach-Faig A, Berry EM, Lairon D, Reguant J, Trichopoulou A, Dernini S, Medina FX, Battino M, Belahsen R, Miranda G, Serra-Majem L; Mediterranean Diet Foundation Expert Group. Mediterranean diet pyramid today. Science and cultural updates. *Public Health Nutr* 2011 Dec;14(12A):2274–84.

24. Sofi F, Abbate R, Gensini GF, Casini A. Accruing evidence on benefits of adherence to the Mediterranean diet on health: An updated systematic review and meta-analysis. *Am J Clin Nutr* 2010 Nov;92(5):1189–96.

25. Gardener H, Wright CB, Gu Y, Demmer RT, Boden-Albala B, et al. Mediterranean-style diet and risk of ischemic stroke, myocardial infarction, and vascular death: The Northern Manhattan Study. *Am J Clin Nutr* 2011;94: 1458–1464.

26. Hoevenaar-Blom MP, Nooyens AC, Kromhout D, Spijkerman AM, Beulens JW, van der Schouw YT, Bueno-de-Mesquita B, Verschuren WM. Mediterranean style diet and 12-year incidence of cardiovascular diseases: The EPIC-NL cohort study. *PLoS One* 2012;7(9):e45458. doi: 10.1371/journal.pone.0045458.

27. Nordmann AJ, Suter-Zimmermann K, Bucher HC, Shai I, Tuttle KR, Estruch R, Briel M. Meta-analysis comparing Mediterranean to low-fat diets for modification of cardiovascular risk factors. *Am J Med* 2011 Sep;124(9):841–51.

28. Estruch R, Ros E, Salas-Salvadó J, et al. Primary prevention of cardiovascular disease with a Mediterranean diet. *N Engl J Med* 2013;368(14):1279–1290.

29. de Lorgeril M, Renaud S, Mamelle N, Salen P, Martin J-L, Monjaud I, Guidollet J, Touboul P, Delaye J. Mediterranean alpha-linolenic acid-rich diet in secondary prevention of coronary heart disease. *Lancet* 1994;143:1454–1459

30. de Lorgeril M, Salen P, Martin JL, Monjaud I, Delaye J, Mamelle N. Mediterranean diet, traditional risk factors, and the rate of cardiovascular complications after myocardial infarction: Final report of the Lyon Diet Heart Study. *Circulation* 1999 Feb 16;99(6):779–85.

31. Champagne CM. Dietary interventions on blood pressure: The Dietary Approaches to Stop Hypertension (DASH) trials. *Nutr Rev* 2006 Feb;64(2 Pt 2):S53–6.

32. Karanja N, Erlinger TP, Pao-Hwa L, Miller ER III, Bray GA. The DASH diet for high blood pressure: From clinical trial to dinner table. *Cleve Clin J Med* 2004 Sep;71(9):745–53.
33. National Heart, Lung, and Blood Institute (NHLBI). *Your Guide to Lowering Your Blood Pressure with DASH* 2006; Washington, DC: U.S. Dept. of Health and Human Services, National Institutes of Health, National Heart, Lung, and Blood Institute.
34. Appel LJ, Moore TJ, Obarzanek E, Vollmer WM, Svetkey LP, Sacks FM, Bray GA, Vogt TM, Cutler JA, Windhauser MM, Lin PH, Karanja N. A clinical trial of the effects of dietary patterns on blood pressure. DASH Collaborative Research Group. *N Engl J Med* 1997 Apr 17;336(16):1117–24.
35. Sacks FM, Svetkey LP, Vollmer WM, Appel LJ, Bray GA, Harsha D, Obarzanek E, Conlin PR, Miller ER III, Simons-Morton DG, Karanja N, Lin PH; DASH-Sodium Collaborative Research Group. Effects on blood pressure of reduced dietary sodium and the Dietary Approaches to Stop Hypertension (DASH) diet. DASH-Sodium Collaborative Research Group. *N Engl J Med* 2001 Jan 4;344(1):3–10.
36. Appel LJ, Champagne CM, Harsha DW, Cooper LS, Obarzanek E, Elmer PJ, Stevens VJ, Vollmer WM, Lin PH, Svetkey LP, Stedman SW, Young DR; Writing Group of the PREMIER Collaborative Research Group. Effects of comprehensive lifestyle modification on blood pressure control: Main results of the PREMIER clinical trial. *JAMA* 2003 Apr 23–30;289(16):2083–93.
37. Chen ST, Maruthur NM, Appel LJ. The effect of dietary patterns on estimated coronary heart disease risk: Results from the Dietary Approaches to Stop Hypertension (DASH) trial. *Circ Cardiovasc Qual Outcomes* 2010 Sep;3(5):484–9.
38. Fung TT, Chiuve SE, McCullough ML, Rexrode KM, Logroscino G, Hu FB. Adherence to a DASH-style diet and risk of coronary heart disease and stroke in women. *Arch Intern Med* 2008 Apr 14; 168(7):713–20.
39. Levitan EB, Wolk A, Mittleman MA. Relation of consistency with the dietary approaches to stop hypertension diet and incidence of heart failure in men aged 45 to 79 years. *Am J Cardiol* 2009 Nov 15;104(10):1416–20.
40. Parikh A, Lipsitz SR, Natarajan S. Association between a DASH-like diet and mortality in adults with hypertension: Findings from a population-based follow-up study. *Am J Hypertens* 2009 Apr;22(4):409–16.
41. Folsom AR, Parker ED, Harnack LJ. Degree of concordance with DASH diet guidelines and incidence of hypertension and fatal cardiovascular disease. *Am J Hypertens* 2007 Mar;20(3):225–32.
42. Fitzgerald KC, Chiuve SE, Buring JE, Ridker PM, Glynn RJ. Comparison of associations of adherence to a Dietary Approaches to Stop Hypertension (DASH)-style diet with risks of cardiovascular disease and venous thromboembolism. *J Thromb Haemost* 2012 Feb;10(2):189–98.
43. Blumenthal JA, Babyak MA, Hinderliter A, Watkins LL, Craighead L, Lin PH, Caccia C, Johnson J, Waugh R, Sherwood A. Effects of the DASH diet alone and in combination with exercise and weight loss on blood pressure and cardiovascular biomarkers in men and women with high blood pressure: The ENCORE study. *Arch Intern Med* 2010 Jan 25;170(2):126–35
44. Obarzanek E, Sacks FM, Vollmer WM, Bray GA, Miller ER III, Lin PH, Karanja NM, Most-Windhauser MM, Moore TJ, Swain JF, Bales CW, Proschan MA; DASH Research Group. Effects on blood lipids of a blood pressure-lowering diet: The Dietary Approaches to Stop Hypertension (DASH) Trial. *Am J Clin Nutr* 2001 Jul;74(1):80–9.
45. Appel LJ, Miller ER III, Jee SH, Stolzenberg-Solomon R, Lin PH, Erlinger T, Nadeau MR, Selhub J. Effect of dietary patterns on serum homocysteine: Results of a randomized, controlled feeding study. *Circulation* 2000 Aug 22;102(8):852–7.
46. Sun B, Williams JS, Svetkey LP, et al. Beta2-adrenergic receptor genotype affects the renin-angiotensin-aldosterone system response to the Dietary Approaches to Stop Hypertension (DASH) dietary pattern. *Am J Clin Nutr* 2010;92(2):444–449.
47. Svetkey LP, Chen YT, McKeown SP, et al. Preliminary evidence of linkage of salt sensitivity in black Americans at the β_2-adrenergic receptor locus. *Hypertension* 1997;29:918–922.
48. Al-Solaiman Y, Jesri A, Zhao Y, et al. Low-sodium DASH reduces oxidative stress and improves vascular function in salt-sensitive humans. *J Hum Hypertens* 2009;23(12):826–835.
49. Omodei D, Fontana L. Calorie restriction and prevention of age-associated chronic disease. *FEBS Lett* 2011 Jun 6;585(11):1537–42.
50. Fontana L. The scientific basis of caloric restriction leading to longer life. *Curr Opin Gastroenterol* 2009 Mar;25(2):144–50.
51. Weiss EP, Fontana L. Caloric restriction: Powerful protection for the aging heart and vasculature. *Am J Physiol Heart Circ Physiol* 2011 Oct;301(4):H1205–19.

52. Brown JE, Mosley M, Aldred S. Intermittent fasting: A dietary intervention for prevention of diabetes and cardiovascular disease? *Br J Diabetes Vasc* 2013;13(2):68–72.
53. Suzuki M, Wilcox BJ, Wilcox CD. Implications from and for food cultures for cardiovascular disease: Longevity. *Asia Pac J Clin Nutr* 2001;10(2):165–71.
54. Willcox BJ, Willcox DC, Todoriki H, Fujiyoshi A, Yano K, He Q, Curb JD, Suzuki M. Caloric restriction, the traditional Okinawan diet, and healthy aging: The diet of the world's longest-lived people and its potential impact on morbidity and life span. *Ann N Y Acad Sci* 2007 Oct;1114:434–55.
55. Willcox DC, Willcox BJ, Todoriki H, Suzuki M. The Okinawan diet: Health implications of a low-calorie, nutrient-dense, antioxidant-rich dietary pattern low in glycemic load. *J Am Coll Nutr* 2009 Aug;28 Suppl:500S–516S.
56. Holloszy JO, Fontana L. Calorie restriction in humans: An update. *Exp. Gerontol* 2007;42:709–712.
57. Varady KA, Hellerstein MK. Alternate-day fasting and chronic disease prevention: A review of human and animal trials. *Am J Clin Nutr* 2007;86(1):7–13.
58. Varady KA, Hudak CS, Hellerstein MK. Modified alternate-day fasting and cardioprotection: Relation to adipose tissue dynamics and dietary fat intake. *Metabolism* 2009;58(6):803–811.
59. Varady KA, Bhutani S, Church EC, et al. Short-term modified alternate-day fasting: A novel dietary strategy for weight loss and cardioprotection in obese adults. *Am J Clin Nutr* 2009;90(5):1138–1143.
60. Varady KA, Bhutani S, Klempel MC, et al. Alternate day fasting for weight loss in normal weight and overweight subjects: A randomized controlled trial. *Nutr J* 2013;12(1):146.
61. Rickman AD, Williamson DA, Martin CK, et al. The CALERIE Study: Design and methods of an innovative 25% caloric restriction intervention. *Contemp Clin Trials* 2011;32(6):874–881.
62. Uribarri J, Woodruff S, Goodman S, Cai W, Chen X, Pyzik R, Yong A, Striker GE, Vlassara H. Advanced glycation end products in foods and a practical guide to their reduction in the diet. *J Am Diet Assoc* 2010 Jun;110(6):911–16.e12.
63. Lin RY, Choudhury RP, Cai W, Lu M, Fallon JT, Fisher EA, Vlassara H. Dietary glycotoxins promote diabetic atherosclerosis in apolipoprotein E-deficient mice. *Atherosclerosis* 2003 Jun;168(2):213–20.
64. Negrean M, Stirban A, Stratmann B, Gawlowski T, Horstmann T, Götting C, Kleesiek K, Mueller-Roesel M, Koschinsky T, Uribarri J, Vlassara H, Tschoepe D. Effects of low- and high-advanced glycation endproduct meals on macro- and microvascular endothelial function and oxidative stress in patients with type 2 diabetes mellitus. *Am J Clin Nutr* 2007 May;85(5):1236–43.
65. Birlouez-Aragon I, Saavedra G, Tessier FJ, Galinier A, Ait-Ameur L, Lacoste F, Niamba CN, Alt N, Somoza V, Lecerf JM. A diet based on high-heat-treated foods promotes risk factors for diabetes mellitus and cardiovascular diseases. *Am J Clin Nutr* 2010 May;91(5):1220–6.
66. Luévano-Contreras C, Garay-Sevilla ME, Wrobel K, Malacara JM, Wrobel K. Dietary advanced glycation end products restriction diminishes inflammation markers and oxidative stress in patients with type 2 diabetes mellitus. *J Clin Biochem Nutr* 2013 Jan;52(1):22–6.
67. Goldberg T, Cai W, Peppa M, Dardaine V, Baliga BS, Uribarri J, Vlassara H. Advanced glycoxidation end products in commonly consumed foods. *J Am Diet Assoc* 2004 Aug;104(8):1287–91.
68. Frassetto L, Morris RC Jr., Sellmeyer DE, Todd K, Sebastian A. Diet, evolution and aging—The pathophysiologic effects of the post-agricultural inversion of the potassium-to-sodium and base-to-chloride ratios in the human diet. *Eur J Nutr* 2001 Oct;40(5):200–13.
69. Remer T, Manz F. Potential renal acid load of foods and its influence on urine pH. *J Am Diet Assoc* 1995 Jul;95(7):791–7.
70. Welch AA, Mulligan A, Bingham SA, Khaw KT. Urine pH is an indicator of dietary acid-base load, fruit and vegetables and meat intakes: Results from the European Prospective Investigation into Cancer and Nutrition (EPIC)–Norfolk population study. *Br J Nutr* 2008 Jun;99(6):1335–43.
71. Murakami K, Sasaki S, Takahashi Y, Uenishi K; Japan Dietetic Students' Study for Nutrition and Biomarkers Group. Association between dietary acid-base load and cardiometabolic risk factors in young Japanese women. *Br J Nutr* 2008 Sep;100(3):642–51.
72. Zhang L, Curhan GC, Forman JP. Diet-dependent net acid load and risk of incident hypertension in United States women. *Hypertension* 2009 Oct;54(4):751–5.
73. Engberink MF, Bakker SJ, Brink EJ, van Baak MA, van Rooij FJ, Hofman A, Witteman JC, Geleijnse JM. Dietary acid load and risk of hypertension: The Rotterdam Study. *Am J Clin Nutr* 2012 Jun;95(6):1438–44.
74. Souto G, Donapetry C, Calviño J, Adeva MM. Metabolic acidosis-induced insulin resistance and cardiovascular risk. *Metab Syndr Relat Disord* 2011 Aug;9(4):247–53.
75. Pizzorno J, Frassetto LA, Katzinger J. Diet-induced acidosis: Is it real and clinically relevant? *Br J Nutr* 2010 Apr;103(8):1185–94.

76. Kanbara A, Miura Y, Hyogo H, Chayama K, Seyama I. Effect of urine pH changed by dietary intervention on uric acid clearance mechanism of pH-dependent excretion of urinary uric acid. *Nutr J* 2012 Jun 7;11:39.

77. Frassetto LA, Schloetter M, Mietus-Synder M, Morris RC Jr, Sebastian A. Metabolic and physiologic improvements from consuming a paleolithic, hunter-gatherer type diet. *Eur J Clin Nutr* 2009 Aug;63(8):947–55.

78. Hu FB, Stampfer MJ, Manson JE, et al. Dietary saturated fats and their food sources in relation to the risk of coronary heart disease in women. *Am J Clin Nutr* 1999;70(6):1001–1008.

79. Halton TL, Willett WC, Liu S, et al. Low-carbohydrate-diet score and the risk of coronary heart disease in women. *N Engl J Med* 2006;355(19):1991–2002.

80. Maki KC, Van Elswyk ME, Alexander DD, Rains TM, Sohn EL, McNeill S. A meta-analysis of randomized controlled trials that compare the lipid effects of beef versus poultry and/or fish consumption. *J Clin Lipidol* 2012;6(4):352–361.

81. Stamler J, Liu K, Ruth KJ, Pryer J, Greenland P. Eight-year blood pressure change in middle-aged men: Relationship to multiple nutrients. *Hypertension* 2002;39(5):1000–1006.

82. Alonso A, Beunza JJ, Bes-Rastrollo M, Pajares RM, Martínez-González MA. Vegetable protein and fiber from cereal are inversely associated with the risk of hypertension in a Spanish cohort. *Arch Med Res* 2006;37(6):778–786.

83. Elliott P, Stamler J, Dyer AR, et al. Association between protein intake and blood pressure: The INTERMAP Study. *Arch Intern Med* 2006;166(1):79–87.

84. Wang YF, Yancy WS Jr, Yu D, Champagne C, Appel LJ, Lin PH. The relationship between dietary protein intake and blood pressure: Results from the PREMIER study. *J Hum Hypertens* 2008;22(11):745–754.

85. Umesawa M, Sato S, Imano H, et al. Relations between protein intake and blood pressure in Japanese men and women: The Circulatory Risk in Communities Study (CIRCS). *Am J Clin Nutr* 2009;90(2):377–384.

86. Altorf-van der Kuil W, Engberink MF, van Rooij FJ, et al. Dietary protein and risk of hypertension in a Dutch older population: The Rotterdam study. *J Hypertens* 2010;28(12):2394–2400.

87. Rebholz CM, Friedman EE, Powers LJ, Arroyave WD, He J, Kelly TN. Dietary protein intake and blood pressure: A meta-analysis of randomized controlled trials. *Am J Epidemiol* 2012;176(suppl 7):S27–S43.

88. He J, Wofford MR, Reynolds K, et al. Effect of dietary protein supplementation on blood pressure: A randomized, controlled trial. *Circulation* 2011;124(5):589–595.

89. Altorf-van der Kuil W, Engberink MF, Vedder MM, Boer JM, Verschuren WM, Geleijnse JM. Sources of dietary protein in relation to blood pressure in a general Dutch population. *PLoS One* 2012;7(2):e30582.

90. Appel LJ, Sacks FM, Carey VJ, et al. Effects of protein, monounsaturated fat, and carbohydrate intake on blood pressure and serum lipids: Results of the Omni Heart randomized trial. *JAMA* 2005;294(19):2455–2464.

91. Altorf-van der Kuil W, Engberink MF, De Neve M, et al. Dietary amino acids and the risk of hypertension in a Dutch older population: The Rotterdam Study. *Am J Clin Nutr* 2013;97(2):403–410.

92. Tuttle KR, Milton JE, Packard DP, Shuler LA, Short RA. Dietary amino acids and blood pressure: A cohort study of patients with cardiovascular disease. *Am J Kidney Dis* 2012;59(6):803–809.

93. Hayes M, Stanton C, Slatter H, et al. Casein fermentate of lactobacillus animalis dpc6134 contains a range of novel propeptide angiotensin-converting enzyme inhibitors. *Appl Environ Microbiol* 2007;73(14):4658–4667.

94. Jauhiainen T, Ronnback M, Vapaatalo H, et al. Long-term intervention with *Lactobacillus helveticus* fermented milk reduces augmentation index in hypertensive subjects. *Eur J Clin Nutr* 2010;64(4):424–431.

95. Larsson SC, Virtamo J, Wolk A. Dietary fats and dietary cholesterol and risk of stroke in women. *Atherosclerosis* 2012;221(1):282–286.

96. Bernstein AM, Pan A, Rexrode KM, Stampfer M, Hu FB, Mozaffarian D, Willett WC. Dietary protein sources and the risk of stroke in men and women. *Stroke* 2012 Mar;43(3):637–44. doi: 10.1161/STROKEAHA.111.633404. Epub 2011 Dec 29.

97. Preis SR, Stampfer MJ, Spiegelman D, Willett WC, Rimm EB. Lack of association between dietary protein intake and risk of stroke among middle-aged men. *Am J Clin Nutr* 2010;91(1):39–45.

98. Anderson JW, Bush HM. Soy protein effects on serum lipoproteins: A quality assessment and meta-analysis of randomized, controlled studies. *J Am Coll Nutr* 2011;30(2):79–91.

99. Wofford MR, Rebholz CM, Reynolds K, et al. Effect of soy and milk protein supplementation on serum lipid levels: A randomized controlled trial. *Eur J Clin Nutr* 2012;66(4):419–425.

100. Campbell SC, Khalil DA, Payton ME, Arjmandi BH. One-year soy protein supplementation does not improve lipid profile in postmenopausal women. *Menopause* 2010;17(3):587–593.
101. Roughead ZK, Hunt JR, Johnson LK, Badger TM, Lykken GI. Controlled substitution of soy protein for meat protein: Effects on calcium retention, bone, and cardiovascular health indices in postmenopausal women. *J Clin Endocrinol Metab* 2005;90(1):181–189.
102. Hodis HN, Mack WJ, Kono N, et al. Isoflavone soy protein supplementation and atherosclerosis progression in healthy postmenopausal women: A randomized controlled trial. *Stroke* 2011; 42(11):3168–3175.
103. Tomatsu M, Shimakage A, Shinbo M, Yamada S, Takahashi S. Novel angiotensin I-converting enzyme inhibitory peptides derived from soya milk. *Food Chem* 2013;136(2):612–616.
104. Rebholz CM, Reynolds K, Wofford MR, et al. Effect of soybean protein on novel cardiovascular disease risk factors: A randomized controlled trial. *Eur J Clin Nutr* 2013;67(1):58–63.
105. Dettmer M, Alekel DL, Lasrado JA, et al. The effect of soy protein beverages on serum cell adhesion molecule concentrations in prehypertensive/stage 1 hypertensive individuals. *J Am Coll Nutr* 2012;31(2):100–110.
106. FitzGerald RJ, Murray BA, Walsh DJ. Hypotensive peptides from milk proteins. *J Nutr* 2004;134(4): 980S–988S.
107. Pins JJ, Keenan JM. Effects of whey peptides on cardiovascular disease risk factors. *J Clin Hypertens* 2006;8(11):775–782.
108. Aihara K, Kajimoto O, Takahashi R, Nakamura Y. Effect of powdered fermented milk with *Lactobacillus helveticus* on subjects with high-normal blood pressure or mild hypertension. *J Am Coll Nutr* 2005;24(4): 257–265.
109. Sousa GT, Lira FS, Rosa JC, et al. Dietary whey protein lessens several risk factors for metabolic diseases: A review. *Lipids Health Dis* 2012;11:67.
110. Berthold HK, Schulte DM, Lapointe JF, Lemieux P, Krone W, Gouni-Berthold I. The whey fermentation product malleable protein matrix decreases triglyceride concentrations in subjects with hypercholesterolemia: A randomized placebo-controlled trial. *J Dairy Sci* 2011;94(2):589–601.
111. de Aguilar-Nascimento JE, Prado Silveira BR, Dock-Nascimento DB. Early enteral nutrition with whey protein or casein in elderly patients with acute ischemic stroke: A double-blind randomized trial. *Nutrition* 2011;27(4):440–444.
112. Pal S, Ellis V. Acute effects of whey protein isolate on blood pressure, vascular function and inflammatory markers in overweight postmenopausal women. *Br J Nutr* 2011;105(10):1512–1519.
113. Tavares T, Contreras Mdel M, Amorim M, et al. Novel whey-derived peptides with inhibitory effect against angiotensin-converting enzyme: In vitro effect and stability to gastrointestinal enzymes. *Peptides* 2011;32(5):1013–1019.
114. Pins J, Keenan J. The antihypertensive effects of a hydrolyzed whey protein supplement. *Cardiovasc Drugs Ther* 2002;16(suppl):68.
115. Mortensen LS, Holmer-Jensen J, Hartvigsen ML, et al. Effects of different fractions of whey protein on postprandial lipid and hormone responses in type 2 diabetes. *Eur J Clin Nutr* 2012;66(7):799–805.
116. Esteves de Oliveira FC, PinheiroVolp AC, Alfenas RC. Impact of different protein sources in the glycemic and insulinemic responses. *Nutr Hosp* 2011;26(4):669–676.
117. Murakami I, Hosono H, Suzuki S, Kurihara J, Itagaki F, Watanabe M. Enhancement or suppression of ace inhibitory activity by a mixture of tea and Foods for Specified Health Uses (FOSHU) that are marketed as "Support For Normal Blood Pressure." *ISRN Pharm* 2011;2011:712196.
118. Petyaev IM, Dovgalevsky PY, Klochkov VA, Chalyk NE, Kyle N. Whey protein lycosome formulation improves vascular functions and plasma lipids with reduction of markers of inflammation and oxidative stress in prehypertension. *Scientific World Journal* 2012;2012:269476.
119. Park K, Mozaffarian D. Omega-3 fatty acids, mercury, and selenium in fish and the risk of cardiovascular diseases. *Curr Atheroscler Rep* 2010;12(6):414–422.
120. Mozaffarian D, Rimm EB. Fish intake, contaminants, and human health: Evaluating the risks and the benefits. *JAMA* 2006;296(15):1885–1899.
121. Li YH, Zhou CH, Pei HJ, et al. Fish consumption and incidence of heart failure: A meta-analysis of prospective cohort studies. *Chin Med J (Engl)* 2013;126(5):942–948.
122. Chowdhury R, Stevens S, Gorman D, et al. Association between fish consumption, long chain omega 3 fatty acids, and risk of cerebrovascular disease: Systematic review and meta-analysis. *BMJ* 2012; 345:e6698.
123. de Goede J, Verschuren WM, Boer JM, Kromhout D, Geleijnse JM. Gender-specific associations of marine n-3 fatty acids and fish consumption with 10-year incidence of stroke. *PLoS One* 2012;7(4):e33866.

124. Pilon G, Ruzzin J, Rioux LE, et al. Differential effects of various fish proteins in altering body weight, adiposity, inflammatory status, and insulin sensitivity in high-fat-fed rats. *Metabolism* 2011; 60(8): 1122–1130.

125. Curtis JM, Dennis D, Waddell DS, MacGillivray T, Ewart HS. Determination of angiotensin-converting enzyme inhibitory peptide Leu-Lys-Pro-Asn-Met (LKPNM) in bonito muscle hydrolysates by LC-MS/MS. *J Agric Food Chem* 2002;50(14):3919–3925.

126. Qian ZJ, Je JY, Kim SK. Antihypertensive effect of angiotensin I converting enzyme-inhibitory peptide from hydrolysates of Bigeye tuna dark muscle, Thunnusobesus. *J Agric Food Chem* 2007;55(21): 8398–8403.

127. Otani L, Ninomiya T, Murakami M, Osajima K, Kato H, Murakami T. Sardine peptide with angiotensin I-converting enzyme inhibitory activity improves glucose tolerance in stroke-prone spontaneously hypertensive rats. *Biosci Biotechnol Biochem* 2009;73(10):2203–2209.

128. Kawasaki T, Seki E, Osajima K, et al. Antihypertensive effect of valyl-tyrosine, a short chain peptide derived from sardine muscle hydrolyzate, on mild hypertensive subjects. *J Hum Hypertens* 2000;14(8):519–523.

129. Wennberg M, Tornevi A, Johansson I, Hörnell A, Norberg M, Bergdahl IA. Diet and lifestyle factors associated with fish consumption in men and women: A study of whether gender differences can result in gender-specific confounding. *Nutr J* 2012;11:101.

130. Sofi F, Fatini C, Sticchi E, et al. Fish intake and LPA 93C>T polymorphism: Gene-environment interaction in modulating lipoprotein (a) concentrations. *Atherosclerosis* 2007;195(2):e147–154.

131. Wang Y, Goodrich JM, Gillespie B, Werner R, Basu N, Franzblau A. An investigation of modifying effects of metallothionein single-nucleotide polymorphisms on the association between mercury exposure and biomarker levels. *Environ Health Perspect* 2012;120(4):530–534.

132. Schläwicke Engström K, Strömberg U, Lundh T, et al. Genetic variation in glutathione-related genes and body burden of methylmercury. *Environ Health Perspect* 2008;116(6):734–739.

133. Valera B, Dewailly E, Poirier P. Association between methylmercury and cardiovascular risk factors in a native population of Quebec (Canada): A retrospective evaluation. *Environ Res* 2013;120:102–108.

134. Valera B, Dewailly E, Poirier P. Environmental mercury exposure and blood pressure among Nunavik Inuit adults. *Hypertension* 2009;54(5):981–986.

135. Choi AL, Weihe P, Budtz-Jørgensen E, et al. Methylmercury exposure and adverse cardiovascular effects in Faroese whaling men. *Environ Health Perspect* 2009;117(3):367–372.

136. Roman HA, Walsh TL, Coull BA, et al. Evaluation of the cardiovascular effects of methylmercury exposures: Current evidence supports development of a dose-response function for regulatory benefits analysis. *Environ Health Perspect* 2011;119(5):607–614.

137. Willett WC. Dietary fats and coronary heart disease. *J Intern Med* 2012;272(1):13–24.

138. Bauman DE, Mather IH, Wall RJ, Lock AL. Major advances associated with the biosynthesis of milk. *J Dairy Sci* 2006;89(4):1235–1243.

139. Ledoux M, Juanéda P, Sébédio JL. Trans fatty acids: Definition and occurrence in foods. *Eur J Lipid Sci Technol* 2007;109(9):891–900.

140. Tasan M, Demirci M. Trans FA in sunflower oil at different steps of refining. *J Am Oil Chem Soc* 2003;80(8):825–828.

141. Lopez-Garcia E, Schulze MB, Meigs JB, et al. Consumption of trans fatty acids is related to plasma biomarkers of inflammation and endothelial dysfunction. *J Nutr* 2005;135(3):562–566.

142. van de Vijver LP, Kardinaal AF, Couet C, et al. Association between trans fatty acid intake and cardiovascular risk factors in Europe: The TRANSFAIR study. *Eur J Clin Nutr* 2000;54(2):126–135.

143. Sun Q, Ma J, Campos H, et al. A prospective study of trans fatty acids in erythrocytes and risk of coronary heart disease. *Circulation* 2007;115(14):1858–1865.

144. Estadella D, da PenhaOller do Nascimento CM, Oyama LM, Ribeiro EB, Dâmaso AR, de Piano A. Lipotoxicity: Effects of dietary saturated and transfatty acids. *Mediators Inflamm* 2013;2013:137579.

145. Mozaffarian D, Katan MB, Ascherio A, Stampfer MJ, Willett WC. Trans fatty acids and cardiovascular disease. *N Engl J Med* 2006;354(15):1601–1613.

146. Wymann MP, Schneiter R. Lipid signalling in disease. *Nat Rev Mol Cell Biol* 2008;9(2):162–176.

147. doNascimento CMO, Ribeiro EB, Oyama LM. Metabolism and secretory function of white adipose tissue: Effect of dietary fat. *Anais da Academia Brasileira de Ciencias* 2009;81(3):453–466.

148. Angelieri CT, Barros CR, Siqueira-Catania A, Ferreira SR. Trans fatty acid intake is associated with insulin sensitivity but independently of inflammation. *Braz J Med Biol Res* 2012;45(7):625–631.

149. Collison KS, Zaidi MZ, Maqbool Z, et al. Sex-dimorphism in cardiac nutrigenomics: Effect of trans fat and/or monosodium glutamate consumption. *BMC Genomics* 2011;12:555.
150. Ganguly R, Pierce GN. Trans fat involvement in cardiovascular disease. *Mol Nutr Food Res* 2012;56(7):1090–1096.
151. Gebauer SK, Chardigny JM, Jakobsen MU, et al. Effects of ruminant trans fatty acids on cardiovascular disease and cancer: A comprehensive review of epidemiological, clinical, and mechanistic studies. *Adv Nutr* 2011;2(4):332–354.
152. Smit LA, Katan MB, Wanders AJ, Basu S, Brouwer IA. A high intake of trans fatty acids has little effect on markers of inflammation and oxidative stress in humans. *J Nutr* 2011;141(9):1673–1678.
153. Siri-Tarino PW, Sun Q, Hu FB, Krauss RM. Meta-analysis of prospective cohort studies evaluating the association of saturated fat with cardiovascular disease. *Am J Clin Nutr* 2010;91(3):535–546.
154. Mensink RP, Zock PL, Kester AD, Katan MB. Effects of dietary fatty acids and carbohydrates on the ratio of serum total to HDL cholesterol and on serum lipids and apolipoproteins: A meta-analysis of 60 controlled trials. *Am J Clin Nutr* 2003;77(5):1146–1155.
155. Hoenselaar R. Saturated fat and cardiovascular disease: The discrepancy between the scientific literature and dietary advice. *Nutrition* 2012;28(2):118–123.
156. Cooper AJ, Forouhi, NG, Ye, Z et al. Fruit and vegetable intake and type 2 diabetes: EPIC-InterAct prospective study and meta-analysis. *Eur J Clin Nutr* 2012 Oct; 66(10): 1082–1092.
157. Siri-Tarino PW, Sun Q, Hu FB, Krauss RM. Saturated fat, carbohydrate, and cardiovascular disease. *Am J Clin Nutr* 2010;91(3):502–509.
158. de Oliveira Otto MC, Mozaffarian D, Kromhout D, et al. Dietary intake of saturated fat by food source and incident cardiovascular disease: The multi-ethnic study of atherosclerosis. *Am J Clin Nutr* 2012;96(2):397–404.
159. Bouchard-Mercier A, Godin G, Lamarche B, Pérusse L, Vohl MC. Effects of peroxisome proliferator-activated receptors, dietary fat intakes and gene-diet interactions on peak particle diameters of low-density lipoproteins. *J Nutrigenet Nutrigenomics* 2011;4(1):36–48.
160. Delgado-Lista J, Garcia-Rios A, Perez-Martinez P, et al. Gene variations of nitric oxide synthase regulate the effects of a saturated fat rich meal on endothelial function. *Clin Nutr* 2011;30(2):234–238.
161. Anton SD, Heekin K, Simkins C, Acosta A. Differential effects of adulterated versus unadulterated forms of linoleic acid on cardiovascular health. *J Integr Med* 2013;11(1):2–10.
162. Mozaffarian D, Micha R, Wallace S. Effects on coronary heart disease of increasing polyunsaturated fat in place of saturated fat: A systematic review and meta-analysis of randomized controlled trials. *PLoS Med* 2010;7(3):e1000252.
163. Mensink RP, Katan MB. Effect of dietary fatty acids on serum lipids and lipoproteins. A meta-analysis of 27 trials. *Arterioscler Thromb* 1992;12(8):911–919.
164. Siri-Tarino PW, Sun Q, Hu FB, Krauss RM. Saturated fatty acids and risk of coronary heart disease: Modulation by replacement nutrients. *Curr Atheroscler Rep* 2010;12(6):384–390.
165. Pischon T, Hankinson SE, Hotamisligil GS, Rifai N, Willett WC, Rimm EB. Habitual of n-3 and n-6 fatty acids in relation to inflammatory markers among US men and women. *Circulation* 2003;108(2):155–160.
166. Harris W. Omega-6 and omega-3 fatty acids: Partners in prevention. *Curr Opin Clin Nutr Metab Care* 2010;13(2):125–129.
167. Lavie CJ, Milani RV, Mehra MR, Ventura HO. Omega-3 polyunsaturated fatty acids and cardiovascular diseases. *J Am Coll Cardiol* 2009;54(7):585–594.
168. Larsson SC, Virtamo J, Wolk A. Dietary protein intake and risk of stroke in women. *Atherosclerosis* 2012;224(1):247–251.
169. Torabian S, Haddad E, Cordero-MacIntyre Z, Tanzman J, Fernandez ML, Sabate J. Long-term walnut supplementation without dietary advice induces favorable serum lipid changes in free-living individuals. *Eur J Clin Nutr* 2010;64(3):274–279.
170. Banel DK, Hu FB. Effects of walnut consumption on blood lipids and other cardiovascular risk factors: A meta-analysis and systematic review. *Am J Clin Nutr* 2009;90(1):56–63.
171. Fukumitsu S, Aida K, Shimizu H, Toyoda K. Flaxseed lignan lowers blood cholesterol and decreases liver disease risk factors in moderately hypercholesterolemic men. *Nutr Res* 2010;30(7):441–446.
172. Barceló-Coblijn G, Murphy EJ, Othman R, Moghadasian MH, Kashour T, Friel JK. Flaxseed oil and fish-oil capsule consumption alters human red blood cell n-3 fatty acid composition: A multiple-dosing trial comparing 2 sources of n-3 fatty acid. *Am J Clin Nutr* 2008;88(3):801–809.
173. Paschos GK, Magkos F, Panagiotakos DB, Votteas V, Zampelas A. Dietary supplementation with flaxseed oil lowers blood pressure in dyslipidaemic patients. *Eur J Clin Nutr* 2007;61(10):1201–1206.

174. Kwak SM, Myung SK, Lee YJ, Seo HG; Korean Meta-analysis Study Group. Efficacy of omega-3 fatty acid supplements (eicosapentaenoic acid and docosahexaenoic acid) in the secondary prevention of cardiovascular disease: A meta-analysis of randomized, double-blind, placebo-controlled trials. *Arch Intern Med* 2012;172(9):686–694.

175. Massaro M, Scoditti E, Carluccio MA, Montinari MR, De Caterina R. Omega-3 fatty acids, inflammation and angiogenesis: Nutrigenomic effects as an explanation for anti-atherogenic and anti-inflammatory effects of fish and fish oils. *J Nutrigenet Nutrigenomics* 2008;1(1–2):4–23.

176. Schmidt S, Stahl F, Mutz KO, Scheper T, Hahn A, Schuchardt JP. Different gene expression profiles in normo- and dyslipidemic men after fish oil supplementation: Results from a randomized controlled trial. *Lipids Health Dis* 2012;11:105.

177. Schmidt S, Stahl F, Mutz KO, Scheper T, Hahn A, Schuchardt JP. Transcriptome-based identification of antioxidative gene expression after fish oil supplementation in normo- and dyslipidemic men. *Nutr Metab (Lond)* 2012;9(1):45.

178. Liang S, Steffen LM, Steffen BT, et al. APOE genotype modifies the association between plasma omega-3 fatty acids and plasma lipids in the Multi-Ethnic Study of Atherosclerosis (MESA). *Atherosclerosis* 2013;228(1):181–187.

179. Mattson FH, Grundy SM. Comparison of effects of dietary saturated, monounsaturated, and polyunsaturated fatty acids on plasma lipids and lipoproteins in man. *J Lipid Res* 1985;26(2):194–202.

180. Jakobsen MU, O'Reilly EJ, Heitmann BL, et al. Major types of dietary fat and risk of coronary heart disease: A pooled analysis of 11 cohort studies. *Am J Clin Nutr* 2009;89(5):1425–1432.

181. Loued S, Berrougui H, Componova P, Ikhlef S, Helal O, Khalil A. Extra-virgin olive oil consumption reduces the age-related decrease in HDL and paraoxonase 1 anti-inflammatory activities. *Br J Nutr* 2013;19:1–13.

182. Martín-Peláez S, Covas MI, Fitó M, Kušar A, Pravst I. Health effects of olive oil polyphenols: Recent advances and possibilities for the use of health claims. *Mol Nutr Food Res* 2013;57(5):760–771.

183. Camargo A, Ruano J, Fernandez JM, et al. Gene expression changes in mononuclear cells in patients with metabolic syndrome after acute intake of phenol-rich virgin olive oil. *BMC Genomics* 2010; 11:253.

184. Baum SJ, Kris-Etherton PM, Willett WC, et al. Fatty acids in cardiovascular health and disease: A comprehensive update. *J Clin Lipidol* 2012;6(3):216–234.

185. Rudel LL, Parks KS, Sawyer JK. Compared with dietary monounsaturated and saturated fat, polyunsaturated fat protects African green monkeys from coronary artery atherosclerosis. *Arterioscler Thromb Vasc Biol* 1995;15:2101–2110.

186. Ma J, Folsom AR, Lewis L, et al. Relation of plasma phospholipid and cholesterol ester fatty acid composition to carotid artery intima-media thickness: The Atherosclerosis Risk in Communities (ARIC) Study. *Am J Clin Nutr* 1997;65:551–559.

187. Degirolamo C, Shelness GS, Rudel LL. Review LDL cholesteryloleate as a predictor for atherosclerosis: Evidence from human and animal studies on dietary fat. *J Lipid Res* 2009;50(suppl):S434–S439.

188. Imamura F, Lemaitre RN, King IB, et al. Long-chain monounsaturated fatty acids and incidence of congestive heart failure in two prospective cohorts. *Circulation* 2013;127(14):1512–1521.

189. Hu T, Mills KT, Yao L, et al. Effects of low-carbohydrate diets versus low-fat diets on metabolic risk factors: A meta-analysis of randomized controlled clinical trials. *Am J Epidemiol* 2012;176(Suppl 7): S44–S54.

190. Nordmann AJ, Nordmann A, Briel M, et al. Effects of low-carbohydrate vs low-fat diets on weight loss and cardiovascular risk factors: A meta-analysis of randomized controlled trials. *Arch Intern Med* 2006;166(3):285–293.

191. Santos FL, Esteves SS, da Costa Pereira A, Yancy WS Jr, Nunes JP. Systematic review and meta-analysis of clinical trials of the effects of low carbohydrate diets on cardiovascular risk factors. *Obes Rev* 2012;13(11):1048–1066.

192. Ma XY, Liu JP, Song ZY. Glycemic load, glycemic index and risk of cardiovascular diseases: Meta-analyses of prospective studies. *Atherosclerosis* 2012;223(2):491–496.

193. Dong JY, Zhang YH, Wang P, Qin LQ. Meta-analysis of dietary glycemic load and glycemic index in relation to risk of coronary heart disease. *Am J Cardiol* 2012;109(11):1608–1613.

194. Neuhouser ML, Schwarz Y, Wang C, et al. A low-glycemic load diet reduces serum C-reactive protein and modestly increases adiponectin in overweight and obese adults. *J Nutr* 2012;142(2):369–374.

195. Kelly KR, Haus JM, Solomon TP, et al. A low-glycemic index diet and exercise intervention reduces TNF (alpha) in isolated mononuclear cells of older, obese adults. *J Nutr* 2011;141(6):1089–1094.

196. Kallio P, Kolehmainen M, Laaksonen DE, et al. Dietary carbohydrate modification induces alterations in gene expression in abdominal subcutaneous adipose tissue in persons with the metabolic syndrome: The FUNGENUT Study. *Am J Clin Nutr* 2007;85(5):1417–1427.
197. Satija A, Hu FB. Cardiovascular benefits of dietary fiber. *Curr Atheroscler Rep* 2012;14(6):505–514.
198. Lee YP, Puddey IB, Hodgson JM. Protein, fibre and blood pressure: Potential benefit of legumes. *Clin Exp Pharmacol Physiol* 2008;35(4):473–476.
199. Chuang SC, Vermeulen R, Sharabiani MT, et al. The intake of grain fibers modulates cytokine levels in blood. *Biomarkers* 2011;16(6):504–510.
200. Johansson-Persson A, Ulmius M, Cloetens L, Karhu T, Herzig KH, Onning G. A high intake of dietary fiber influences C-reactive protein and fibrinogen, but not glucose and lipid metabolism, in mildly hyper-cholesterolemic subjects. *Eur J Nutr* 2014;53(1):39–48.
201. Tighe P, Duthie G, Vaughan N, et al. Effect of increased consumption of whole-grain foods on blood pressure and other cardiovascular risk markers in healthy middle-aged persons: A randomized controlled trial. *Am J Clin Nutr* 2010;92(4):733–740.
202. Bazzano LA, Thompson AM, Tees MT, Nguyen CH, Winham DM. Non-soy legume consumption lowers cholesterol levels: A meta-analysis of randomized controlled trials. *Nutr Metab Cardiovasc Dis* 2011;21(2):94–103.
203. Larsson SC, Männistö S, Virtanen MJ, Kontto J, Albanes D, Virtamo J. Dietary fiber and fiber-rich food intake in relation to risk of stroke in male smokers. *Eur J Clin Nutr* 2009;63(8):1016–1024.
204. Bray GA. Energy and fructose from beverages sweetened with sugar or high-fructose corn syrup pose a health risk for some people. *Adv Nutr* 2013;4(2):220–225.
205. Mucci L, Santilli F, Cuccurullo C, Davì G. Cardiovascular risk and dietary sugar intake: Is the link so sweet? *Intern Emerg Med* 2012;7(4):313–322.
206. Johnson RK, Appel LJ, Brands M, et al. Dietary sugars intake and cardiovascular health: A scientific statement from the American Heart Association. *Circulation* 2009;120(11):1011–1020.
207. Sievenpiper JL, Chiavaroli L, de Souza RJ, et al. "Catalytic" doses of fructose may benefit glycaemic control without harming cardiometabolic risk factors: A small meta-analysis of randomised controlled feeding trials. *Br J Nutr* 2012;108(3):418–423.
208. Livesey G, Taylor R. Fructose consumption and consequences for glycation, plasma triacylglycerol, and body weight: Meta-analyses and meta-regression models of intervention studies. *Am J Clin Nutr* 2008;88(5):1419–1437.
209. Le MT, Lobmeyer MT, Campbell M, et al. Impact of genetic polymorphisms of SLC2A2, SLC2A5, and KHK on metabolic phenotypes in hypertensive individuals. *PLoS One* 2013;8(1):e52062.
210. Feig DI, Soletsky B, Johnson RJ. Effect of allopurinol on blood pressure of adolescents with newly diagnosed essential hypertension: A randomized trial. *JAMA* 2008;300:924–932.
211. Nguyen S, Choi HK, Lustig RH, Hsu CY. Sugar-sweetened beverages, serum uric acid, and blood pressure in adolescents. *J Pediatr* 2009;154:807–813.
212. Bremer AA, Auinger P, Byrd RS. Relationship between insulin resistance-associated metabolic parameters and anthropometric measurements with sugar-sweetened beverage intake and physical activity levels in US adolescents: Findings from the 1999–2004 National Health and Nutrition Examination Survey. *Arch Pediatr Adolesc Med* 2009;163:328–335.
213. Dhingra R, Sullivan L, Jacques PF, et al. Soft drink consumption and risk of developing cardiometabolic risk factors and the metabolic syndrome in middle-aged adults in the community. *Circulation* 2007;116(5):480–488.
214. Lê KA, Tappy L. Metabolic effects of fructose. *Curr Opin Clin Nutr Metab Care* 2006;9:469–475.
215. Stanhope KL, Schwarz JM, Keim NL, et al. Consuming fructose-sweetened, not glucose-sweetened, beverages increases visceral adiposity and lipids and decreases insulin sensitivity in overweight/obese humans. *J Clin Invest* 2009;119:1322–1334.
216. Fried SK, Rao SP. Sugars, hypertriglyceridemia, and cardiovascular disease. *Am J Clin Nutr* 2003;78:873S–880S.
217. Bantle JP, Raatz SK, Thomas W, Georgopoulos A. Effects of dietary fructose of plasma lipids in healthy subjects. *Am J Clin Nutr* 2000;72:1128–1134.
218. Chong MF, Fielding BA, Frayn KN. Mechanisms for the acute effect of fructose of postprandial lipemia. *Am J Clin Nutr* 2007;85:1511–1520.
219. Teff KL, Elliott SS, Tschöp M, et al. Dietary fructose reduces circulating insulin and leptin, attenuates postprandial suppression of ghrelin, and increases triglycerides in women. *J Clin Endocrinol Metab* 2004;89:2963–2972.

220. Jang W, Jeoung NH, Cho KH. Modified apolipoprotein (apo) A-I by artificial sweetener causes severe premature cellular senescence and atherosclerosis with impairment of functional and structural properties of apoA-I in lipid-free and lipid-bound state. *Mol Cells* 2011;31(5):461–470.

221. Ortega R. Importance of functional foods in the Mediterranean diet. *Public Health Nutr* 2006 Dec;9(8A):1136–40.

222. Hasler CM, Kundrat S, Wool D. Functional foods and cardiovascular disease. *Curr Atheroscler Rep* 2000 Nov;2(6):467–75.

223. Esfahani A, Jenkins DJ, Kendall CW. Session 4: CVD, diabetes and cancer: A dietary portfolio for management and prevention of heart disease. *Proc Nutr Soc* 2010 Feb;69(1):39–44.

224. Dauchet L, Amouyel P, Hercberg S, Dallongeville J. Fruit and vegetable consumption and risk of coronary heart disease: A meta-analysis of cohort studies. *J Nutr* 2006;136(10):2588–2593.

225. Dauchet L, Amouyel P, Hercberg S, Dallongeville J. Fruit and vegetable consumption and risk of coronary heart disease: A meta-analysis of cohort studies. *J Nutr* 2006 Oct;136(10):2588–93.

226. McCall DO, McGartland CP, McKinley MC, Patterson CC, Sharpe P, McCance DR, Young IS, Woodside JV. Dietary intake of fruits and vegetables improves microvascular function in hypertensive subjects in a dose-dependent manner *Circulation* 2009;119(16):2153–2560.

227. Flock MR, Kris-Etherton PM. Dietary Guidelines for Americans 2010: Implications for cardiovascular disease. *Curr Atheroscler Rep* 2011 Dec;13(6):499–507.

228. Holt EM, Steffen LM, Moran A, et al. Fruit and vegetable consumption and its relation to markers of inflammation and oxidative stress in adolescents. *J Am Diet Assoc* 2009;109(3):414–421.

229. Bhupathiraju SN, Tucker KL. Coronary heart disease prevention: Nutrients, foods, and dietary patterns. *Clin Chim Acta* 2011;412(17–18):1493–1514.

230. Bazzano LA, He J, Ogden LG, et al. Legume consumption and risk of coronary heart disease in US men and women: NHANES I Epidemiologic Follow-up Study. *Arch Intern Med* 2001;161(21):2573–2578.

231. Anderson JW. Whole grains protect against atherosclerotic cardiovascular disease. *Proc Nutr Soc* 2003;62(1):135–142.

232. Ye EQ, Chacko SA, Chou EL, Kugizaki M, Liu S. Greater whole-grain intake is associated with lower risk of type 2 diabetes, cardiovascular disease, and weight gain. *J Nutr* 2012;142(7):1304–1313.

233. Katcher HI, Legro RS, Kunselman AR, et al. The effects of a whole grain-enriched hypocaloric diet on cardiovascular disease risk factors in men and women with metabolic syndrome. *Am J Clin Nutr* 2008;87(1):79–90.

234. Sabaté J, Ang Y. Nuts and health outcomes: New epidemiologic evidence. *Am J Clin Nutr* 2009; 89(5):1643S–1648S.

235. Kris-Etherton PM, Hu FB, Ros E, Sabaté J. The role of tree nuts and peanuts in the prevention of coronary heart disease: Multiple potential mechanisms. *J Nutr* 2008;138(9):1746S–1751S.

236. Ros E. Health benefits of nut consumption. *Nutrients* 2010;2(7):652–682.

237. Mattes RD, Kris-Etherton PM, Foster GD. Impact of peanuts and tree nuts on body weight and healthy weight loss in adults. *J Nutr* 2008 Sep;138(9):1741S–1745S.

238. Salas-Salvadó J, Fernández-Ballart J, Ros E, Martínez-González MA, Fitó M, Estruch R, Corella D, Fiol M, Gómez-Gracia E, Arós F, Flores G, Lapetra J, Lamuela-Raventós R, Ruiz-Gutiérrez V, Bulló M, Basora J, Covas MI; PREDIMED Study Investigators. Effect of a Mediterranean diet supplemented with nuts on metabolic syndrome status: One-year results of the PREDIMED randomized trial. *Arch Intern Med* 2008 Dec 8;168(22):2449–58.

239. Guasch-Ferré M, Bulló M, Martínez-González MÁ, et al. Frequency of nut consumption and mortality risk in the PREDIMED nutrition intervention trial. *BMC Med* 2013;11:164.

240. Bao Y, Han J, Hu FB, et al. Association of nut consumption with total and cause-specific mortality. *N Engl J Med* 2013;369(21):2001–2011.

241. Rafehi H, Ververis K, Karagiannis TC. Mechanisms of action of phenolic compounds in olive. *J Diet Suppl* 2012;9(2):96–109.

242. Visioli F, Bernardini E. Extra virgin olive oil's polyphenols: Biological activities. *Curr Pharm Des* 2011;17(8):786–804.

243. Lou-Bonafonte JM, Arnal C, Navarro MA, et al. Efficacy of bioactive compounds from extra virgin olive oil to modulate atherosclerosis development. *Mol Nutr Food Res* 2012;56(7):1043–1057.

244. Bermudez B, Lopez S, Ortega A, et al. Oleic acid in olive oil: From a metabolic framework toward a clinical perspective. *Curr Pharm Des* 2011;17(8):831–843.

245. Buckland G, Mayén AL, Agudo A, et al. Olive oil intake and mortality within the Spanish population (EPIC-Spain). *Am J Clin Nutr* 2012;96(1):142–9.

246. Moreno-Luna R, Muñoz-Hernandez R, Miranda ML, et al. Olive oil polyphenols decrease blood pressure and improve endothelial function in young women with mild hypertension. *Am J Hypertens* 2012;25(12):1299–304.
247. Corti R, Flammer AJ, Hollenberg NK, Lüscher TF. Cocoa and cardiovascular health. *Circulation* 2009;119(10):1433–1441.
248. Buitrago-Lopez A, Sanderson J, Johnson L, et al. Chocolate consumption and cardiometabolic disorders: Systematic review and meta-analysis. *BMJ* 2011;343:d4488.
249. Hooper L, Summerbell CD, Thompson R, et al. Reduced or modified dietary fat for preventing cardiovascular disease. *Cochrane Database Syst Rev* 2012;5:CD002137.
250. Bøhn SK, Ward NC, Hodgson JM, Croft KD. Effects of tea and coffee on cardiovascular disease risk. *Food Funct* 2012 Jun;3(6):575–91.
251. Shen L, Song LG, Ma H, Jin CN, Wang JA, Xiang MX. Tea consumption and risk of stroke: A dose-response meta-analysis of prospective studies. *J Zhejiang Univ Sci B* 2012 Aug;13(8):652–62.
252. Hodgson JM, Puddey IB, Woodman RJ, et al. Effects of black tea on blood pressure: A randomized controlled trial. *Arch Intern Med* 2012;172(2):186–188.
253. Cornelis MC, El-Sohemy A, Kabagambe EK, et al. Coffee, CYP1A2 genotype, and risk of myocardial infarction. *JAMA* 2006;295(10):1135–1141.
254. Palatini P, Ceolotto G, Ragazzo F, et al. CYP1A2 genotype modifies the association between coffee intake and the risk of hypertension. *J Hypertens* 2009;27(8):1594–1601.
255. Giordano P, Scicchitano P, Locorotondo M, et al. Carotenoids and cardiovascular risk. *Curr Pharm Des* 2012;18(34):5577–5589.
256. Riccioni G, Speranza L, Pesce M, Cusenza S, D'Orazio N, Glade MJ. Novel phytonutrient contributors to antioxidant protection against cardiovascular disease. *Nutrition* 2012 Jun;28(6):605–10.
257. Karppi J, Kurl S, Mäkikallio TH, Ronkainen K, Laukkanen JA. Serum β-carotene concentrations and the risk of congestive heart failure in men: A population-based study. *Int J Cardiol* 2013;168(3):1841–1846.
258. Buscemi S, Rosafio G, Arcoleo G, et al. Effects of red orange juice intake on endothelial function and inflammatory markers in adult subjects with increased cardiovascular risk. *Am J Clin Nutr* 2012;95(5):1089–1095.
259. Xaplanteris P, Vlachopoulos C, Pietri P, et al. Tomato paste supplementation improves endothelial dynamics and reduces plasma total oxidative status in healthy subjects. *Nutr Res* 2012;32(5):390–394.
260. Chun OK, Chung SJ, Song WO. Estimated dietary flavonoid intake and major food sources of U.S. adults. *J Nutr* 2007 May;137(5):1244–52.
261. Middleton E Jr, Kandaswami C, Theoharides TC. The effects of plant flavonoids on mammalian cells: Implications for inflammation, heart disease, and cancer. *Pharmacol Rev* 2000 Dec;52(4):673–751.
262. Chun OK, Chung SJ, Claycombe KJ, Song WO. Serum C-reactive protein concentrations are inversely associated with dietary flavonoid intake in U.S. adults. *J Nutr* 2008;138(4):753–760.
263. McCullough ML, Peterson JJ, Patel R, Jacques PF, Shah R, Dwyer JT. Flavonoid intake and cardiovascular disease mortality in a prospective cohort of US adults. *Am J Clin Nutr* 2012 Feb;95(2):454–64.
264. Habauzit V, Morand C. Evidence for a protective effect of polyphenols-containing foods on cardiovascular health: An update for clinicians. *Ther Adv Chronic Dis* 2012;3(2):87–106.
265. Machha A, Schechter AN. Dietary nitrite and nitrate: A review of potential mechanisms of cardiovascular benefits. *Eur J Nutr* 2011;50(5):293–303.
266. Gilchrist M, Shore AC, Benjamin N. Inorganic nitrate and nitrite and control of blood pressure. *Cardiovasc Res* 2011;89(3):492–498.
267. Kapil V, Haydar SM, Pearl V, et al. Physiological role for nitrate-reducing oral bacteria in blood pressure control. *Free Radic Biol Med* 2013;55:93–100.
268. Oplander C, Volkmar CM, Paunel-Gorgulu A, et al. Whole body UVA irradiation lowers systemic blood pressure by release of nitric oxide from intracutaneous photolabile nitric oxide derivates. *Circ Res* 2009;105(10):1031–1040.
269. Ysart G, Miller P, Barrett G, Farrington D, Lawrance P, Harrison N. Dietary exposures to nitrate in the UK. *Food Addit Contam* 1999;16:521–532.
270. Bondonno CP, Yang X, Croft KD, et al. Flavonoid-rich apples and nitrate-rich spinach augment nitric oxide status and improve endothelial function in healthy men and women: A randomized controlled trial. *Free Radic Biol Med* 2012;52(1):95–102.
271. Coles LT, Clifton PM. Effect of beetroot juice on lowering blood pressure in free-living, disease-free adults: A randomized, placebo-controlled trial. *Nutr J* 2012;11:106.

272. Sobko T, Marcus C, Govoni M, Kamiya S. Dietary nitrate in Japanese traditional foods lowers diastolic blood pressure in healthy volunteers. *Nitric Oxide* 2010;22(2):136–140.

273. Hord NG, Tang Y, Bryan NS. Food sources of nitrates and nitrites: The physiologic context for potential health benefits. *Am J Clin Nutr* 2009;90(1):1–10.

274. Kumar M, Nagpal R, Kumar R, Hemalatha R, Verma V, Kumar A, Chakraborty C, Singh B, Marotta F, Jain S, Yadav H. Cholesterol-lowering probiotics as potential biotherapeutics for metabolic diseases. *Exp Diabetes Res* 2012;2012:902917.

275. Mohan JC, Arora R, Khalilullah M. Preliminary observations on effect of Lactobacillus sporogenes on serum lipid levels in hypercholesterolemic patients. *Indian J Med Res* 1990 Dec;92:431–2.

276. Naruszewicz M, Johansson ML, Zapolska-Downar D, Bukowska H. Effect of Lactobacillus plantarum 299v on cardiovascular disease risk factors in smokers. *Am J Clin Nutr* 2002 Dec;76(6):1249–55.

277. Salminen SJ, Gueimonde M, Isolauri E. Probiotics that modify disease risk. *J Nutr.* 2005 May;135(5):1294–8.

278. Mallappa RH, Rokana N, Duary RK, Panwar H, Batish VK, Grover S. Management of metabolic syndrome through probiotic and prebiotic interventions. *Indian J Endocrinol Metab* 2012 Jan;16(1):20–7.

279. Vulevic J, Juric A, Tzortzis G, Gibson GR. A mixture of trans-galactooligosaccharides reduces markers of metabolic syndrome and modulates the fecal microbiota and immune function of overweight adults. *J Nutr* 2013 Mar;143(3):324–31.

280. Cani PD, Delzenne NM. The gut microbiome as therapeutic target. *Pharmacol Ther* 2011; 130(2):202–212.

281. Ried K, Frank OR, Stocks NP, Fakler P, Sullivan T. Effect of garlic on blood pressure: A systematic review and meta-analysis. *BMC Cardiovasc Disord* 2008;8:13.

282. Eilat-Adar S, Sinai T, Yosefy C, Henkin Y. Nutritional recommendations for cardiovascular disease prevention. *Nutrients* 2013;5(9):3646–3683.

283. Reinhart KM, Coleman CI, Teevan C, Vachhani P, White CM. Effects of garlic on blood pressure in patients with and without systolic hypertension: A meta-analysis. *Ann Pharmacother* 2008;42(12):1766–1771.

284. Ried K, Toben C, Fakler P. Effect of garlic on serum lipids: An updated meta-analysis. *Nutr Rev* 2013;71(5):282–299.

285. Watz LB, Kulling SE, Möseneder J, Barth SW, Bub A. A 4-wk intervention with high intake of carotenoid-rich vegetables and fruit reduces plasma C-reactive protein in healthy, nonsmoking men. *Am J Clin Nutr* 2005;82(5):1052–1058.

286. Joshipura KJ, Hu FB, Manson JE, et al. The effect of fruit and vegetable intake on risk for coronary heart disease. *Ann Intern Med* 2001;134(12):1106–1114.

287. Chang WH, Liu JF. Effects of kiwifruit consumption on serum lipid profiles and antioxidative status in hyperlipidemic subjects. *Int J Food Sci Nutr* 2009;60(8):709–716.

288. Basu A, Fu DX, Wilkinson M. Strawberries decrease atherosclerotic markers in subjects with metabolic syndrome. *Nutr Res* 2010;30(7):462–469.

289. Morand C, Dubray C, Milenkovic D, et al. Hesperidin contributes to the vascular protective effects of orange juice: A randomized crossover study in healthy volunteers. *Am J Clin Nutr* 2011;93(1):73–80.

290. Ignarro LJ, Byrns RE, Sumi D, deNigris F, Napoli C. Pomegranate juice protects nitric oxide against oxidative destruction and enhances the biological actions of nitric oxide. *Nitric Oxide* 2006; 15(2):93–102.

291. Rodriguez-Mateos A, Rendeiro C, Bergillos-Meca T, et al. Intake and time dependence of blueberry flavonoid-induced improvements in vascular function: A randomized, controlled, double-blind, crossover intervention study with mechanistic insights into biological activity. *Am J Clin Nutr* 2013;98(5):1179–1191.

292. Ellis CL, Edirisinghe I, Kappagoda T, Burton-Freeman B. Attenuation of meal-induced inflammatory and thrombotic responses in overweight men and women after 6-week daily strawberry (Fragaria) intake. A randomized placebo-controlled trial. *J Atheroscler Thromb* 2011;18(4):318–327.

293. Anderson JW, Major AW. Pulses and lipaemia, short- and long-term effect: Potential in the prevention of cardiovascular disease. *Br J Nutr* 2002;88(suppl 3):S263–S271.

294. Winham DM, Hutchins AM, Johnston CS. Pinto bean consumption reduces biomarkers for heart disease risk. *J Am Coll Nutr* 2007;26(3):243–249.

295. Pittaway JK, Ahuja KD, Cehun M, et al. Dietary supplementation with chickpeas for at least 5 weeks results in small but significant reductions in serum total and low-density lipoprotein cholesterols in adult women and men. *Ann Nutr Metab* 2006;50(6):512–518.

296. Larsson SC, Orsini N, Wolk A. Long-chain omega-3 polyunsaturated fatty acids and risk of stroke: A meta-analysis. *Eur J Epidemiol* 2012;27(12):895–901.

297. Bulliyya G. Influence of fish consumption on the distribution of serum cholesterol in lipoprotein fractions: Comparative study among fish-consuming and non-fish-consuming populations. *Asia Pac J Clin Nutr* 2002;11(2):104–111.
298. Myhrstad MC, Retterstø LK, Telle-Hansen VH, et al. Effect of marine n-3 fatty acids on circulating inflammatory markers in healthy subjects and subjects with cardiovascular risk factors. *Inflamm Res* 2011;60(4):309–319.
299. Lankinen M, Schwab U, Erkkilä A, et al. Fatty fish intake decreases lipids related to inflammation and insulin signaling: A lipidomics approach. *PLoS One* 2009;4(4):e5258.
300. Xun P, Hou N, Daviglus M, et al. Fish oil, selenium and mercury in relation to incidence of hypertension: A 20-year follow-up study. *J Intern Med* 2011;270(2):175–186.
301. Campbell F, Dickinson HO, Critchley JA, Ford GA, Bradburn M. A systematic review of fish-oil supplements for the prevention and treatment of hypertension. *Eur J Prev Cardiol* 2013;20(1):107–120.
302. Higdon J. Essential Fatty Acids. Retrieved from http://lpi.oregonstate.edu/infocenter/othernuts/omega3fa/>.
303. Mayo Clinic. Omega-3 in fish: How eating fish helps your heart. Retrieved from http://www.mayoclinic.com/health/omega-3/HB00087.
304. Does smoked fish contain heart-healthy omega-3 fats? The Harvard Heart Letter explains. April 2011. Retrieved from http://www.health.harvard.edu/press_releases/does-smoked-fish-contain-heart-healthy-omega-3-fats
305. Perona JS, Cabello-Moruno R, Ruiz-Gutierrez V. The role of virgin olive oil components in the modulation of endothelial function. *J Nutr Biochem* 2006;17(7):429–445.
306. Tripoli E, Giammanco M, Tabacchi G, DiMajo D, Giammanco S, LaGuardia M. The phenolic compounds of olive oil: Structure, biological activity and beneficial effects on human health. *Nutr Res Rev* 2005;18(1):98–112.
307. Lucas L, Russell A, Keast R. Molecular mechanisms of inflammation. Anti-inflammatory benefits of virgin olive oil and the phenolic compound oleocanthal. *Curr Pharm Des* 2011;17(8):754–768.
308. Raederstorff D. Antioxidant activity of olive polyphenols in humans: A review. *Int J Vitam Nutr Res* 2009;79(3):152–165.
309. Ruano J, López-Miranda J, delaTorre R, et al. Intake of phenol-rich virgin olive oil improves the postprandial prothrombotic profile in hypercholesterolemic patients. *Am J Clin Nutr* 2007;86(2):341–346.
310. Ferrara LA, Raimondi AS, d'Episcopo L, Guida L, DelloRusso A, Marotta T. Olive oil and reduced need for antihypertensive medications. *Arch Intern Med* 2000;160(6):837–842.
311. Alonso A, Martínez-González MA. Olive oil consumption and reduced incidence of hypertension: The SUN study. *Lipids* 2004;39(12):1233–1238.
312. Ruíz-Gutiérrez V, Muriana FJ, Guerrero A, Cert AM, Villar J. Plasma lipids, erythrocyte membrane lipids and blood pressure of hypertensive women after ingestion of dietary oleic acid from two different sources. *J Hypertens* 1996;14(12):1483–1490.
313. Marrugat J, Covas MI, Fitó M, et al. Effects of differing phenolic content in dietary olive oils on lipids and LDL oxidation: A randomized controlled trial. *Eur J Nutr* 2004;43(3):140–147.
314. LiT Y, Brennan AM, Wedick NM, Mantzoros C, Rifai N, HuF B. Regular consumption of nuts is associated with a lower risk of cardiovascular disease in women with type 2 diabetes. *J Nutr* 2009;139(7):1333–1338.
315. Aguilera CM, Mesa MD, Ramirez-Tortosa MC, Nestares MT, Ros E, Gil A. Sunflower oil does not protect against LDL oxidation as virgin olive oil does in patients with peripheral vascular disease. *Clin Nutr* 2004;23(4):673–681.
316. Pérez-Jiménez F, Ruano J, Perez-Martinez P, Lopez-Segura F, Lopez-Miranda J. The influence of olive oil on human health: Not a question of fat alone. *Mol Nutr Food Res* 2007;51(10):1199–1208.
317. Cicerale S, Conlan XA, Sinclair AJ, Keast RS. Chemistry and health of olive oil phenolics. *Crit Rev Food Sci Nutr* 2009;49(3):218–236.
318. Blomhoff R, Carlsen MH, Andersen LF, Jacobs DR Jr. Health benefits of nuts: Potential role of antioxidants. *Br J Nutr* 2006;96(suppl 2):S52–S60.
319. Kris-Etherton PM, Zhao G, Binkoski AE, Coval SM, Etherton TD. The effects of nuts on coronary heart disease risk. *Nutr Rev* 2001;59(4):103–111.
320. O'Neil CE, Keast DR, Nicklas TA, Fulgoni VL 3rd. Nut consumption is associated with decreased health risk factors for cardiovascular disease and metabolic syndrome in U.S. adults: NHANES 1999–2004. *J Am Coll Nutr* 2011;30(6):502–510.
321. Albert CM, Gaziano JM, Willett WC, Manson JE. Nut consumption and decreased risk of sudden cardiac death in the Physicians' Health Study. *Arch Intern Med* 2002;162(12):1382–1387.

322. Sabaté J, Fraser GE, Burke K, Knutsen SF, Bennett H, Lindsted KD. Effects of walnuts on serum lipid levels and blood pressure in normal men. *N Engl J Med* 1993;328(9):603–607.
323. Sabaté J, Oda K, Ros E. Nut consumption and blood lipid levels: A pooled analysis of 25 intervention trials. *Arch Intern Med* 2010;170(9):821–827.
324. Griel AE, Cao Y, Bagshaw DD, Cifelli AM, Holub B, Kris-Etherton PM. A macadamia nut-rich diet reduces total and LDL-cholesterol in mildly hypercholesterolemic men and women. *J Nutr* 2008;138(4):761–767.
325. Sabaté J, Haddad E, Tanzman JS, Jambazian P, Rajaram S. Serum lipid response to the graduated enrichment of a Step I diet with almonds: A randomized feeding trial. *Am J Clin Nutr* 2003;77(6):1379–1384.
326. Good D, Lavie CJ, Ventura HO. Dietary intake of nuts and cardiovascular prognosis. *Ochsner J* 2009 Spring;9(1):32–36.
327. Jenkins DJ, Kendall CW, Marchie A, et al. Dose response of almonds on coronary heart disease risk factors: Blood lipids, oxidized low-density lipoproteins, lipoprotein(a), homocysteine, and pulmonary nitric oxide: A randomized, controlled, crossover trial. *Circulation* 2002;106(11):1327–1332.
328. Griel AE, Kris-Etherton PM. Tree nuts and the lipid profile: A review of clinical studies. *Br J Nutr* 2006;96(suppl 2):S68–S78.
329. Hudthagoso LC, Haddad EH, McCarthy K, Wang P, Oda K, Sabaté J. Pecans acutely increase plasma postprandial antioxidant capacity and catechins and decrease LDL oxidation in humans. *J Nutr* 2011;141(1):56–62.
330. López-Uriarte P, Bulló M, Casas-Agustench P, Babio N, Salas-Salvadó J. Nuts and oxidation: A systematic review. *Nutr Rev* 2009;67(9):497–508.
331. West SG, Krick AL, Klein LC, et al. Effects of diets high in walnuts and flax oil on hemodynamic responses to stress and vascular endothelial function. *J Am Coll Nutr* 2010;29(6):595–603.
332. Kelly JH Jr, Sabaté J. Nuts and coronary heart disease: An epidemiological perspective. *Br J Nutr* 2006;96(suppl 2):S61–S67.
333. Schmitzer V, Slatnar A, Veberic R, Stampar F, Solar A. Roasting affects phenolic composition and antioxidative activity of hazelnuts (*Corylus avellana* L.). *J Food Sci* 2011;76(1):S14–S19.
334. Garrido I, Monagas M, Gómez-Cordovés C, Bartolomé B. Polyphenols and antioxidant properties of almond skins: Influence of industrial processing. *J Food Sci* 2008;73(2):C106–C115.
335. Seeram NP, Zhang Y, Henning SM, et al. Pistachio skin phenolics are destroyed by bleaching resulting in reduced antioxidative capacities. *J Agric Food Chem* 2006;54(19):7036–7040.
336. Seal CJ. Whole grains and CVD risk. *Proc Nutr Soc* 2006;65(1):24–34.
337. Liu S, Sesso HD, Manson JE, Willett WC, Buring JE. Is intake of breakfast cereals related to total and cause-specific mortality in men? *Am J Clin Nutr* 2003;77(3):594–599.
338. Jacobs DR Jr, Gallaher DD. Whole grain intake and cardiovascular disease: A review. *Curr Atheroscler Rep* 2004;6(6):415–423.
339. Flint AJ, Hu FB, Glynn RJ, et al. Whole grains and incident hypertension in men. *Am J Clin Nutr* 2009;90(3):493–498.
340. Newby PK, Maras J, Bakun P, Muller D, Ferrucci L, Tucker KL. Intake of whole grains, refined grains, and cereal fiber measured with 7-d diet records and associations with risk factors for chronic disease. *Am J Clin Nutr* 2007;86(6):1745–1753.
341. Zhang J, Li L, Song P, et al. Randomized controlled trial of oatmeal consumption versus noodle consumption on blood lipids of urban Chinese adults with hypercholesterolemia. *Nutr J* 2012;11:54.
342. Andersson KE, Hellstrand P. Dietary oats and modulation of atherogenic pathways. *Mol Nutr Food Res* 2012;56(7):1003–1013.
343. Othman RA, Moghadasian MH, Jones PJ. Cholesterol-lowering effects of oat β-glucan. *Nutr Rev* 2011;69(6):299–309.
344. Reyna-Villasmil N, Bermúdez-Pirela V, Mengual-Moreno E, et al. Oat-derived beta-glucan significantly improves HDLC and diminishes LDLC and non-HDL cholesterol in overweight individuals with mild hypercholesterolemia. *Am J Ther* 2007;14(2):203–212.
345. Queenan KM, Stewart ML, Smith KN, et al. Concentrated oat beta-glucan, a fermentable fiber, lowers serum cholesterol in hypercholesterolemic adults in a randomized controlled trial. *Nutr J* 2007;6:6.
346. Kristensen M, Jensen MG, Aarestrup J, et al. Flaxseed dietary fibers lower cholesterol and increase fecal fat excretion, but magnitude of effect depend on food type. *Nutr Metab (Lond)* 2012;9:8.
347. Pan A, Yu D, Demark-Wahnefried W, Franco O H, Lin X. Meta-analysis of the effects of flaxseed interventions on blood lipids. *Am J Clin Nutr* 2009;90(2):288–297.

348. Bassett CM, Rodriguez-Leyva D, Pierce GN. Experimental and clinical research findings on the cardiovascular benefits of consuming flaxseed. *Appl Physiol Nutr Metab* 2009;34(5):965–974.
349. Bassett CM, Rodriguez-Leyva D, Pierce GN. Experimental and clinical research findings on the cardiovascular benefits of consuming flaxseed. *Appl Physiol Nutr Metab* 2009;34(5):965–974.
350. Wang CZ, Ma XQ, Yang DH, et al. Production of enterodiol from defatted flaxseeds through biotransformation by human intestinal bacteria. *BMC Microbiol* 2010;10:115.
351. Adolphe JL, Whiting SJ, Juurlink BH, Thorpe LU, Alcorn J. Health effects with consumption of the flax lignan secoisolariciresinol diglucoside. *Br J Nutr* 2010;103(7):929–938.
352. Faintuch J, Bortolotto LA, Marques PC, Faintuch JJ, França JI, Cecconello I. Systemic inflammation and carotid diameter in obese patients: Pilot comparative study with flaxseed powder and cassava powder. *Nutr Hosp* 2011;26(1):208–213.
353. Lucas EA, Wild RD, Hammon dLJ, et al. Flaxseed improves lipid profile without altering biomarkers of bone metabolism in postmenopausal women. *J Clin Endocrinol Metab* 2002;87(4):1527–1532.
354. vanDam RM, Naidoo N, Landberg R. Dietary flavonoids and the development of type 2 diabetes and cardiovascular diseases: Review of recent findings. *Curr Opin Lipidol* 2013;24(1):25–33.
355. Tokede OA, Gaziano JM, Djoussé L. Effects of cocoa products/dark chocolate on serum lipids: A meta-analysis. *Eur J Clin Nutr* 2011;65(8):879–886.
356. Hooper L, Kroon PA, Rimm EB, et al. Flavonoids, flavonoid-rich foods, and cardiovascular risk: A meta-analysis of randomized controlled trials. *Am J Clin Nutr* 2008;88(1):38–50.
357. Ried K, Sullivan TR, Fakler P, Frank OR, Stocks NP. Effect of cocoa on blood pressure. *Cochrane Database Syst Rev* 2012;8:CD008893.
358. Almoosawi S, Tsang C, Ostertag LM, Fyfe L, Al-Dujaili EA. Differential effect of polyphenol-rich dark chocolate on biomarkers of glucose metabolism and cardiovascular risk factors in healthy, overweight and obese subjects: A randomized clinical trial. *Food Funct* 2012;3(10):1035–1043.
359. Sarriá B, Mateos R, Sierra-Cinos JL, Goya L, García-Diz L, Bravo L. Hypotensive, hypoglycaemic and antioxidant effects of consuming a cocoa product in moderately hypercholesterolemic humans. *Food Funct* 2012;3(8):867–874.
360. Grassi D, Desideri G, Necozione S, et al. Protective effects of flavanol-rich dark chocolate on endothelial function and wave reflection during acute hyperglycemia. *Hypertension* 2012;60(3):827–832.
361. Bøhn SK, Ward NC, Hodgson JM, Croft KD. Effects of tea and coffee on cardiovascular disease risk. *Food Funct* 2012;3(6):575–591.
362. Mineharu Y, Koizumi A, Wada Y, et al. Coffee, green tea, black tea and oolong tea consumption and risk of mortality from cardiovascular disease in Japanese men and women. *J Epidemiol Community Health* 2011;65(3):230–240.
363. Kuriyama S, Shimazu T, Ohmori K, et al. Green tea consumption and mortality due to cardiovascular disease, cancer, and all causes in Japan: The Ohsaki study. *JAMA* 2006;296(10):1255–1265.
364. Nakachi K, Matsuyama S, Miyake S, Suganuma M, Imai K. Preventive effects of drinking green tea on cancer and cardiovascular disease: Epidemiological evidence for multiple targeting prevention. *Biofactors* 2000;13(1–4):49–54.
365. Hartley L, Flowers N, Holmes J, et al. Green and black tea for the primary prevention of cardiovascular disease. *Cochrane Database Syst Rev* 2013;6:CD009934.
366. Hodgson JM, Croft KD, Woodman RJ, et al. Black tea lowers the rate of blood pressure variation: A randomized controlled trial. *Am J Clin Nutr* 2013;97(5):943–950.
367. Nagao T, Hase T, Tokimitsu I. A green tea extract high in catechins reduces body fat and cardiovascular risks in humans. *Obesity* (SilverSpring) 2007;15(6):1473–1483.
368. Babu PV, Liu D. Green tea catechins and cardiovascular health: An update. *Curr Med Chem* 2008;15(18):1840–1850.
369. Basu A, Lucas EA. Mechanisms and effects of green tea on cardiovascular health. *Nutr Rev* 2007;65 (8 Pt 1):361–375.
370. DiCastelnuovo A, diGiuseppe R, Iacoviello L, deGaetano G. Consumption of cocoa, tea and coffee and risk of cardiovascular disease. *Eur J Intern Med* 2012;23(1):15–25.
371. Hodgson JM, Puddey IB, Burke V, Beilin LJ, Jordan N. Effects on blood pressure of drinking green and black tea. *J Hypertens* 1999;17(4):457–463.
372. Lorenz M, Stang K, Stang V. Vascular effects of tea are suppressed by soy milk. *Atherosclerosis* 2009;206(1):31–32.

373. Lorenz M, Jochmann N, von Krosigk A, et al. Addition of milk prevents vascular protective effects of tea. *Eur Heart J* 2007;28(2):219–223.
374. Cheng TO. All teas are not created equal: The Chinese green tea and cardiovascular health. *Int J Cardiol* 2006;108(3):301–308.
375. Marnewick JL, Rautenbach F, Venter I, et al. Effects of rooibos (*Aspalathus linearis*) on oxidative stress and biochemical parameters in adults at risk for cardiovascular disease. *J Ethnopharmacol* 2011;133(1):46–52.
376. Persson IA, Persson K, Hägg S, Andersson RG. Effects of green tea, black tea and Rooibos tea on angiotensin-converting enzyme and nitric oxide in healthy volunteers. *Public Health Nutr* 2010; 13(5):730–737.

7 Potential of Diet and Dietary Supplementation to Ameliorate the Chronic Clinical Perturbations of Metabolic Syndrome

Harry G. Preuss and Dallas Clouatre

CONTENTS

INTRODUCTION

Throughout the world, many elements comprising metabolic syndrome (MS) such as diabetes, obesity, hypertension, and dyslipidemia are becoming alarmingly common. Although many etiological factors may be involved in this situation, one hypothesis is that a well-recognized increased consumption of sugars and refined carbohydrates (CHO) such as sucrose and high fructose corn syrup (HFCS) plays a pivotal role in the increase of these unwanted entities. Overindulgence, coupled with a rapid absorption (high glycemic load) and, in some cases, excess fructose content of these foods are believed to be important contributors to insulin resistance/type 2 diabetes (IR/T2D) that may be the responsible, shared factor behind the increased incidence of obesity, hypertension, dyslipidemias, and coagulation perturbations. If this scenario is correct to any extent, then suitable lifestyle changes could be to some extent corrective. However, dietary restrictions and enhanced exercise programs are not easy alternatives for too many people. Accordingly, drugs, particularly antidiabetic drugs, have been tried as preventatives. Although drugs seem to have some benefit while in use, long-term use is somewhat limited due to their poor history of serious adverse reactions. Fortunately, many safe, inexpensive dietary supplements exist that have been shown to beneficially influence IR/T2D, and thus, may favorably influence other elements present in the MS.

To sum up, the major purpose of this chapter is to bring to light the possibility that effective and safe dietary supplements should be examined to aid in the quest to ameliorate the different elements of the MS that currently trouble individuals, especially during the aging process.

ASSOCIATION OF DIETARY SUGARS AND REFINED CARBOHYDRATES WITH METABOLIC SYNDROME

BACKGROUND

The alarming increased incidence of many chronic human maladies, especially those occurring most frequently during aging, such as glucose–insulin disturbances (IR/T2D), overweight/obesity, hypertension, and dyslipidemia (hypertriglyceridemia and low circulating levels of high-density lipoprotein cholesterol [HDL-C]) presents a significant health problem for the United States as well as countries throughout the world.[1-6] These prominent chronic disorders along with other perturbations, such as a prothrombic state caused by increased levels of fibrinogen/plasminogen activator inhibitor in the blood and a high proinflammatory state indicated by elevated C-reactive protein in the blood, are commonly lumped together as the "metabolic syndrome (MS)" because of their repeated association[7,8] (see Table 7.1). In the past, this collection of pathological conditions was also referred to as "syndrome X."[9,10]

In addition to the physical harm caused by MS, the monetary costs stress personal and national financial reserves. A good estimate regarding the overall adult population in the United States toward the end of the first decade of the twenty-first century is that 8.3% were diabetic,[11] 34.9% were obese,[12] 18%–32%—depending on age—were hypertensive,[5] and overall 31% possessed high circulating triglyceride levels.[6] Unfortunately, none of these approximations have shown a noticeable downward movement; instead, most reliable observers believe the trends may be increasing.

PATHOGENESIS

Because of the frequent common occurrence among components of the syndrome, many believe that a shared underlying pathogenesis exists, at least for many of the cases. The perturbation most widely favored as underlying the development of the many components of the MS is IR.[9,10,13] IR is a disorder in which peripheral tissues such as muscle and fat do not respond adequately to circulating insulin, and so with IR, it takes much more of insulin to bring about a normal effect.[13] A common result is development of both hyperglycemia and compensatory hyperinsulinemia.

TABLE 7.1
Diagnosis of Metabolic Syndrome

Criteria vary slightly among different groups. According to guidelines from the National Heart, Lung, and Blood Institute (NHLBI) and the American Heart Association (AHA), metabolic syndrome is diagnosed when a patient has at least three of the following four conditions:

1. Insulin resistance/type 2 diabetes mellitus
   Fasting glucose ≥100 mg/dL (or receiving drug therapy for hyperglycemia)
2. Elevated blood pressure
   BP ≥130/85 mmHg (or receiving drug therapy for hypertension)
3. Dyslipidemia
   Triglycerides ≥150 mg/dL (or receiving drug therapy for hypertriglyceridemia)
   HDL-C < 40 mg/dL in men or <50 mg/dL in women (or receiving drug therapy for reduced HDL-C)
4. Central overweight/obesity
   Waist circumference ≥40 in. in men or 35 in. in women; if Asian-American, ≥35 in. in men or 32 in. in women

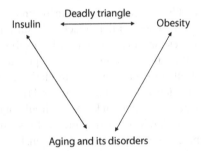

FIGURE 7.1 Figure depicting a relationship between insulin resistance and obesity and disorders of aging.

IR is relatively ubiquitous possibly due, at least in part, to its close association with obesity, a disorder like other elements of MS that is increasing in epidemic proportions.[8,14–22] Fat accumulation, particularly in the abdomen and liver (nonalcoholic fatty liver disease, [NAFLD]), has received considerable attention over the last few years as a principal causative factor.[10] In the past, we have presented at lectures a slide with the title of "A Deadly Triangle" depicted in Figure 7.1. This figure suggests that a reasonable way to ameliorate the various elements of MS is to prevent IR and/or obesity. It may be that fat accumulation only exacerbates the events caused by IR as the incidence of cardiovascular disease (CVD) or T2D does not generally increase in obese individuals without some evidence for the presence of IR.[10,23,24] Therefore, ameliorating IR and obesity could slow the development of the other age-related maladies, such as hypertension and dyslipidemia. IR, like MS itself, has been linked to the hypercoagulable state and increased cytokine levels (Figure 7.1).[22]

Accordingly, it is not too surprising that preventing and/or ameliorating IR/T2D and overweight/obesity are important measures in the current therapeutic efforts, although it remains somewhat controversial whether and to what extent overweight/obesity causes IR.[10] Suffice it to say, natural lifestyle measures that enhance insulin sensitivity and/or decrease fat mass such as proper diet and exercise have shown promise against the components of MS.[25] The addition of "weight loss" and antidiabetic drugs to lifestyle changes may provide further help; however, the extra benefits derived from such pharmaceutical regimens generally disappear when these regimens are discontinued.[26–35]

The eventual removal of a drug often is carried out as a precaution based on an established history of the use of such weight loss and antidiabetic drugs being implicated with significant adverse reactions.[36–39]

Assuming that IR is an important factor in the increasing occurrence of the many components that constitute the MS, we believe the so-called "Western diet," which is high in refined CHO such as sugars and low in fibers, is a significant contributor to the current deteriorating state of American health. Consumption of sugars, especially sucrose and HFCS, is increasing worldwide. Excess sugar consumption is closely tied to IR based on at least two known mechanisms. First, excess sugar consumption provides unneeded calories that cause increased fat accumulation that in turn indirectly influences glucose–insulin metabolism and other hormonal systems unfavorably. Second, excess sugar intake itself perturbs many hormonal systems, particularly the glucose–insulin system, by directly inducing IR, i.e., a diet high in sugar(s) alters liver function and influences peripheral tissues, both fat and muscle, to respond inadequately to insulin.

Practically speaking, averting the MS by merely avoiding dietary sugars in modern Western diets through conscious effort may be very difficult to achieve. There are many reasons for this. Sugars and refined CHO components today are cheap and readily available ingredients—ubiquitous in food processing. For another, most individuals of all ages love sweets. Some experts have even proposed the existence of an addiction to refined foods, especially to sugars.[40]

INSULIN RESISTANCE AND TYPE 2 DIABETES MELLITUS

Insulin was discovered and isolated by the Banting group in Toronto, Canada, in the early 1920s.[41–44] With this discovery, most physicians reasoned that a lack of insulin production and/or release was responsible for all diagnosed diabetes mellitus. Consequently, insulin replacement became the treatment of choice for this disease. With time, however, a more prevalent pathophysiological process behind diabetes was uncovered. Rather than a dearth of circulating insulin being primarily responsible for most cases of hyperglycemia, it was found that peripheral tissues, including fat and muscle, do not respond appropriately to adequate or even high levels of circulating insulin.[45,46] When circulating glucose levels rise into a range considered "diabetic," medical researchers characterized this more prevalent form of persistent hyperglycemia as T2D to distinguish it from the originally described type 1 diabetes caused by insufficient circulating insulin.[47–50] The lack of proper response on the part of peripheral tissues and organs came to be termed "IR." In the initial course, a mild degree of IR may not produce the markedly elevated circulating concentrations of glucose necessary for a diagnosis of T2D.[51–53] However, the glucose–insulin disturbance during this period is still harmful and is associated with the eventual development of many cardiovascular risks.[52,53] Most experts believe that this "prediabetic" stage is the best moment in time for instituting prevention/treatment. Suffice it to say that while IR is a major component in the development of T2D, it also has been linked to the pathophysiology of the components that constitute the MS.[51–55] For the purpose of this review, it is not necessary to decide conclusively whether IR is the underlying driver of MS or merely a component.

HISTORICAL EVIDENCE LINKING DIETARY SUGARS TO VARIOUS COMPONENTS OF METABOLIC SYNDROME, ESPECIALLY GLUCOSE–INSULIN PERTURBATIONS

During the First World War, the incidence of diabetes mellitus and arteriosclerotic heart disease dramatically decreased in countries where the food supply was inadequate. Paton[56] attributed this to a lack of dietary sugar. However, Aschoff favored an alternative hypothesis.[57] He believed that low fat availability rather than low sugar availability during the war was the primary reason behind diminution of cardiovascular disorders. Subsequently, Himsworth preferred the latter assumption,[58] whereas Yudkin favored the Paton proposal.[59] Hence, two different points of view arose as to which was the more important factor. Data from the Second World War failed to solve the debate as to whether sugars or fats were more important in the lessening of diabetes mellitus and atherosclerotic heart disease because, once again, both low sugar and low fat intakes preceded the decreased occurrence.[60] Obviously, both may have contributed, but was one a more important source?

Starting in 1957, John Yudkin authored a series of articles championing the theory that consumption of sugars is largely responsible for the increasing incidence of T2D and coronary heart disease.[54,61–63] To strengthen his contentions, he emphasized that the findings are clear that a higher consumption of sucrose raises blood pressure and both circulating triglycerides and insulin levels. In 1974, while assessing an increased incidence of hypertension in the Western world, the researcher Ahrens reported, "the most striking recent dietary change has been the sevenfold increase in consumption of sucrose."[60]

By 1973, strong links between sugar intake, diabetes, obesity, and heart disease had begun to trouble many perceptive individuals. This prompted a select committee led by Senator George McGovern to question whether excess intake of dietary sugars was largely responsible for the fact that since 1970 the obesity rates had more than doubled, coinciding with a tripling incidence of diabetes.[49,64,65] In 1983, Israel et al. stated that sensitive individuals could be adversely affected by high levels of sucrose present in a number of modern diets.[66] When 24 CHO-sensitive individuals consumed 5%, 18%, or 33% w/w sucrose in a crossover design, diastolic blood pressure increased with augmented sucrose intake, thus supporting Ahren's contention that dietary sucrose plays a major role in the increasing incidence of hypertension.[60,66–68] In addition, a case was made for a prominent role for excess sugar ingestion over the long term in the increased IR reported in the aging process.[69–71] Nevertheless, a call to decrease sucrose consumption did not occur immediately despite the evidence. In fact, the general recommendation to the public by important health sources was to restrict dietary saturated fats that resulted in replacement of lost calories with refined CHO.

What is the status of sugar consumption presently? Today, the majority of sugar calories are derived from processed foods. These include popular sources such as breads, cakes, jams, and ice cream.[72] Less obvious to the casual observer is the fact that sugar is present in significant amounts in foods such as tomato sauces, salad dressings, and cereals. Sodas and sugar-containing drinks presently are coming under very careful scrutiny because they supply roughly one-third of calories in the diet that are derived from added sugars. Since 1970, it is estimated that the daily consumption of calories from "sugary drinks" has at least doubled. Two unfortunate coinciding events of this excess are a decreased intake of micronutrients[73,74] and increased body weight.[75] Although the dietary Guidelines for Americans 2010 recommends that no more than 5%–15% calories should come from solid fats and sugars combined, approximately 13% adult total calories between 2005 and 2010 came from added sugars alone.[76] Matters have continued to deteriorate since that time. Today, it is estimated that children and adolescents derive roughly 16% of their calories from added sugars.[77]

CORRELATION OF FAT ACCUMULATION WITH INSULIN RESISTANCE AND METABOLIC SYNDROME

In the not too distant past, many individuals began consuming too many calories in the form of refined CHO. Much of this occurred when the public was encouraged to avoid saturated fats to prevent cardiovascular disorders, but the replacement was predominantly CHO calories that caused more body fat accumulation along with IR as discussed in the "Historical Evidence" section. Excess body fat accumulation from consuming too many calories increases the probability for developing T2D, and IR is associated with T2D[14–21]: more than 80% of T2D in the United States are obese, and 10% of obese patients are diabetic.[78] The accumulation of mesenteric (abdominal) fat has especially been linked to IR and various disorders associated with the MS.[14,19]

The prevalence of diabetes and levels of fasting glucose, insulin, c-peptide and HbA1c in the NHANES study between 1999 and 2006 were examined across different weight classes.[79] The prevalence of diabetes was greater in the heavier weight classes. Consequently, it is not surprising that losing weight is one important way to prevent, delay, and ameliorate the development of diabetes.[21]

CARBOHYDRATES AND THEIR METABOLISM

BASICS

It seems reasonable in any regimen designed to prevent IR/T2D, to reduce caloric intake when over-weight/obesity is present. Certainly, consistent intake of too many calories from fats as well as sugars could be responsible. However, some have contended that there are "special calories"—those coming from refined CHO such as sugars—that particularly need to be avoided for reasons in addition to calorie count.[70] Sweet and refined CHO have the potential to further worsen IR directly.[69,70] Interestingly, the addition of excess sugar to the diet will increase IR and systolic blood pressure in rats without increasing body weight.[80,81] The point to be emphasized is that reducing calories to reduce body fat is important, but that some CHO exhibit additional factors that make their role in the MS more pronounced.

Over a span covering many years, several different research groups have consistently reported that isocaloric consumption of sucrose compared to starch perturbs glucose tolerance.[82,83] In 1978, a review article by Yudkin published in the *Journal of the Royal Society of Medicine* stated clearly his reasoning behind the different responses between sucrose and starch: "Present evidence suggests that most of the effects of sucrose are due in small part to its ease of digestion and absorption compared with starch, also in small part to its being a disaccharide, but chiefly to the fructose released when sucrose is digested."[84] Accordingly, Yudkin proposed over 30 years ago two important pathophysiological principles favored even today, namely, that the harm from caloric sweeteners such as sucrose and HFCS lies in both their high glycemic indices (rapid absorption) and the presence of fructose.[84,85]

GLYCEMIC INDEX AND LOAD

CHO are absorbed at different rates—some relatively quickly (high glycemic index) and some relatively slowly (low glycemic index).[85,86] The absorption rate with consideration of the amount taken in (glycemic load) can affect the insulin system greatly—rapidly absorbed CHO in enough quantity are associated with IR and many chronic health maladies.[85,86]

CHO absorption reflects principles of structure and basic metabolism. CHO are characteristically classified by size.[87] The smallest units are monosaccharides (single units, such as glucose) and disaccharides (two bound units, such as sucrose, composed of glucose and fructose). These smaller units are commonly referred to as sugars. Larger units consist of oligosaccharides (3–9 units) and polysaccharides (>10 units). Starches are polysaccharides in which the polymers consisting of glucose units are bound covalently either by alpha-(1,4) or alpha-(1,6) linkages.

To be absorbed, CHO must be broken down into monosaccharides. At a minimum, two major enzymes are involved in this process. Alpha-amylase from saliva and pancreatic juice decomposes starches into monosaccharide, disaccharide, trisaccharide, and oligosaccharide units. Alpha-glucosidases bound in the brush border of the small intestines further divide the remaining larger units into monosaccharides.[87] To give an example, sucrose, commonly referred to as "table sugar," is a disaccharide of linked glucose and fructose. Sucrase, an alpha-glucosidase, breaks down sucrose into glucose and fructose. Different monosaccharides are absorbed by different transport mechanisms.[87] As a general principal, the smaller the CHO molecule, the more rapid is the absorption (high glycemic index). This rapid absorption has been connected to the harm that excess sugar intake (high glycemic load) induces.[84,85]

In recent decades, sucrose consumption in the United States has diminished as table sugar has been gradually replaced by an ingredient called "high fructose corn syrup (HFCS)." The latter is a stable product that is cheaper than sucrose. In HFCS, the glucose and fructose are free rather than bound, as is the case for sucrose. Two major forms of HFCS exist. The ratio of glucose to fructose is either 42:53 or 55:42, not the 50:50 ratio seen with sucrose. Suffice it to say, the consumer still receives a good supply of each monosaccharide in the switch from table sugar to HFCS, but no sucrase activity is necessary for absorption of the latter. Both substances exhibit a high glycemic index and, because the population favors their consumption, dietary sucrose and HFCS typically provide a high glycemic load, as well.

The presence of viscous fiber slows down absorption of sugars. This is one reason that it is unfortunate that the typical Western diet is low in fiber, yet high in rapidly absorbable sugars. Drugs such as acarbose and natural supplements like L-arabinose restrain the activity of alpha-glucosidases—sucrase being an example. Other natural products, such as bean and hibiscus extracts, also can effectively slow down CHO absorption via inhibition of alpha-amylase activity. Thus, there are a number of means by which to slow the absorption of CHO via inhibition of enzymes involved in digestion.[88]

Much of the information about the role of excess sugar consumption in many metabolic perturbations has been derived from animal studies. Since the late 1970s, our laboratory has consistently added sucrose to regular rodent feed to bring out various aspects of the MS, such as IR and hypertension, that are in turn associated with disturbances in the glucose–insulin, renin–angiotensin, and nitric oxide systems.[80,81,89,90] Most of our findings from earlier animal studies have been confirmed in clinical investigations. For example, after 30 years, the conclusion derived from rat studies that a heavy ingestion of sucrose and fructose elevates blood pressure has been born out in clinical studies.[80,91] It is important to repeat that in animal models, however, body weight increases have not been a key factor in the development of these disorders, including IR.[80,81,89,90] Rather, this speaks to hormonal disturbances not directly linked to an accumulation of fat mass, but, instead, via the direct influences of excess sugar intake.

Fructose

Various findings have suggested that excess dietary fructose, in particular, is associated with numerous health problems. Hepatic metabolism of fructose favors *de novo* lipogenesis, and subsequent hepatic steatosis has been connected to many aspects of IR and the MS.[92–96] Other data suggest that excess fructose consumption from high sugar consumption can play a role in heart failure.[97–99] In addition, the unique ability of fructose intake to increase uric acid levels has been proposed as a major mechanism through which fructose produces cardiorenal disease[100,101] and elevates blood pressure.[100,102] Sucrose ingestion is associated with retinal capillary damage,[103–105] and the fructose moiety appears to be the culprit.[106–108] Fructose has been linked to obesity. It is reported that beverages high in fructose produce smaller increases in satiety hormones and feelings of satiety than drinks sweetened with comparable amounts of glucose.[109] To add insult to injury, fructose consumption may exacerbate diverse abnormalities already present in obese subjects.[109]

It is generally accepted that over the last few years there has been an increased consumption of soft drinks as well as breakfast cereals, deserts, and baked goods sweetened with sucrose and HFCS.[110] Countries with a higher availability of HFCS also have a higher prevalence of T2D independent of obesity.[111,112] It is important to note that individuals on average obtain even more fructose (about 10%) on average from HFCS (containing 55% fructose) than that from sucrose.[112] Accordingly, fructose consumption makes up a significant proportion of all energy intake in the American diet. The bottom line is that in recent decades the upsurge in fructose consumption corresponds chronologically with the increased prevalence of obesity and diabetes.

Fructose does not initially stimulate insulin secretion nor enhance leptin production—important afferent signals regulating food intake and body weight. Thus, there is less insulin response compared to glucose intake with fructose ingestion.[93] As a result of lesser insulin response to meals, circulating leptin levels are also decreased because insulin has a significant role in leptin production.[93,96,100] These actions may have deleterious long-term effects on the regulation of energy intake and body adiposity that depend on these two hormones to quell appetite when appropriate. In addition, fructose interferes with the normal transport of and signaling by leptin. Overconsumption of fructose has been reported to lead to leptin resistance, and leptin resistance has been shown to cause excess weight gain in rats when combined with a high-fat, high-calorie diet.[113] Leptin produces satiety and reduces dopamine signaling, hence decreases the pleasure derived from food.[114] Although fructose alone does not in the beginning augment circulating insulin concentrations, subsequent development of IR will eventually give rise to hyperinsulinemia.

Sources of fructose such as sucrose and HFCS are linked to numerous chronic conditions other than obesity.[100] In rodents, fructose consumption induces elevated systolic blood pressure, IR, impaired glucose tolerance, hyperinsulinemia, and hypertriglyceridemia.[115–119] In monkeys, fructose rapidly causes liver damage that relates to the duration of fructose consumption and total calories consumed.[120] Similar data obtained from humans are not readily available.

The implication that fructose is significantly involved in "sugar-induced chronic diseases" is not unanimously acknowledged. Sievenpiper discussed a series of his investigations in which fructose substituted for other CHO to maintain the isocaloric state and did not find that fructose caused pathology, i.e., substitution of fructose for other sources of CHO did not increase body weight, circulating lipids, blood pressure, uric acid, and even improved glycemic control.[121] More precisely, this group did not find evidence that supports the proposition that fructose is harmful at typical intakes. "High levels of exposure and excess energy appear to be the dominant considerations for harm." These investigators, however, did mention that larger, longer, and higher quality studies are needed. Moreover, if one mechanism of dysfunction introduced by high fructose intake is lessened regulatory control over consumption, relatively short-term tests performed under isocaloric conditions likely obscure the actions of fructose in an unregulated diet.

SUGAR-SWEETENED BEVERAGES

Sugar-sweetened beverages (SSBs) such as soft drinks and fruit juices are significant sources of sugars in the American diet.[111,122] In addition to supplying excess calories leading to body-fat accumulation associated with IR, SSBs also make available those rapidly absorbed sugars (sucrose and/or HFCS) that directly encourage development of IR/T2D.[123] Numerous recent studies performed in various settings have shown in both adults and children that the rising level of obesity and T2D has paralleled a concomitant rise in the consumption of SSBs.[92,124,125] Three supporting examples are given below.

In 51,603 females from the Nurses' Health Care Study, higher consumption of SSBs was associated with a greater degree of weight gain and greater risk for developing diabetes.[126] Differently, diet sodas were not linked to an augmented risk of diabetes. The authors hypothesized that augmented weight gain from excess calories and the large amount of absorbable sugars in SSBs was mainly responsible despite the fact that other influences could have contributed, such as less physically activity, smoking, and more alcohol intake. This investigation brought up an intriguing question. Do liquid sources of sugars differ from solid sources? A suggestion was made that sugar-sweetened soft drinks and fruit punches caused low satiety and did relatively little to lessen caloric intake from solid foods.[127–129]

In a different report examining 43,960 African–American women, researchers evaluated the risk of developing T2D in individuals who provided a comprehensive dietary history and weight information and were free of diabetes at the beginning of the investigation.[130] An important finding was that the development of diabetes was more prevalent in those with the greater intake of both sugar-sweetened soft drinks and fruit drinks. It appeared that perturbations were mediated mainly through increased body mass index (BMI). Similarly to the study performed on nurses,[126] the consumption of "straight" orange and grapefruit juices and diet soda did not increase the rate of developing diabetes as did the sugar-sweetened products. In yet another study, Duffey et al. examined data obtained from 2,774 adults in the CARDIA study over 7 years and found that SSB consumption was associated with higher waist circumference, and increased LDL cholesterol and triglycerides, as well as blood pressure.[131]

ROLE OF LOW CARBOHYDRATE DIETS IN PREVENTING VARIOUS COMPONENTS OF METABOLIC SYNDROME

One way to determine the effects of rapidly absorbed sugars and the relationship of the consumption of refined CHO to the MS is to make these items components of the diet.[80] The past several decades in the United States might be characterized as a great, uncontrolled experiment in just this type of dietary intervention. Contrarily, the effects of simple CHO can be explored by testing diets that are the reverse of the currently popular one, which is to say, by testing diets that are "low" in CHO rather than "high" in CHO.[132,133]

In 2003, 132 severely obese subjects (mean BMI 43) with a proclivity for diabetes (39%) were given either a CHO-restricted diet (low-carb) or a calorie- and fat-restricted diet (low-fat).[134] After 6 months, the low-carb group as compared to the low-fat group had lost statistically significantly more weight; mean −5.8 kg vs. −1.9 kg ($p = .002$). Greater improvements in insulin sensitivity and circulating triglyceride levels were found in the low-carb group even after adjustment for weight loss. A follow-up report in 2004 based on results after 1 year revealed a mean decrease in body weight that did not prove to be statistically significantly different this time, mean −5.1 vs. −3.1 kg.[135] Nevertheless, in the same study, hemoglobin A1C and triglyceride levels improved more in the low-carb group. The dropout rate was high (34%), leading the investigators to report suboptimal dietary adherence.

Other studies have confirmed various findings from the 2003 trial. In 2005, 96 IR women with BMI exceeding 27 kg/m² were assigned to one of three dietary interventions: a high-CHO/high-fiber (HC) diet, a high-fat (HF) Atkins diet, or a high-protein (HP) Zone diet.[136] Body weight, waist circumference, triglycerides, and insulin levels decreased with all diets, but with the exception of circulating insulin levels, the changes were significantly greater in the HF and HP groups compared to the HC group.

Nordmann et al. in 2006 examined data from five trials composed of 447 individuals with a BMI exceeding 25 kg/m² to compare effects of low-CHO diets without caloric restriction vs. low-fat, caloric-restricted diets.[132] By 6 months, those individuals consuming the low-CHO diets lost significantly more scale weight than subjects following the low-fat, caloric-restricted regimens (weighted mean difference was −3.3 kg). However, the difference did not reach statistical significance after 12 months (weighted mean difference −1.0 kg). Nevertheless, triglyceride and HDL changed more favorably in the low-CHO group, whereas LDL levels were more favorable in the low-fat group.

Six randomized control trials involving 202 participants were studied to determine the effects of low glycemic index or load diets on weight loss in overweight/obese individuals.[133] Compared to diets with a higher glycemic loads, overweight/obese subjects lost more weight and total fat mass consuming lower glycemic loads and had more improvement in their lipid profiles. Another systematic review focused on data from randomized controlled trials of low-CHO diets compared with low-fat/low-calorie ones.[137] The reviewers arrived at results similar to others: low-CHO/high-protein diets are more effective at 6 months and are as effective for up to 1 year as low-fat diets in reducing weight and CVD.

Sacks et al. examined the possible advantages in respect to weight loss from diets that featured different macronutrient contents of proteins, fats, and CHO.[138] A total of 811 overweight adults were assigned to one of four diets containing different levels of the macronutrients. All the reduced calorie diets resulted in significant weight loss—it did not matter which macronutrient was emphasized in the diet.

The objective of a recently reported study by Krebs was to assess the value of a low-CHO diet in obese patients with T2D.[139] The principal end points were insulin sensitivity, glycemic control, and risk factors for CVD. Measurements in 14 obese patients were made at baseline and at 12 and 24 weeks. The diet was well tolerated, and the subjects achieved statistically significant weight loss over 24 weeks. The weight loss was associated with a voluntary reduction in calorie intake. Glycemic control, measured by various means, improved significantly.

CLINICAL STUDIES EXAMINING PREVENTION OF GLUCOSE-INSULIN PERTURBATIONS SUCH AS IR/T2D

On the basis of the generally accepted principal that IR plays a significant role in the development of MS, it seems reasonable that any plan for prevention would attack that perturbation.[9,10] To date, successful interventions that prevent IR/T2D have primarily included lifestyle changes such as modification of diet and exercise.[140,141] Some trials have included antidiabetic drugs to gain further benefits. A review of several of these studies quickly reveals overlapping elements of success.

In one trial, 41 male subjects, 47–49 years of age with early-stage T2D and 181 subjects with impaired glucose tolerance (IGT) were followed to assess whether long-term, lifestyle changes could avert diabetes.[142] After 6 years, body weights were reduced 2.3%–3.7%, and 50% of patients experienced signs of diabetic remission. For example, blood pressure, circulating lipid levels, and hyperinsulinemia were significantly reduced. Because improvement in glucose tolerance correlated with weight reduction, the clinicians concluded that chronic intervention with proper diet and exercise was effective even after several years.

Results from the Da Qing IGT (impaired glucose tolerance) and Diabetes Study were reported in 1997 based on data gathered in 1986 from 33 health-care clinics in the city of Da Qing.[143] A total of 577 subjects with IGT had been divided into four groups, i.e., control and three treatment groups. Treatment groups comprised a diet-only group, an exercise-only group, and a diet-plus exercise group. The health professionals found that all three treatments compared to control led to a statistically significantly greater decrease in the development of diabetes over a 6-year period: 68% in control, 44% in diet-only, 41% in exercise-only, and 46% in diet plus exercise. The authors concluded that diet and exercise led to a significant decrease in the incidence of diabetes among individuals with impaired glucose tolerance over a 6-year period that ended in 1992.

Question subsequently arose as to how long the benefits from the above study would last beyond the period of active intervention.[144] In 2006, 14 years after intervention, participants were reevaluated in order to define the lasting effects of the earlier intervention. Whereas the average annual incidence of diabetes was 7% for the intervention group, it was 11% for the control. Participants in the intervention group continued for an average of 3.6 fewer years without diabetes compared to control. A change in cardiovascular status could not be determined.

In 2001, Tuomilehto et al. arbitrarily allocated 172 male and 350 female subjects with reduced glucose tolerance (IGT), mean age of 55 years and a mean BMI of 31, to either an intervention or control group.[145] The intervention group received individualized counseling aimed at reducing weight, intake of total fat, and saturated fat while increasing the intake of fiber and physical activity. An oral glucose tolerance test was performed annually during a 3.2-year duration of follow-up. Weight loss after 1 and 2 years was 4.2% and 3.5% in the intervention group as compared to 0.8% and 0.8%, respectively, in the control group ($p < .001$ for both periods). The rate of diabetes averaged 11% in the intervention group and 23% in control by the end of study ($p < .001$). Four years after the end of study, the participants who remained free of diabetes were followed another 3 years after discontinuation of active counseling for a total study time of 7 years.[146] The occurrence of T2D was 4.3% and 7.4%, respectively, in the intervention and control groups. Thus, sustained good lifestyle practices leading to a reduction in disease incidence continued to be practiced even after active counseling was discontinued.

Added drug interventions have been tested similarly to diet and exercise interventions alone to determine if such regimens can yield benefits in the form of reduced incidence of diabetes. Chiasson et al. randomly assigned patients with impaired glucose tolerance to receive 100 mg acarbose ($n = 714$) or placebo ($n = 715$) three times daily.[26] Acarbose, an antidiabetic agent in common use, decreases the absorption of CHO in the small intestines. A total of 221 (32%) patients receiving acarbose and 285 (42%) in the placebo group eventually developed diabetes. At the end of protocol, treatment with placebo for 3 months was followed by an increased conversion of impaired glucose tolerance to diabetes. The most frequent side effects with acarbose were flatulence and diarrhea. The authors concluded that taking acarbose could delay T2D in those with impaired glucose tolerance.

In the so-called TRIPOD study (Troglitazone in Prevention of Diabetes), Buchanan et al. randomized women with gestational diabetes to the insulin sensitizer troglitazone (400 mg/day) ($n = 133$) or to placebo ($n = 133$).[27] During a follow-up of 30 months, the average incidence rate for T2D was 5.4% in the troglitazone treatment group compared to 12.1% in the placebo group ($p < .01$). Accordingly, treating women with troglitazone was deemed to delay and perhaps prevent the onset of T2D. Women who completed the TRIPOD study were offered participation in the PIPOD study (Pioglitazone in the Prevention of Diabetes).[28] The risk of diabetes found at 4.6% per year in PIPOD was similar to that found in those taking troglitazone in TRIPOD. The conclusion from both studies was that thiazolidinedione drugs could favorably delay the onset of diabetes in Hispanic women with prior gestational diabetes.

The hypothesis of the Diabetes Prevention Program (DPP) study published in 2002 was that a lifestyle intervention program that incorporated lowering elevated glucose levels, reducing overweight, living a more active lifestyle, or taking the antidiabetic drug metformin would ameliorate the severity of, delay the onset of, and/or avert diabetes.[29] The investigators assigned 3234 nondiabetic subjects with elevated fasting blood glucose, mean age 51 years, and mean BMI 34.0 to three groups: a placebo group, a metformin group (850 mg twice daily), or a lifestyle modification program that had a 7% weight loss target and a minimum of 150 minutes of exercise per week as goals. The incidence of diabetes was 11.0%, 7.8%, and 4.8%, respectively, after a mean 2.8-year follow-up. The results suggested that persons at risk for diabetes might avoid or delay onset of diabetes by reducing modest amounts of excess weight through diet and exercise. The group participants in the lifestyle intervention decreased risk of developing diabetes by 58%. The lifestyle intervention regimen proved statistically significantly more effective than use of metformin. Nevertheless, metformin use proved effective compared to placebo. Of note, although lifestyle intervention was helpful for all age groups, metformin therapy became less so with age—being no different than placebo in patients over the age of 60.

Troglitazone was used initially in a separate grouping in the DPP study described earlier. However, it was discontinued later when the drug was shown to be hepatotoxic.[29] An article published in 2005 evaluated both the short-term results while the trial was active and the long-term results after troglitazone use was discontinued with the other trial groups.[30] The troglitazone group ceased functioning after a mean of 0.9 years: at that time, the diabetes incident rate was 3.0 cases per 100 patient-years compared to 12.0 (placebo), 6.7 (metformin), and 5.1 (intensive lifestyle intervention) cases per 100 person-years in the other three groups. However, 3 years later after troglitazone withdrawal, the incidence rate for diabetes was no different than the placebo group. Therefore, troglitazone appeared effective only during the shortened period of actual use.

When the DPP study was completed, 88% of the enrolled patients entered a 10-year follow-up phase.[31] In this phase, all three groups (placebo, lifestyle intervention, and metformin) were now offered only lifestyle intervention. At the end of the study, diabetes incidence rates were similar between groups—(5.9/100 person-years for the original lifestyle group, 4.9 for the metformin group, and 5.6 for the placebo group). The investigators believed based on the original numbers for the placebo group the findings implied that prevention or delay of diabetes through lifestyle intervention could persist for at least 10 years.

Torgerson et al. in 2004 reasoned that addition of a weight-loss drug (Orlistat) to a lifestyle regimen change would be even more effective than a lifestyle change alone.[32] This postulate was based on the close link between obesity and T2D. A total of 3305 subjects were assigned to a lifestyle regimen change plus either Orlistat 120 mg or placebo three times daily. In a 4-year double blind prospective study, participants were required to have a BMI exceeding 30 kg/m². In an assessment of glucose tolerance among the subjects, 79% were normal and 21% showed impaired glucose tolerance. Unfortunately, the dropout figures were large—only 52% of the Orlistat-treated group and 34% of the placebo group completed the 4-year study. The cumulative incidence of diabetes was 9.0% in the placebo group and 6.2% in those taking Orlistat. Average weight loss in the treated group, which was comparable in both the impaired and normal glucose tolerance subgroups, exceeded that of the placebo group—5.8 vs. 3.0 kg ($p < .001$). Of note, only subjects with impaired glucose tolerance showed greater diabetes prevention relative to placebo. The investigators concluded that Orlistat contributed to diabetes prevention in a setting of lifestyle change.

Kosaka et al. in 2005 examined whether a concentrated lifestyle intervention that attempts to achieve and maintain ideal body weight would be beneficial in subjects with impaired glucose tolerance.[147] The intensive intervention group contained 102 individuals, whereas the control group consisted of 356 individuals. Control subjects were urged to maintain a BMI < 24.0 kg/m^2 and the intervention subjects were urged to maintain a BMI < 22.0 kg/m^2. Importantly, the cumulative 4-year incidence of diabetes in the control group was 9.3% compared to 3.0% in the intervention group ($p < .001$). The trial was associated with body weight decrease of 0.39 kg in control compared to 2.18 kg in the intervention group ($p < .001$). This study provides evidence that lifestyle intervention aimed at achieving ideal body weight in men with impaired glucose tolerance can be successful.

In 2006, Gerstein et al. designed a study to determine the ability of rosiglitazone to prevent T2D in individuals at high risk of developing this entity.[33] The subjects were aged 30 years or more and had impaired fasting glucose or impaired glucose tolerance or both. The subjects, who up to the initiation of the study were without evidence of CVD, were assigned to receive rosiglitazone (8 mg daily) or placebo for a median of 3 years. End points were the development of diabetes or death. 11.6% subjects receiving rosiglitazone in contrast to 26.0% given placebo developed diabetes. About 50.5% of treated subjects and 30.3% receiving placebo eventually became normoglycemic ($p < .001$). Cardiovascular event rates were the same in both groups, although congestive heart failure (0.5% compared to 0.1%) may have been greater in the rosiglitazone group. Therefore, rosiglitazone was effective in preventing T2D under the conditions of study.

In a 2009 article, Kawamori et al. examined high-risk Japanese patients eating standard diets, taking regular exercise, and exhibiting impaired glucose tolerance.[34] Subjects were randomly assigned to placebo ($n = 883$) or oral voglibose, a CHO inhibitor similar to acarbose, 0.2 mg three times a day ($n = 897$). Subjects in the voglibose group had a lower risk of progression to diabetes compared to placebo (50 vs. 106) ($p < .0014$). The conclusion was that voglibose is able to help prevent diabetes.

DeFronzo et al. frequently assessed 602 patients who received pioglitazone or placebo for a medium follow up of 2.4 years.[35] As compared to placebo, pioglitazone reduced the risk for conversion of impaired glucose tolerance to T2D by 72%. Other benefits included a reduced rate of carotid intimal thickening, a lowered diastolic blood pressure, and an increased level of HDL. However, pioglitazone was associated with significant weight gain, increased plasma volume, and edema. McCowen and Fajtova, in a letter to the editor that followed, noted the parallel rise in HbA1c between the placebo and pioglitazone groups once the drug was stopped and suggested that the drug only had short-term effects.[148] In other words, evidence that prevention remained after stopping the drug was weak.

The foregoing studies were designed to assess ways to avoid or at least ameliorate the ramifications of IR/T2D and to some extent overweight/obesity. Many consider these entities to be the driving forces behind many important aspects of the MS.[10] The regimens to date include lifestyle changes such as modification of diet and exercise as well as use of antidiabetic drugs. The success in one study using Orlistat was attributed to weight loss. With the development of various classes of antidiabetic agents, it commonly has been hypothesized that each one could be used early on to prevent development of further glucose-insulin perturbations. In the above studies, metformin, thiazolidinediones, and alpha-glucosidase inhibitors were all associated with favorable effects over the period of use. However, the benefits derived from drugs seemed to dissipate once they were stopped. Also, it is unclear as to at what length of intervention brings out side effects, such as the weight gain associated with pioglitazone and related drugs.

DIETARY SUPPLEMENTS TO PREVENT AND/OR AMELIORATE THE MS: THERAPEUTIC POTENTIAL

PERSPECTIVE

As discussed earlier, in addition to lifestyle intervention alone, drugs have been used along with lifestyle changes in various research protocols designed to examine IR/T2D prevention.[26–35] However, many believe that overcoming glucose–insulin perturbations would also benefit other components of the MS.[9,10,13] Although inclusion of drugs in the various regimens appears to have some added merit, by and large, their removal eventually causes loss of prior positive gains.[148] Nevertheless, there is obviously hesitancy to use drug therapy over the long term to prevent or lessen manifestations of IR/T2D.[26–35] No doubt the major fear leading to avoidance of prolonged drug use is the potential for adverse reactions.[149,150]

In contrast to drugs, natural dietary substances with a long history of safety have not been used extensively in major clinical studies despite their potential to overcome IR, promote weight loss, lower elevated blood pressure, and produce a more healthful lipid profile (see Table 7.2). As a general rule, natural dietary supplements compared to drugs are less potent, but also have fewer and less severe adverse reactions. The major reasons behind the paucity of cogent clinical research performed on natural dietary supplements compared to drugs are simple. For one, the typical manufacturer of natural agents has meager cash available to sponsor definitive research compared to manufacturers of pharmaceuticals. In addition, difficulties in patenting natural substances play a role.

TABLE 7.2

Supplements to Ameliorate Metabolic Syndrome

1. Digestion and absorption blockers
   a. Carbohydrate blockers
      i. Phase two—*alpha*-amylase inhibitor and *alpha*-glucosidase inhibitor
      ii. In-Sea 2—*alpha*-amylase and *alpha*-glucosidase inhibitor
      iii. L-arabinose—inhibits sucrose absorption via enzyme blockage
      iv. HCA—inhibits pancreatic alpha-amylase and intestinal alpha-glucosidase, reduces rate of glucose uptake from gut (Na exchange inhibitor?)
      v. *Salacia oblonga* (alpha glucosidase inhibitor)
      vi. Green coffee/chlorogenic acid—reduces rate of glucose uptake from gut (reduces sodium electrochemical gradient in the brush border membrane vesicles)
   b. Fat blockers
      i. Chitosan—fat binder
      ii. Opuntia—fat binder
      iii. Fenugreek fiber—fat binder
      iv. *Cassia nomame*—lipase inhibitor
      v. Green tea—lipase inhibitor
      vi. Green coffee bean extract—inhibit pancreatic lipase
      vii. Grape seed extract and pine bark–lipase inhibitors
      viii. Low-molecular weight pectin—lipase inhibitor
2. Insulin sensitizers and mimetics (blood sugar and insulin)
   a. Chromium
   b. Cinnamon
   c. HCA—binds to cellular insulin, cortisol and FXR receptors; inhibits ATP:citrate lyase
   d. Biotin, vanadium
   e. *Gymnema sylvestre*
   f. Banaba leaf extract/corosolic acid/phenolic compounds
   g. Fenugreek (4 hydroxy-isoleucine)
   h. Alpha-lipoic acid
   i. Bitter melon/wild bitter melon
   j. Ginseng berry extract
   k. *Salacia oblonga* (alpha-glucosidase inhibitor)
   l. Green coffee bean extract—Inhibits hepatic glucose-6-phosphatase activity
   m. Green tea—May mildly increase expression of GLUT 4
   n. Fiber

(Continued)

TABLE 7.2   (Continued)

Supplements to Ameliorate Metabolic Syndrome

3. Metabolic enhancers
   a. Activate fatty acid release and oxidation
      i. Green tea/EGCG with caffeine—reduces norephinephrine degradation
      ii. Bitter orange—Beta-3 agonist (synephrine, octopamine, tyramine, n-methyl tyramine)
      iii. Coleus forskohlii
      iv. Caffeine, theobromine, guarana, yerba mate
      v. Cayenne, black pepper extracts
      vi. Ginger extracts
      vii. Evodiamine
      viii. Yohimbe
   b. Increase general metabolism/basal metabolic rate/prevent downregulation
      i. Bitter orange extract
      ii. 7-Keto DHEA
      iii. Cordyceps
   c. Thyroid enhancers
      i. Guggulsterones
      ii. Phosphate salts
      iii. 7-Keto DHEA

Major antidiabetic drugs can be classified as insulin stimulators that increase production and release of insulin (sulfonylureas and meglitinides), compounds that block the gastrointestinal absorption of CHO (acarbose, voglibose), remedies that reduce hepatic glucose production (biguanides), and preparations that improve insulin action peripherally (thiazolidinediones and biguanides).[36,37,149,150] In many instances, the natural dietary supplements that have a beneficial effect on glucose-insulin metabolism do so via multiple mechanisms. For instance, both the (–)-hydroxy-citric acid in *Garcinia cambogia* and the chlorogenic acids in green coffee bean extract help to regulate varying degrees of CHO digestion and absorption, liver gluconeogenesis, and insulin sensitivity as well as other mechanisms.[151] Despite all difficulties, we will attempt to compare the working of natural dietary supplements with drugs used to treat IR/T2D.

As a first approximation, attempts to classify natural supplements in the same manner as drugs might look like this: compounds that augment insulin production and/or release (*Gymnema sylvestre*, fenugreek, garlic)[152,153]; ingredients that beneficially decrease and delay gut absorption of CHO (soluble fibers and carb blockers such as bean extract and L-arabinose)[88,154,155]; substances that reduce hepatic glucose production (biotin)[156]; and items that improve insulin action peripherally (trivalent chromium, cinnamon, maitake mushroom SX fraction, and bitter melon).[157–161]

We will highlight only a few of the most popular natural supplements below such as soluble fibers, white bean extract, and L arabinose that lessen CHO absorption in the small intestines and thus lower the glycemic index like acarbose[88]; biotin that can lessen hepatic glucose formation and release like metformin,[156] trivalent chromium that is basically an insulin sensitizer such as thiazolidenediones,[157] and *Garcinia cambogia* that is among other things an appetite suppressor and can decrease fat accumulation and thus obviate IR.[151]

NATURAL MEANS TO BENEFICIALLY INFLUENCE CARBOHYDRATE GUT ABSORPTION

Overview: Accepting that diets high in sugars and other refined CHO are major factors in the various pathologies of the MS such as IR/T2D, overweight/obesity, and other contributing entities comprising the MS,[9,10] the most direct form of therapy would be simply to reduce the oral intake of sugars, especially fructose, and/or slow their absorption to lower the glycemic index and load.

Benefits realized from reducing dietary intake via low CHO diets have been summarized earlier.[132–139,162–165] Nevertheless, many individuals are not prepared to adopt such necessary dietary changes. Issues ranging from advisability of replacing CHO with fats to the palatability of CHO-depleted meals have led to hesitancy. Nevertheless, the ongoing emergence of data strengthening the positive correlation between excess intake of rapidly absorbed CHO such as fructose, glucose, and sucrose with obesity has challenged many nutritionists to seek more practical means to duplicate results found with the rigorous removal of refined CHO from the diet. Two general approaches commonly are suggested to help overcome this challenge. First, more fiber can be added to the diet to take advantage of the findings that various viscous fibers slow CHO absorption and have beneficial effects on weight loss.[166–168] Second, enzymes necessary for CHO absorption, such as amylase and sucrase, can be inhibited to reduce the rate of gastrointestinal processing of CHO.[88,169]

Fiber intake: If a reasonable portion of CHO will remain in the diet of many for the sake of palatability and reducing fat intake, the addition of soluble, viscous fibers can still provide some therapeutic relief, because soluble fibers slow the absorption of refined CHO. Nutritionists long have implored the public to eat more dietary fiber, especially soluble fiber.[170,171] In carefully controlled animal studies, the ability of soluble fiber to delay sugar absorption is associated with the lowering of elevated blood pressures, a major cardiovascular risk factor.[172,173] Unfortunately, the general public has significantly resisted increasing dietary fiber intake, probably for taste reasons and because of perturbations created in the gastrointestinal tract—gas, cramps, and frequent bowel movements.

Carbohydrate blockers: Many preparations have been developed to block major enzymes involved in CHO digestion and absorption, including *alpha*-amylase and glucosidase.[88,169] Two of the most popular and well-studied such compounds are a bean extract to primarily inhibit *alpha*-amylase and L-arabinose to inhibit sucrase. The discussion on CHO blockers in the "Specific Carbohydrate Blockers" section will focus on these two preparations. Using effective inhibitors of digestive enzymes involved in CHO absorption would allow an individual to maintain a more reasonable dietary proportion of CHO while lessening or at least slowing absorption of sugars and refined CHO with relatively high glycemic indices. For decades, it has been recognized that extracts from certain beans inhibit *alpha*-amylase activity.[88,169,174–176] In addition to the potential to lower caloric intake and prevent IR secondary to rapid CHO absorption, the ability to convert some CHO into resistant starches that are subsequently fermented in the large bowel is another advantage of CHO blockers.[177]

Resistant starches: Starches that escape enzymatic digestion in the small intestines and pass into the large bowel are characteristically referred to as "resistant starches." A good estimate is that under usual circumstances 10% of consumed starches pass through the gastrointestinal tract undigested.[178] There are many reasons for nondigestion. Starches located in the cell walls of plants may not be available for enzymatic action. Also, because of crystalline structure and size, raw starch granules are often unavailable. Some fibers such as cellulose, hemicelluloses, pectins, mucilages, and gums escape digestion, because humans lack the necessary enzymes. An important aspect of resistant starches is that after passage into the colon, they can be fermented into short-chain fatty acids, organic acids, carbon dioxide, and hydrogen.[177] The fermented, undigested starches are associated with weight loss, improved blood lipid status, better glycemic control, and improved antioxidant protection.[85,179–181]

Specific Carbohydrate Blockers

Phaseolus vulgaris–White Kidney Bean Extract

Many excellent reviews detail early work carried out in the 1970s and 1980s on bean extract inhibitors.[88,174,175,182,183] A number of crude bean amylase inhibitors were marketed as "carb blockers" in the early 1980s. However, early clinical trials designed to show efficacy were generally disappointing.[184–186] As a result, the Food and Drug Administration (FDA) suspended sales of the products in

1982. Subsequently, Layer et al. pointed out that many preparations examined earlier showed insufficient antiamylase activity, which explains the failures of these early trials.[187] With the development of better preparations having greater capability to inhibit amylase, later clinical studies began to report more promise.[188–192]

The most popular current bean preparation is a water extract of the white kidney bean—*Phaseolus vulgaris*. The extract has been shown to be relatively free of toxic metabolites and safe for human consumption.[184] Animal studies (rats and pigs) on the more recent bean extract provided the initial indication that it would be a clinically useful tool to inhibit starch absorption in vivo.[193–196] In both acute and subchronic studies on rats, Preuss et al. examined the capability of *Phaseolus vulgaris* and other CHO blockers to inhibit the absorption of rice starch and sucrose.[195,196] To estimate CHO absorption, groups of rats were fed with water or water plus rice starch and/or sucrose; circulating glucose subsequently was measured at timed intervals. After the ingestion of bean extract, glucose elevations above baseline over the 4 hours following a rice starch challenge as estimated by area-under-curve (AUC) were 40% of that of the internal control.[195] Unexpectedly, bean extract also inhibited sucrose absorption. In contrast, although L-arabinose effectively blocked sucrose absorption, it did not influence rice starch absorption. Giving either natural inhibitor without a CHO challenge led to no significant changes in circulating glucose concentrations. This suggests no major effects on overall metabolism from the bean extract and confirms that the lowered circulating glucose levels were secondary to blocked absorption.

A subchronic study was undertaken to determine whether inhibitors of gastrointestinal starch and sucrose absorption remained effective with continued use. As a secondary gain, metabolic influences after prolonged intake were examined.[196] Rats were intubated twice daily over 9 weeks with either water or an equal volume of water containing a formula that comprised both the bean extract and L-arabinose. No toxic effects (hepatic, renal, hematologic) were evident. Blood chemistries revealed significantly lower circulating glucose levels and a trend toward decreased HbA1C in the nondiabetic rats receiving the carb blockers compared to control. Subchronic administration of enzyme inhibitors was also linked to many metabolic changes that included lowered systolic blood pressure and altered fluid-electrolyte balance.

Vinson et al. carried out two single-dose human studies with the primary purpose of determining whether bean extract inhibited human CHO absorption.[197] In the first, they challenged eleven fasting subjects with white bread and margarine with and without 1.5 g bean extract. In estimating AUC, the investigators found that glucose absorption was decreased by 66%. In the second full-meal study, this time performed with seven subjects who received 0.75 g bean extract, the trend again was inhibited absorption as indicated by a 28%–41% diminution in CHO uptake.

Thom, in 2000, published results from a randomized, double-blind, placebo-controlled trial performed in Norway that utilized a test product containing white kidney bean extract, inulin, chicory root, and *Garcinia cambogia*.[198] Forty healthy, overweight subjects with a BMI between 27.5 and 39 took two tablets of the test product before all meals for 12 weeks. Subjects were also instructed to follow a 1200 kcal low-fat diet. After 12 weeks, the active group lost an average of 3.5 kg (7.7 lb) ($p = .001$), whereas the placebo group lost 1.3 kg (2.86 lb) ($p > .05$). Between-group statistical differences were not calculated. Percent body fat (as measured by bioelectrical impedance) decreased by 2.3% ($p = .01$) in the active group in contrast to 0.7% ($p > .05$) in the placebo. No adverse events were reported.

A study performed by Celleno et al. in Italy utilized a bean extract for weight reduction.[199] In a randomized, double-blinded, placebo-controlled clinical trial consisting of a 30-day run-in phase followed by a 30-day active phase, 60 subjects between ages 20 and 45 were chosen. Subjects were 5–15 kg overweight, but their weight had been stable during the preceding 6 months. Through the run-in phase, subjects were educated on the importance of maintaining a test diet that included a 2000- to 2200-calorie diet with complex CHO intake concentrated in one of the two daily meals. Subjects were given either 450 mg of bean extract or placebo before the main CHO-containing meal of the day. Considering the major end point, the active group lost an average of 2.93 kg (6.45 lb) in 30 days compared with an average of 0.35 kg (0.77 lb) in the placebo group ($p < .001$). The active group demonstrated a 10.45% reduction in body fat compared with a 0.16% reduction in the placebo group ($p < .001$). Waist and hip circumferences in the test group showed 2.93 and 1.48 cm reductions, respectively, compared with 0.46 and 0.11 cm reductions in the placebo group ($p < .001$). No adverse events were reported.

In a randomized, double-blinded, placebo-controlled study performed by the Udani group, 39 obese subjects (BMI 30–43) received either 1500 mg of bean extract or placebo.[200] Twenty-seven subjects completed the study. The pills were taken with at least 8 oz of water daily with lunch and dinner for 8 weeks. The treatment group lost an average of 3.79 lb compared with the placebo group that lost an average of 1.65 lb ($p = .35$). Triglyceride levels in the treatment group were reduced by an average of 26.3 mg/dL compared to the 8.2 mg/dL in the placebo group ($p = .07$). Energy level (as measured by a 10-point Likert scale) demonstrated a 14% increase in the treatment group in contrast to a 1% decrease in the placebo group. However, this difference did not approach statistical significance ($p > .05$). No significant adverse events were associated with the active product.

Roughly 3 years later, Udani and Singh carried out a separate 4-week, randomized, double-blind, placebo-controlled study involving 25 healthy subjects consuming 1000 mg of proprietary fractionated white bean extract or an identical placebo twice a day before meals.[201] Both active and control group lost weight and waist inches—active group, −6.0 lb ($p = .0002$) and −2.2 in ($p = .0050$) and the placebo group −4.7 lb ($p = .0016$) and −2.1 in ($p = .0001$). There was no statistical difference in these parameters between the two groups. When the subjects were stratified by total dietary CHO intake, comparing the tertiles consuming the most CHO did show statistically significant differences between the active and placebo groups (body weight −8.7 vs. −1.7 lb, $p = .04$ and waist circumference −3.3 vs. −1.3 inches, $p = .01$).

In an 8-week, open-label study performed by Koike et al. in 10 subjects receiving white bean extract, a 2.4% reduction in weight, a 5.9% reduction in body fat, a 5.2% reduction in waist circumference, and a 2.9% reduction in hip circumference were found.[202] All differences were statistically significant and no adverse events took place.

Wu et al. performed a randomized, double-blinded, placebo-controlled study on 101 volunteers with a BMI between ages 25 and 40.[203] Volunteers received either placebo or the active substance. For 60 consecutive days, two capsules containing *Phaseolus vulgaris* extract (1000 mg) or placebo were taken 15 minutes before each meal. Body weights, waist and hip measurements, and blood for chemical analysis were obtained. After 60 days, the 51 subjects receiving *Phaseolus vulgaris* extract compared to a placebo group of 50 subjects exhibited clinical and statistically significantly greater average reduction of body weight (−1.9 vs. −0.4 kg [$p < .001$])and waist circumference (−1.9 vs. −0.4 cm [$p < .001$]), but no difference in the changes of average hip circumference (−0.3 vs. −0.3 cm [$p = .84$]). These results indicate that *Phaseolus vulgaris* extract can bring about clinically and statistically significant decrements in body weight and waist circumference.

Examination of the safety and efficacy of *Phaseolus vulgaris* extract on weight management was carried out by Grube et al.[204] Importantly, the investigation was carried out in two phases: first, a double-blind, weight loss phase in which subjects adhered to a mildly hypocaloric diet for 12 weeks; and second, an open-label weight maintenance trial in which participants energy intake was ad libitum over 24 weeks. In the first phase, there were 123 subjects, ages 18–60 years with a BMI between 25 and 35 kg/m^2 assigned to a treatment and placebo group. In the treatment group, subjects received 1.0 g of bean extract three times a day—at mealtime, while the placebo group received the same number of dummy pills containing inactive ingredients on the same schedule. At the end of study (12 weeks), the treatment group lost a mean of 2.91 ± 2.63 kg in body weight compared to 0.92 ± 2.00 kg for the placebo group ($p < .001$). Changes in impedance and waist circumference indicated that much of the weight transformation was secondary to fat loss. After completion of the first phase, 49 subjects from both the active and placebo arms who had lost at least 3% of body weight participated in the open-label 24-week extension period. During this phase, 36 out of 49 subjects (73.5%) maintained their weight to within 1.0% of their mass at initiation of the second phase. No serious adverse events were noted over the entire 36 weeks of study.

As suggested above, no major adverse reactions related to *Phaseolus vulgaris* extract have been reported to date.[205,206] Theoretically, gastrointestinal complaints such as gas, cramping, and so on should accompany use, but these problems seem much less severe with natural carb blockers than with drugs or fiber. In some early studies, ingesting CHO blockers led to gas and bloating. However, Boivin reported that this could be ameliorated using lower dosing.[190]

Brudnak carefully examined the safety of bean extracts because kidney bean lectins can present serious problems.[176] Fortunately, the commonly used extraction process for the bean extract employed in the clinical studies described above frees the extract of lectins. Using the same extract, thorough acute and subchronic laboratory studies on rats have shown no toxicity.[195,196]

L-Arabinose

Concerning alpha-glucosidase inhibitors, much work has been performed on L-arabinose.[155,195,196] L-arabinose is a naturally occurring compound that has been shown to have specific inhibitory activity on the digestive enzyme sucrase.[207–209] The effects of sucrase inhibition have been found to be extensive after sucrose challenge to rats—ranging from suppressing increases in blood glucose to thwarting the initiation of lipogenic enzyme activity.[208] A clinical study[209] reported that consuming L-arabinose caused a significant suppression of serum glucose levels after a sucrose challenge and attenuated sucrose-induced hyperglycemia in diabetic and nondiabetic subjects when L-arabinose was ingested in conjunction with sucrose. It is important to realize that L-arabinose should not influence absorption of HFCS. HFCS, a mixture of free glucose and fructose, does not require sucrase for absorption.

Other Potential Carbohydrate Blockers

Other choices exist that influence gastrointestinal absorption of CHO via inhibition of various digestive enzymes. In previous rat studies, hibiscus extract proved to be as effective and as safe as white bean extract.[210–212] Although further studies are indicated, hibiscus alone or combined with other ingredients appears to be quite effective.[195,196] A stereoisomer related to hibiscus acid, (–)-hydroxycitric acid (HCA), which commonly is extracted from *Garcinia cambogia* and related species, inhibits pancreatic alpha-amylase and intestinal alpha-glucosidase as well as directly delaying glucose uptake from the small intestine.[213,214] Yet other natural compounds are known to be active. In 1998, Lankisch et al. reported on the use of an amylase inhibitor extracted from wheat.[215] They found that the inhibitor delayed CHO absorption and reduced peak postprandial plasma glucose concentrations.

In the near future, formulas may be developed from a wide array of natural CHO blockers. *Gymnema sylvestre*,[216,217] apple extract (phloridzin)[218] and green coffee bean extract (chlorogenic and related acids) have been reported to inhibit glucose transport.[219] In the case of coffee extracts, components other than chlorogenic acid *per se* exhibit benefits and, at least in the liver, there may be some benefits in relation to fructose consumption.[220] Among proposed mechanisms of action, glucose transport may be inhibited by flavonoids via effects on the Glut 2 sugar transporter.[221] Fructose transport is influenced by eucalyptus leaf.[222]

INSULIN SENSITIZERS

Trivalent Chromium

Perhaps the best-examined natural supplement, insulin sensitizer, is trivalent chromium.[223–225] Nearly 60 years ago, Schwarz and Mertz discovered that an extract derived from pork kidney restored glucose tolerance in rats[226] and 2 years later reported that chromium was a major component of the so-called glucose tolerance factor (GTF).[227] Connections of GTF to human health first arose from studies in individuals receiving total parenteral nutrition (TPN), a procedure at that time in which chromium was absent in the replacement fluid.[228–230] In the initial reports, patients eventually showed characteristic signs and symptoms of chromium deficiency,[231] namely high circulating glucose levels, a need for insulin replacement, elevated circulating lipids, and even peripheral neuropathy and encephalopathy that improved after trivalent chromium replacement.[228-230] Largely through the investigations of Richard Anderson at the USDA, much knowledge has been gained concerning many aspects of chromium metabolism.[225,231]

Various facets of MS, particularly IR and hypertension, can be brought out in rats by addition of sucrose in diets—even at levels comparable to those consumed in the Western diet.[80,108,232] Importantly, the addition of chromium can overcome these sucrose-induced conditions. Interestingly, in one study examining the effects of trivalent chromium on insulin sensitivity and hypertension, although lower levels of chromium supplementation ameliorated IR and lowered the sucrose-induced elevations of blood pressure initially, over time these effects dissipated and both parameters returned to control baseline.[232] In this case, increasing the chromium dose returned the favorable effects. These findings raised two possibilities that (1) it took longer to bring about sugar-induced chromium deficiency under conditions of low but insufficient chromium intake or (2) chromium was not working entirely through a replacement of any deficiency in body chromium and more was needed to maintain effects.

A major difficulty with chromium replacement is bioavailability.[223-225] It appears that all forms of trivalent chromium are not equal in bioavailability according to many laboratory and clinical studies.[224,225,233,234] Initially, the most popular form of supplementation was chromium chloride, but as early as 1989 Evans pointed out the poor absorption of chromium chloride (inorganic ligand) when compared to chromium picolinate (organic ligand).[224] The normal absorption for chromium chloride is only 0.4%–1.0% of the oral dose.[225] This fact led to the development of more bioavailable, organic forms of chromium, for instance, having nicotinate, picolinate, and histidinate as ligands.[224,225,233,234] Seaborn and Stoecker performed a series of studies showing the effects of CHO, acids, and agents affecting prostaglandin metabolism to alter absorption.[235-237]

Although the hexavalent form of chromium is toxic, little evidence suggests the same for the trivalent form.[223] Trivalent chromium, such as the nicotinic, picolinic, and histidinate forms, appears to be quite safe, yet still effective.[238,239] Early studies that indicated possible mutagenic effects of chromium picolinate today seem to lack relevance[240] inasmuch as further studies with both animals and humans have failed to corroborate toxic effects.[241,242]

Clinical studies have supported claims of benefits from oral organic trivalent chromium compounds. Anderson et al. performed the most convincing of these studies in China.[157] A group of 180 men and women with T2D were randomly divided into three groups: placebo, chromium 200 mcg daily, and chromium 1000 mcg daily. Subjects did not change their normal medications, eating habits, or living habits. Those individuals in the higher chromium dose group showed the earliest and greatest benefits, although the group receiving the lower dose also profited. After 4 months, HbA1C, fasting blood glucose, circulating insulin levels, and plasma total cholesterol levels improved in the active arms. Of note, the beneficial effects in the individuals with diabetes occurred at levels of chromium exceeding the upper limit of the Estimated Safe and Adequate Daily Dietary Intake.

Martin et al. examined subjects with T2D who had received glipizide and placebo for a three month run-in period.[243] For another six months, 12 continued with the sulfonylurea and placebo regimen, whereas 17 were given 1000 mcg of chromium picolinate in addition to glipizide. Relative to the placebo group, subjects in the chromium group showed significant improvements in insulin sensitivity and glucose control. At the same time, this group displayed less body-weight gain and visceral fat accumulation.

Accordingly, many believe that chromium supplementation could be an excellent tool to overcome and/or ameliorate IR/T2D rather than more toxic drugs.[244,245] Linday commented in 1997 on the Diabetes Prevention Program developed to determine whether T2D can be prevented or delayed in persons with impaired glucose tolerance.[244] Noting that drugs such as metformin and troglitazone had been used, the author questioned why trivalent chromium with its ability to ameliorate IR as well as an acceptable adverse action profile and reasonable costs had not been included as one arm of the study. Preuss and Anderson came to the same conclusions regarding the use of chromium to overcome many of the chronic conditions associated with IR.[245]

SUBSTANCES THAT REDUCE HEPATIC GLUCOSE PRODUCTION AND OUTPUT

Biotin: Biotin, a B vitamin, administered in high doses improves glycemic control in several animal models while showing no evidence of toxicity.[246–248] In one study, 26 diabetic KK mice that were moderately hyperglycemic and insulin resistant received saline (control) or different doses of biotin.[246] Biotin treatment, compared to control, lowered postprandial glucose levels, improved tolerance to glucose, and lessened IR. In a second study, oral glucose tolerance testing was performed in an animal model of spontaneous non-insulin-diabetes—Otsuka Long-Evans Tokushima Fatty rat. The rats received different doses of biotin. Biotin corrected impaired glucose tolerance, and insulin secretion decreased leading to lower circulating insulin levels.[247] In a third study carried out in streptozotocin-induced diabetic rats, impaired glucose tolerance improved after intraperitoneal biotin was given even though the poor insulin secretion did not improve.[248] Relatively low glucokinase and hexokinase activities were found in liver and pancreas of the diabetic rats. However, both liver and pancreas values increased into the normal range after the biotin application. These results demonstrate that injected biotin can improve glucose handling without increasing insulin secretion in streptozotocin-induced diabetic rats.

Much of these findings have been duplicated in clinical studies.[249,250] When people with type 1 diabetes were given 16 mg of oral biotin per day for 1 week, their fasting blood sugars dropped by 50%.[249] In a larger study, 43 patients with noninsulin-dependent diabetics showed lower serum biotin levels than 64 healthy controls.[250] Serum biotin levels inversely correlated with fasting blood sugars. Perhaps not a surprise, 9 mg of biotin given daily corrected hyperglycemia with virtually no change in insulin levels. As elevated levels of pyruvate and lactate decreased into normal ranges, the investigators postulated that biotin enhances the activity of the biotin-dependent enzyme, pyruvate carboxylase, and is the reason behind improvement.

McCarty wrote an interesting article in the *Journal Medical Hypotheses*.[156] On the basis of the earlier work, he hypothesized that biotin enhances glucokinase activity, which has a key role for normal glucose-stimulated insulin secretion, postprandial hepatic glucose uptake, and the appropriate suppression of hepatic glucose output and gluconeogenesis by elevated plasma glucose levels. Secondary effects on pyruvate kinase and phosphoenolpyruvate carboxykinase lowered hepatic glucose output. Suffice it to say, biotin decreases hepatic glucose production and output, as the drug metformin. Of interest, biguanides like metformin that have similar effects on hepatic output of glucose, have been shown to increase longevity in rodents.[251,252] Could biotin mimic this effect in humans?

HCA AND MULTIPLE MECHANISMS REGULATING GLUCOSE METABOLISM

(–)-Hydroxycitric Acid—*Garcinia* spp. Extract: (–)-Hydroxycitric acid (HCA), a naturally occurring substance found chiefly in fruits of the species of *Garcinia*, is a totally unexpected regulator of multiple pathways that influence glucose uptake and metabolism. Indeed, for 30 years after its discovery, it was universally considered to be a source of gluconeogenesis that, at best, would exercise no impact on blood glucose and insulin levels and, at worst, would seriously elevate serum glucose in diabetics. It and several synthetic derivatives of citric acid have been investigated extensively in regard to their ability to inhibit the production of fatty acids from CHO, to suppress appetite, and to inhibit weight gain.[253] Weight-loss benefits were first ascribed to HCA, its salts, and its lactone in United States Patent 3,764,692 granted to John M. Lowenstein in 1973.

The proposed mechanisms of action for HCA, most of which were originally put forth by researchers at the pharmaceutical firm of Hoffmann-La Roche, have been summarized in numerous publications since that time. The primary mechanism according to general agreement in the field is HCA's reduction of the conversion of CHO calories into fats by competitively inhibiting the actions of adenosine 5'-triphosphate (ATP) citrate lyase, the enzyme that catalyzes the extramitochondrial cleavage of citrate to oxaloacetate and acetyl CoA. ATP citrate lyase is the enzyme that initiates the conversion of citrate into fatty acids and cholesterol in the primary pathway of fatty acid synthesis in the body[254] HCA increases the production and storage of glycogen (which is found in the liver, small intestine, and muscles of mammals) while reducing both appetite and weight gain.[255]

HCA serves to disinhibit fatty acid oxidation. The compound malonyl CoA, which is activated as the first committed step in the biosynthesis of fatty acids in the body, also is a negative regulator of fatty acid metabolism for energy. In other words, if the body is synthesizing fatty acids from carbohydrates at the same time, it is inhibiting the oxidation of fats for energy. The prevalent orthodoxy in the end of the 1990s was that HCA acts to unleash fatty acid oxidation by negating the effects of malonyl CoA while promoting gluconeogenesis.[256]

Quite surprisingly, a beneficial effect of HCA on blood sugar regulation was never suggested in the early literature on the topic and only was discovered in 2000. The original pharmaceutical research on HCA performed at Hoffman-La Roche failed to find significant changes in either blood glucose levels or blood insulin levels, undoubtedly in part due to the fact that almost all of that research used diets that consisted largely of glucose (e.g., 70% glucose diets were typically employed to encourage lipogenesis) or fructose. Reviews published as late as 2000 continued to indicate that the use of HCA as a component in the nutritional therapy for diabetes should focus entirely upon a reduction in serum free fatty acids with a likely increase in gluconeogenesis that must be counterbalanced by the ingestion of items such as chromium, biotin or metformin.[257] However, by 2003, the first of many publications confirmed, initially in animal models, that HCA seemingly directly influences the glucose–insulin system, among others.[242,258]

Clouatre-Preuss added to the experimental body of knowledge in this area and reviewed the current literature in an article published in 2008.[259] By that time, animal models had confirmed the impact upon the glucose–insulin system. For instance, using female mice consuming a low-fat diet consisting of 3.3% liquid *Garcinia cambogia* extract (60% HCA) and supplemented with 10% sucrose water for 4 weeks, it was found that HCA significantly reduced serum insulin without influencing serum glucose.[260] One major surprise from the 2008 article was the striking differences in efficacy of different HCA salts in affecting the glucose–insulin axis.[259] The potassium and potassium–magnesium hydroxycitrate salts experimentally were quite active in maintaining normal serum blood sugar with the aid of insulin levels that were only one-half of those in the placebo animals, but at the relatively low levels of intake used in this study, the potassium–calcium salt exercised no influence on the insulin system.[259]

Others have found differences in the efficacy of the HCA salts in influencing insulin sensitivity. As one example, in a short-term experiment involving a high-glucose diet supplemented with 3% dietary HCA as potassium–calcium hydroxycitrate following a period of restrictive feeding, blood glucose levels were significantly reduced; but, as in the 2008 study, there was no significant effect on insulin with the potassium–calcium HCA salt.[261] In published work, potassium–calcium HCA has influenced serum insulin only when given at levels considerably above those used in the 2008 study (i.e., HCA from a potassium–calcium salt equivalent to 120 mg or higher in rats vs. a maximum dose of 84 mg of the potassium–magnesium HCA salt) and in an animal model (mouse) that the Roche-era studies showed to be much more sensitive to the effects of HCA than is the rat.[262] Quite typical in the literature are reports of effects on the insulin system only with experimental dosages of potassium–calcium hydroxycitrate delivering HCA-free acid equivalents of roughly five or more times the required dosages from potassium and potassium–magnesium hydroxycitrate. Several unpublished pilot trials involving diabetics ingesting potassium and potassium–magnesium hydroxycitrate salts have confirmed that these salts are significantly active in humans, whereas at normally acceptable dosages the potassium–calcium salts are not (D.L. Clouatre and J.M. Dunn with G. Jackson of Drew University Medical School, 1999, data in US Patents 6,207,714; 6,476,071; and 7,015,250. Also D.L. Clouatre and D.E. Clouatre with Novel Bisyir of Jakarta, Indonesia, 2006).

Experiments employing a potassium hydroxycitrate salt (the Regulator) at a very high dose (310 mg/kg body weight, HCA concentration unclear) showed a reduced insulin response to an intragastric glucose load, but no impact on insulin or glucose with an intravenous glucose tolerance test.[263] In a later publication by the same researchers, HCA treatment was found to delay the intestinal absorption of enterally administered glucose at the level of the small intestinal mucosa in rats and to strongly attenuate postprandial blood glucose levels after both intragastric ($p < .01$) and intraduodenal ($p < .001$) glucose administration.[264] The explanation offered is that HCA delays the entry of glucose into the blood from the gut and that the effect on insulin is secondary to this action.[264] At best, this can be only a partial explanation. An effect on glucose entry into the blood from the gut under acute conditions does not explain (1) lower insulin with stable serum glucose with chronic ingestion of HCA for several weeks, i.e., lower insulin with stable serum glucose under conditions not tied to immediate food intake, (2) glucose challenge data in which animals were not given HCA immediately before the test and the glucose was delivered intraperitoneally, or (3) the response to a direct test with insulin injection, which demonstrated better early glucose clearance. Only improved insulin sensitivity or actual insulin mimesis would appear to explain these findings, especially the glucose tolerance and insulin challenge testing in the second experiment in the Clouatre-Preuss article.[259] Moreover, the glucose challenge approach via intragastric and intraduodenal administration does not address yet another mechanism that has been identified for HCA's intervention in carbohydrate digestion, to wit, HCA inhibits pancreatic alpha-amylase and intestinal alpha-glucosidase.[213]

Experiments have begun to hint at unsuspected mechanisms of action for HCA in glucose–insulin metabolism. Unpublished in vitro work with cardiomyocytes and hepatocytes challenged with glucose (Faiyaz Ahmed using a modification of the method of Ravi et al., 2009) quite surprisingly has revealed that the potassium–magnesium salt tested directly induces the uptake of glucose by these cells even in the complete absence of insulin.[265] This effect is considerably stronger in hepatocytes than in the cardiomyocytes (using glucose concentrations of 5–25 mM). Interestingly, there is an additive effect with insulin in the latter, but not the former. An appealing explanation for these findings comes from computational docking studies, which serve as direct measures of the affinity of ligands for receptors. One such study performed by students of S. Karthi of the Bioinformatics programs of The University of Texas (El Paso) and SASTRA University (India) posted in 2012 found that HCA exhibits its highest affinity for the insulin receptor followed by the 11-β-hydroxysteroid dehydrogenase and farnesoid X receptors.

Although the picture is hardly complete, it is intriguing that this compound that initially was thought to exert no effect at all on glucose–insulin metabolism, over the last decade and a half has begun to reveal some of its secrets with significant implications for future research. Mechanism include, among others, inhibition of pancreatic *alpha*-amylase and intestinal *alpha*-glucosidase, a delay in the absorption of glucose from the small intestine (involving a sodium pump?), direct action on the cellular insulin receptor and, quite possibly, action on the cellular uptake of glucose that is not dependent on insulin. Fortunately, for a compound that is this metabolically active, extensive recent safety reviews have not found properly manufactured HCA to be the source of any major adverse reaction.[266]

CONCLUSIONS

Although the concept that refined CHO like sugars in the diet can be hazardous to health when consumed in excess was proposed many years ago,[54,56,60–63,67,69,71] it is only relatively recently that a general acceptance has become apparent.[2,25,114] The most favored, current hypothesis is that the harm from sugars arise from their ability to bring on perturbations in the glucose–insulin system,[9,54] as well other regulatory systems such as the renin–angiotensin system important for normal existence.[81,89,90] Although we need insulin, too much may present a problem.[9,54,71] Lifestyle changes that overcome the responsible factors offer one solution. However, carrying out these changes presents a challenge to most individuals' ability to comply. Although long-term use of antidiabetic pharmaceuticals has been commonly avoided probably because of possible adverse reactions, the use of safer dietary supplements has been virtually ignored.[244,245] Table 7.2 provides a list of numerous natural agents that have the potential to ameliorate the effects of too much sugar consumption. We believe these should be further investigated.

REFERENCES

1. Ford ES, Giles WH, Dietz WH. Prevalence of metabolic syndrome among US adults: Findings from the third National Health and Nutrition Examination Survey. *JAMA* 2002;287:356–359.
2. Weiss R, Bremer AA, Lustig RH. What is metabolic syndrome, and why are children getting it? *Ann NY Acad Sci* 2013;1281:123–140.
3. Smyth S, Heron Smyth SA. Diabetes and obesity: The twin epidemics. *Nat Med* 2005;12:75–80.
4. Emery N. The global diabetes epidemic brought to you by global development. *The Atlantic*, July 2, 2012. http://www.theatlantic.com/health//07/diabetes-epidemic/259305/ (accessed December 4, 2014).
5. Dreisbach AW, Batuman V. Epidemiology of hypertension (Updated July 11, 2013) http://emedicine.medscape.com/article/1928048-overview#aw2aab6b3 (accessed April 4, 2014).
6. Miller M, Stone NJ, Ballantyne C et al. Triglycerides and cardiovascular disease, a scientific statement from the American Heart Association. *Circulation* 2011;123:2293–2294.
7. Bjorntorp P. Body fat distribution, insulin resistance and metabolic diseases. *Nutrition* 1997; 13:795–803.
8. Wilborn C, Beckham J, Campbell B et al. Obesity: Prevalence, theories, medical consequences, management and research directions. *J Inter Soc Sports Nutr* 2005;2:4–31.
9. Reaven GM. Banting Lecture 1988. Role of insulin resistance in human disease. *Diabetes* 1988;37:1595–1607.
10. Reaven GM. The individual components of metabolic syndrome: Is there a raison d'etre? *J Amer Coll Nutr* 2007;6:191–195.
11. Center for Disease Control and Prevention, National Diabetes Fact Sheet. http://www.cdc.gov/diabetes/pubs/estimates11.htm (accessed April 4, 2014)
12. Center for Disease Control and Prevention, National Diabetes Fact Sheet. http://www.cdc.gov/nchs/data/databriefs/db131.htm (accessed April 4, 2014).
13. Jornayvaz FR, Samuel VT, Shulman GI. The role of muscle insulin resistance in the pathogenesis of atherogenic dyslipidemia and nonalcoholic fatty liver disease associated with metabolic syndrome. *Ann Rev Nutr* 2010;30:273–290.
14. Beck-Nielsen H, Hother-Nielsen O. Obesity in non-insulin-dependent diabetes mellitus. In: LeRoith D, Taylor SI, Olefsky J, editors. *Diabetes Mellitus: A Fundamental & Clinical Text*. Philadelphia, PA: Lippincott-Raven; 1996, pp. 475–484.
15. Ohlson LO, Larsson B, Svardsudd K et al. The influence of body fat distribution on the incidence of diabetes mellitus. 13.5 years of follow-up of the participants in the study of men born in 1913. *Diabetes* 1985;34:1055–1058.
16. Lundgren H, Bengtsson C, Blohme G et al. Adiposity and adipose tissue distribution in relation to the incidence of diabetes in women. Results from a prospective study in Gothenburg, Sweden. *Int J Obes* 1989;13:413–423.
17. Colditz GA, Willett WC, Rotnitzky A, Manson JE. Weight gain as a risk factor for clinical diabetes mellitus in women. *Ann Intern Med* 1995;122:481–486.
18. Resnick HE, Valsania P, Halter JB, Lin X. Relation of weight gain and weight loss on subsequent diabetes risk in overweight adult. *J Epidemiol Community Health* 2000;54:596–602.
19. Mokdad AH, Ford ES, Bowman BA et al. Prevalence of obesity, diabetes, and obesity-related health risk factors, 2001. *JAMA* 2003;289:76–79.
20. Snijder MB, Dekker JM, Visser M et al. Associations of hip and thigh circumferences independent of waist circumference with the incidence of type 2 diabetes. The Hoorn Study. *Am J Clin Nutr* 2003; 77:1192–1197.
21. Aucott LS. Influences of weight loss on long-term diabetes outcome. *Proc Nutr Soc* 2008;67:54–59.
22. http://en.wikipedia.org/wiki/insulin-resistance (accessed December 4, 2014).
23. Ninomiya JK, L'Italien G, Criqui MH et al. Association of metabolic syndrome with history of myocardial infarction and stroke in the Third National Health and Nutrition Examination Survey. *Circulation* 2004;109:42–46.
24. Meigs JB, Wilson P, Fox CS et al. Body mass index, metabolic syndrome and risk of type 2 diabetes or cardiovascular disease. *J Clin Endo Metab* 2006;91:2906–2912.
25. Bremer AA, Mietus-Snyder M, Lustig RH. Toward a unifying hypothesis of metabolic syndrome. *Pediatrics* 2012;129:557–570.
26. Chiasson JL, Josse RG, Gornis R et al. Acarbose for prevention of type 2 diabetes mellitus: The STOP-NIDDM randomized trial. *Lancet* 2002;359:2072–2077.

27. Buchanan TA, Xiang AH, Peters RK et al. Preservation of pancreatic beta-cell function and prevention of type 2 diabetes by pharmacological treatment of insulin resistance in high-risk Hispanic women. *Diabetes* 2002;51:2796–2803.
28. Xiang AH, Peters RK, Kios SL et al. Effect of pioglitazone on pancreatic beta-cell function and diabetes risk in Hispanic women with prior gestational diabetes. *Diabetes* 2006;55:517–522.
29. Knowler WC, Barrett-Connor E, Fowler SB et al. Reduction in the incidence of type 2 diabetes with life-style intervention or metformin. *New Engl J Med* 2002;346:393–403.
30. Knowler WC, Hamman RF, Edelstein SL et al. Prevention of type 2 diabetes with troglitazone in the Diabetes Prevention Program. *Diabetes* 2005;54:1150–1156.
31. Knowler WC, Fowler SE, Hamman RF et al. 10-year follow-up of diabetes incidence and weight loss in the Diabetes Prevention Program outcomes Study. *Lancet* 2009;374:1677–1686.
32. Torgerson JS, Hauptman J, Boldrin MN, Sjostrom L. Xenical in the prevention of diabetes in obese subjects (XENDOS) study: A randomized study of orlistat as an adjunct to life-style changes for the prevention of type 2 diabetes in obese patients. *Diabetes Care* 2004;27:155–161.
33. Gerstein HC, Yusuf S, Bosch J et al. Effect of rosigliazone on the frequency of diabetes in patients with impaired glucose tolerance or impaired fasting glucose: A randomised controlled study. *Lancet* 2006;368:1096–1105.
34. Kawamori R, Tajima N, Iwamoto Y et al. Voglibose for prevention of type 2 diabetes mellitus: A randomized, double-blind trial in Japanese individuals with impaired glucose tolerance. *Lancet* 2009;373:1607–1614.
35. DeFronzo RA, Tripathy D, Schwenke DC et al. (Act Now Study): Pioglitazone for diabetes prevention in impaired glucose tolerance. *N Eng J Med* 2011;364:1104–1115.
36. Krentz AJ, Bailey CJ. Oral antidiabetic agents: Current role in type 2 diabetes mellitus. *Drugs* 2005;65:385–411.
37. Ketz J. Review of Oral Antidiabetic Agents. https://www.clevelandclinicmeded.com/medicalpubs/pharmacy/MayJune2001/oral_antidiabetic.htm (accessed December 4, 2014).
38. Gangji AS, Cukierman T, Gerstein HC et al. A systematic review and meta-analysis of hypoglycemia and cardiovascular events: A comparison of glyburide with other secretagogues and with insulin. *Diabetes Care* 2007;30:389–394.
39. Fonseca V. Effect of thiazolidinediones on body weight in patients with diabetes mellitus. *Am J Med* 2003;115(suppl 8A):42S–48S.
40. Ifland JR, Sheppard K, Preuss HG et al. Refined food addiction: A classic substance use disorder. *Med Hypotheses* 2009;72:518–526.
41. No Author Listed. Frederick Grant Banting (1891–1941), co-discoverer of insulin. *JAMA* 1966;198:660–661.
42. Rafuse J. Seventy-five years later, insulin remains Canada's major medical-research coup. *Canad Med Assoc J* 1996;155:1306–1308.
43. Preuss HG. The insulin system in health and disease (Editorial). *J Amer Coll Nutr* 1997;16:393–394.
44. Rosenfeld L. Insulin: Discovery and controversy. *Clin Chemistry* 2002;48:2270–2288.
45. Himsworth H. Diabetes mellitus: A differentiation into insulin-sensitive and insulin-insensitive types. *Lancet* 1936;1:127–130.
46. Ginsberg H, Kimmerling G, Olefsky JM, Reaven GM. Further evidence that insulin resistance exists in patients with chemical diabetes. *Diabetes* 1974;23:674–678.
47. Olefsky JM. Diabetes mellitus. In: Wyngaarden JB, Smith LH Jr, Bennett JC, editors. *Cecil Textbook of Medicine*, 19th Ed. Philadelphia, PA: WB Saunders;1992, pp 1291–1310.
48. King H, Aubert RE, Herman WH. Global burden of diabetes, 1995-2025: Prevalence, numerical estimates, and projections. *Diabetes Care* 1998;22:1414–1431.
49. Wild S, Roglic G, Green A et al. Global prevalence of diabetes: Estimates for the year 2000 and projections for 2030. *Diabetes Care* 2004;27:1047–1053.
50. Winer N, Sowers JR. Epidemiology of diabetes. *J Clin Pharmacol* 2004;44:397–405.
51. Broughton DL, Taylor RL. Review: Deterioration of glucose tolerance with age: The role of insulin resistance. *Age Aging* 1991;20:221–225.
52. DeFronzo RA, Ferrannini E. Insulin resistance. A multifaceted syndrome responsible for NIDDM, obesity, hypertension, dyslipidemia, and atherosclerotic cardiovascular disease. *Diabetes Care* 1991;14:173–194.
53. Haffner SM, Stern MP, Hazuda HP et al. Cardiovascular risk factors in confirmed diabetic individuals: Does the clock start ticking before the onset of clinical diabetes? *JAMA* 1990;263:2893–2898.
54. Yudkin J. Sucrose, coronary heart disease, diabetes and obesity. Do hormones provide a link? *Am Heart J* 1988;115:493–498.

55. Ferrannini E, Natali A, Bell P et al. Insulin resistance and hypersecretion in obesity. *J Clin Invest* 1997;100:1166–1173.
56. Paton JH. Relation of excessive carbohydrate ingestion to catarrhs and other diseases. *Brit Med J* 1933;1:738.
57. Aschoff L. Observations concerning the relationship between cholesterol metabolism and vascular disease. *Br Med J* 1932;2:1131–1134.
58. Himsworth HP. Diet and the incidence of diabetes mellitus. *Clin Sci* 1935;2:117–148.
59. Yudkin J. Patterns and trends in carbohydrate consumption and their relation to disease. *Proc Nutr Soc* 1964;23:149–162.
60. Ahrens RA. Sucrose, hypertension, and heart disease: An historical perspective. *Am J Clin Nutr* 1974;27:403–422.
61. Yudkin J. Sucrose and cardiovascular disease. *Proc Nutr Soc* 1972;31:331–337.
62. Yudkin J, Morland J. Sugar and myocardial infarction. *Am J Clin Nutr* 1964;20:503–506.
63. Yudkin J, Szanto SS. Hyperinsulinism and atherogenesis. *Br Med J* 1971;1:349.
64. American Diabetic Association: Diabetes statistics. http//www.diabetes.org/diabetes-basics/diabetes-statistics/ (accessed December 4, 2014).
65. National Diabetes Information Clearinghouse (NDIC). National Diabetes Statistics, 2011. http//www.CDC.gov/diabetes/pubs/statsreport14/national-diabetes-report-web.pdf (accessed December 4, 2014).
66. Israel KD, Michelis OE 4th, Reiser S, Keeney M. Serum uric acid, inorganic phosphorus, and glutamic-oxalacetic transaminase and blood pressure in carbohydrates-sensitive adults consuming three different levels of sucrose. *Ann Nutr Metab* 1983;27:425–435.
67. Preuss HG, Fournier RD. Effects of sucrose ingestion on blood pressure. *Life Sci* 1982;30:879–886.
68. Preuss HG, Gondal JA, Lieberman SL. Association of macronutrients and energy intake with hypertension. *J Amer Coll Nutr* 1996;15:21–35.
69. Preuss HG, Echard B, Bagchi D et al. Anti-aging nutraceuticals. In: Klatz R, Goldman R, editors. *Anti-Aging Therapeutics*. Chicago, IL: A4M Publications; 2008, pp 219–224.
70. Preuss HG, Bagchi D, Clouatre D. Insulin resistance: A factor of aging. In: Ghen MJ, Corso N, Joiner-Bey H, Klatz R, Dratz A, editors. *The Advanced Guide to Longevity Medicine*, Landrum SC: Ghen; 2001, pp 239–250.
71. Preuss HG. Effects of glucose/insulin perturbations on aging and chronic disorders of aging: The evidence. *J Am Coll Nutr* 1997;16:397–403.
72. Ervin RB, Ogden CL. Consumption of added sugars among US adults, 2005–2010. NCHS data brief, no 122. Hyattsville, MD: National Center for Health Statistics. May 2013.
73. Marriott BP, Olsho L, Hadden L, Conner P. Intake of added sugars and selected nutrients in the United States, National Health and Nutrition Examination Survey (NHANES) 2003–2006. *Crit Rev Food Sci Nutr* 2010;50:228–258.
74. Bowman SA. Diets of individuals based on energy intakes from added sugars. *Fam Econ Nutr Rev* 1999;12:31–38.
75. Vartanian LR, Schwartz MB, Brownell KD. Effects of soft drink consumption on nutrition and health. A systematic review and meta-analysis. *Am J Public Health* 2007;97:667–675.
76. US Department of Agriculture and US Department of Health and Human Services. Dietary Guidelines for Americans, 2010. 7th Ed. Washington, DC: US Government Printing Office, 2010.
77. Ervin RB, Kit BK, Carroll MD, Ogden CL. Consumption of added sugars among US children and adolescents, 2005–2008. NCHS data brief, no 87. Hyattsville, MD: National Center for Health Statistics, 2013.
78. Harris MI, Hadden WC, Knowler WC, Bennett PH. Prevalence of diabetes and impaired glucose tolerance and plasma glucose levels in US population aged 20–74 yr. *Diabetes* 1987; 36:523–534.
79. Nguyen NT, Nguyen XM, Lane J, Wang P. Relationship between obesity and diabetes in a US adult population: Findings from the National Health and Nutrition Examination Survey, 1999–2006. *Obes Surg* 2011;21:351–355.
80. Preuss MB, Preuss HG. Effects of sucrose on the blood pressure of various strains of Wistar rats. *Lab Invest* 1980;43:101–107.
81. Preuss HG, Montamarry S, Echard B et al. Long-term effects of chromium, grape seed extract, and zinc on various metabolic parameters of rats. *Mol Cell Biochem* 2001;223:95–102.
82. Cohen AM, Teitelbaum A, Balogh M, Groen JJ. Effect of interchanging bread and sucrose as main source of carbohydrate in a low fat diet on the glucose tolerance curve of healthy volunteer subjects. *Am J Clin Nutr* 1966;19:59–62.
83. Hallfrisch J, Lazar D, Jorgensen C, Reiser S. Insulin and glucose responses in rats fed sucrose or starch. *Am J Clin Nutr* 1979;32:787–793.

84. Yudkin J. Carbohydrate confusion. *J Royal Soc Med* 1978;71:551–556.
85. Jenkins DJA, Srichaikul K, Mirrahimi A et al. Glycemic index. In Bagchi D, Preuss HG, editors. *Obesity: Epidemiology, Pathophysiology, and Prevention*, 2nd Ed. Boca Raton, FL: CRC Press; 2012, pp 212–238.
86. Erik E, Aller JG, Abete I et al. Starches, sugars, and obesity. *Nutrients* 2011;3:341–369.
87. Sanders LM, Lupton JR. Carbohydrates. In: JW Erdman Jr, IA Macdonald, SH Zeisel, editors. Present Knowledge in Nutrition, 10th Ed. Ames, IA: Wiley-Blackwell; 2012, pp 83–96.
88. Preuss HG. Bean amylase inhibitor and other carbohydrate absorption blockers: Effects on diabesity and general health. *J Amer Coll Nutr* 2009;28:266–276.
89. Preuss HG, Echard B, Bagchi D, Perricone NV. Maitake mushroom extracts ameliorate progressive hypertension and other chronic metabolic perturbations in aging female rats. *Int J Med Sci* 2010;7:169–180.
90. Preuss HG, Echard MT, Bagchi D, Perricone NV. Effects of astaxanthin on blood pressure and insulin sensitivity are not directly interdependent. *Int J Med Sci* 2011;8:126–138.
91. Chen L, Caballero B, Mitchell DC et al. Reducing consumption of sugar-sweetened beverages is associated with reduced blood pressure: A prospective study among U.S. adults. *Circulation* 2010;121:2398–2406.
92. Malik VS, Popkin BM, Bray GA et al. Sugar-sweetened beverages, obesity, type 2 diabetes mellitus, and cardiovascular disease risk. *Circulation* 2010;121:1356–1364.
93. Elliott SS, Keim NL, Stern JS et al. Fructose, weight gain, and the insulin resistance syndrome. *Am J Clin Nutr* 2002;76:911–922.
94. Havel PJ. Control of energy homeostasis and insulin action by adipocyte hormones: Leptin acylation stimulating protein, and adiponectin. *Curr Opin Lipidol* 2002;13:51–59.
95. Havel PJ. Dietary fructose: Implications for dysregulation of energy homeostasis and lipid/carbohydrate metabolism. *Nutr Rev* 2005;63:133–157.
96. Tappy L, Le KA, Tran C, Paquot N. Fructose and metabolic diseases: New findings, new questions. *Nutrition* 2010;26:1044–1049.
97. Sen S, Kundu BK, Wu HC-J et al. Glucose regulation of load-induced mTor signaling and ER stress in mammalian heart. Doi:10.1161/JAHA.113.004796.
98. Wiernsperger N, Geloen A, Rapin J-R. Fructose and cardiometabolic disorders: The controversy will, and must, continue. *Clinics* 2010;65:729–738.
99. Teff KL, Grudziak J, Townsend RR et al. Endocrine and metabolic effects of consuming fructose- and glucose-sweetened beverages with meals in obese men and women: Influence of insulin resistance on plasma triglyceride responses. *J Clin Endocrinol Metab* 2009;94:1562–1569.
100. Johnson RJ, Segal MS, Sautin Y et al. Potential role of sugar (fructose) in the epidemic of hypertension, obesity, and metabolic syndrome, diabetes, kidney disease, and cardiovascular disease. *Am J Clin Nutr* 2007;86:899–906.
101. Cox L. Stanhope KL, Schwarz JM et al. Consumption of fructose- but not glucose-sweetened beverages for 10 weeks increases circulating concentrations of uric acid, retinol binding protein-4, and gamma-glutamyl transferase activity in overweight/obese humans. *Nutr Metab* 2012;9(1):68. doi: 10.1186/1743-7075-9-68.
102. Jalal DL, Smits G. Increased fructose associates with elevated blood pressure. *J Am Soc Nephrol* 2010;21:1543–1549.
103. Cohen AM, Michaelson IC, Yanko L, Retinopathy in rats with disturbed carbohydrate metabolism following a high sucrose diet. *Am J Ophthalmol* 1972;73:863–869.
104. Papachristodoulou D, Heath H. Ultrastructural alterations during the development of retinopathy in sucrose-fed and streptozotocin-diabetic rats. *Exp Eye Res* 1977;25:371–384.
105. Thornber JM, Eckhert CD. Protection against sucrose-induced retinal capillary damage in the Wistar rat. *J Nutr* 1984;114:1070–1075.
106. Boot-Handford R, Hezath H. Identification of fructose as the retinopathic agent associated with the ingestion of sucrose-rich diets in the rat. *Metabolism* 1980;29:1247–1252.
107. More NS, Rao NA, Preuss HG. Early sucrose-induced retinal vascular lesions in SHR and WKY rats. *Ann Lab Clin Sci* 1986;16:419–426.
108. Preuss HG, Fournier RD, Chieuh CC et al. Refined carbohydrates affect blood pressure and retinal vasculature in SHR and WKY. *J Hypertension* 1986;4:S459–S462.
109. Page KA, Chan O, Arora J et al. Effects of fructose vs glucose on regional cerebral blood flow in brain regions involved with appetite and reward pathways. *JAMA* 309:63–70.
110. Drewnowski A, Rehm CD. Energy intakes of US children and adults by food purchase location and by specific food sources. *Nutr J* 2013;12:59. doi:10.1186/1475-2891-12-59.
111. Bray GA, Nielsen SJ, Popkin BM. Consumption of high-fructose corn syrup in beverages may play a role in the epidemic of obesity. *Am J Clin Nutr* 2004;79:537–543.

112. Goran MI, Ulijaszek SJ, Ventura EE. High fructose corn syrup and diabetes prevalence: A global perspective. *Global Pub Health* 2013;8:55–64.
113. Shapiro A, Mu W, Roncal C et al. Fructose-induced leptin resistance exacerbates weight gain in response to subsequent high-fat feeding. *Am J Physiol* 2008;295:R21370–1375.
114. Lustig RH, Schmidt LA, Brindis CD. The toxic truth about sugar. *Nature* 2012;482:27–29.
115. Tobey TA, Nondon CE, Zavaroni I, Reaven GM. Mechanism of insulin resistance in fructose-fed rats. *Metabolism* 1982;31:608–612.
116. Reaven GM. Effects of fructose on lipid metabolism. *Am J Clin Nutr* 1982;35:627.
117. Fournier RD, Chiueh CC, Kopin IJ et al. The interrelationship between excess CHO ingestion, blood pressure and catecholamine excretion in SHR and WKY. *Am J Physiol* 1986;250:E381–385.
118. Preuss HG, Fournier RD, Preuss J et al. Effects of different refined carbohydrates on the blood pressure of SHR and WKY Rats. *J Clin Biochem Nutr* 1988;5:9–20.
119. Reaven GM, Ho H, Hoffman BB. Effects of a fructose-enriched diet on plasma insulin and triglyceride concentration in SHR and WKY rats. *Horm Metab Res* 1990;22:363–365.
120. Kavanagh K, Wylie AT, Tucker KL et al. Dietary fructose induces endotoxemia and hepatic injury in calorically controlled primates. *Am J Clin Nutr* 2013;98(2):349–357.
121. Sievenpiper JL. Fructose: Where does the truth lie? *J Am Coll Nutr* 2012;31:149–151.
122. Johnson RK, Appel LJ, Brands M et al. Dietary sugars intake and cardiovascular health: A scientific statement from the American Heart Association. *Circulation* 2009;120:1011–1020.
123. Akgun S, Ertel NH. The effects of sucrose, fructose, and high-fructose corn syrup meals on plasma glucose and insulin in non-insulin-dependent diabetic subjects. *Diabetes Care* 1985;88:279–283.
124. Putnam JJ, Allshouse JE. Food Consumption, Prices, and Expenditures 1970–97. Washington DC: Food and Rural Economics Division, Economic Research Service. US Department of Agriculture: 1999. Statistical Bulletin No. 965.
125. French SA, Lin BH, Guthrie JF. National trends in soft drink consumption among children and adolescents age 6 to 17 years: Prevalence, amounts, and sources, 1977/1978 to 1994/1998. *J Amer Diet Assoc* 2003;103:1326–1331.
126. Schulze MB, Manson JE, Ludwig DS et al. Sugar-sweetened beverages, weight gain, and incidence of type 2 diabetes in young and middle-aged women. *JAMA* 292:927–934.
127. Mattes RD. Dietary compensation by humans for supplemental energy provided as ethanol or carbohydrates in fluids. *Physiol Behav* 1996;59:179–187.
128. DiMeglio DP, Mattes RD. Liquid versus solid carbohydrates: Effects on food intake and body weight. *Int J Obes Relat Metab Disord* 2000;24:794–800.
129. DeCastro JM. The effects of the spontaneous ingestion of particular foods or beverages on the meal pattern and overall nutrient intake of humans. *Physiol Behav* 1993;53:1133–1144.
130. Palmer JR, Boggs DA, Krishnan S et al. Sugar-sweetened beverages and incidence of type 2 diabetes mellitus in African American women. *Arch Intern Med* 2008;168:1487–1492.
131. Duffey KJ, Gordon-Larsen P, Steffen LM et al. Drinking caloric beverages increases the risk of adverse cardiometabolic outcomes in the Coronary Risk Development in Young Adults (CARDIA) study. *Am J Clin Nutr* 2010;92:954–959.
132. Nordmann AJ, Nordmann A, Briel M et al. Effects of low-carbohydrate vs. low-fat diets on weight loss and cardiovascular risk factors: A meta-analysis of randomized controlled trials. *Arch Intern Med* 2006;166:285–293.
133. Thomas DE, Elliott EJ, Baur L. Low glycaemic index or low glycaemic load diets for overweight and obesity. *Cochrane Database Syst Rev* 2007;(3):CD005105.
134. Samaha FF, Iqbal N, Seshadri P et al. A low-carbohydrate as compared with a low-fat diet in severe obesity. *N Eng J Med* 2003;348:2074–2081.
135. Stern L, Iqbal N, Seshadri P et al. The effects of low-carbohydrate versus conventional weight loss diets in severely obese adults: One-year follow-up of a randomized trial. *Ann Int Med* 2004;18:778–785.
136. McAuley KA, Hopkins CM, Smith KJ et al. Comparison of high-fat and high-protein diets with a high-carbohydrate diet in insulin-resistant obese women. *Diabetologia* 48:8–16.
137. Hession M, Rolland C, Kulkarni U et al. Systematic review of randomized controlled trials of low-carbohydrate vs. low-fat/low-calorie diets in the management of obesity and its comorbidities. *Obes Rev* 2009;10:36–50.
138. Sacks FM, Bray GA, Carey VJ et al. Comparison of weight-loss diets with different compositions of fat, protein, and carbohydrates. *N Engl J Med* 2009;360:859–873.
139. Krebs JD, Bell D, Hall R et al. Improvements in glucose metabolism and insulin sensitivity with a low-carbohydrate diet in obese patients with type 2 diabetes. *J Amer Coll Nutr* 2013;32:11–17.

140. Shin J-A, Lee J-H, Kim H-S et al. Prevention of diabetes: A strategic approach for individual patients. *Diabetes Metab Res Rev* 2012;28:79–84.

141. American Diabetes Association. Diabetes mellitus and exercise. *Diab Care* 2002;25:S64–S70.

142. Eriksson K-F, Lindgarde F. Prevention of type 2 (non-insulin-dependent) diabetes mellitus by diet and physical exercise. The 6-year Malmo feasibility study. *Diabetologia* 1991;34:891–898.

143. Pan XR, Li GW, Hu YH et al. Effects of diet and exercise in preventing NIDDM in people with impaired glucose tolerance. The Da Qing IGT and diabetes study. *Diab Care* 1997;20:537–544.

144. Li G, Zhang P, Wang J et al. The long-term effect of life-style interventions to prevent diabetes in the China Da Qing Diabetes Prevention Study: A 20-year follow-up study. *Lancet* 2008;371:1783–1789.

145. Tuomilehto J, Lindstrom J, Eriksson JG et al. Prevention of type 2 diabetes mellitus by changes in lifestyle among subjects with impaired glucose tolerance. *N Engl J Med* 2001;344:1343–1350.

146. Lindstrom J, Ilanne-Parikka P, Peltonen M et al. Sustained reduction in the incidence of type 2 diabetes by life-style intervention: Follow-up of the Finnish Diabetes Prevention Program. *Lancet* 2006;368:1673–1679.

147. Kosaka K, Noda M, Kuzuya T. Prevention of type 2 diabetes by life-style intervention. A Japanese trial in IGT males. *Diabetes Res Clin Pract* 2005;67:152–162.

148. McCowen KC, Fajtova VT. Pioglitazone for diabetes prevention. *N Eng J Med* 2011;365:182–183.

149. Okayasu S, Kitaichi K, Hori A et al. The evaluation of risk factors associated with adverse drug reactions by metformin in type 2 diabetes mellitus. *Biol Pharm Bull* 2012;35:933–937.

150. Stein SA, Lamos EM, Davis SN. A review of the efficacy and safety of oral antidiabetic drugs. *Expert Opin Drug Saf* 2013;12:153–175.

151. Bagchi D, Zafra-Stone S, Bagchi M, Preuss HG. Overview on (-) hydroxycitric acid in weight management. In: Bagchi D, Preuss HG, editors. *Obesity: Epidemiology, Pathophysiology, and Prevention.* Boca Raton, FL: CRC Press; 2013, pp 511–534.

152. Al-Romaiyan A, King AJ, Persaud SJ, Jones PM. A novel extract of *Gymnema sylvestre* improves glucose tolerance in vivo and stimulates insulin secretion and synthesis *in vitro*. *Phytother Res* 2013;27:1006–1011.

153. Rizvi SIO, Mishra N. Traditional Indian medicines used for the management of diabetes mellitus. *J Diabetes Res* 2013;2013:712092. doi: 10.1155/2013/7120-92.

154. Udani JK, Singh BB, Barrett ML, Preuss HG. Lowering the glycemic index of white bread using a white bean extract. *Nutr J* 2009;8:52.

155. Kaats GR, Keith SC, Keith PL et al. A combination of L-arabinose and chromium lowers circulating glucose and insulin levels after acute oral sucrose challenge. *Nutr J* 2011;10:42. doi: 10.1186/1475-2891-10-42.

156. McCarty MF. High-dose biotin, an inducer of glucokinase expression, may synergize with chromium picolinate to enable a definitive nutritional therapy for type II diabetes. *Med Hypotheses* 1999;52:401–406.

157. Anderson RA, Cheng N, Bryden N et al. Elevated intakes of supplemental chromium improve glucose and insulin variables in individuals with type 2 diabetes. *Diabetes* 1997;46:1786–1791.

158. Qin B, Panickar KS, Anderson RA. Cinnamon: Potential role in the prevention of insulin resistance, metabolic syndrome, and type 2 diabetes. *J Diabetes Sci Technol* 2010;4:685–693.

159. Preuss HG, Echard B, Polansky MM, Anderson R. Whole cinnamon and aqueous extracts ameliorate sucrose-induced blood pressure elevations in spontaneously hypertensive rats. J Am Coll Nutr 25: 144–150, 2006.

160. Preuss HG, Echard B, Bagchi D et al. Enhanced insulin-hypoglycemic activity in rats consuming a specific glycoprotein extracted from maitake mushroom. *Mol Cell Biochem* 2007;306:105–113.

161. Clouatre D, Echard B, Preuss HG. Effects of bitter melon extracts in diabetic and normal rats on blood glucose and blood pressure regulation. *J Med Foods* 2011;14:1496–1504.

162. Gardner DC, Kiazand A, Alhassan S et al. Comparison of the Atkins, Zone, Ornish, and LEARN diets for change in weight and related risk factors among overweight premenopausal women; the A to Z weight loss study: A randomized trial. *JAMA* 297:969–977.

163. Pawlak DB, Kushner JA, Ludwig DS. Effects of dietary glycaemic index on adiposity, glucose homeostasis, and plasma lipids in animals. *Lancet* 364:778–785.

164. Brehm BJ, Seeley RJ, Daniels SR, D'Allessio DA. A randomized trial comparing a very low carbohydrate diet and a calorie-restricted low fat diet on body weight and cardiovascular risk factors in healthy women. *J Fam Pract* 52:515–516.

165. Meckling KA, Gauthier M, Grubb R, Sanford J. Effects of a hypocaloric, low carbohydrate diet on weight loss, blood lipids, blood pressure, glucose tolerance, and body composition in free-living overweight women. *Canad J Physiol Pharmacol* 2002;80:1095–1105.

166. Ganji V, Kies CV. Psyllium husk fiber supplementation to soybean and coconut oil diets of humans: Effect of fat digestibility and faecal fatty acid excretion. *Eur J Clin Nutr* 1994;48:595–597.

167. Wadstein J, Thom E, Heldman E et al. Biopolymer L112, a chitosan with fat binding properties and potential as a weight reducing agent. In: Muzzarelli RAA, editor. *Chitosan Per Os: From Dietary Supplement to Drug Carrier*. Grottammare, Italy: Atec; 2000, pp 65–76.

168. Preuss HG, Kaats GR. Chitosan as a dietary supplement for weight loss. A review. *Curr Nutr Rev* 2006;2:297–311.

169. Preuss HG, Gottlieb B. Lower your carbs: Without a low-carb diet. In: Preuss HG, Gottlieb B. editors. *The Natural Fat-Loss Pharmacy*. New York, NY: Broadway Books; 2007, pp 105–124.

170. Fukagawa NK, Anderson JW, Hageman G et al. High-carbohydrate, high-fiber diets increase peripheral insulin sensitivity in healthy young and old adults. *Am J Clin Nutr* 1990;52:524–528.

171. Jenkins DJ, Kendall CW, Marchie A et al. Type 2 diabetes and the vegetarian diet. *Am J Clin Nutr* 2003;78(3 Suppl):610S–616S.

172. Zein M, Areas J, Knapka J et al. Influence of oat bran on sucrose-induced blood pressure elevations in SHR. *Life Sci* 1990;47:1121–1128.

173. Preuss HG, Gondal JA, Bustos E et al. Effect of chromium and guar on sugar-induced hypertension in rats. *Clin Neph* 1995;44:170–177.

174. Udani J, Hardy M, Kavoussi B. Dietary supplement carbohydrate digestion inhibitors: A review of the literature. In: Bagchi D, Preuss HG, editors. *Obesity: Epidemiology, Pathophysiology, and Prevention*. Boca Raton, FL: CRC Press; 2007, pp 279–298.

175. Meiss DE. *Phaseolus vulgaris* and alpha amylase inhibition. In: Bagchi D, Preuss HG, editors. *Obesity: Epidemiology, Pathophysiology, and Prevention*. CRC Press, Boca Raton, FL; 2007, pp 423–432.

176. Brudnak MA. Weight-loss drugs and supplements: Are there safer alternatives? *Med Hypotheses* 2002;58:28–33.

177. Andoh A, Tsujikawa T, Fujiyama Y. Role of dietary fiber and short chain fatty acids in the colon. *Curr Pharm Des* 2003;9:347–358.

178. Guyton AC, Hall JE. *Textbook of Medical Physiology*, 9th Ed. Philadelphia, PA: WB Saunders, 1996.

179. Higgins JA, Higbee DR, Donahoo WT et al. Resistant starch consumption promotes lipid oxidation. *Nutr Metab* 2004;87:761–768.

180. Keenan MJ, Zhou J, McCutcheon KL et al. Effects of resistant starch, a non digestible fermentable fiber, on reducing body fat. *Obesity* 2006;14:1523–1534.

181. Grabitske HA, Slavin JL. Low-digestible carbohydrates in practice. *J Am Diet Assoc* 2008;108:1677–1681.

182. Obiro WC, Zhang T, Jiang B. The nutraceutical role of the *Phaseolus vulgaris* a-amylase inhibitor. *Br J Nutr* 2008;100:1–12.

183. Barrett ML, Udani JK. A proprietary alpha-amylase inhibitor from white bean (*Phaseolus vulgaris*): A review of clinical studies on weight loss and glycemic control. *Nutr J* 2011;10:24.

184. Hollenbeck CB, Coulston AM Quan R et al. Effects of a commercial starch blocker preparation on carbohydrate digestion and absorption: In vivo and in vitro studies. *Am J Clin Nutr* 1983;38:498–503.

185. Garrow JS, Scott PF, Heels S et al. A study or "starch blockers" in many using ¹³C-enriched starch as a tracer. *Hum Nutr Clin Nutr* 1983;37:301–305.

186. Carlson GL, Li BU, Bass P, Olsen WA. A bean alpha-amylase inhibitor formulation (starch blocker) is ineffective in man. *Science* 1983;219:393–395.

187. Layer P, Carlson GL, DiMagno EP. Partially purified white bean amylase inhibitor reduces starch digestion in vitro and inactivates intraduodenal amylase in humans. *Gastroenterology* 1985;88:1895–1902.

188. Layer P, Rizza RA, Zinsmeister AR et al. Effect of a purified amylase inhibitor on carbohydrate tolerance in normal subjects and patients with diabetes mellitus. *Mayo Clin Proc* 1986;61:442–447.

189. Brugge WR, Rosenfeld MS. Impairment of starch absorption by a potent amylase inhibitor. *Am J Gastroenterol* 1987;82:718–722.

190. Boivin M, Zinsmeister AR, Go VL, DiMagno EP. Effect of a purified amylase inhibitor on carbohydrate metabolism after a mixed meal in healthy humans. *May Clin Proc* 1987;62:249–255.

191. Jain NK, Boivin M, Zinsmeister AR et al. Effect of ileal perfusion of carbohydrates and amylase inhibitor on gastrointestinal hormones and emptying. *Gastroenterology* 1989;96:377–387.

192. Boivin M, Flourie B, Rizza RA et al. Gastrointestinal and metabolic effects of amylase inhibition in diabetics. *Gastroenterology* 1988;94:387–394.

193. Tormo MA, Gil-Exojo I, Romero de Tejada A, Campillo JE. Hypoglycemic and anorexigenic activities of an alpha-amylase inhibitor from white kidney beans (*Phaseolus vulgaris*) in Wistar rats. *Br J Nutr* 2004;92:785–790.

194. Deglaire A, Moughan PJ, Bos C, Tome D. Commercial *Phaseolus vulgaris* extract (starch stopper) increases ileal endogenous amino acid and crude protein losses in the growing rat. *J Agric Food Chem* 2006;54:5197–5202.

195. Preuss HG, Echard B, Talpur N et al. Inhibition of starch and sucrose gastrointestinal absorption in rats by various dietary supplements alone and combined. Acute studies *Int J Med Sci* 2007;4:196–202.

196. Preuss HG, Echard B, Talpur N et al. Inhibition of starch and sucrose gastrointestinal absorption in rats by various dietary supplements alone and combined. Subchronic studies. *Int J Med Sci* 2007;4:209–215.

197. Vinson JA, Al Kharrat H, Shuta D. Investigation of an amylase inhibitor on human glucose absorption after starch consumption. Open Nutraceuticals J 2009;2:88–91.

198. Thom E. A randomized, double-blind, placebo-controlled trial of a new weight-reducing agent of natural origin. *J Int Med Res* 2000;28:229–233.

199. Celleno L, Perricone NV, Preuss HG. Effect of a dietary supplement containing standardized *Phaseolus vulgaris* extract on the body composition of overweight men and women. *Int J Med Sci* 2007;4:45–52.

200. Udani J, Hardy M, Madsen DC. Blocking carbohydrate absorption and weight loss: A clinical trial using Phase 2 brand proprietary fractionated white bean extract. *Altern Med Rev* 2004;9:63–69.

201. Udani J, Singh BB. Blocking carbohydrate absorption and weight loss: A clinical trial using a proprietary fractionated white bean extract. *Altern Ther Health Med* 2007;13:32–37.

202. Koike T, Koizumi Y, Tang L et al. The anti-obesity effect and the safety of taking "Phaseolamin ™1600 diet." *J New Rem Clin* 2005;54:1–16.

203. Wu X, Xu X, Shen J, Preuss HG. Enhanced weight loss from a dietary supplement containing standard-ized *Phaseolus vulgaris* extract in overweight men and women. *J Appl Res* 2010;10:73–79.

204. Grube B, Chong WF, Chong PW, Riede L. Weight reduction and maintenance with IQP-PV-101: A 12 week randomized controlled study with a 24-week open label period. *Obesity* 2014;22:645–651.

205. Chokshi D. Toxicity studies of Blokal, a dietary supplement containing Phase 2 starch neutralizer (Phase 2), standardized extract of the common white kidney bean (*Phaseolus vulgaris*). *Int J Toxicol* 2006;25:361–371.

206. Chokshi D. Subchronic oral toxicity of a standardized white kidney bean (*Phaseolus vulgaris*) extract in rats. *Food Chem/Toxicol* 2007;45:32–40.

207. Seri K, Sanai K, Matsuo N et al. L-arabinose selectively inhibits intestinal sucrase in an uncompetitive man-ner and suppresses glycemic response after sucrose ingestion in animals. *Metabolism* 1996;45:1368–1374.

208. Osaki S, Kimura T, Sugimoto T et al. L-arabinose feeding prevents increases due to dietary sucrose in lipogenic enzymes and triacylglycerol levels in rats. *J Nutr* 2001;131:796–799.

209. Inoue S, Sanai K, Seri K. Effect of L-arabinose on blood glucose level after ingestion of sucrose-containing food in humans. *J Jpn Soc Nutr Food Sci* 2000;53:243–247.

210. Hansawasdi C, Kawabata J, Kasai T. Alpha-amylase inhibitors from roselle (*Hibiscus sabdariffa* Linn.) tea. *Biosci Biotechnol Biochem* 2000;64:1041–1043.

211. Hansawadi C, Kawabata J, Kasai T. Hibiscus acid as an inhibitor of starch digestion in the Caco-2 cell model system. *Biosci Biotechnol Biochem* 2001;65:2087–2089.

212. Sachdewa A, Khemani LD. Effects of *Hibiscus rosa sinensis* Linn. ethanol flower extract on blood glu-cose and lipid profile in streptozotocin induced diabetes in rats. *J Ethnopharmacol* 2003;89, 61–66.

213. Yamada T, Hida H, Yamada Y. Chemistry, physiologic properties, and microbial production of hydroxy-citric acid. *Appl Microbiol Biotechnol* 2007;75:977–982.

214. Wielinga PY, Wachters-Hagedoorn RE, Bouter B et al. Hydroxycitric acid delays intestinal glucose absorption in rats. *Am J Physiol Gastrointest Liver Physiol* 2005;288:1144–1149.

215. Lankisch M, Layer P, Rizza RA, DiMagno EP. Acute postprandial gastrointestinal and metabolic effects of wheat amylase inhibitor (WAI) in normal, obese, and diabetic humans. *Pancreas* 1998;17:176–181.

216. Yoshikawa M, Muarakami T, Kadoya M et al. The inhibitors of glucose absorption from the leaves of *Gymnema sylvestre* R. BR. (Asclepiadaceae): Structures of gymnemosides a and b. *Chem Pharm Bull* 1997;45:1671–1676.

217. Shimizu K, Iino A, Nakajima J, Tanaka K et al. Suppression of glucose absorption by some fractions extracted from *Gymnema sylvestre* leaves. *J Vet Med Sci* 1997;59:245–251.

218. Hirsh AJ, Yao SY, Young JD, Cheeseman CI. Inhibition of glucose absorption in the rat jejunum: A novel action of alpha-D-glucosidase inhibitors. *Gastroenterology* 1997;113:205–211.

219. Meng S, Cao J, Feng Q et al. Roles of chlorogenic acid on regulating glucose and lipids metabolism: A review. *Evid Based Complement Alternat Med* 2013;2013:801457.

220. Ochiai R, Sugiura Y, Shioya Y et al. Coffee polyphenols improve peripheral endothelial function after glucose loading in healthy male adults. *Nutr Res* 2014;34:155–159.

221. Kwon O, Eck P, Chen S et al. Inhibition of the intestinal glucose transporter GLUT2 by flavonoids. *FASEB J* 2007;21:366–377.
222. Sugimoto K, Suzuki J, Nakagawa K et al. Eucalyptus leaf extract inhibits intestinal fructose absorption, and suppresses adiposity due to dietary sucrose in rats. *Br J Nutr* 2005;93:957–963.
223. Mertz W. Chromium. History and nutritional importance. *Biol Trace Element Res* 1992;32:3–8.
224. Evans GW. The effect of chromium picolinate on insulin controlled parameters in humans. *Int J Biosocial Med Res* 1989;11:163–180.
225. Anderson RA. Nutritional factors influencing the glucose/insulin system: Chromium. *J Am Coll Nutr* 1997;16:404–410.
226. Schwartz K, Mertz W. A glucose tolerance factor and its differentiation from factor 3. *Arch Biochem Biophy* 1957;72:515–518.
227. Schwartz K, Mertz W. Chromium (III) and the glucose tolerance factor. *Arch Biochem Biophys* 1959;85:292–295.
228. Jeejeebhoy KN, Chu RC, Marliss EB et al. Chromium deficiency, glucose intolerance, and neuropathy reversed by chromium supplementation in a patient receiving long-term total parenteral nutrition. *Am J Clin Nutr* 1977;30:531–538.
229. Freund H, Atamian S, Fischer JE. Chromium deficiency during total parenteral nutrition. *JAMA* 1979;241:496–498.
230. Brown RO, Forloines-Lynn S, Cross RE, Heizer WD. Chromium deficiency after long-term parenteral nutrition. *Dig Dis Sci* 1986;31:661–664.
231. Anderson RA. Chromium as an essential nutrient for humans. *Regul Toxicol Pharmacol* 1997;26:S35–S41.
232. Perricone NV, Bagchi D, Echard B, Preuss HG. Long-term metabolic effects of different doses of niacin-bound chromium on Sprague-Dawley rats. *Mol Cell Biochem* 2009;338:91–103.
233. Preuss HG, Echard B, Perricone NV et al. Comparing metabolic effects of six different commercial trivalent chromium compounds. *J Inorg Biochem* 2008;102:1986–1990.
234. Anderson RA, Polansky MM, Bryden NA. Stabilitiy and absorption of chromium histidinate complexes by humans. *Biol Trace Elem Res* 2004;101:211–218.
235. Seaborn CD, Stoecker BJ. Effects of starch, sucrose, fructose on chromium absorption and tissue concentrations in obese and lean mice. *J Nutr* 1989;119:1444–1451.
236. Seaborn CD, Stoecker BJ. Effects of antacid or ascorbic acid on tissue accumulation of ^{51}chromium. *Nutr Res* 1989;10:1401–1407.
237. Seaborn CD, Stoecker BJ. Effects of ascorbic acid depletion and chromium status on retention and urinary excretion of ^{51}chromium. *Nutr Res* 1992;12:1229–1234.
238. Anderson RA, Bryden NA, Polansky MM. Lack of toxicity of chromium chloride and chromium picolinate in rats. *J Am Coll Nutr* 1997;18:273–279.
239. Lamson DW, Plaza SM. The safety and efficacy of high-dose chromium. *Altern Med Rev* 2002;7:218–235.
240. Stearns DM, Wise JP Sr, Patierno SR, Wetterhahn KE. Chromium (III) picolinate produces chromosome damage in Chinese hamster ovary cells. *FASEB J* 1995;9:1643–1648.
241. Hininger I, Benaraba R, Osman M et al. Safety of trivalent chromium complexes: No evidence for DNA damage in human HaCaT keratinocytes. *Free Radic Biol Med* 2007;42:1759–1765.
242. Talpur N, Echard B, Yasmin D et al. Effects of niacin-bound chromium, maitake mushroom fraction SX and a novel (-)-hydroxycitric acid extract on metabolic syndrome in aged diabetic Zucker Fatty Rats. *Molec Cell Biochem* 2003;252:369–377.
243. Martin J, Wang ZQ, Zhang XH et al. Chromium picolinate supplementation attenuates body weight gain and increases insulin sensitivity in subjects with type 2 diabetes. *Diabetes Care* 2006;29(8):1826–1832.
244. Linday LA. Trivalent chromium and the diabetes prevention program. *Med Hypotheses* 1997;49:47–49.
245. Preuss H, Anderson RA. Chromium update: Examining recent literature 1997–1998. *Clin Nutr Metab Care* 1998;1:509–512.
246. Reddi A, DeAngelis B, Frank O et al. Biotin supplementation improves glucose and insulin tolerance in genetically diabetic KK mice. *Life Sci* 1988;42:1323–1330.
247. Zhang H, Osada K, Maebashi M et al. A high biotin diet improves the impaired glucose tolerance of long-term spontaneously hyperglycemic rats with non-insulin-dependent diabetes mellitus. *J Nutr Sci Vitaminol* (Tokyo) 1996;42:517–526.
248. Zhang H, Osada K, Sone H, Furukawa Y. Biotin administration improves the impaired glucose tolerance of streptozotocin-induced diabetic Wistar rats. *J Nutr Sci Vitaminol* (Tokyo) 1997;43:271–280.
249. Coggeshall JC, Heggers JP, Robson MC, Baker H. Biotin status and plasma glucose in diabetics. *Ann NY Acad Sci* 1985;447:387–392.

250. Maebashi M, Makino Y, Furukawa Y et al. Therapeutic evaluation of the effect of biotin on hyperglycemia in patients with non-insulin dependent diabetes mellitus. *J Clin Biochem Nutr* 1993;14:211–218.
251. Dilman VM, Anisimov VN. Effect of treatment with phenformin, dyphenylhydantoin, or L-DOPA on lifespan and tumor incidence in C3H/Sn mice. *Gerontology* 1980;26:241–245.
252. Anisimov VN, Semenchenko AV, Yashin AI. Insulin and longevity: Antidiabetic biguanides as geroprotectors. *Biogerontology* 2003;4:297–307.
253. Sullivan C, Triscari J. Metabolic regulation as a control for lipid disorders. I. Influence of (—)-hydroxycitrate on experimentally induced obesity in the rodent. *Am J Clin Nutr* 1977;30:767–776.
254. Lowenstein JM, Brunengraber H. Hydroxycitrate. *Methods Enzymol* 1981;72:486–497.
255. Greenway F. Garcinia. *Encyclopedia of Dietary Supplements*, 2010, pp 307–313.
256. McCarty MF. Promotion of hepatic lipid oxidation and gluconeogenesis as a strategy for appetite control. *Med Hypotheses* 1994;42:215–225.
257. McCarty MF. Toward a wholly nutritional therapy for type 2 diabetes. *Med Hypotheses* 2000;54:483–487.
258. Clouatre D, Talpur N, Talpur F et al. Comparing metabolic and inflammatory parameters among rats consuming different forms of hydroxycitrate. *J Am Coll Nutr* 2005;24:429 (Abstract).
259. Clouatre D, Preuss HG. Potassium magnesium hydroxycitrate at physiologic levels influences various metabolic parameters and inflammation in rats. *Curr Top Nutraceutical Res* 2008;6:201–210.
260. Hayamizu K, Hirakawa H, Oikawa D et al. Effect of Garcinia cambogia extract on serum leptin and insulin in mice. *Fitoterapia* 2003;74:267–273.
261. Leonhardt M, Balkan B, Langhans W. Effect of hydroxycitrate on respiratory quotient, energy expenditure, and glucose tolerance in male rats after a period of restrictive feeding. *Nutrition* 2004;20:911–915.
262. Kim KY, Lee HN, Kim YJ, Park T. *Garcinia cambogia* extract ameliorates visceral adiposity in C57BL/6J mice fed on a high-fat diet. *Biosci Biotechnol Biochem* 2008;72:1772–1780.
263. Wielinga PY, Klunder JW, Bouter B et al. Hydroxycitrate (HCA) reduces the insulin response to an intragastric glucose load. *Appetite* 2003;40:369.
264. Wielinga PY, Wachters-Hagedoorn RE, Bouter B et al. Hydroxycitric acid delays intestinal glucose absorption in rats. *Am J Physiol Gastrointest Liver Physiol* 2005;28:G1144–1149.
265. Ravi S, Sadashiva CT, Tamizmani T et al. In vitro glucose uptake by isolated rat hemi-diaphragm study of Aegle marmelos Correa root. *Bangladesh J Pharmacol* 2009;4:65–68.
266. Clouatre DL, Preuss HG: Hydroxycitric acid does not promote inflammation or liver toxicity. *World J Gastroenterol* 2013;19:8160–8162.

8 Naturopathic Medicine and the Prevention and Treatment of Cardiovascular Disease

Drew Sinatra

CONTENTS

INTRODUCTION

As specialists in natural and complementary medicines, naturopathic doctors (NDs) offer many treatment options for patients with cardiovascular disease (CVD). Because our visits are longer than most primary care providers, we have time to educate patients about dietary and lifestyle practices that are supportive to optimal health. We acknowledge and support the body's inherent healing mechanisms and use nutrition, herbal and nutraceutical medicines, hydrotherapy, acupuncture, detoxification, stress management therapies, and counseling to help shift disease back into health. We recognize when the body requires additional support through medications and surgery and utilize these modalities when necessary. Above all, we work with cardiologists and other specialists to provide the best care for the patient.

We know that most cases of CVD are preventable through proper diet and lifestyle modification. Many physicians, however, do not have enough time during office visits to give specific nutritional advice or to discuss healthy living habits with their patients. A visit with an ND typically lasts 30–60 minutes, and plenty of time is allocated to discussing which diet is appropriate for a particular cardiovascular condition. Awareness of healthy eating options is essential for proper meal planning, so we strive to empower patients by teaching them which foods to eat and which foods to avoid. As discussed later, a seemingly healthy vegetarian diet, touted by many to be heart healthy, may do more harm than good if improper food choices are made.

Learning to identify and address the root cause of cardiovascular dysfunction, such as high blood pressure, is essential for healing to occur. Hypertension can be due to many factors including stress, hormone imbalance, environmental toxin exposure, lack of exercise, medications, obesity, and/or nutritional deficiencies. Lowering a surrogate marker such as blood pressure using diuretics, angiotensin-converting enzyme (ACE) inhibitors, β-blockers, or other medications never truly addresses the cause, which if left unchecked will result in additional physiological change and damage. Moreover, putting patients on medications is a lot easier than taking them off. Therefore, when addressing CVD, physicians must look at all causative factors before recommending treatment options and start with the safest therapies first.

Some statistics show that 60%–90% of doctor visits are stress related. What can we do for patients to help minimize stress in their lives?[1] What treatments or techniques can we offer for quick and easy stress reduction? What effect can yoga, deep breathing, meditation, or biofeedback have on cardiovascular end points? We will always have stress in our lives because mortgages, demanding jobs, sick family members, or living in constant fear or worry are difficult to avoid. Learning how to manage these stressors is critical for sound health. Asking your patients about the stress in their lives and teaching them methods to reduce it are extremely important considerations in naturopathic medicine.

In this chapter, we will investigate the multidisciplinary role the naturopath has in the prevention and treatment of CVD. Lifestyle optimization through diet, mind body medicines, targeted nutritional supplements, exercise, fasting, grounding, and detoxification techniques will be discussed as appropriate adjunctive therapies in not only the prevention of CVD and hypertension but also the overall management.

VEGETARIAN, PALEOLITHIC, AND WESTERN DIETS: FOOD AS MEDICINE

Epidemiological research has looked into the cardioprotective benefits of vegetarian, Mediterranean, and Paleolithic diets.[2-6] These diets all focus on the consumption of fresh fruits and vegetables, nuts, and heart-healthy oils (olive and coconut). They differ in how much, or little, meat, fish, legumes, dairy, and eggs are consumed. In this section, modified vegetarian and Paleolithic diets are recommended as medically appropriate diets for preventing and treating heart disease because they eliminate or avoid grains containing gluten.[7] They both are very practical diets that improve not only the health of the cardiovascular system but also vitality in general. It is very important to know how to implement and eat healthy vegetarian and Paleolithic diets, as unhealthy versions are common without proper guidance.

The definition of a vegetarian is one who eats most foods except meat products. There are varying levels of vegetarianism, however, as some vegetarians choose to eat fish (pesco-vegetarians) and/or dairy products and eggs (lacto-ovo vegetarians). There is a wide range of what is considered a health-promoting vegetarian diet, as some vegetarians may choose to avoid fish and dairy products but eat in abundance highly refined, processed, and sugary foods that may promote inflammation in the body. Avoiding processed, high-sugar, and high-glycemic foods such as wheat is key for supporting cardiovascular health outcomes.[8,9]

Studies show that eating a vegetarian diet does lead to a reduction in CVD. A cohort study comparatively looked at 67 vegetarians and 134 omnivores (consumers of plant and animal origin) and assessed the risk of CVD. The vegetarians had a marked reduction in the following measures: blood pressure, body mass index (BMI), waist to hip ratio, fasting blood glucose, and elevated total cholesterol.[10] In the Oxford Vegetarian Study, 6000 vegetarians and vegans were compared with 5000 omnivores. The authors proposed that eating a lifelong vegetarian diet reduced the incidence of ischemic heart disease by as much as 24%, whereas the incidence was 57% lower among lifelong vegans, who strictly avoid all animal products including dairy and eggs. The vegans in this study had the lowest low-density lipoprotein (LDL) cholesterol and the fish eaters the highest high-density lipoprotein (HDL) cholesterol.[11]

It is important to note that high consumption of fruits, vegetables, and fiber is the foundation of a healthy vegetarian diet and thus contributes to lowered risk of heart disease.[12] Eating a vegetarian diet high in fruits and vegetables and moderately high in fish, eggs, nuts, oils, and gluten-free grains is conducive to superior heart health. For patients who want to eat a whole foods diet and consume animal products, high-quality lean meats such as grass-fed beef, buffalo, bison, and pasture-raised chicken are healthy options. This type of gluten- and diary-free diet that promotes high-quality meats is known as the Paleolithic or hunter–gatherer diet.

The Paleolithic diet is based on what our ancestors ate before the agricultural revolution 10,000 years ago. Genetically, we are practically identical to our Paleolithic ancestors, yet the Western diet is drastically different in macro- and micronutrients; phytonutrients; electrolytes; and composition of fats, proteins, and particularly carbohydrates.[13] Some say that the preagricultural diet should be the standard for contemporary human nutrition considering the genetic similarity to our Paleolithic ancestors.[14]

The typical hunter–gatherer culture consumed sweet and ripe fruits and berries, shoots, flowers, buds and young leaves, meat, bone marrow, organ meats, fish, shellfish, insects, larvae, eggs, roots, bulbs, nuts, and nongrass seeds.[6] These hunter–gatherers relied on finding food rather than cultivating it. Grains and diary were not available and thus were not consumed.[13] In fact, Dr. David Permutter, author of *Grain Brain*, reports that humans have eaten gluten free for 99.9% of our existence.[15] This statistic puts into perspective why so many people feel better on gluten-free diets; we have been eating gluten free for the majority of our time on the earth.

It is thought that hunter–gatherers had greater metabolic output due to their mobile nature and greater caloric intake compared to modern man.[14,16] The high nutrient content of wildly harvested foods and game helped sustain their greater metabolic needs. Considering the high carbohydrate intake of modern man coupled with no to minimal exercise, it is no wonder why the obesity epidemic is out of control.[17] Low-fat diets rarely seem to work well for weight loss, as more carbohydrates (sugars) are consumed in place of fats. The Paleolithic diet selects low-sugar carbohydrates and allows consumption of high-quality fats.

Traditional hunter–gatherers who eat a Paleo-type diet have shown exceptionally favorable levels of serum cholesterol, blood pressure, and other cardiovascular risk factors.[6] In a 12-week study where pigs were fed a Paleo-type diet or cereal diet, the pigs eating Paleo had lower C-reactive protein (CRP), lower blood pressure, and higher insulin sensitivity. The authors of this study suggest that diseases of affluence may be attributable to insufficient evolutionary adaptation to grains.[18]

If we compare the Paleolithic diet to the Western diet, we see stark differences in nutrient composition, antioxidants, fiber, and sugar intake. Overall, hunter–gatherers consumed less sodium and more potassium, riboflavin, folate, thiamin, carotene, vitamin A, vitamin C, and vitamin E.[19] They also consumed more fiber (100–150 vs. 24 g/day), more meat (45%–60% vs. 12% total calories), more cholesterol (520 vs. 430 mg/day), and fewer carbohydrates (22%–46% vs. 50% total calories).

One of the most shocking differences between Paleolithic diet and Western diet is the consumption of refined sugar. Because refined sugar did not exist in hunter–gatherer societies, 0 kg/year were consumed compared to 69.1 kg/year in the United States in 2000.[19] This translates to 152 lb of refined sugar being consumed by Americans every year. According to Dr. Staffan Lindeberg, "roughly three-fourth of the calories in Western countries is today provided by foods that were practically unavailable during human evolution: wheat and other cereal grains, dairy foods, refined fats, and sugar."

When you consider the proinflammatory nature of refined sugar,[20] it comes as no surprise why chronic disease is rising steadily and why CVD is the number one cause of mortality in the United States. As a culture, Americans are consuming too much sugar and too many carbohydrate calories sourced from grains. According to a small randomized clinical trial, consuming sugar-sweetened beverages (SSBs) for 3 weeks led to increases in waist to hip ratio, fasting blood glucose, and hs-CRP levels. The researches also noted a decrease in LDL particle size.[20] People need to be aware that sugar is very toxic for the body even in socially acceptable portion sizes (12 oz. soda), and that drinking these sugar beverages regularly can increase the risk for CVD.

Underlying chronic inflammation is emerging as the pivotal risk factor in the genesis of CVD. Sugar and highly refined foods are thought to cause inflammation in the body particularly in the endothelial lining (or innermost membrane) of blood vessels. To say it bluntly, sugar and subsequent insulin surges are the most endothelial unfriendly components that promote oxidative stress. As a rise in blood sugar leads to inflammation in the endothelial lining, the body reacts by depositing cholesterol along the walls of the blood vessels as a protective mechanism to stabilize and strengthen the vessel. This is the inflammatory cascade that leads to atherosclerosis, one of the most common contributors to heart disease. By removing or at least dramatically decreasing sugar from a diet, you are eliminating a key player in the inflammatory response to heart disease.

WHEAT (GLUTEN), BLOOD SUGAR, AND INFLAMMATION

One of the biggest players responsible for this inflammation is a grain hidden in almost all packaged or processed foods: wheat. It is found in breads, bagels, pastas, pizzas, pastries, pretzels, wraps, crackers, candy bars, soy sauce, and other foods. For decades, the medical establishment has supported consuming a moderate intake of grains including wheat. If you browse grocery store aisles and analyze the endless array of processed foods, you may see an endorsement from the American Diabetes Association or American Heart Association. We are taught from a very young age that grains including wheat are good for us.

Over the years, wheat has dominated the market in processed foods that are convenient, inexpensive, and long lasting. The wheat found in most foods these days, however, is not the same wheat that was around decades ago, nor is it healthy for you. According to Dr. William Davis, author of *Wheat Belly*, modern wheat genes have been spliced over 50,000 times to make it more desirable (i.e., pest or drought resistant, higher gluten content, etc.), but in the process a toxic form of wheat has been created. The gene splicing has transformed the wheat species into one of the highest glycemic index foods that humans consume, a glycemic index higher than that of even table sugar.[21]

Higher glycemic index foods, like wheat, are broken down into sugar. Sugar raises insulin levels, and high insulin levels are proinflammatory, accelerating the aging process. Higher blood sugars in combination with proteins and lipids in the plasma create advanced glycation end products (AGEs).[22] AGEs not only accelerate aging but also cause enormous oxidative stress in the body at the same time. Never in the history of modern man has diabetes, insulin resistance, and metabolic syndrome been expressed in the population at such an accelerating rate, largely due to our modern industrial food production. Flooding the body with sugar is only going to aggravate preexisting heart disease and make it more challenging to reverse.

Gluten consumption may not only contribute to inflammation in the arteries but also lead to inflammation in the intestines. In a landmark study out in *The Lancet*, Dr. Alessio Fasano discovered an intestinal protein called zonulin elevated in people with celiac disease. In the small intestine, zonulin induces tight junction disassembly, which leads to an increase in intestinal permeability.[23]

In other words, gluten consumption can cause leaky gut syndrome. The intestines become inflamed, and "leaky" contents of the intestinal tract including bacterium and undigested food proteins are allowed to pass through the intestinal epithelium into the bloodstream.[24] Chronically, this can lead to an overactivation of the immune system that may set the stage for autoimmune disease and other chronic inflammatory conditions. Surprisingly, even individuals who do not have celiac disease are susceptible to zonulin elevations. Gliadin, one of the proteins found in gluten, can trigger zonulin release temporarily regardless of whether someone has celiac disease or not.[25] Therefore, all of us are susceptible to the increased intestinal permeability due to gluten consumption.

Hypertension can be caused by oxidative stress, inflammation, and autoimmune dysfunction.[26] Because there is a connection between leaky gut syndrome, inflammation in the intestines, and autoimmune disease, could gluten consumption be a contributing factor for the emergence of hypertension? Clinically, I have seen better blood pressure control after putting patients on gluten-free diets. Although the exact mechanism of action for this finding is unknown, could regulating blood sugar and decreasing intestinal inflammation be responsible for reducing oxidative stress in blood vessels, leading to a decrease in blood pressure? Further study will perhaps shed more light on this theory.

KNOW THY FOOD SOURCE

When choosing to eat a vegetarian diet, it is very important to limit or completely eliminate gluten and to make sure that particular vitamins are replenished. Unhealthy vegetarians are those who typically consume high quantities of gluten and sugar products in place of meat products. They too suffer from most of the modern world's chronic diseases that are highly preventable through healthy eating. Many wheat-free (gluten-free) grains are beneficial to consume, and these include quinoa, amaranth, millet, and buckwheat. Legumes such as lentils and beans can also be eaten in moderation to provide additional fiber, B vitamins, calcium, and iron.

Although vegetarian diets are high in fiber, vitamin C, vitamin E, folic acid, magnesium, and potassium, strict vegetarians and vegans have been known to be deficient in vitamin B12, vitamin D, zinc, and long-chain ω-3 fatty acids.[27,28] Low levels of vitamin B12, found in meat and eggs, cause an increase in plasma homocysteine, an amino acid linked with heart disease.[29] It is therefore important for vegetarians to supplement with vitamin B12, folate, and vitamin B6 to help metabolize methionine more efficiently, thus lowering homocysteine.[30] Because meat and eggs are consumed regularly on a Paleolithic diet, most Paleo followers do not need to take additional B vitamins, carnitine, α-lipoic acid, and coenzyme Q10 as these nutrients are found in abundance in the animal kingdom.

It can be challenging to find high-quality meat sources. The majority of red meat and chicken in the United States is factory farmed. Factory-farmed animals eat genetically modified soy and corn, are housed in extremely inhumane quarters, and fed and injected with antibiotics to treat and prevent infection. When choosing to eat a Paleolithic type diet, it is important to select the meats wisely. Typically, local farmers markets and health food stores sell grass-fed beef or pasture-raised chickens and eggs. Although the cost of pasture-raised meat is slightly higher compared to factory-farmed meats, trans fat levels are lower, whereas ω-3 fatty acid levels are significantly higher.[31–33]

Choosing to eat a whole foods diet, whether vegetarian or Paleolithic, will help promote healthy eating habits and help reduce risk for CVD.[6,10] Both diets thrive on eating lots of fruits and vegetables (raw and cooked), and in moderation, nuts, seeds, eggs, and fish. Paleolithic diets include meats, and I recommend sourcing high-quality grass-fed or pasture-raised local meats when possible to optimize healthy fats. Vegetarian diets do include grains, but I suggest eliminating gluten-containing grains, particularly wheat, to minimize sugar intake. In summary, I recommend either diet depending on one's personal preference but cannot emphasize the importance of gluten (wheat) elimination and choice of high-quality meats without chemicals and pesticides.

Care should be taken in those with moderate to severe diabetes as blood sugar levels may drop when beginning a Paleolithic or vegetarian diet. Make sure your diabetic patients are closely monitoring blood sugar, as hypoglycemia is not uncommon. Remember that radically shifting a diet from highly refined, processed, and sugary foods/drinks to one of healthy whole foods can dramatically affect body physiology, so be watchful and check in regularly with your patients.

NATUROPATHIC APPROACH TO TREATING HYPERTENSION

In the United States, nearly half of all Americans have elevated blood pressures in the prehypertensive (systolic blood pressure [SBP] 120–139 or diastolic blood pressure [DBP] 80–89) to hypertensive (SBP > 140 or DBP > 90) range.[34] This statistic is alarming considering the deleterious effects of high blood pressure and negative sequelae including stroke, CVD, and kidney disease. Although antihypertensive medications are effective in the reduction of blood pressure, adherence is often poor and cost is high.[34] Additionally, side effects are common with antihypertensive medications and include hypokalemia, insomnia, depression, dry mouth, bronchospasm, impotence, and headaches.[35] It is therefore suggested that prehypertensive and hypertensive patients pursue complementary therapies including diet and lifestyle modifications, and mind–body medicines, to assist in blood pressure control.[34]

There is overwhelming evidence supporting the use of lifestyle measures to reduce blood pressure. Most physicians, however, are quick to prescribe pharmaceuticals before addressing a patient's diet and lifestyle. Health care in the United States is more like disease care, with an emphasis on drugs and surgery and a lack of attention for prevention. A naturopath's goal is to help change prescription pad readiness into education and self-responsibility. Patients need to be exposed to the most up-to-date evidence-based medicines possible and to be able to make informed decisions about their treatment plan. In this section on hypertension, evidence-based diet and lifestyle modifications including nutraceuticals that reduce blood pressure without the use of pharmaceuticals are addressed.

One of the foundations of medicine is learning how to identify and treat the cause of disease. Often we focus too much attention on treating the symptom, which will only alleviate the problem temporarily. For acute conditions like a myocardial infarction, treating the symptom such as acute coronary syndrome or unstable angina with nitroglycerine is necessary to reduce pain and perfuse blood-starved heart muscle. It is not the ideal time or place for dietary recommendations or stress reduction management. Knowing how and when to address the cause is a fine art, and it takes time and effort to uncover. Help your patients learn why they have a symptom or disease.

For most patients with essential hypertension, there is an underlying cause that can be identified with proper questions and insight. If we think of hypertension like an alarm going off in a burning building, prescribing a diuretic, an ACE inhibitor, a β-blocker, or an ARB is analogous to turning off the alarm without addressing the fire. We need to know where the alarm is going off, why it is making noise, and how to turn it off. Once we investigate the source of the fire, we can treat it using proper lifestyle measures like a noninflammatory diet, stress control, and targeted nutraceuticals. Occasionally, the fire may be burning out of control and require immediate attention with medication. This is usually a hypertensive crisis where blood pressure is higher than 180/110 mmHg, or when renal function is impaired.

Learning how to treat hypertension with natural medicines takes patience, time, and effort. In my clinical practice, many factors go into deciding whether a medication is required to lower blood pressure. The most important ones are blood pressure levels, family and past medical history, age, exercise, diet, stress level, smoking, environmental toxin exposure, oxidative stress, comorbidities (e.g., diabetes and autoimmune disease), medications, and motivation to make changes. Unfortunately, there is no simple algorithm to help you decide whether to use medication or not. There are over a dozen recommendations in this section for natural ways to lower blood pressure. Although some interventions only lower blood pressure modestly, cumulatively these treatments can have a profound impact on the cardiovascular system.

Identifying and treating the etiology of hypertension can be challenging as many causes can overlap and create confusion. For instance, the following commonly contribute to hypertension cases: nutritional deficiencies, stress, endocrine dysfunction (e.g., hyperthyroidism), obesity, lack of exercise, smoking, alcohol, and prescription medications (e.g., NSAIDS and birth control). Other causes need to be ruled out as well such as renal disease, hyperaldosteronism, Cushing's disease, coarctation of the aorta, and white-coat hypertension. How do you truly know what is contributing to the patient's elevated blood pressure?

As an ND, I cannot emphasize the importance of spending ample time questioning your patient about his or her current and past health. Without hesitation, ask your patients about their diet and nutrient intake, weight, exercise, lifestyle (i.e., smoking, alcohol intake), stress, and prescription drug use. What foods and fluids are they regularly consuming? What is their home and work life like? Are they shift workers? What is their level of emotional stress? Are they unhappy or unfulfilled? Asking these types of questions can not only help unravel a complex case but also build a strong patient–doctor relationship, which is an important step for healing to occur. If there is no obvious cause after an in-depth intake, basic laboratories (CBC, TSH, BUN, GFR, CR, aldosterone, and cortisol) and imaging (renal ultrasound and echocardiogram) may help to determine the cause.

The bottom line is to spend time with your patients, ask appropriate questions, and thoroughly investigate their case. Even if the cause is very challenging to determine and treat, always address diet and lifestyle. You may learn from reviewing a simple diet diary that your hypertensive patient eats a bag of potato chips at night because she is angry with a coworker. The high sodium and trans fat intake coupled with sustained cortisol release from chronic stress is setting the stage for CVD including hypertension. Instead of prescribing a diuretic, talk about the patient's stress and offer suggestions to alleviate emotional toxicity and thus emotional eating.

DIET, LIFESTYLE, AND HYPERTENSION

How many times have you heard that healthy eating, exercise, restricted salt intake, and stress reduction are supportive for blood pressure control? Why are these therapies often overlooked, and why do doctors willingly reach for the prescription pad so quickly? I believe it is important to know quantitatively how much these lifestyle factors can influence SBP and DBP. One of the roles of a physician is to educate patients about the risk/benefit ratio of a treatment plan, and this includes lifestyle changes as well as medications. Learn to become familiar with other therapies besides medications, which takes time and patience. In medicine, it is easy to get caught up in treating numbers (blood pressure) when ultimately we are treating people.

For hypertensive patients, I generally recommend a whole food diet similar to the modified Paleolithic and vegetarian diets discussed earlier. This type of diet includes fresh fruits, vegetables, nuts, seeds, heart healthy oils (olive and coconut), pasture-raised eggs and lean meats, fish, non-gluten grains (i.e., brown rice, quinoa, and amaranth), and legumes (lentils and beans). This means eating little to no processed and fast foods, as these "foods" contain mainly sugar, toxic fats, genetically modified organisms (GMOs), preservatives, food colorings, and a whole list of other chemicals. Hippocrates, the father of Western medicine, once said, "let food be thy medicine and medicine be thy food." In other words, eat real foods to support, nourish, and heal the body.

The Dietary Approach to Stop Hypertension (DASH) diet contains the foods mentioned plus low-fat dairy. Research shows that it can lower SBP and DBP by 5.5 and 3.3 mmHg, respectively.[36] Some large randomized controlled trials (RCTs) looking at the DASH diet show even greater reductions in SBP of approximately 11 mmHg and DBP of 5 mmHg.[37] For reducing blood pressure, I do support a DASH-type diet. Overall, I believe that it is a very healthy diet and very similar to the Mediterranean diet. I do make minor modifications, however, that include a reduction in gluten-containing grains, a preference for full-fat organic dairy products, and a smarter option for cooking oils.

I find that too many servings of grains particularly wheat can contribute to fluctuations in blood sugar and insulin levels, and therefore fluctuations in blood pressure. Remember, wheat is a grain consumed in excess these days due to the prevalence of packaged and fast foods and has a very high glycemic index. High glycemic index foods turn into sugar in the body. In a prospective study looking at the sugar content of SSBs, reducing the intake of 1 SSB a day lead to a clinically significant drop in blood pressure of 1.1–1.8 mmHg over 18 months.[38] As an added bonus, weight can also drop from eliminating this extraneous sugar source. Therefore, when possible reduce wheat and grain consumption as lowering intake will invariably lead to better glycemic control, and thus reduced blood pressure.

On the DASH diet, low-fat dairy products are recommended. There is moderate research suggesting an inverse relationship between dairy consumption and blood pressure, although more clinical research is needed to delineate a casual relationship.[39] If choosing to consume dairy, try to buy organic full-fat products instead, as low-fat products typically contain more sugar and other additives that may not be conducive to optimal blood pressure control. Studies show that cows fed grass instead of grains have higher levels of ω-3 fatty acids in their milk.[40] If available, consume organic grass fed dairy products as the fatty acid profile is more desirable. Also, organic dairy products should not contain any hormone by-products, which may lead to oxidative stress in the body.

The DASH diet suggests consuming two to three servings a day of fats and oils including vegetable oil and/or margarine. I do not recommend these oils because they may contain trans fats and may promote free radical oxidation in the body, particularly the blood vessels. Instead, I like olive and coconut oil for supporting cardiovascular health. Studies on olive oil show promising reductions in blood pressure when consumed in upward of 60 g (4 tbsp) a day.[41] The oleic acid present in olive oil may be responsible for the blood pressure–lowering effect. Coconut oil is a very stable oil and great to use for high-heat cooking. In a recent study, virgin coconut oil fed to rats helped prevent blood pressure elevation, which the authors suggest may be due to a reduction in vasoconstriction of the endothelium.[42] Therefore, do not hesitate to use olive and coconut oils with your food as they exert cardioprotective qualities.

With regard to fluids, I recommend consuming mainly filtered water and avoiding excessive alcohol and caffeine intake. In a meta-analysis of 15 randomized controlled trials, reducing alcohol intake lowered SBP and DBP by 3.31 and 2.04 mmHg, respectively.[43] Caffeine intake mainly from coffee elicits very minor increases in blood pressure, so I suggest coffee in moderation.[44] Remember, blood sugar swings can contribute to fluctuations in blood pressure. Minimally consume desserts and highly refined carbohydrates and sugary foods, as sugar will also trigger a neurohormonal response leading to an elevation in blood pressure.

In addition to consuming filtered water, some studies show promising reductions in blood pressure with the use of hibiscus tea. Hibiscus flowers contain anthocyanins, which are thought to exhibit blood pressure–lowering effects through mild ACE inhibitor and diuretic actions. In a randomized, double blind, and placebo-controlled trial, 3240 mL servings per day of hibiscus tea were administered for 6 weeks to prehypertensive and mildly hypertensive adults. Compared to placebo, those consuming hibiscus tea had lower SBP and DBP by 7.2 and 3.1 mmHg, respectively.[45] In two other RCTs (one of them double blinded), hibiscus tea was almost comparable to the ACE inhibitors lisinopril and captopril in lowering blood pressure with a wide margin of tolerability and safety.[46,47]

Patients commonly ask me about salt and whether they can add it to meals. Excessive salt intake is associated with an elevation in blood pressure[48] and an increased risk for CVD, renal disease, and stroke.[49] In a meta-analysis of 34 trials, researchers found that a reduction in salt intake of 4 g/day led to reductions in SBP and DBP of 4.18 and 2.06 mmHg, respectively, in normotensive and hypertensive individuals. They propose that reducing salt intake to 4 to 5 g/day can have a major effect on blood pressure and that lowering it to 3 g/day offers the most cardioprotective benefits.[50] As reference, 3 g of sodium a day is just over 1 tsp of salt.

The main source of salt in the standard American diet is processed food products such as canned goods, fast foods, pickles, chips, candies, and processed meats. If the aforementioned foods are consumed infrequently, it is okay in moderation to add high-quality sea salt (a "pinch") to meals as this can actually benefit digestion and provide essential trace minerals.

It should be noted that increasing potassium in the diet or via a supplement can lower the risk of stroke[51] and help reduce blood pressure.[52] According to research, if 4.7 g/day of dietary potassium are consumed, SBP and DBP can decrease by 8.0 and 4.1 mmHg, respectively. A potassium-induced reduction in blood pressure can offer other cardiovascular benefits including a reduction in myocardial infarction and coronary heart disease.[53] In a large prospective study of 43,738 men, greater potassium intake through diet resulted in a lowered incidence of stroke.[51] If supplemental potassium is administered, care should be taken in those patients taking potassium-sparing medications or with renal disease.[53]

EXERCISE AND HYPERTENSION

Regular exercise can reduce blood pressure in hypertensive and normotensive individuals. In a meta-analysis of 54 randomized controlled trials, aerobic exercise could lower SBP and DBP by 3.84 and 2.58 mmHg, respectively.[54] One study had participants exercise three to four times per week for 1 hour at 75%–85% of their initial heart rate (HR) reserve, and then this group was compared to an exercise and weight management group. The participants in the exercise and weight management group had the greatest reductions in SBP and DBP of 7 and 5 mmHg, respectively.[55] The lesson to learn from this study is exercise coupled with weight loss promotes greater blood pressure control than exercise alone.

Research reports that modest increases in exercise of 61–90 min/week can decrease blood pressure in a sedentary hypertensive population.[56] One study indicated that 10,000 steps per day, regardless of duration or intensity, are effective in lowering blood pressure and reducing sympathetic nerve activity.[57] Walking for most people is a simple form of exercise that can benefit the cardiovascular system. I recommend exercise that is practical, convenient, and enjoyable, and for most people a 20-minute walk in the neighborhood will suffice. It also provides time to walk with a loved one or pet or enjoy the quiet solitude of nature.

STRESS, BREATHING, AND HYPERTENSION

One of the most important, and often neglected, lifestyle measures to address with your patients is stress. Stress exists in many forms and may include situational (e.g., car accident), mental (e.g., anxiety), emotional (e.g., fear, guilt), physical (e.g., chronic back pain), chemical (e.g., pesticides), oxidative (e.g., heavy metals and electromagnetic radiation [EMR]) and psycho-spiritual (e.g., relationship and career). We all manage stress on a daily basis whether it is paying bills, sitting in traffic, caring for a sick family member, or constantly connecting through social media. These stressors have a cumulative effect that can result in chronic stimulation of the sympathetic nervous system.

An overactive sympathetic nervous system may lead to chronically elevated vasoconstrictive stress hormones that set the stage for hypertension.[58] When under chronic stress, the hypothalamic–pituitary–adrenal axis overproduces glucocorticoid and catecholamine hormones. These "fight or flight" hormones include cortisol, epinephrine, and norepinephrine and can elevate blood sugar and blood pressure, causing significant neurohormonal changes including immune system dysfunction. Acutely activating this fight or flight system is advantageous because heart rate, respiratory rate, and blood flow increase and our ability to react to stimuli is enhanced. We desperately need these hormones to survive, but balancing them in a chronically stressful environment is key to supporting cardiovascular health.

One method to calm an overactive sympathetic nervous system is to increase parasympathetic tone. Many mind–body therapies including tai chi, qigong, yoga, biofeedback, and meditation and/or slow belly breathing help reduce stress by activating parasympathetic pathways.

When practiced regularly, these therapies can have a profound impact on quality of life and can reduce blood pressure as well.[59-65] These mind–body therapies have a common denominator: meditation through habitual breathing. Learning how to breathe, and building awareness around breathing exercises, is likely why these therapies are beneficial for lowering blood pressure; breathing encourages parasympathetic tone in the body, which in turn supports heart rate variability. Increasing heart rate variability is a major prognosticator in protecting cardiovascular health.[66]

Biofeedback can be used to slow breathing rate and, therefore, help lower blood pressure. In a small RCT, 22 menopausal women with prehypertension were assigned to either a control group (slow abdominal breathing) or an experimental group. The experimental group performed ten 25-minute sessions of slow abdominal breathing (six cycles per minute) combined with frontal electromyographic biofeedback training and daily home practice. The biofeedback training involved muscle relaxation techniques and guided imagery. The experimental group showed the greatest reductions in SBP and DBP of 8.4 and 3.9 mmHg, respectively. The control group experienced a small drop in SBP of 4.3 mmHg but no significant drop in DBP. The researchers conclude that slow breathing at six cycles a minute coupled with biofeedback training is an effective intervention to manage prehypertension.[67]

In addition to biofeedback, breathing devices can also help regulate blood pressure. In a randomized double blind placebo-controlled study, participants were able to lower their blood pressure using a breathe with interactive music (BIM) device for 10 minutes every evening. The BIM device guided users on how to breathe slowly and regularly using sound patterns. A control group listened to a walkman with quiet music. At the end of the 8-week study, BIM participants lowered SBP and DBP by 15.2 and 10 mmHg, respectively, and control group participants by 11.3 and 5.6 mmHg, respectively. These findings suggest that a calming cardiovascular response opposite to that caused by mental stress is responsible for the decrease in blood pressure in both groups. The lower blood pressure in the BIM group is further attributed to breathing modulation.[68] These BIM devices produced reductions in blood pressure similar to those found by commonly prescribed antihypertensives.

In an RCT of 79 patients using device-guided breathing exercises (DGBE), hypertensive medicated participants spent 15 min/day practicing deep breathing at home. Blood pressures were measured at home and in office over an 8-week period. By the end of the study, the participants using DGBE had a reduction in SBP of 5.5 mmHg and DBP of 3.6 mmHg.[69] These results from the previous two studies show that breathing devices, commonly available to patients, can help lower blood pressure by assisting with deep breathing exercises. Moreover, reductions in blood pressure can be seen weeks after cessation of treatment.

Many of these aforementioned studies use machines to guide breathing. Other practices such as yoga or tai chi focus on breathing as well. It is important to understand that it is not the machine that is lowering blood pressure but the habitual practice of breathing. One of the reasons why yoga is so popular is because the practice not only supports the musculoskeletal system with stretching and posture alignment but also teaches people to breathe properly. Effectively learning how to breathe can take time and practice. Fortunately, biofeedback and breathing machines, breathing exercises, teachers, or group work can help develop awareness about how to breathe.

Out of all the meditation practices, Transcendental Meditation (TM) seems to offer the greatest blood pressure–lowering effect.[70] TM is a nonreligious meditation technique that focuses on mantra repetition for 20 minutes two times a day. It is thought to promote relaxation and can bring the meditator into a deeper state of consciousness. In a meta-analysis of nine randomized controlled trials looking at TM and its effect on blood pressure, regular practice of TM has the potential to approximately lower SBP and DBP by 4.7 and 3.2 mmHg, respectively.[71] In one RCT, 298 university students were assigned to a TM program or wait list control. The students in the TM program exhibited lower SBP and DBP, and improvements were noted in total psychological stress, anxiety, depression, anger/hostility, and coping.[72]

BREATHING TECHNIQUE AND HYPERTENSION

For people who want to practice breathing on their own, I teach a simple breathing exercise that takes 15 minutes to complete. First, I recommend that patients sit down on the edge of a chair to help align the spine. Lying supine in the *shavasana* yoga pose is another option. Then I tell patients to imagine a balloon in their lower abdomen inflating and deflating with each breath. This helps to develop belly breathing instead of chest breathing, which we are more inclined to do when under stress. Now start breathing. Breathe in for two counts and then breathe out for two counts. Do this for a couple of cycles and increase to three counts in and three counts out. Repeat for a couple of cycles and increase to four counts in and four counts out. Again, repeat and breathe in for five counts and breathe out for five counts. This breathing pattern typically results in five to six breaths per minute. It may take a few days or a week to settle at five to six breaths a minute, so be patient.

This technique of slow deep breathing is very useful because it helps to focus our attention away from stress and reduce ruminating thoughts by allowing the mind to be in the present moment. Slow deep breathing will invariably lower blood pressure as well. The goal of this breathing exercise is to habituate natural functional breathing by slowing it down and making it deeper. One study having participants breathe at six cycles per minute showed an increase in baroreceptor sensitivity and a decrease in sympathetic activity and chemoreflex activation, which are potential beneficial effects for treating hypertension.[73] Regardless of what breathing technique you suggest to your patients, persistence is the foundation for success. Structured breathing every day will achieve positive results and may help take your patient to another level in their meditation practice.

TARGETED NUTRITIONAL SUPPLEMENTS, BOTANICAL MEDICINES, AND ACUPUNCTURE AND HYPERTENSION

Although there is no question that hypertensive medications significantly lower blood pressure, and reduce CVD events and stroke, side effects are common and cost can be prohibitive. Many patients these days are searching for a more holistic approach to treating hypertension and demand alternatives for drug therapy. When blood pressure elevation is mild to moderate (prehypertension to stage I hypertension), diet and lifestyle interventions should be addressed first as these treatments are fundamental to sound health. In addition to diet and lifestyle changes (e.g., exercise, fasting, and meditation), targeted nutritional supplements, botanical medicines, and acupuncture can further lower blood pressure. These natural medicine treatments may be necessary to get blood pressure under control quickly while diet and lifestyle measures take effect and can help wean patients off certain hypertensive medications. Although there are multiple targeted supplements to choose from, I have had the most success with coenzyme Q10, magnesium, ω-3 fatty acids, garlic, and rauwolfia to name a few.

Coenzyme Q10 (which is discussed in detail in Chapter 12) is a powerful antioxidant found in all human cells. It helps to support adenosine triphosphate turnover in the mitochondria, is a membrane stabilizer, and can help reduce inflammatory markers.[74,75] Although the exact mechanism is unknown in humans for reducing blood pressure, CoQ10 does reduce peripheral resistance through nitric oxide preservation and acts as a potent free radical scavenger helping to reduce free radical stress.[76] Whereas some studies show mixed results with CoQ10 for blood pressure control, other studies show a moderate reduction in blood pressure. One randomized, double blind, and placebo controlled trial found a mean reduction in SBP of 17.8 mmHg.[77] In a Cochrane meta-analysis of three double-blinded, placebo-controlled studies, mean decreases in SBP and DBP were 11 and 7 mmHg, respectively. It should be noted that the authors of this analysis were concerned about the quality of blinding, and author credibility.[78] The typical dose for CoQ10 supplementation is 100–200 mg a day. Side effects are rarely seen.

Magnesium is a mineral involved in over 300 enzymatic reactions in the body. It may help reduce blood pressure due to the mild smooth muscle relaxation and Ca^{2+} ion antagonizing effects. A recent meta-analysis of 22 trials showed that 410 mg (mean dosage) of magnesium can reduce SBP by 3–4 mmHg and DBP by 2–3 mmHg.[79–81] As many people are deficient in magnesium because of decreasing soil concentrations and poor dietary habits including excessive caffeine and alcohol intake, it may be worthwhile to measure magnesium red blood cell levels and supplement if low levels are found. Magnesium is available in many different forms (citrate, chloride, glycinate, oxide, and aspartate), and the doses can range from 200 to 600 mg/day. Side effects may include diarrhea or abdominal cramping if dosed too high, and magnesium should not be given to patients with renal insufficiency.

There are many studies on fish oil supplementation and increased fish intake for the treatment of blood pressure for medicated and unmedicated hypertensive patients. Some studies show modest reductions in blood pressure. In a recent meta-analysis of 17 studies, researches concluded that reductions in SBP of 2.56 mmHg and DBP of 1.47 mmHg were found with fish oil supplementation. Varying doses of fish oil including docosahexaenoic acid (DHA) and eicosapentaenoic acid (EPA) were used in this analysis. Although a small reduction in blood pressure was found, the researchers state that a 2-mmHg reduction in SBP can lower mortality by 10% for strokes and mortality by 7% for ischemic heart disease.[82] Typical doses for fish oil are 2–3 g/day. Side effects may include burping and abdominal discomfort.

Garlic as a food-based supplement is very helpful for reducing blood pressure. In one meta-analysis of 10 trials, participants with hypertension (SBP > 140 mmHg) experienced reductions in SBP and DBP by 16.3 and 9.3 mmHg, respectively. There was no clinically significant drop in SBP or DBP in normotensive participants, however.[83] Similar results were found in another meta-analysis of hypertensive participants where reductions in SBP of 8.4 and in DBP 7.3 of mmHg were observed.[84] These findings suggest that garlic supplementation may help reduce blood pressure in hypertensive individuals. It should be noted that many forms of garlic were used in these studies and that the average dose was 600–900 mg/day providing 3.6–5.4 mg of allicin, the active compound in garlic.[84] As a side note, garlic cloves generally contain 5–9 mg of allicin, so they may be used in cooking to achieve some hypotensive benefits. Garlic may interact with some pharmaceuticals such as coumadin, so make sure you look up possible herb–drug interactions before initializing treatment.

There are many other food-based supplements and nutraceuticals that help reduce blood pressure. According to Dr. Mark Houston, who recently published an article summarizing nonpharmacological approaches to treating hypertension, the following can also assist in blood pressure control: taurine; L-arginine; vitamins E, C, D, and B6; flavonoids; quercetin; α-lipoic acid; N-acetyl cysteine; melatonin; grape seed extract; pomegranate juice; black and green tea; chocolate; sesame; and seaweed.[85] Many of these vitamins and nutrients can be found in whole foods, which brings us back to the notion of food as medicine. They can also be taken in supplement form. In Chapter 9, the reader will investigate foods and supplements in more detail.

Traditionally, botanical medicines have been used to lower blood pressure and support the heart. Many naturopathic physicians and herbalists compound antihypertensive botanical formulas that may contain the following herbs: hawthorn, rauwolfia, rosemary, dandelion leaf, mistletoe, coleus forskohlii, and arjuna. Although there is some research to support their use, a physician must intensely study these herbs and interactions to feel confident enough to prescribe them. Most herbal medicines are very safe to use, but caution must be taken particularly if patients are taking multiple hypertensive pharmaceuticals concurrently.

NDs often use botanical formulas to wean a patient off a pharmaceutical while addressing diet and lifestyle changes.[86] The aforementioned herbs, especially rauwolfia, have been used with great success. When prescribing rauwolfia, however, you must be careful about potential drug interactions including MAO inhibitors. Severe depression and Parkinson's disease are contraindications. Because rauwolfia contains the alkaloid reserpine, side effects are not uncommon, so care needs to be taken when prescribing this herb.

Acupuncture is a system of medicine that has been around for thousands of years and can help treat hypertension. Although research does support its use for reducing blood pressure, many of the trials have unclear methodological quality and most are in other languages other than English (i.e., Chinese and Russian). In a recent meta-analysis of 35 studies, acupuncture significantly reduced SBP by 7.47 mmHg and DBP by 4.22 mmHg. The authors of this analysis conclude, however, that the results are limited by methodological flaws in the studies. They suggest further large-scale studies be done to confirm these results. In my practice, I frequently use acupuncture to help reduce stress. I take blood pressures before and after treatment and on average notice drops of 2–3 mmHg SPB and 1–2 mmHg DBP. My personal belief is that acupuncture helps to reduce blood pressure through stress-relieving qualities.

FASTING AND HYPERTENSION

Fasting has been shown to lower blood pressure and reduce the prevalence of coronary artery disease.[87,88] In one study, 174 hypertensive adults participated in extended water-only fasting, which averaged 10 to 11 days in length. At the end of the study, 90% of the participants were normotensive with an average reduction in SBP and DBP of 37 and 13 mmHg, respectively. The greatest reduction in blood pressure occurred in those with stage III hypertension with an average reduction of 60/17 mmHg (systolic/diastolic). This study suggests that medically supervised water-only fasting is a safe and effective treatment for hypertension.[88]

One anecdotal case that made a lasting impression on my practice involved a 69-year-old male with stage I/II hypertension. Timothy asked me to supervise a 10-day water-only fast for his elevated blood pressure, which was slowly creeping up into the 175/80 mmHg range. While fasting, he agreed to rest as much as possible allowing himself to venture into his garden for a couple of hours each day.[89] Timothy also agreed to be in close contact with me over the phone and through e-mail to update me regularly about his condition.

After 5 days of fasting, his blood pressure dropped to 128/66 mmHg. He wanted to continue with the fast, and by the end of the 15th day (10 days of fasting and 5 days of proper food reintroduction) his blood pressure had reached 100/55 mmHg. During the fast, he experienced weight loss (14 lb) and moderate to severe fatigue. He also developed a mild anemia with lowered red blood cells, hematocrit, and hemoglobin, which returned to normal 6 weeks post fast. Timothy said "although this fast lowered my blood pressure tremendously, it did lower my chi (energy), which took many weeks to build again."

Timothy returned again 1 year later with mildly elevated blood pressure (160/80 mmHg) and commented that his blood pressure remained low throughout the year but started to slowly rise about 6 months post fast. This rise in blood pressure, he commented, was likely due to life stressors as his diet (Paleolithic) and exercise (running 28 km/week) remained unchanged. The life stressors included taking on more housework, caring for his wife who has multiple sclerosis, and commuting longer hours to visit his grandchildren. He also suspects that rising blood pressure is related to aging.

I learned a valuable lesson from this experience; water-only fasting is an excellent treatment option to lower blood pressure in highly motivated patients who desire nondrug approaches. Remarkably, Timothy wants to fast again this upcoming spring. Currently, I have him taking aged garlic, CoQ10, fish oils, and magnesium to manage his elevated blood pressure. If his blood pressure does not decrease significantly using these nutraceuticals, I have given Timothy clearance for a 5-day water-only fast in the spring or summer. I feel a 5-day fast (compared to a 10-day fast) is medically more appropriate and safe with his history of moderate to severe fatigue and development of anemia.

GROUNDING AND HYPERTENSION

There is research emerging showing a positive cardiovascular benefit from connecting our bodies to the surface of the earth.[90] This technique is known as grounding or earthing, and it can improve heart rate variability, reduce blood viscosity, lower nighttime cortisol, reduce pain, increase ζ potential, and increase parasympathetic activity.[91–93] The simplest way to ground our bodies is to walk barefoot in the grass. For most of our existence, humans have walked barefoot or with conductive footwear (e.g., leather) and have slept close to the earth. With the introduction of rubber and plastic sole shoes, however, people are rarely in contact with the earth. When the skin touches the earth's electron rich surface, there is a free flow of negative charge into the body, which may help neutralize free radicals or reactive oxygen species. This may be a possible mechanism of action for the physiological benefits attributed through grounding. Although there are case reports of grounding lowering blood pressure, more research needs to be done to suggest this as a treatment for hypertension.[93]

IMPORTANCE OF DETOXIFICATION IN SUPPORTING THE CARDIOVASCULAR SYSTEM

INTRODUCTION

Considering the enormous toxin burden we are facing today, detoxification must become a way of life or toxin accumulation will inadvertently affect our health and, more importantly, the health of future generations. Since the Industrial Revolution and the introduction of chemical fertilizers and pesticides, the level of toxins present in air, water, and soil has skyrocketed to unprecedented levels. Heavy metals such as mercury, pesticides such as dichlorodiphenyltrichloroethane (DDT), and xenoestrogens such as phthalates found in plastics have infiltrated the environment and ultimately our bodies. The amount of chemicals used for agriculture alone has increased tremendously over the last half decade, and some of these pesticides originally deemed as safe are proving to be carcinogenic.[94] This massive increase in environmental toxins has put tremendous strain on our cell's detoxification mechanisms and, consequently, toxins are being stored rather than properly excreted.[95–97]

EFFECTS OF ENVIRONMENTAL TOXINS ON BLOOD PRESSURE AND THE CARDIOVASCULAR SYSTEM

Many studies have looked at the effects of environmental toxins on blood pressure and CVD. It is known that heavy metals including mercury, arsenic, cadmium, and lead; cigarette smoke; and pesticides can cause elevations in blood pressure.[98,99] In one study looking at residents living near a Monsanto chemical plant, those with high polychlorinated biphenyl (PCB) exposure had elevations in SBP and DBP. PCBs are manmade chemicals banned in the United States in 1979 due to their high level of toxicity. Although the exact mechanism of how PCBs affect blood pressure is unclear, it is thought that they promote endothelial dysfunction through their proinflammatory nature. PCBs have been shown to induce oxidative stress in endothelial cells, which may be an underlying mechanism for the development of atherosclerosis and hypertension.[100] Sadly, PCBs are still showing up in our food supply, and subsequently our bodies, as they continue to be dumped into the environment and have a considerably long half-life (www.EPA.gov).

There is speculation that exposure to pesticides before birth may lead to greater susceptibility to hypertension in adulthood. DDT is a pesticide that was banned in the United States decades ago, but it is still used worldwide for indoor malaria vector control, and as a pesticide in countries outside the United States. Today, DDT is still found in our soil and indoor air samples and continues to infiltrate our bodies due to its long half-life and semivolatility. In a birth cohort study following women into their fifth decade of life, prenatals exposed to DDT were found to be at higher risk for developing hypertension in adulthood.[101] The implications of this study are enormous considering the plethora of toxins found in prenatals today.

In a recent monumental study looking at environmental chemical levels in 268 pregnant women, many chemicals known to have detrimental effects on health (e.g., carcinogenic compounds) were positively identified. In fact, some of these chemicals were found in 99%–100% of the samples tested, and they included PCBs, organochlorine pesticides, perfluoroalkyl chemicals (PFCs), phenols, polybrominated diphenyl ethers (PBDEs), phthalates, polycyclic aromatic hydrocarbons, and perchlorate.[102] According to research, exposure to PCBs,[103] PBDEs, PFCs, and phthalates leads in an increased risk of developing hypertension and other CVDs.[104–107] When you consider the ubiquitous nature of some of these chemicals such as phthalates, found in food and commercial plastics, it is no surprise that exposure is increasing.

Considering the high level of prenatal exposure to chemicals in the womb, including the ones listed earlier, physicians should implement detoxification into every parent's preconception plan. Detoxification treatments for future parents may develop into a specialty in the future. Health professionals must protect the unborn and newborn from the onslaught of chemicals in the environment. Ideally, detoxification should be prioritized as important as prenatal vitamins and folate support. My wife, also an ND, specializes in prenatal, perinatal, and postnatal care. She has noticed a staggering increase in infertility over the years, which she believes is largely due to environmental toxicants and EMR exposure. Treating disease does not begin once a symptom or disease develops but starts before the fertilization of an egg.

The aforementioned Woodruff study elucidates that we are all vulnerable to toxin exposure even before birth. What happens to physiological processes in the body after years of exposure? In one study looking at the biological mechanisms of ambient air pollution on cardiovascular health, chronic exposure to air pollution can increase rates of hypertension, coronary artery disease (CAD), CVD, and thromboembolism.[108–112] It is thought that particulate matter in air pollution activates inflammatory pathways and hemostasis factors, produces reactive oxygen species due to elevated oxidative stress, alters vascular tone, and decreases heart rate variability.[108] Normally, healthy endothelial cells secrete endothelial-derived relaxing factor (EDRF), which helps relax vascular smooth muscle. Oxidative stress via exposure to particulate matter is thought to damage endothelial cells, thus preventing the release of EDRF, which could contribute to systemic hypertension. Additionally, white blood cells adhere to the endothelium in response to tissue damage from oxidative stress, which sets the stage for atherosclerosis to develop. Atherosclerotic disease can be a sequela of hypertension.[112]

Research shows that reductions in particulate matter exposure over a few years does lower cardiovascular mortality rates.[110] Although many of us live in urban centers and are exposed to ever increasing levels of particulate matter and air pollution, we can reduce our risk of CVD by reducing exposure. The best way to reduce our exposure to toxins is avoidance of them in the first place. Additionally, we can support the body's detoxification pathways by helping to mobilize and eliminate toxins that have been stored. Working in concert together, the organ systems are able to effectively remove toxins that we accumulate through the air, water, and soil.

Detoxification is a systematic lifestyle practice to enhance optimal functioning of body physiology.[113] It is absolutely necessary to detoxify on a daily basis considering the overabundance of environmental toxins, and our increasing levels of exposure. Toxins are natural and foreign substances found in the environment and are normal by-products of cell metabolism. In the section on "Reducing Toxic Exposure with Simple and Easy Interventions," I present a general overview of detoxification therapies and how they can be utilized every day to minimize toxin exposure and accumulation. Although the emphasis is on supporting overall health, additional benefits for the cardiovascular system are discussed as well.

REDUCING TOXIC EXPOSURE WITH SIMPLE AND EASY INTERVENTIONS

Sauna Therapy

Any method to increase circulation will support detoxification pathways. For basic detoxification support, try walking at least 20 minutes each and every day. If walking or light exercise is not an option due to arthritis or injury, sauna therapy is another great method to increase circulation. Finnish saunas have been studied the most because of their extensive use in Europe and popularity in North America. A Finnish sauna is usually constructed of wood walls and benches and uses radiant heat to warm the air from 176°F to 194°F.[90] Infrared saunas are another option for sauna therapy. They are typically heated to 110°F–130°F using infrared rays, and some patients fare better in infrared saunas due to the lower temperature and humidity. Both the Finnish and the infrared saunas can be used for detoxification purposes.

Saunas can improve hemodynamics through vasodilation of arteries, which can support the mobilization of fat-soluble xenobiotics.[114] Although there are few studies looking at heavy metal removal with sauna therapy, we do know that mercury, cadmium, antimony, lead, and nickel are released through sweat. Sauna therapy can increase left ventricular ejection fraction in patients with heart failure and increase peripheral circulation by 5%–10%, accounting for 50%–70% of cardiac output. Also, some studies report moderate reductions in blood pressure with sauna therapy.[114,115]

Most people, including cardiac patients with stable coronary heart disease or a history of myocardial infarction, can safely use saunas.[115] Contraindications include unstable angina, aortic stenosis, and recent myocardial infarction. Relative contraindications include heart arrhythmias and decompensated heart failure.[115] If the goal of sauna therapy is to lower blood pressure, only 15-minute sessions are recommended. If optimizing detoxification is the primary outcome, longer sessions at lower temperatures (140°F) are recommended.[116] Remember to drink plenty of fluids and electrolytes before, during, and after treatment to help mobilize toxins and prevent dehydration. Ginger/yarrow tea is another drink commonly consumed before saunas to increase vasodilation, and thus diaphoresis.

If saunas are not an option, hot yoga is another excellent form of detoxification therapy to promote toxin release via sweating. Typically, rooms are heated at 104°F with 40%–60% humidity. Practicing yoga in this temperature and humidity promotes profuse sweating and improves flexibility and strength.[117] In a recent study on Bikram yoga, a popular form of hot yoga, older adults who practiced three times per week for 90 minutes had improved insulin sensitivity by the end of the 8-week study.[118] I recommend that patients go one to two times per week for general detoxification and musculoskeletal support.

HIGH-FIBER PHYTONUTRIENT-RICH DIETS OF ORGANIC FRUITS AND VEGETABLES

Eating a high-fiber predominately plant-based diet of organic vegetables and fruits provides protection for the cardiovascular system.[119] Fruits and vegetables are loaded with antioxidants, vitamins, and minerals, which can neutralize free radical stress, and contain high levels of fiber to move toxins out of the digestive tract. The average American consumes 11–18 g of fiber a day,[120] but we should consume greater than 50 g/day to maintain optimal colon health. Eating a combination of raw and cooked vegetables is best. If buying organic foods is not an option, at the very least try to avoid the "dirty dozen" fruits and vegetables known to have higher levels of pesticides: celery, peaches, strawberries, apples, hot peppers, sweet bell peppers, nectarines, spinach, cherry tomatoes, potatoes, cherries, and grapes. Avoiding these dirty dozen foods will decrease your pesticide exposure tremendously.

The fruits and vegetables with the lowest levels of pesticide residues include onion, avocado, sweet corn, pineapple, mango, sweet peas, asparagus, kiwi, cabbage, eggplant, cantaloupe, mushrooms, papaya, grapefruit, and sweet potato. You can print out a handy, wallet-sized chart of the least and most toxic fruits and vegetables at http://www.foodnews.org/fulllist.php. The dirty dozen can fluctuate over time, so it is a good idea to update your list regularly. More useful information about the Environmental Working Group, which strives to educate the public about environmental toxicants, may be found at www.ewg.org and www.foodnews.org.

Children who eat organic fruits and vegetables have lower detectable levels of organophosphorus pesticides in their urine. This finding came out from a study conducted in Mercer Island, Washington. Children were fed conventional foods for 4 days, then all organic foods for 5 days, and then again conventional foods for 6 days. Malathion and chlorpyrifos were the organophosphorus pesticides detected in daily urine samples. Median levels of these two pesticides significantly dropped to nondetectable levels immediately after the introduction of the organic diets and remained nondetectable until the conventional foods were reintroduced again.[121]

Consuming organic fruits and vegetables is important because pesticides may damage the cardiovascular system. Pesticides including organophosphates have been shown to induce lipid peroxidation, stimulate free radical production, and disturb the total antioxidant capability of the body.[122] In a study where rats were exposed to varying levels of the organophosphate pesticide chlorpyrifos (the same pesticide tested for in the aforementioned Washington study), blood pressure elevations were recorded and strongly correlated with increasing doses of the pesticide. The authors of this study propose that chlorpyrifos, which is an irreversible acetylcholinesterase inhibitor, causes cholinergic stimulation.[123] Acute central nervous system stimulation can lead to elevations in SBP and DBP.

LIVER AND GASTROINTESTINAL SUPPORTIVE FOODS AND BOTANICAL MEDICINES

We can alleviate the burden that toxins put on our cardiovascular system by supporting two very important elimination pathways (organs): the liver and gastrointestinal tract. The liver is responsible for metabolizing drugs, toxins, hormones, and other endogenous and exogenous substances into metabolites that are then excreted through the skin, kidneys, or gastrointestinal tract. Any substance (food, vitamin, nutraceutical, etc.) that supports liver detoxification pathways will enhance removal of toxins. Once these toxins enter the small intestine, they need support getting out properly, and this is where a healthy gastrointestinal tract comes into play. There is a saying in medicine that when in doubt treat the liver and gastrointestinal tract; if detoxification pathways are impaired, the body literally becomes too toxic to function optimally.

There are various foods that you can eat on a daily basis to support the liver and gastrointestinal tract. Root vegetables (artichokes, carrots, dandelion, and beets), sulfur-containing foods (eggs, garlic, and onions), water-soluble fibers (pears, oat bran, apples, and beans), and cabbage family vegetables (broccoli, brussels sprouts, and cabbage) all optimize healthy liver and intestine function. You can also juice many of the aforementioned fruits and vegetables, which also aids in the detoxification process by supplying live enzymes. Avoiding sugary foods will also help your body detox, which may help you think twice about reaching for that midafternoon cookie. Instead, eat a handful of raisins and almonds, or dip an apple slice into a freshly made hummus.

Other foods that you should try to implement into your diet to support the liver and gastrointestinal tract include fermented foods and drinks. Fermented foods and drinks include kimchi, sauerkraut, pickled ginger, beet kvass, kombucha, miso, tempeh, natto, yogurt, raw cheese, and kefir. There are many other food and drinks including high-quality beers and wines that are considered fermented. Fermented food and drinks supply a natural source of probiotics to the gastrointestinal tract, which help to digest foods, improve immune function, and prevent "bad" microorganisms (*Escherichia coli*) from causing infection. Many cultures around the world consume fermented foods and drinks with every meal. When looking for a high-quality fermented food or drink, check to see if excess heating has been used, which destroys the natural fermentation process. I highly recommend making these foods and drinks at home, as quality is increased with smaller production. Check out the book *Wild Fermentation* by Sandor Ellix Katz for more information and home recipes.

There are many botanical medicines that support liver function and therefore augment liver detoxification pathways. Some of these botanicals include milk thistle seed, schisandra seed, dandelion root, burdock root, turmeric root, and artichoke leaf. These herbs can be ingested in foods, tinctures, teas, or pills. They have different functions (e.g., hepatoprotective, antioxidant, and alterative), depending on how they are prescribed, and can be combined in formulas to create synergistic effects. Generally, they are very safe in lower doses; however, consult with an experienced practitioner before using these botanicals.

Skin Brushing

To improve the functioning of the skin and lymphatic system, try incorporating skin brushing into a daily routine. Skin brushing has been practiced in many cultures over the years to improve skin hygiene. By keeping the skin free from dry, dead skin cells, waste removal from the body is greatly enhanced, blood flow is increased, and buildup of bacteria is decreased. The best time to skin brush is before a shower or before bed. Using a natural vegetable bristle or loofah brush, start at the feet using gentle, quick strokes and move upward toward the heart covering most of the body. This is the direction of lymph and venous blood flow. It is completely normal for the skin to feel slightly tingly, but be sure to avoid harsh brushing and brushing over open wounds, the face, or over any lymphatic malignancies.

Castor Oil Applications

One of the most important detoxification treatments that I offer to my patients is the castor oil pack.[124] Castor oil is an anti-inflammatory agent that when absorbed through the skin promotes increased circulation, decreased constipation symptoms, elimination of toxins, and stimulation of white blood cells.[125–127] The castor oil pack should be done five to seven times a week for a month to promote optimal detoxification of the liver, intestines, and lymphatic system. It can be done whenever you are feeling run down, or want to improve the functioning of the gastrointestinal tract and immune system. It is now known that approximately 60%–70% of our immune system is found around our intestines as a vast network of gut-associated lymphatic tissue (GALT). According to one study looking at the immunomodulation effects of topical castor oil, a 2-hour application led to a significant increase in blood lymphocytes.[125]

The easiest method to use a castor oil pack is to apply about 1 to 2 tbsp of castor oil to a flannel cloth and place it on the abdomen and upper right quadrant so that the oil is in contact with the skin. The castor oil should form a thin layer on the skin and not be dripping. Then place an old towel on top (castor oil can stain) and a hot water bottle over the towel to help drive the castor oil into the skin. A hot water bottle or other heating device is not required, but most people report feeling more relaxed when it is used. The heat should be strong enough that you feel a warm gentle heat on your abdomen, but avoid burning. During the next 45–60 minutes, try meditating, reading, or listening to calming music.

This is a great opportunity to devote a small part of your day to healing and relaxing. You can even go to sleep! The castor oil pack affects many systems of the body, and you may feel like you sleep better, have more energy, or experience more regular bowel movements. After the castor oil pack is completed, you can either wash off the excess oil with water and soap or baking soda, or leave it on your skin. Store the flannel cloth in a plastic bag and use repeatedly, applying less castor oil as the cloth becomes more saturated with frequent use.

Contrast Hydrotherapy

Contrast hydrotherapy has been used for centuries to improve circulation, immune system function, and remove toxins.[128–130] Ever visit a spa and notice that a cold pool for immersion is usually next to a sauna or whirlpool? When the body is exposed to heat, blood vessels vasodilate to improve nutrient/waste transfer and blood flow. This is what causes us to sweat. Quickly jumping into a cold plunge causes vasoconstriction, which drives the oxygen-rich blood to the vital organs. Research shows that hydrotherapy tonifies the immune system by increasing the migration of white blood cells.[131] In one study, men who were submerged in warm baths or exercised prior to cold immersion showed an increase in the migration of leukocytes, monocytes, and granulocytes.[132] Most of us do not have cold plunges in our homes, but contrast hydrotherapy can be practiced in the shower. After taking a warm shower, try ending with a 30-second cool water spray starting with the extremities and ending with the abdominal area and low back.

THERAPEUTIC FASTING

One of the most ancient, powerful, and cost-effective methods of cleansing is fasting. Historically, religious and spiritual people have fasted to cleanse the body, mind, and spirit of impurities.[133] From a purely physical perspective, fasting enables the body to rest and work more efficiently. Fasting induces metabolic and hormonal changes by improving insulin sensitivity, enhancing enzyme status, recalibrating taste sensation (e.g., salt), promoting weight loss, and reducing leaky gut. Though fasting is indicated for loss of appetite, acute illness, and chronic illness; to accelerate healing and change behaviors (e.g., quit smoking); and for its psycho-spiritual effect, not everyone is a candidate for fasting.[88] Please consult with a health-care professional before choosing to do a fast.

ELECTROMAGNETIC RADIATION

There is another environmental toxicant that is slowly emerging as a threat to our health, and it is not a heavy metal, chemical, or pesticide.[133] This invisible toxin is the increasing expansion and use of wireless technologies that emit radio frequencies. EMR, or wireless radiation, is a frequency that we cannot see, feel, hear, taste, or smell, and as such we do not realize when we are exposed. These devices include cell phones and cell phone antennas, cordless phones, Wi-Fi routers, microwave ovens, smart meters, baby monitors, tablets, computers, and any other device that utilizes wireless technology. Unfortunately, radio frequency devices were not rigorously tested before market release, and some say our safety regulations are obsolete.

There are many harmful nonthermal biological effects caused by wireless radiation that have emerged via recent research, but standards continue to stay the same.[134] For instance, we do know that wireless radiation induces oxidative damage,[135] but the magnitude of oxidative damage caused by radio frequencies is unknown. Also, there have been no long-term studies on radio frequency safety or analysis of the cumulative effect of using multiple wireless technologies at once over an extended period of time. The best way to reduce exposure to these technologies is to avoid them. This entails talking on cellular speakerphone, using wires instead of wireless whenever possible (i.e., corded phone or Ethernet) and refusing to use a smart meter for your electrical utility meter. There are radio frequency–protective clothing, fabrics, and devices available as well if wireless use is necessary.

Be particularly careful if you are pregnant or carrying a young one as their tiny bodies and developing brains are more susceptible to radiation exposure.[136] Remember, we should not sacrifice safety for convenience, and the effect of lifelong exposure to these frequencies is unknown. Any couple trying to conceive should avoid using wireless devices. A recent study showed that men who use laptops with Wi-Fi had a significant decrease in sperm motility and an increase in sperm DNA fragmentation.[137,138] Since Wi-Fi is currently used in many homes and businesses, avoidance is tricky, but it can be done. It should be noted that many public libraries in France have removed Wi-Fi due to health concerns, and Germany has warned its citizens to use corded connections (Ethernet) as often as possible.

SUMMARY

It is important to remember that although we live in a toxic world where exposure to chemicals, industry by-products, and pollution is common, our bodies are intelligently designed to protect us from toxin exposure. We can optimize organ function and detoxification mechanisms by following these simple-to-implement strategies: drink plenty of filtered water; consciously breathe; exercise; encourage sweating; eat foods that are low in pesticide residue, are fermented, and support the liver and gastrointestinal tract; apply castor oil packs; practice skin brushing and hydrotherapy; and reduce wireless radiation exposure. Try incorporating some or all of these suggestions into your daily regimen and see how you feel.

A word of caution when starting to detoxify is you may feel worse before you feel better, particularly if you have a history of toxin exposure. Moreover, when beginning to eat healthier foods the body may begin detoxifying more efficiently, so detoxification reactions are common. Symptoms may include headaches, nausea, joint pain, fatigue, insomnia, irritability, anxiety, depression, and changes in bowel habits. These reactions may happen because you are eliminating toxins that have been stored in your body for years.

Many techniques and treatments discussed here minimize adverse reactions by optimizing the body's detoxification pathways. Special care and support need to be given to the key organs of elimination, which include the liver, intestines, lungs, kidneys, skin, and lymphatic system. After implementing some of the aforementioned detoxification strategies for a couple of weeks or months, you may notice increased vitality, improved sleep and energy, elevated mood, and fewer signs and symptoms. These changes indicate that your organs of elimination are functioning well and properly detoxifying your body. It may take some time and effort to feel better though. For many NDs, detoxification therapies are one of the most important modalities offered to patients. If we could visibly see what we are exposed to on a daily basis, detoxification would become standard of care for every person on this planet.

CONCLUSION

In medicine, there are many ways to achieve an outcome. I find that practicing individualized medicine is the foundation for optimal health. Every patient is different due to genetics, diet and lifestyle choices, comorbidities, stress, overall toxic burden, gender, age, and other factors. Empower your patients by increasing their awareness and consciousness about health. Teach your patients about healthy diet and lifestyle measures, mind–body medicines including breathing and meditation, nutraceuticals, botanical medicines, therapeutic fasting, detoxification techniques, and grounding. All of these modalities will strengthen your practice as more and more people are searching for nonpharmacological ways to stay healthy. Remember to spend time with your patients, ask questions about their current and past health, listen to their concerns, and investigate the true cause of their suffering.

REFERENCES

1. Perkins A. Saving money by reducing stress. *Harvard Business Review* 1994;72(6):12.
2. Kok FJ, Kromhout D. Atherosclerosis—epidemiological studies on the health effects of a Mediterranean diet. *Eur J Nutr* 2004;43(suppl 1):1/2–5.
3. Lindeberg S, Eliasson M, Lindahl B, Ahren B. Low serum insulin in traditional Pacific Islanders—the Kitava Study. *Metabolism* 1999;48(10):1216–1219.
4. Lindeberg S, Nilsson-Ehle P, Terent A, Vessby B, Schersten B. Cardiovascular risk factors in a Melanesian population apparently free from stroke and ischaemic heart disease: The Kitava study. *J Intern Med* 1994;236(3):331–340.
5. Huang T, Yang B, Zheng J, Li G, Wahlgvist ML, Li D. Cardiovascular disease mortality and cancer incidence in vegetarians: A meta-analysis and systematic review. *Ann Nutr Metab* 2012;60(4):223–240.
6. Lindeberg S. Paleolithic diets as a model for prevention and treatment of Western disease. *Am J Hum Biol* 2012;24(2):110–115.
7. Osterdahl M, Kocturk T, Koochek A, Wandell PE. Effects of a short-term intervention with a paleolithic diet in healthy volunteers. *Euro J Clin Nutr* 2008;62(5):682–5.
8. Davis W. *Wheat Belly*. Emmaus, PA: Rodale Books, Pennsylvania; 2011.
9. De Punder, K, Pruimboom, L. The dietary intake of wheat and other cereal grains and their role in inflammation. *Nutrients* 2013;5(3):771–787.
10. Teixeira RC, Molina Mdel C, Zandonade E, Mill JG. Cardiovascular risk in vegetarians and omnivores: A comparative study. *Arg Bras Cardiol* 2007;89(4):237–244.
11. Appleby PN, Thorogood M, Mann JI, Key TJ. The Oxford Vegetarian Study: An overview. *Am J Clin Nutr* 1999;70(3 suppl):525S–531S.

12. Segasothy M, Phillips PA. Vegetarian diet: Panacea for modern lifestyle diseases? *QJM* 1999;92(9):531–544.
13. Neustadt J. Western diet and inflammation. *Integr Med* 2006;5(4):14–18.
14. Eaton SB, Eaton SB 3rd, Konner MJ. Paleolithic nutrition revisited: A twelve-year retrospective on its nature and implications. *Eur J Clin Nutr* 1997;51(4):207–216.
15. Permutter D. *Grain Brain: The Surprising Truth about Wheat, Carbs, and Sugar—Your Brain's Silent Killers.* New York, NY: Little, Brown, and Company, 2013.
16. Eaton SB, Eaton SB III, Konner MJ. Paleolithic nutrition revisited: A twelve-year retrospective on its nature and implications. *Eur J Clin Nutr* 1997;51(4):207–216.
17. Traube, G. Why We Get Fat: And what to do about it. New York, NY: Anchor Books; 2011.
18. Jonsson T, Ahren B, Pacini G et al. A Paleolithic diet confers higher insulin sensitivity, lower C-reactive protein and lower blood pressure than a cereal-based diet in domestic pigs. *Nutr Metab (Lond)* 2006;2(3):39.
19. Neustadt J. Western diet and inflammation. *Integr Med* 2006;5(4):14–18.
20. Aeberli I, Gerber PA, Hochuli M et al. Low to moderate sugar-sweetened beverage consumption impairs glucose and lipid metabolism and promotes inflammation in healthy young men: A randomized controlled trial. *Am J Clin Nutr* 2011;94(2):479–485.
21. Davis W. *Wheat Belly.* Emmaus, PA: Rodale Books, 2011.
22. Goldin A, Beckman JA, Schmidt AM, Creager MA. Advanced glycation end products: Sparking the development of diabetic vascular injury. *Circulation* 2006;114(6):597–605.
23. Fasano A, Not T, Wang W et al. Zonulin, a newly discovered modulator of intestinal permeability, and its expression in coeliac disease. *Lancet* 2000;335(9214):1518–1519.
24. Segersten A. *Nourishing Meals Cookbook.* Bellingham, WA: Whole Life Press, 2012.
25. Visser J, Rozing J, Sapone A, Lammers K, Fasano A. Tight junctions, intestinal permeability, and autoimmunity: Celiac disease and type I diabetes paradigms. *Ann NY Acad Sci* 2009;1165:195–205.
26. Houston M. Nutrition and nutraceutical supplements for the treatment of hypertension: Part I. *J Clin Hypertens (Greenwich)* 2013;15(10):752–757.
27. Craig WJ. Health effects of vegan diets. *Am J Clin Nutr* 2009;89(5):1627S–1633S.
28. Key TJ, Abbleby PN, Rosell MS. Health effects of vegetarian and vegan diets. *Proc Nutr Soc* 2006;65(1):35–41.
29. Humphrey LL, Fu R, Rogers K, Freeman M, Helfand M. Homocysteine level and coronary heart disease incidence: A systematic review and meta-analysis. *Mayo Clin Proc* 2008;83(11):1203–1212.
30. Schnyder G, Roffi M, Flammer Y, Pin R, M. Hess O. Effect of homocysteine-lowering therapy with folic acid, vitamin B12, and vitamin B6 on clinical outcome after percutaneous coronary intervention: The Swiss Heart study: A randomized controlled trial. *JAMA* 2002;288(8):973–979.
31. Cordain L, Watkins BA, Florant GL, Kelher M, Rogers L, Li Y. Fatty acid analysis of wild ruminant tissues: Evolutionary implications for reducing diet-related chronic disease. *Eur J Clin Nutr* 2002;56:181–191.
32. Ponnampalam EN, Mann NJ, Sinclair AJ. Effect of feeding systems on omega-3 fatty acids, conjugated linoleic acid and trans fatty acids in Australian beef cuts: Potential impact on human health. *Asia Pac J Clin Nutr* 2006;15(1):21–29.
33. Daley CA, Abbott A, Doyle PS, Nader GA, Larson S. A review of fatty acid profiles and antioxidant content in grass-fed and grain-fed beef. *Nutr J* 2010;10:9–10.
34. Goldstein CM, Josephson R, Xie S, Hughes JW. Current perspectives on the use of meditation to reduce blood pressure. *Int J Hypertens* 2012;2012:1–11.
35. Ram CV. Antihypertensive drugs: An overview. *Am J Cardiovasc Drugs* 2002;2(2):77–79.
36. Bacon SL, Sherwood A, Hinderliter A, Blumenthal JA. Effects of exercise, diet and weight loss on high blood pressure. *Sports Med* 2004;34(5):307–316.
37. Conlin PR, Chow D, Miller ER 3rd et al. The effect of dietary patterns on blood pressure control in hypertensive patients: Results from the Dietary Approaches to Stop Hypertension (DASH) trial. *Am J Hypertens* 2000;13(9):949–955.
38. Chen L, Caballero B, Mitchell DC et al. Reducing consumption of sugar-sweetened beverages is associated with reduced blood pressure: A prospective study among United States adults. *Circulation* 2010;121(22):2398–2406.
39. Park KM, Cifelli CJ. Dairy and blood pressure: A fresh look at the evidence. *Nutr Rev* 2013; 71(3):149–157.
40. Hebeisen DF, Hoeflin F, Reusch HP, Junker E, Lauterburg BH. Increased concentrations of omego-3 fatty acids in milk and platelet rich plasma of grass-fed cows. *Int J Vitam Nutr Res* 1993;63(3):229–233.

41. Perona JS, Canizares J, Montero E et al. Virgin olive oil reduces blood pressure in hypertensive elderly subjects. *Clin Nutr* 2004;23(5):1113–1121.

42. Badlishah S, Kamisah Y, Kamsiah J, Oodriyah HM. Virgin coconut oil prevents blood pressure elevation and improves endothelial functions in rats fed with repeatedly heated palm oil. *Evid Based Complement Alternat Med* 2013;2013:7.

43. Xin X, He J, Frontini MG, Ogden LG, Motsamai OI, Whelton PK. Effects of alcohol reduction on blood pressure: A meta-analysis of randomized controlled trials. *Hypertension* 2001;38(5):1112–1117.

44. Noordzij M, Uiterwaal CS, Arends LR, Kok FJ, Grobbee DE, Geleijnse JM. Blood pressure response to chronic intake of coffee and caffeine: A meta-analysis of randomized controlled trials. *J Hypertens* 2005;23(5):921–928.

45. McKay DL, Chen CY, Saltzman E, Blumberg JB. Hibiscus sabdariffa L. tea (tisane) lowers blood pressure in prehypertensive and mildly hypertensive adults. *J Nutr* 2010;140(2):298–303.

46. Herrera-Arellano A, Miranda-Sanchez J, Avila-Castro P et al. Clinical effects produced by a standardized herbal medicinal product of Hibiscus sabdariffa on patients with hypertension: A randomized, double blind, lisinopril controlled clinical trial. *Plana Med* 2007;73(1):6–12.

47. Herrera-Arellano A, Flores-Romero S, Chavez-Soto MA, Tortoriello J. Effectiveness and tolerability of a standardized extract from Hibiscus sabdariffa in patients with mild to moderate hypertension: A controlled and randomized clinical trial. *Phytomedicine* 2004;11(5):375–382.

48. He FJ, MacGregor GA. Salt, blood pressure and cardiovascular disease. *Curr Opin Cardiol* 2007;22(4):298–305.

49. Kotchen TA, McCarron DA. Dietary electrolytes and blood pressure: A statement for healthcare professionals from the American Heart Association Nutrition Committee. *Circulation* 1998;98(6):613–617.

50. He FJ, Li J, Macgregor GA. Effect of longer-term modest salt reduction on blood pressure. *Cochrane Database Syst Rev* 2013;30:4:CD004937.

51. Ascherio A, Rimm EB, Hernan MA et al. Intake of potassium, magnesium, calcium, and fiber and risk of stroke among US men. *Circulation* 1998;98(12):1198–1204.

52. Whelton PK, He J, Cutler JA. Effects of oral potassium on blood pressure. Meta-analysis of randomized controlled clinical trials. *JAMA* 1997;28(20):1624–1632.

53. Houston M. Nutrition and nutraceutical supplements for the treatment of hypertension: Part II. *J Clin Hypertens (Greenwich)* 2013; Nov;15(11):845–51.

54. Whelton SP, Chin A, Xin X, He J. Effect of aerobic exercise on blood pressure: A meta-analysis of randomized, controlled trials. *Ann Intern Med* 2002;136(7):493–503.

55. Blumenthal JA, Sherwood A, Gullette EC et al. Exercise and weight loss reduce blood pressure in men and women with mild hypertension: Effects on cardiovascular, metabolic, and hemodynamic functioning. *Arch Intern Med* 2000;160(13):1947–1958.

56. Ishikawa TK, Ohta T, Tanaka H. How much exercise is required to reduce blood pressure in essential hypertensives: A dose-response study. *Am J Hypertens* 2003;16(8):629–633.

57. Iwane M, Arita M, Tominoto S et al. Walking 10,000 steps/day or more reduces blood pressure and sympathetic nerve activity in mild essential hypertension. *Hypertens Res* 2000;23(6):573–580.

58. Kulkarni S, O'Farrell I, Erasi M, Kochar MS. Stress and hypertension. *WMJ* 1998;97(11):34–38.

59. LI G, Yuan H, Zhang W. Effects of Tai Chi on health related quality of life in patients with chronic conditions: A systematic review of randomized controlled trials. *Complement There Med* 2014;22(4):743–55.

60. Tsai JC, Wang WH, Chan P, Lin LJ, Wang CH, Tomlinson B, Hsieh MH, Yang HY, Liu JC. The beneficial effects of Tai Chi Chuan on blood pressure and lipid profile and anxiety status in a randomized controlled trial. *J Altern Complement Med* 2003;9(5):747–54.

61. Ho TJ, Christiani DC, Ma TC, Jang TR, Lieng CH, Yeh YC, Lin SZ, Lin JG, Lai JS, Lan TY. Effect of Qigong on quality of life: A cross-sectional population-based comparison study in Taiwan. *BMC Public Health* 2011;11:546.

62. Lee MS, Pittler MH, Guo R, Ernst E. Qigong for hypertension: A systematic review of randomized clinical trials. *J Hypertens* 2007;25(8):1525–32.

63. Cheung BM, Lo JL, Fong DY, Chan MY, Wong SH, Wong VC, Lam KS, Lau CP, Karlberg JP. Randomized controlled trial of Qigong in the treatment of mild essential hypertension. *J Hum Hypertens* 2005;19(9):697–704.

64. Hjelland IE, Svebak S, Berstad A, Flatabo G, Hausken T. Breathing exercises with vagal biofeedback may benefit patients with functional dyspepsia. *Scand J Gastroenterol* 2007;42(9):1054–62.

65. Mason HJ, Serrano-Ikkos E, Kamm MA. Psychological state and quality of life in patients having behavioral treatment (biofeedback) for intractable constipation. *Am J Gastroenterol* 2002;97(12):3154–9.

66. Thayer JF, Yamamoto SS, Brosschot JF. The relationship of autonomic imbalance, heart rate variability and cardiovascular disease risk factors. *Int J Cardiol* 2010;141(2):122–131.
67. Wang SZ, Li S, Xu XY et al. Effect of slow abdominal breathing combined with biofeedback on blood pressure and heart rate variability in prehypertension. *J Alternat Complement Med* 2010; 16(10):1039–1045.
68. Schein MH, Gavish B, Herz M et al. Treating hypertension with a device that slows and regularizes breathing: A randomized, double-blind controlled study. *J Hum Hypertens* 2001;15(4):271–278.
69. Meles E, Giannattasio C, Failla M, Gentile G, Capra A, Mancia G. Nonpharmacologic treatment of hypertension by respiratory exercise in the home setting. *Am J Hypetens* 2004;17(4):370–374.
70. Goldstein CM, Josephson R, Xie S, Hughes JW. Current perspectives on the use of meditation to reduce blood pressure. *Int J Hypertens* 2012;2012:578397.
71. Anderson JW, Liu C, Kryscio RJ. Blood pressure response to Transcendental Meditation: A meta-analysis. *Am J Hypertens* 2008;21(3):310–316.
72. Nidich SI, Rainforth MV, Haaga DA et al. A randomized controlled trial on effects of the Transcendental Meditation program on blood pressure, psychological distress, and coping in young adults. *Am J Hypertens* 2009;22(12):1326–1331.
73. Chacko JN, Porta C, Casucci G et al. Slow breathing improves arterial baroreflex sensitivity and decreases blood pressure in essential hypertension. *Hypertension* 2005;46:714–718.
74. Lee BJ, Huang YC, Chen SJ, Lin PT. Effects of coenzyme Q10 supplementation on inflammatory markers (high-sensitivity C-reactive protein, interleukin-6, and homocysteine) in patients with coronary artery disease. *Nutrition* 2012;28(7–8):767–772.
75. Greenberg S, Frishman WH. Co-Enzyme Q10: A new drug for cardiovascular disease. *J Clin Pharmacol* 1990;30(7):596–608.
76. Salvatore P, Marasco SF, Haas SJ, Sheeran FL, Krum H, Rosenfeldt FL. Coenzyme Co$_{10}$ in cardiovascular disease. *Mitrochondrion* 2012;7:154–167.
77. Burke BE, Neuenschwander R, Olson RD. Randomized, double-blind, placebo-controlled trial of coenzyme Q10 in isolated systolic hypertension. *South Med J* 2001;94(11):1112–1117.
78. Ho MJ, Bellusci A, Write JM. Blood pressure lowering efficacy of coenzyme Q10 for primary hypertension. *Cochrane Database Syst Rev* 2009;(4):CD007435.
79. Kass L, Weekes J, Carpenter L. Effect of magnesium supplementation on blood pressure: A meta-analysis. *Eur J Clin Nutr* 2012;66(4):411–418.
80. Swaminathan R. Magnesium metabolism and its disorders. *Clin Biochem Rev* 2003;24(2):47–66.
81. Johnson S. The multifaceted and widespread pathology of magnesium deficiency. *Med Hypotheses* 2001;56(2):163–70.
82. Campbell F, Dickinson HO, Critchlev JA, Ford GA, Bradburn M. A systematic review of fish-oil supplements for the prevention and treatment of hypertension. *Eur J Prev Cardiol* 2013;20(1):107–120.
83. Reinhart KM, Coleman CI, Teevan C, Vachhani P, White CM. Effects of garlic on blood pressure in patients with and without systolic hypertension: A meta-analysis. *Ann Pharmacother* 2008;42(12): 1766–1771.
84. Reid K, Oliver FR, Stocks NP, Fakler P, Sullivan T. Effect of garlic on blood pressure: A systematic review and meta-analysis. *BMC Cardiovasc Disord* 2008;8:13.
85. Houston M. Nutrition and nutraceutical supplements for the treatment of hypertension: Part III. *J Clin Hypertens (Greenwich)* 2013;15(12):931–937.
86. Valkil R. Rauwolfia Serpentina in the treatment of high blood-pressure. *Lancet* 1954;264(6841):726–727.
87. Horne BD, Muhlestein JB, Lappe DL et al. Randomized cross-over trial of short-term water-only fasting: Metabolic and cardiovascular consequences. *Nutr Metab Cardiovasc Dis* 2013;23(11):1050–1057.
88. Goldhamer A, Lisle D, Parpia B, Anderson SV, Campbell TC. Medically supervised water-only fasting in the treatment of hypertension. *J Manipulative Physiol Ther* 2001;24(5):335–339.
89. Longo VD, Mattson MP. Fasting: Molecular mechanisms and clinical applications. *Cell Metab* 2014;19(2):181–92.
90. Chevalier G, Sinatra ST. Emotional stress, heart rate variability, grounding, and improved autonomic tone: Clinical applications. *Integr Med: A Clin J* 2011;10(3):16–21.
91. Ghaly M, Teplitz D. The biologic effects of grounding the human body during sleep as measured by cortisol levels and subjective reporting of sleep, pain, and stress. *J Altern Complement Med* 2004; 10(5):767–776.
92. Chevalier G, Sinatra ST, Oschman JL, Delany RM. Earthing (grounding) the human body reduces blood viscosity-a major factor in cardiovascular disease. *J Altern Complement Med* 2013;19(2):102–110.

93. Chevalier G, Sinatra ST, Oschman JL, Sokal K, Sokal P. Earthing: Health implications of reconnecting the human body to the Earth's surface electrons. *J Environ Public Health* 2012;2012:291541.
94. Alavanja MCR. Pesticides use and exposure extensive worldwide. *Rev Environ Health* 2009;24(4):303–309.
95. Jandacek RJ, Tso P. Factors affecting the storage and excretion of toxic lipophilic xenobiotics. *Lipids* 2001;36(12):1289–305.
96. Bose-O'Reilly S, McCarty K, Steckling N, Lettmeier B. Mercury exposure and children's health. *Curr Probl Pediatr Adolesc Health Care* 2010;40(8):186–215.
97. Goncharov A, Bloom M, Pavuk M, Birman I, Carpenter DO. Blood pressure and hypertension in relation to levels of serum polychlorinated biphenyls in residents of Anniston, Alabama. *J Hypertens* 2010;28(10)2053–60.
98. Goncharov A, Pavuk M, Foushee HR, Carpenter DO. Blood pressure in relation to concentrations of PCB congeners and chlorinated pesticides. *Environ Health Perspect* 2011;119(3):319–325.
99. Rahman M, Tondel M, Ahmad SA, Chowdhury IA, Faruquee MH, Axelson O. Hypertension and arsenic exposure in Bangladesh. *Hypertension* 1999;33(1):74–78.
100. Hennig B, Meerarani P, Slim R et al. Proinflammatory properties of coplanar PCB's: In vitro and in vivo evidence. *Toxicol Appl Pharmacol* 2002;181(3):174–183.
101. La Merrill M, Cirillo PM, Terry MB, Krigbaum NY, Flom JD, Cohn BA. Prenatal exposure to the pesticide DDT and hypertension diagnosed in women before age 50: A longitudinal birth cohort study. *Environ Health Perspect* 2013;121(5):594–599.
102. Woodruff TJ, Zota AR, Schwartz JM. Environmental chemicals in pregnant women in the United States: NHANES 2003-2004. *Environ Health Perspect* 2011;119(6):878–885. 10.1289/ehp.1002727.
103. EPA. Basic Information: Polychlorinated Bisphenyl (PCB). http://www.epa.gov/wastes/hazard/tsd/pcbs/about.htm (accessed September 15, 1013)
104. Everett CJ, Mainous AG 3rd, Frithsen IL, Player MS, Matheson EM. Association of polychlorinated biphenyls with hypertension in the 1999–2002 National Health and Nutrition Examination Survey. *Environ Res* 2008;108(1):94–97.
105. Trasande L, Sathyanarayana S, Spanier AJ, Tractman H, Attina TM, Urbina EM. Urinary phthalates are associated with higher blood pressure in childhood. *J Pediatr* 2013;163(3):747–753.e.1.
106. Shankar A, Xiao J, Ducatman A. Perfluoroalky chemicals and elevated serum uric acid in US adults. *Clin Epidemiol* 2011;3:251–258.
107. Min JY, Lee KJ, Park JB, Min KB. Perfluorooctanoic acid exposure is associated with elevated homocysteine and hypertension in US adults. *Occup Environ Med* 2012;69(9):658–662. 10.1136/oemed-2011-100288.
108. Franchini M, Mannucci PM. Thrombogenicity and cardiovascular effects of ambient air pollution. *Blood* 2011;118(9):2405–2412.
109. Dyonch JT, Kannan S, Schultz AJ et al. Acute effects of ambient particulate matter on blood pressure: Differential effects across urban communities. *Hypertension* 2009;53(5):853–859.
110. Brook RD, Rajagopalan S, Pope CA 3rd et al. Particulate matter air pollution and cardiovascular disease: An update to the scientific statement from the American Heart Association. *Circulation* 2010;121(21):2331–2378.
111. Bhatnangar A. Environmental cardiology: Studying mechanistic links between pollution and heart disease. *Circ Res* 2006;99:692–705.
112. Taylor A. Cardiovascular effects of environmental chemicals. *Otolaryngol Head Neck Surg* 1996;114(2):209–211.
113. Rogers, Sherry. *Detoxify or Die*. Sarasota, FL: Sand Key Company; 2002.
114. Crinnion W. Sauna as a valuable clinical tool for cardiovascular, autoimmune, toxicant-induced and other chronic health problems. *Altern Med Rev* 2011;16(3):215–225.
115. Hannuksela M, Samer E. Benefits and risks of sauna bathing. *Am J Med* 2001;110(2):118–126.
116. Crinnion W Components of practical clinical detox programs—sauna as a therapeutic tool. *Altern Ther Health Med* 2007;13(2):S154–S156.
117. Tracy BL, Hart CE. Bikram yoga training and physical fitness in healthy young adults. *J Strength Cond Res* 2013;27(3):822–830.
118. Hunter SD, Dhindsa MS, Cunningham E, Tarumi T, Alkatan M, Nualnim N, Tanaka H. The effect of Bikram yoga on arterial stiffness in young and older adults. *J Altern Complement Med* 2013; 19(12):930–4.
119. Worthington V. Nutritional quality of organic versus conventional fruits, vegetables, and grains. *J Altern Complement Med* 2001;7(2):161–173.

120. King DE, Mainous AG 3rd, Labourne CA. Trends in dietary fiber intake in the United States, 1999–2008. *J Acad Nutr Diet* 2012;112(5):642–648.

121. Lu C, Toepel K, Irish R, Fenske RA, Barr DB, Bravo R. Organic diets significantly lower children's dietary exposure to organophosphorus pesticides. *Environ Health Perspect* 2006;114(2):260–263.

122. Abdollahi M, Ranjbar A, Shadnia S, Nikfar S, Rezaie A. Pesticides and oxidative stress: A review. *Med Sci Monit* 2004;10(6):RA141–RA147.

123. Gordon CJ, Padnos BK. Prolonged elevation in blood pressure in the unrestrained rat exposed to chlorpyrifos. *Toxicology* 2000;146(1):1–13.

124. McGarey, William. *Oil That Heals: A Physician's Successes with Castor Oil Applications.* Virginia Beach, VA: A.R.E. Press; 2002.

125. Grady H. Immunomodulation through castor oil packs. *J Naturopathic Med* 1999;7(1):84–89.

126. Arslan GG, Eser I. An examination of the effect of castor oil packs on constipation in the elderly. *Complement Ther Clin Pract* 2011;17(1):58–62.

127. Vieira C, Fetzer S, Sauer SK et al. Pro- and anti-inflammatory actions of ricinoleic acid: Similarities and differences with capsaicin. *Naunyn Schmiedebergs Arch Phamacol* 2001;364(2):87–95.

128. Nasermoaddeli A, Kagamimori S. Balneotherapy in medicine: A review. *Environ Health Prev Med* 2005;10(4):171–9.

129. Routh HG, Bhowmik KR, Parish LC, Witkowski JA. Balneology, mineral water, and spas in historical perspective. *Clin Dermatol* 1996;14(6):551–4.

130. Falagas ME, Zarkadoulia E, Rafailidis PL. The therapeutic effect of balneotherapy: Evaluation of the evidence from randomised controlled trials. *Int J Clin Pract* 2009;63(7):1068–84.

131. Jansky L, Pospisilova D, Honzova S et al. Immune system of cold-exposed and cold-adapted humans. *Eur J Appl Physiol Occup Physiol* 1996;72(5–6):445–450.

132. Brenner IK, Castellani JW, Gabaree C et al. Immune changes in humans during cold exposure: Effects of prior heating and exercise. *J Appl Physiol (1985)* 1998;87(2):699–710.

133. Crofton K. *A Wellness Guide for the Digital Age.* 2014. Victoria, BC, Canada: Global Well Being Books; 2014.

134. Khurana VG, Hardell L, Everaet J, Bortkiewicz A, Carlberg M, Ahonen M. Epidemiological evidence for a health risk from mobile phone base stations. *Int J Occup Environ Health* 2010;16(3):263–267.

135. Naviroglu M, Cig B, Dogan S, Uguz AC, Dilek S, Faouzi D. 2.45-Gz wireless devices induce oxidative stress and proliferation through cytosolic Ca^{2+} influx in human leukemia cancer cells. *Int J Radiat Biol* 2012;88(6):449–456.

136. Crofton K. *Radiation Rescue.* Victoria, BC, Canada: Global Well Being Books; 2010.

137. Avendano C, Mata A, Sanchez Sarmiento CA, Doncel GF. Use of laptop computers connected to internet through Wi-Fi decreases human sperm motility and increases sperm DNA fragmentation. *Fertil Steril* 2012;97(1):39–45.

138. Atasoy HI, Gunal MY, Atasoy P, Elgun S, Bugdayci G. Immunohistopathologic demonstration of deleterious effects on growing rat testes of radiofrequency waves emitted from conventional Wi-Fi devices. *J Pediatr Urol* 2013;9(2):223–229.

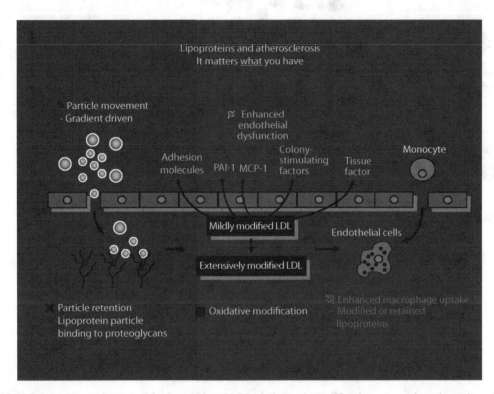

FIGURE 5.1 The various steps in the uptake of LDL cholesterol, modification, macrophage ingestion with scavenger receptors, foam cell formation, oxidative stress, inflammation, and autoimmune cytokines and chemokine production.

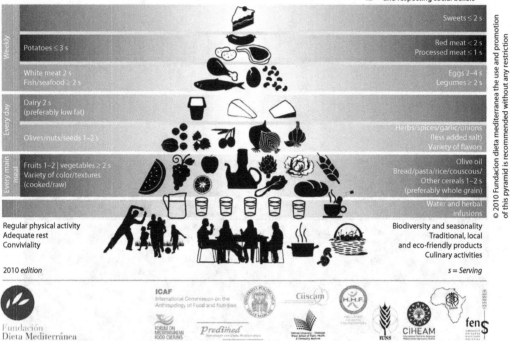

FIGURE 6.1 The Mediterranean diet pyramid.

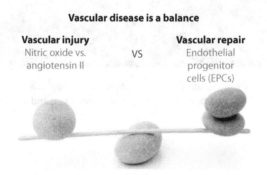

Vascular disease is a balance

Vascular injury		**Vascular repair**
Nitric oxide vs. angiotensin II	VS	Endothelial progenitor cells (EPCs)

FIGURE 9.1 Vascular health is a balance of injury and repair.

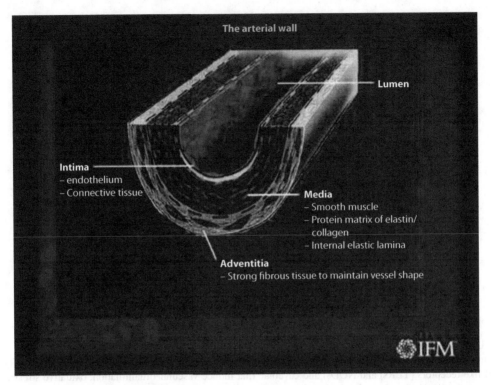

FIGURE 9.2 The blood vessel structure. (Modified from Ross, R, *N Eng J Med*, 340, 115–126, 1999; Mulvany, MJ, *Physiol Rev*, 70, 921–961, 1990.)

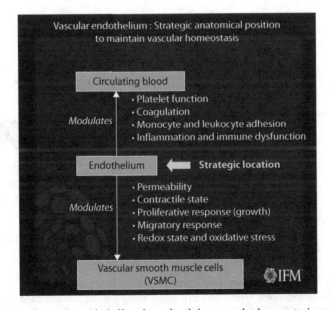

FIGURE 9.3 The role of vascular endothelium in maintaining vascular homeostasis and health.

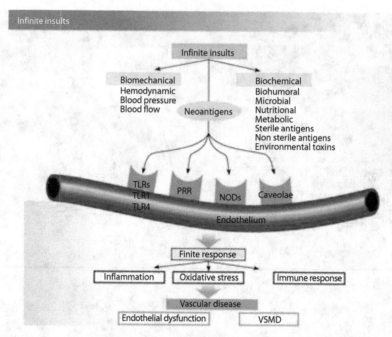

FIGURE 9.4 Infinite insults with three finite vascular responses.
Biomechanical insults such as hypertension result in stimulation of pattern recognition receptors (PRRs) (toll-like receptors [TLRs] and NODs) and caveolae that induce vascular inflammation, oxidative stress and immune dysfunction, endothelial dysfunction, and vascular and cardiac smooth muscle dysfunction.

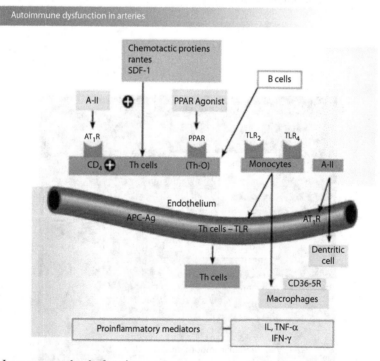

FIGURE 9.5 Immune vascular dysfunction.
Stimulation of angiotensin receptor type 1 (ATR1), peroxisome proliferator-activated receptor (PPAR), and toll-like receptor (TLR), and direct stimulation of T cells on the endothelium and vascular smooth muscle lead to immune dysfunction, inflammation, and oxidative stress.

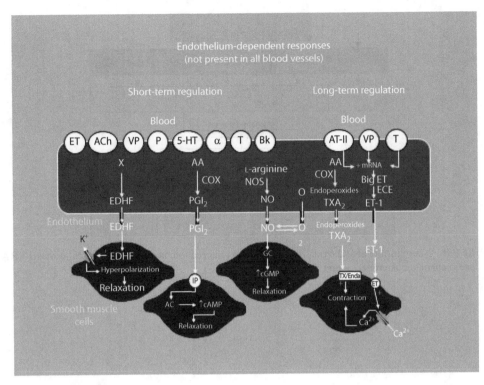

FIGURE 9.6 Stimulation of angiotensin receptor type 1 increases the production of superoxide anion, which neutralizes NO and also forms additional downstream radical oxygen species (ROSs) and radical nitrogen species (RNSs) that increase vascular oxidative stress.

The cytotoxic reactive oxygen species and the natural defense mechanisms

Reactive oxygen species		Antioxidant defense mechanisms	
Free radicals		*Enzymatic scavengers*	
$O_2 \bullet$	Superoxide anion radical	SOD	Superoxide dismutase
OH $\bullet$	Hydroxyl radical		$2O_2 \bullet^- + 2H^+ \rightarrow H_2O_2 + O_2$
ROO $\bullet$	Lipid peroxide (peroxyl)	CAT	Catalase (peroxisomal-bound)
RO $\bullet$	Alkoxyl		$2H_2O_2 \rightarrow O_2 + H_2O$
RS $\bullet$	Thiyl	GTP	Glutathione peroxidase
NO $\bullet$	Nitric oxide		$2GSH + H_2O_2 \rightarrow GSSG + 2H_2O$
$NO_2 \bullet$	Nitrogen dioxide		$2GSH + ROOH \rightarrow GSSG + ROH + 2H_2O$
$ONOO^-$	Peroxynitrite		
$CCl_3 \bullet$	Trichloromethyl	*Nonenzymatic scavengers*	
		Vitamin A	
Non-radicals		Vitamin C (ascorbic acid)	
H_2O_2	Hydrogen peroxide	Vitamin E (α-tocopherol)	
HOCl	Hypochlorous acid	β-carotene	
$ONOO^-$	Peroxynitrite	Cysteine	
$^1O_2$	Singlet oxygen	Coenzyme Q	
		Uric acid	
		Flavonoids	
		Sulfhydryl group	
		Thioether compounds	

The superscripted bold dot indicates an unpaired electron and the negative charge indicates a gained electron. GSH, reduced glutathione; GSSG, oxidized glutathione; R, lipid chain. Singlet oxygen is an unstable molecule due to the two electrons present in its outer orbit spinning in opposite directions.

FIGURE 9.7 Oxidative Stress Induces ED, Vascular Disease, and Hypertension. Note: Host-protective factors include enzymatic and nonenzymatic defenses influenced by diet and nutrients.

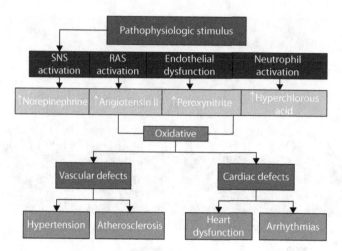

FIGURE 9.8 Neurohormonal and oxidative stress system interaction on cardiac and vascular muscle. RAS, renin angiotensin (aldosterone) system.

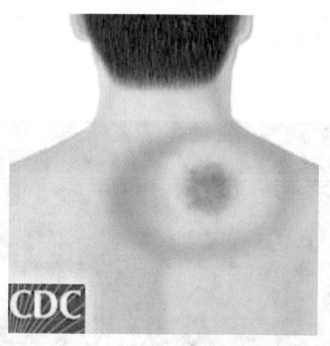

FIGURE 11.1 Typical erythema migrans (EM) rash of Lyme borreliosis. (Courtesy of Centers for Disease Control and Prevention website.)

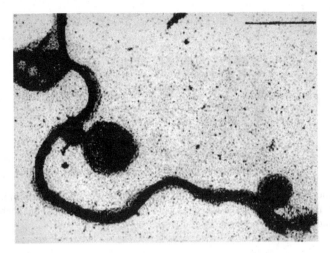

FIGURE 11.2 *Borrelia* spirochete–forming granules soon after antibiotic exposure. (From Kersten A et al., *Antimicrob Agents Chemother*, 39, 5, 1127–1133, 1995. With permission.)

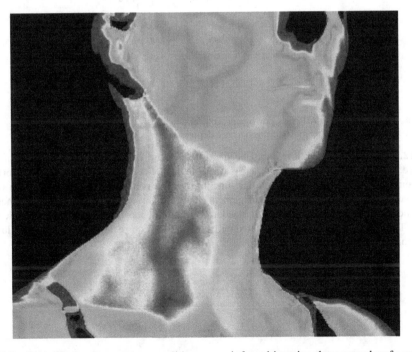

FIGURE 11.3 Probable jugular venous vasculitis seen on infrared-imaging thermography of a woman with borreliosis and chronic headaches. (Courtesy of D. Hickey, unpublished data. With permission.)

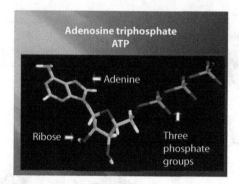

FIGURE 12.1 Adenosine triphosphate (ATP) is composed of D-ribose, adenine, and three phosphate groups. Breaking the chemical bond attaching the last phosphate group to ATP releases the chemical energy that is converted to mechanical energy to perform cellular work.

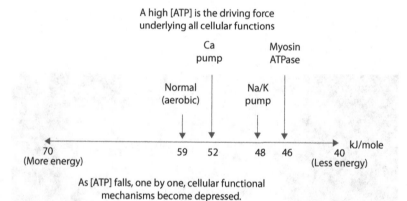

FIGURE 12.5 Cellular energy levels can be measured as the free energy of hydrolysis of adenosine triphosphate, or the amount of chemical energy available to fuel cellular function. Healthy, normal hearts contain enough energy to fuel all the cellular functions with a contractile reserve for use in emergency. Cellular mechanisms used in calcium management and cardiac relaxation require the highest level of available energy. Sodium/potassium pumps needed to maintain ion balance are also significant energy consumers. The cellular mechanisms associated with contraction require the least amount of cellular energy. (Adapted from several sources.)

9 Nutrition and Nutraceutical Supplements for the Treatment of Hypertension

Mark Houston

CONTENTS

INTRODUCTION

Vascular disease is a balance between vascular injury and repair (Figure 9.1). The endothelium is in a strategic location between the blood and the vascular smooth muscle and secretes various substances to maintain vascular homeostasis and health (Figures 9.2 and 9.3). Various insults that

Vascular disease is a balance

Vascular injury		**Vascular repair**
Nitric oxide vs. angiotensin II	VS	Endothelial progenitor cells (EPCs)

FIGURE 9.1   **(See color insert.)** Vascular health is a balance of injury and repair.

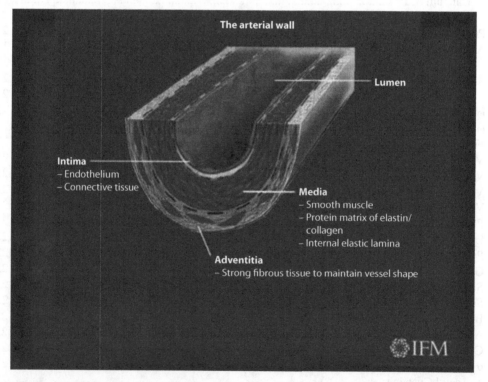

FIGURE 9.2   **(See color insert.)** The blood vessel structure. (Modified from Ross, R, *N Eng J Med*, 340, 115–126, 1999; Mulvany, MJ, *Physiol Rev*, 70, 921–961, 1990.)

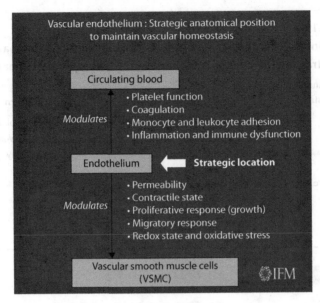

FIGURE 9.3 **(See color insert.)** The role of vascular endothelium in maintaining vascular homeostasis and health.

damage the endothelium lead to endothelial dysfunction (ED) and may induce hypertension and other cardiovascular diseases (CVDs). Hypertension may be a hemodynamic marker of injured endothelium and vascular smooth muscle related to finite responses of inflammation, oxidative stress and immune dysfunction of the arteries leading to ED, vascular and cardiac smooth muscle dysfunction, loss of arterial elasticity with reduced arterial compliance, and increased systemic vascular resistance. Hypertension is a consequence of the interaction of genetics and environment. Macronutrients and micronutrients are crucial in the regulation of blood pressure (BP) and subsequent target organ damage (TOD). Nutrient–gene interactions, subsequent gene expression, epigenetics, oxidative stress, inflammation, and autoimmune vascular dysfunction have positive or negative influences on vascular biology in humans. Endothelial activation with ED and vascular smooth muscle dysfunction (VSMD) initiate and perpetuate essential hypertension.

In my opinion, macronutrient and micronutrient deficiencies are very common in the general population and may be even more common in patients with hypertension and CVD due to genetics, environmental causes, and prescription drug use. These deficiencies will have an enormous impact on present and future cardiovascular health outcomes such as hypertension, myocardial infarction (MI), stroke, and renal disease. The diagnosis and treatment of these nutrient deficiencies will reduce BP and improve vascular health, ED, vascular biology, and cardiovascular events.

EPIDEMIOLOGY

Epidemiology underscores the etiologic role of diet and associated nutrient intake in hypertension. The transition from Paleolithic diet to our modern diet of high sugar and carbohydrate foods has produced an epidemic of nutritionally related diseases (Table 9.1). Hypertension, atherosclerosis, coronary heart disease (CHD), MI, congestive heart failure (CHF), cerebrovascular accidents (CVAs), renal disease, type 2 diabetes mellitus (T2DM), metabolic syndrome (MS), and obesity are some of these diseases.[1,2] Table 9.1 contrasts intake of nutrients involved in BP regulation during the Paleolithic era and modern times. Evolution from a preagricultural, hunter–gatherer milieu to an agricultural, refrigeration society has imposed an unnatural and unhealthful nutritional selection process. In my opinion, diet has changed more than our genetics can adapt.

TABLE 9.1

Dietary Intake of Nutrients Involved in Vascular Biology: Comparing and Contrasting the Diet of Paleolithic and Contemporary Humans

Nutrients and Dietary Characteristics	Paleolithic Intake	Modern Intake
Sodium	<50 mmol/day (1.2 g)	175 mmol/day (4 g)
Potassium	>10,000 mEq/day (256 g)	150 mEq/day (6 g)
Sodium/potassium ratio	<0.13/day	>0.67/day
Protein	37%	20%
Carbohydrate	41%	40%–50%
Fat	22%	30%–40%
P/S fat ratio	1.4	0.4
Fiber	>100 g/day	9 g/day

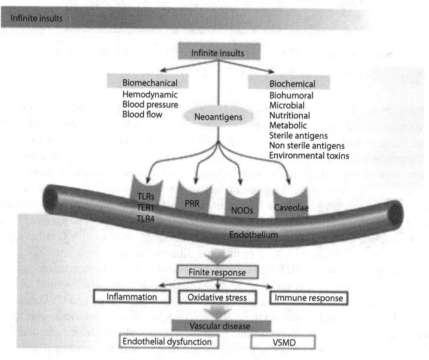

FIGURE 9.4 **(See color insert.)** Infinite insults with three finite vascular responses. Biomechanical insults such as hypertension result in stimulation of pattern recognition receptors (PRRs) (toll-like receptors [TLRs] and nucleotide-binding oligomerization domain receptors [NODs]) and caveolae that induce vascular inflammation, oxidative stress and immune dysfunction, endothelial dysfunction, and vascular and cardiac smooth muscle dysfunction.

The human genetic makeup is 99.9% that of our Paleolithic ancestors, yet our nutritional, vitamin, and mineral intakes are vastly different.[3] The macronutrient and micronutrient variations; oxidative stress from radical oxygen species (ROS) and radical nitrogen species (RNS); and inflammatory mediators such as cell adhesion molecules (CAMs), cytokines, signaling molecules, and autoimmune vascular dysfunction of T cells and B cells contribute to the higher incidence of hypertension and other CVDs through complex nutrient–gene interactions, epigenetic and nutrient–caveolae interactions and nutrient reactions with pattern recognition receptors (PRRs) (toll-like receptors [TLRs] and nod-like receptors [NLRs]) in the endothelium[4–9] (Figure 9.4). A reduction in nitric oxide bioavailability and an increase in angiotensin II (A-II) and endothelin coupled with endothelial activation initiate vascular and cardiac dysfunction and hypertension. Poor nutrition, coupled with obesity and a sedentary lifestyle, has resulted in an exponential increase in nutritionally related diseases. In particular, the high Na^+/K^+ ratio of modern diets has contributed to hypertension, CVAs, CHD, MI, CHF, and renal disease,[3,10] as have the relatively low intake of ω-3 polyunsaturated fatty acids (PUFAs), increase in ω-6 PUFAs, saturated fat, and trans fatty acids.[11]

PATHOPHYSIOLOGY

Vascular biology assumes a pivotal role in the initiation and perpetuation of hypertension and cardiovascular TOD.[1] Oxidative stress (ROS and RNS), inflammation (increased expression of redox-sensitive proinflammatory genes, CAMs, and recruitment migration and infiltration of circulating cells), and autoimmune vascular dysfunction (T cells and B cells) are the primary pathophysiologic and functional mechanisms that induce vascular disease[1,12–14] (Figure 9.5). All three of these are closely interrelated and establish a deadly combination that leads to ED, vascular smooth muscle and cardiac dysfunction, hypertension, vascular disease, atherosclerosis, and CVD. Hypertension is not a disease but the correct and chronically dysregulated response with an exaggerated outcome of the infinite insults to the blood vessel with subsequent environmental–genetic expression patterns and downstream disturbances in which the vascular system is the innocent bystander. This becomes a maladaptive vascular response that was initially intended to provide vascular defense to

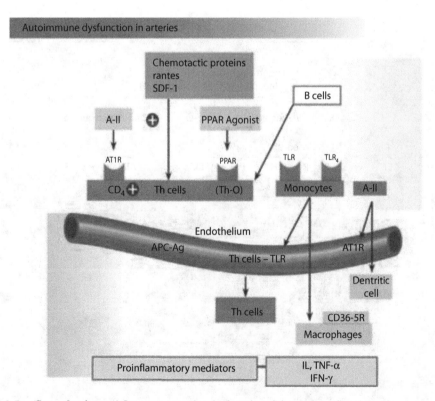

FIGURE 9.5 (**See color insert.**) Immune vascular dysfunction. Stimulation of angiotensin receptor type 1 (ATR1), peroxisome proliferator-activated receptor (PPAR), and toll-like receptor (TLR), and direct stimulation of T cells on the endothelium and vascular smooth muscle lead to immune dysfunction, inflammation, and oxidative stress.

the endothelial insults.[1,13–15] Hypertension is a vasculopathy characterized by ED, structural remodeling, vascular inflammation, increased arterial stiffness, reduced distensibility, and loss of elasticity.[13] These insults are biomechanical (BP, pulse pressure, blood flow, oscillatory flow, turbulence, augmentation, pulse wave velocity, and reflected waves) and biohumoral or biochemical, which includes all the nonmechanical causes such as metabolic, endocrine, nutritional, toxic, infectious, and other etiologies[1] (Figure 9.6). In addition to the very well-established connections for endocrine and nutritional causes of hypertension, toxins and infections also increase BP.[16–20] Various toxins such as polychlorinated biphenyls (PCBs), mercury, lead, cadmium, arsenic, and iron also increase BP and CVD.[16,17] Numerous microbial organisms have been implicated in hypertension and CHD.[18–20] All of these insults lead to impaired microvascular structure and function, which manifests clinically as hypertension.[12–14] The level of BP may not give an accurate indication of the microvascular involvement and impairment in hypertension. Hypertensive patients have abnormal microvasculature in the form of inward eutrophic remodeling of the small resistance arteries leading to impaired vasodilatory capacity, increased vascular resistance, increased media to lumen ratio, decreased maximal organ perfusion, and reduced flow reserve, especially in the heart with decreased coronary flow reserve (CFR).[12–14] Significant functional and structural microvascular impairment occurs even before the BP begins to rise in normotensive offspring of hypertensive parents evidenced by ED, impaired vasodilation, forearm vascular resistance, diastolic dysfunction, increased left ventricular mass index, increased septal and posterior wall thickness, and left ventricular hypertrophy.[12,15] Thus, the cellular processes underlying the vascular perturbations constitute a vascular phenotype of hypertension that may be determined by early life programming and imprinting, which is compounded by vascular aging.[12–14]

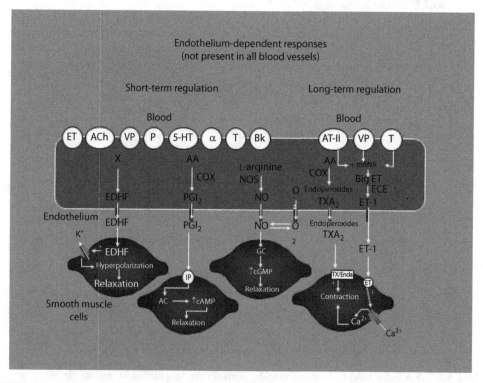

FIGURE 9.6 **(See color insert.)** Stimulation of angiotensin receptor type 1 increases the production of superoxide anion, which neutralizes NO and also forms additional downstream radical oxygen species (ROSs) and radical nitrogen species (RNSs) that increase vascular oxidative stress.

Oxidative Stress

Oxidative stress, with an imbalance between ROS and RNS and the antioxidant defense mechanisms, contributes to the etiology of hypertension in animals[21] and humans.[22,23] ROSs and RNSs are generated by multiple cellular sources, including NADPH oxidase, mitochondria, xanthine oxidase, uncoupled endothelium-derived NO synthase (U-eNOS), cyclo-oxygenase, and lipo-oxygenase.[22] Superoxide anion is the predominant ROS produced by these tissues, which neutralizes NO and also leads to downstream production of other ROSs (Figure 9.3). Hypertensive patients have impaired endogenous and exogenous antioxidant defense mechanisms,[24] an increased plasma oxidative stress, and an exaggerated oxidative stress response to various stimuli.[24,25] Hypertensive subjects also have lower ferric reducing ability of plasma (FRAP), lower vitamin C levels, and increased plasma 8-isoprostanes correlate with both an increase in systolic blood pressure (SBP) and diastolic blood pressure (DBP). Various single-nucleotide polymorphisms (SNPs) in genes that codify for antioxidant enzymes are directly related to hypertension.[26] These include NADPH oxidase, xanthine oxidase, superoxide dismutase (SOD) 3, catalase, GPx 1 (glutathione peroxidase), and thioredoxin. Antioxidant deficiency and excess free radical production have been implicated in human hypertension in numerous epidemiologic, observational, and interventional studies[24,25,27] (Figure 9.7). ROSs directly damage endothelial cells; degrade NO; influence eicosanoid metabolism; oxidize low-density lipoprotein (LDL), lipids, proteins, carbohydrates, DNA, and organic molecules; increase catecholamines; damage the genetic machinery; and influence gene expression and transcription factors.[1,22–25] The interrelations of neurohormonal systems, oxidative stress, and CVD are shown in Figure 9.8. The increased oxidative stress, inflammation, and autoimmune vascular dysfunction in human hypertension result from a combination of increased generation of ROSs and RNSs, an exacerbated response to ROSs and RNSs, and a decreased antioxidant reserve.[24–29] Increased oxidative stress in the rostral ventrolateral medulla (RVLM) enhances glutamatergic excitatory inputs and attenuates γ-aminobutyric acid (GABA)-ergic inhibitory inputs to the RVLM, which contributes to increased sympathetic nervous system (SNS) activity from the paraventricular nucleus.[30] Activation of AT1R in the RVLM increases NADPH oxidase and increases oxidative stress and superoxide

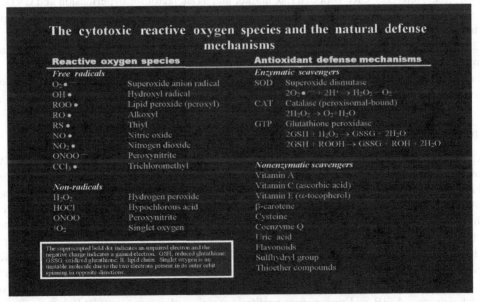

FIGURE 9.7 **(See color insert.)** Oxidative stress induces ED, vascular disease, and hypertension. Note: Host-protective factors include enzymatic and nonenzymatic defenses influenced by diet and nutrients.

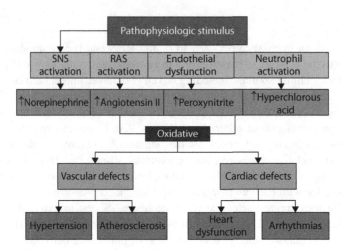

FIGURE 9.8   (**See color insert.**) Neurohormonal and oxidative stress system interaction on cardiac and vascular muscle. RAS, renin angiotensin (aldosterone) system.

anion and increases SNS outflow causing an imbalance of SNS/parasympathetic nervous system (PNS) activity with elevation of BP, increased heart rate, and alterations in heart rate variability and heart rate recovery time, which can be blocked by AT1R blockers.[30,31]

INFLAMMATION

The link between inflammation and hypertension has been suggested in both cross-sectional and longitudinal studies.[32] Increases in high-sensitivity C-reactive protein (HS-CRP) as well as other inflammatory cytokines such as interleukin 1B (IL-1B), interleukin 6 (IL-6), tumor necrosis factor-α (TNF-α), and chronic leukocytosis occur in hypertension and hypertension-related TOD, such as increased carotid intimal medial thickness.[33] HS-CRP predicts future cardiovascular events.[32,33] Elevated HS-CRP is both a risk marker and a risk factor for hypertension and CVD.[34,35] Increases in HS-CRP of over 3 μg/mL may increase BP in just a few days, which is directly proportional to the increase in HS-CRP.[34,35] Nitric oxide and eNOS are inhibited by HS-CRP.[34,35] AT2R, which normally counterbalances AT1R, is downregulated by HS-CRP.[34,35] A-II upregulates many of the cytokines, especially IL-6, CAMs, and chemokines, by activating nuclear factor κB (NFκB) leading to vasoconstriction. These events, along with the increases in oxidative stress and endothelin-1, elevate BP.[32]

AUTOIMMUNE DYSFUNCTION

Innate and adaptive immune responses are linked to hypertension and hypertension-induced CVD through at least three mechanisms: cytokine production, central nervous system (CNS) stimulation, and renal damage. This includes salt-sensitive hypertension with increased renal inflammation as a result of T cell imbalance, dysregulation of CD4 and CD8 lymphocytes, and chronic leukocytosis with increased neutrophils and reduced lymphocytes.[36–38] Leukocytosis, especially increased neutrophils and decreased lymphocyte count, increases BP in blacks by 6/2 mmHg in the highest versus the lowest tertile.[38] Macrophages and various T-cell subtypes regulate BP, invade the arterial wall, activate TLRs, and induce autoimmune vascular damage.[38,39] A-II activates immune cells (T cells, macrophages, and dendritic cells) and promotes cell infiltration into target organs.[39] CD4 + T lymphocytes express AT1R and peroxisome proliferator-activated receptor-γ (PPARγ) receptors and release TNF-α, interferons, and interleukins within the vascular wall when activated[39] (Figure 9.5). Interleukin 17 (IL-17) produced by T cells may play a pivotal role in the genesis of hypertension caused by A-II.[39] Hypertensive patients have significantly higher TLR 4 mRNA in monocytes compared to normals.[40] Intensive reduction in BP to SBP less than 130 mmHg versus SBP to only 140 mmHg lowers the TLR 4 more.[40] A-II activates the TLR expression leading to inflammation and activation of the innate immune system. When TLR 4 is activated, there is downstream macrophage activation and migration and increase in metalloproteinase 9 (MMP 9), vascular remodeling, collagen accumulation in the artery, left ventricular hypertrophy (LVH), and cardiac fibrosis.[40] The autonomic nervous system is critical in either increasing or decreasing immune dysfunction and inflammation.[41] Efferent cholinergic anti-inflammatory pathways via the vagal nerve innervate the spleen, nicotine acetylcholine receptor subunits, and cytokine-producing immune cells to influence vasoconstriction and BP.[41] Local CNS inflammation or ischemia may mediate vascular inflammation and hypertension.[39]

Aldosterone is associated with increased adaptive immunity and autoimmune responses with CD4+T cell activation and Th 17 polarization with increased IL-17, transforming growth factor (TGF)-β, and TNF-α, which modulate over 30 inflammatory genes.[42,43] Increased serum aldosterone is an independent risk factor for CVD and CHD through nonhemodynamic effects as well as through increased BP.[42,43] Blockade of mineralocorticoid receptors in the heart, brain, blood vessels, and immune cells reduces cardiovascular risk even with the persistence of hypertension.[42,43]

TREATMENT

Many of the natural compounds in food, certain nutraceutical supplements, vitamins, antioxidants, or minerals function in a similar fashion to a specific class of antihypertensive drugs. Although the potency of these natural compounds may be less than that of the antihypertensive drugs, when used in combination with other nutrients and nutraceutical supplements, the antihypertensive effect is additive or synergistic. Table 9.2 summarizes these natural compounds into the major antihypertensive drug classes such as diuretics, β-blockers, central α agonists, direct vasodilators, calcium channel blockers (CCBs), angiotensin-converting enzyme inhibitors (ACEIs), angiotensin receptor blockers (ARBs), and direct renin inhibitors (DRIs).

DASH DIETS

The Dietary Approaches to Stop Hypertension (DASH) I and II diets conclusively demonstrated significant reductions in BP in borderline and stage I hypertensive patients.[44,45] In DASH I, untreated hypertensive subjects with SBP < 160 mmHg and DBP = 80–95 mmHg were placed on one of three diets for 4 weeks, control diet, fruit and vegetable diet (F+V), and combined diet that added F+V and low-fat dairy.[44] DASH II added progressive sodium restriction in each group.[45] The control diet consisted of sodium at 3 g/day; potassium, magnesium, and calcium at 25% of the U.S. average; macronutrients at the U.S. average of 4 servings per day; a sodium to potassium ratio of 1.7; and fiber at 9 g/day. The F+V diet increased the potassium, magnesium, and calcium to 75%; macronutrients to greater than the U.S. average; a sodium to potassium ratio of 0.7; 31 g of fiber; and 8.5 servings of fruits and vegetables per day. The combined diet was similar to the F+V diet but added low-fat dairy. At 2 weeks, the BP was decreased by 10.7/5.2 mmHg in the hypertensive patients in DASH I and by 11.5/6.8 mmHg in the hypertensive patients in DASH II. These reductions persisted as long as the patients were on the diet. The DASH diet increases plasma renin activity (PRA) and serum aldosterone levels in response to the BP reductions.[46,47] The mean increase in PRA was 0.37 ng·mL/h.[47] The A allele of G46A had a greater BP reduction and blunted PRA and aldosterone. The AA genotype had the best response, and the GG genotype had no response. Adding an ARB, an ACEI, or a DRI improved BP response to the DASH diet in the GG group due to blockade of the increase in PRA. A low-sodium DASH diet decreases oxidative stress (urine F2-isoprostanes), improves vascular function (augmentation index), and lowers BP in salt-sensitive subjects.[48] In addition, plasma nitrite increased and pulse wave velocity decreased at week 2 on the DASH diet.[49]

TABLE 9.2
Natural Antihypertensive Compounds Categorized by Antihypertensive Class

Antihypertensive Therapeutic Class (Alphabetical Listing)	Foods and Ingredients Listed by Therapeutic Class	Nutrients and Other Supplements Listed by Therapeutic Class
ACEIs	Egg yolk	Melatonin
	Fish (specific):	ω-3 Fatty acids
	Bonito	Pomegranate
	Dried salted fish	Pycnogenol
	Fish sauce	Zinc
	Sardine muscle/protein	
	Tuna	
	Garlic	
	Gelatin	
	Hawthorn berry	
	Milk products (specific):	
	Casein	
	Sour milk	
	Whey (hydrolyzed)	
	Sake	
	Sea vegetables (kelp)	
	Seaweed (wakame)	
	Wheat germ (hydrolyzed)	
	Zein (corn protein)	
ARBs	Celery	Coenzyme Q10
	Fiber	GLA
	Garlic	NAC
	MUFA	Oleic acid
		Resveratrol
		Potassium
		Taurine
		Vitamin C
		Vitamin B6 (pyridoxine)
β-Blockers	Hawthorn berry	
CCBs	Celery	ALA
	Garlic	Calcium
	Hawthorn berry	Magnesium
	MUFA	NAC
		Oleic acid
		ω-3 Fatty acids:
		EPA
		DHA
		Taurine
		Vitamin B6
		Vitamin C
		Vitamin E
Central α-agonists (reduce SNS activity)	Celery	Coenzyme Q10
	Fiber	GLA
	Garlic	Potassium
	Protein	Restriction of sodium
		Taurine

TABLE 9.2 (*Continued*)
Natural Antihypertensive Compounds Categorized by Antihypertensive Class

Antihypertensive Therapeutic Class (Alphabetical Listing)	Foods and Ingredients Listed by Therapeutic Class	Nutrients and Other Supplements Listed by Therapeutic Class
		Vitamin C
		Vitamin B6
		Zinc
DRIs		Vitamin D
Direct vasodilators	Celery	ALA
	Cooking oils with	Arginine
	MUFAs	Calcium
	Fiber	Flavonoids
	Garlic	Magnesium
	MUFA	ω-3 Fatty acids
	Soy	Potassium
		Taurine
		Vitamin C
		Vitamin E
		Calcium
Diuretics	Celery	Coenzyme Q10
	Hawthorn berry	Fiber
	Protein	GLA
		L-carnitine
		Magnesium
		Potassium
		Taurine
		Vitamin B6
		Vitamin C
		Vitamin E: high γ-/δ-tocopherols and tocotrienols

Sodium (Na⁺) Reduction

The average sodium intake in the United States is 5,000 mg/day, with some areas of the country consuming 15,000–20,000 mg/day.[50] However, the minimal requirement for sodium is probably about 500 mg/day.[50] Epidemiological, observational, and controlled clinical trials demonstrate that an increased sodium intake is associated with higher BP as well as an increased risk for CVD, CVA, LVH, CHD, MI, renal insufficiency, proteinuria, and overactivity of the SNS.[1,50] A reduction in sodium intake in hypertensive patients, especially the salt-sensitive patients, will significantly lower BP by 4–6/2 to 3 mmHg that is proportional to the degree of sodium restriction and may prevent or delay hypertension in high-risk patients and reduce future cardiovascular events.[51–53]

Salt sensitivity (≥10% increase in mean arterial pressure (MAP) with salt loading) occurs in about 51% of hypertensive patients and is a key factor in determining the cardiovascular, cerebrovascular, renal, and BP responses to dietary salt intake.[54] Cardiovascular events are more common in the salt-sensitive patients than in the salt-resistant ones, independent of BP.[55] An increased sodium intake has a direct positive correlation with BP and the risk of CVA and CHD.[56] The risk is independent of BP for CVA with a relative risk of 1.04–1.25 from the lowest to the highest quartile.[56] In addition, patients will convert to a nondipping BP pattern with increases in nocturnal BP as the sodium intake increases.[56]

Increased sodium intake has a direct adverse effect on endothelial cells.[57–61] Sodium promotes cutaneous lymphangiogenesis; increases endothelial cell stiffness; reduces size, surface area, volume, cytoskeleton, deformability, and pliability; reduces eNOS and NO production; and increases asymmetric dimethyl arginine (ADMA), oxidative stress, and TGF-β. All of these abnormal vascular responses are increased in the presence of aldosterone.[57–61] These changes occur independent of BP and may be partially counteract by dietary potassium.[57–61] The endothelial cells act as vascular salt sensors.[62] Endothelial cells are targets for aldosterone, which activate epithelial sodium channels and have a negative effect on the release of NO and on endothelial function. The mechanical stiffness of the cell plasma membrane and the submembranous actin network (endothelial glycocalyx) ("shell") serve as a "firewall" to protect the endothelial cells and are regulated by serum sodium, potassium, and aldosterone within the physiological range.[62] Changes in shear stress–dependent activity of the endothelial NO synthase located in the caveolae regulate the viscosity in this shell.[62] High plasma sodium gelates the shell of the endothelial cell, whereas the shell is fluidized by high potassium. These communications between extracellular ions and intracellular enzymes occur at the plasma membrane barrier, whereas 90% of the total cell mass remains uninvolved in these changes. Blockade of the epithelial sodium channel (ENaC) with spironolactone (100%) or amiloride (84%) minimizes or stops many of these vascular endothelial responses and increases NO.[60,63] Nitric oxide release follows endothelial nanomechanics and not vice versa and membrane depolarization decreases vascular endothelial cell stiffness, which improves flow-mediated nitric oxide–dependent vasodilation.[64,65] In the presence of vascular inflammation and increased HS-CRP, the effects of aldosterone on ENaC is enhanced further increasing vascular stiffness and BP.[66] High sodium intake also abolishes the AT2R-mediated vasodilation immediately, with complete abolition of endothelial vasodilation within 30 days.[67] Thus, it is clear that increased dietary sodium has adverse effects on the vascular system, BP, and CVD by altering the endothelial glycocalyx, which is a negatively charged biopolymer that lines the blood vessels and serves as a protective barrier against sodium overload, increased sodium permeability, and sodium-induced TOD.[68] Certain SNPs of salt-inducible kinase I (SIK1) that alter Na^+/K^+ ATPase determine sodium-induced hypertension and LVH.[69]

The sodium intake per day in hypertensive patients should be between 1500 and 2000 mg. Sodium restriction improves BP reduction in those patients who are on pharmacological treatment, and the decrease in BP is additive with restriction of refined carbohydrates.[70,71] Reducing dietary sodium intake may reduce damage to the brain, heart, kidney, and vasculature through mechanisms dependent on the small BP reduction as well as those independent on the decreased BP.[72–74]

A balance of sodium with other nutrients, especially potassium, magnesium, and calcium, is important not only in reducing and controlling BP but also in decreasing cardiovascular and cerebrovascular events.[3,70,71] An increase in the sodium to potassium ratio is associated with a significantly increased risk of CVD and all-cause mortality.[72] The Yanomamo Indians consume and excrete only 1 mEq of sodium in 24 hours and consume and excrete 152 mEq of potassium in 24 hours.[75] The Na^+ to K^+ ratio is 1/152 and is associated with elevated PRA, but BP does not increase with age. At the age of 50 years, the average BP in the Yanomamo is 100–108/64–69 mmHg.[75]

Potassium

The average U.S. dietary intake of potassium (K^+) is 45 mmol/day with a potassium to sodium (K^+/Na^+) ratio of less than 1:2.[10,73] The recommended intake of K^+ is 4700 mg a day (120 mmol) with a K^+/Na^+ ratio of about 4 to 5 to 1.[10,73] Numerous epidemiological, observational, and clinical trials have demonstrated a significant reduction in BP with increased dietary K^+ intake in both normotensive and hypertensive patients.[10,73,76] The average BP reduction with a K^+ supplementation of 60–120 mmol/day is 4.4/2.5 mmHg in hypertensive patients but may be as much as 8/4.1 mmHg with 120 mmol/day (4700 mg).[10,73,76–78] In hypertensive patients, the linear dose–response relationship is 1.0 mmHg reduction in SBP and 0.52 mmHg reduction in DBP per 0.6 g/ day increase in dietary potassium intake, which is independent of baseline dietary potassium ingestion.[78] The response depends on race (black > white) and sodium, magnesium, and calcium intakes.[10] Those on a higher sodium intake have a greater reduction in BP with potassium.[10] Alteration of the K^+/Na^+ ratio to a higher level is important for both antihypertensive and cardiovascular and cerebrovascular effects.[77,78] High potassium intake reduces the incidence of cardiovascular accidents (CHD and MI) and CVAs independent of the BP reduction.[10,73,76–78] There are also reductions in CHF, LVH, diabetes mellitus (DM), and cardiac arrhythmias.[10,78] If the serum potassium is less than 4.0 mEq/dL, there is an increased risk of CVD mortality, ventricular tachycardia, ventricular fibrillation, and CHF.[10,78] Red blood cell potassium is a better indication of total body stores and CVD risk than serum potassium.[10] Gu et al.[77] found that potassium supplementation at 60 mmol of KCl per day for 12 weeks significantly reduced SBP, –5.0 mm Hg (range: –2.13 to –7.88 mmHg) ($p < .001$), in 150 Chinese men and women aged 35–64 years.

Potassium increases natriuresis, modulates baroreflex sensitivity, vasodilates, decreases the sensitivity to catecholamines and A-II, increases sodium potassium ATPase and DNA synthesis in vascular smooth muscle cells, and decreases SNS activity in cells with improved vascular function.[10,78] In addition, potassium increases bradykinin and urinary kallikrein; decreases NADPH oxidase, which lowers oxidative stress and inflammation; improves insulin sensitivity; decreases ADMA; reduces intracellular sodium; and lowers the production of TGF-β.[10,78]

Each 1000 mg increase in potassium intake per day reduces all-cause mortality by approximately 20%. Potassium intake of 4.7 g/day is estimated to decrease CVA by 8%–15% and MI by 6%–11%.[78] Numerous SNPs such as nuclear receptor subfamily 3 group C (NR3C2), angiotensin II type receptor (AGTR1), and hydroxysteroid 11 β-dehydrogenase (HSD11B1 and B2) determine an individual's response to dietary potassium intake.[79] Each 1000 mg decrease in sodium intake per day will decrease all-cause mortality by 20%.[72,78] A recent analysis suggested a dose-related response to CVA with urinary potassium excretion.[80] There was a relative risk reduction (RRR) of CVA of 23% at 1.5–1.99 g, 27% at 2.0–2.49 g, 29% at 2.5–3 g, and 32% over 3 g/day of potassium urinary excretion.[80] The recommended daily dietary intake for patients with hypertension is 4.7–5.0 g of potassium and less than 1500 mg of sodium.[10,78] Potassium in food or from supplementation should be reduced or used with caution in those patients with renal impairment or those on medications that increase renal potassium retention such as ACEI, ARB, DRI, and serum aldosterone receptor antagonists (SARAs).[10,78]

Magnesium (Mg^{++})

A high dietary intake of magnesium of at least 500–1000 mg/day reduces BP in most of the reported epidemiological, observational, and clinical trials, but the results are less consistent than those seen with Na^+ and K^+.[73,81] In most epidemiological studies, there is an inverse relationship between dietary magnesium intake and BP.[73,81,82] A study of 60 essential hypertensive subjects given magnesium supplements showed a significant reduction in BP over an 8-week period documented by 24-hour ambulatory BP, home and office blood BP.[73,81,82] The maximum reduction in clinical trials has been 5.6/2.8 mmHg, but some studies have shown no change in BP.[83] The combination of high potassium and low sodium intake with increased magnesium intake had additive antihypertensive effects.[83] Magnesium also increases the effectiveness of all antihypertensive drug classes.[83]

Magnesium competes with Na^+ for binding sites on vascular smooth muscle and acts as a direct vasodilator, like a CCB. Magnesium increases prostaglandin E (PGE); regulates intracellular calcium, sodium, potassium, and pH; increases nitric oxide; improves endothelial function; reduces oxLDL; and reduces HS-CRP, TBxA2, A-II, and norepinephrine. Magnesium also improves insulin resistance, glucose, and MS; binds in a necessary cooperative manner with potassium, inducing endothelial vasodilation (EVD) and BP reduction; reduces CVD and cardiac arrhythmias;

decreases carotid IMT; lowers cholesterol; lowers cytokine production; inhibits NFκB; reduces oxidative stress; and inhibits platelet aggregation to reduce thrombosis.[73,81–87]

Magnesium is an essential cofactor for the δ-6-desaturase enzyme that is the rate-limiting step for the conversion of linoleic acid (LA) to γ-linolenic acid (GLA)[73,81–86] needed for synthesis of the vasodilator and platelet inhibitor prostaglandin E_1 (PGE_1). Altered TRPM7 channels, which are the transporters for magnesium, occur in many hypertensive patients.[84]

A meta-analysis of 241,378 patients with 6,477 strokes showed an inverse relationship of dietary magnesium to the incidence of ischemic stroke.[85] For each 100 mg of dietary magnesium intake, ischemic stroke was decreased by 8%. The proposed mechanism include inhibition of ischemia-induced glutamate release, n-methyl-D-aspartate (NMDA) receptor blockade, CCB actions, mitochondrial calcium buffering, decrease in ATP depletion, and vasodilation of cerebral arteries.[85] A meta-analysis showed reductions in BP of 3–4 mmHg/2–3 mmHg in 22 trials of 1173 patients.[88]

Intracellular level of magnesium (RBC) is more indicative of total body stores and should be measured in conjunction with serum and urinary magnesium.[83] Magnesium may be supplemented in doses of 500–1000 mg/day. Magnesium formulations chelated to an amino acid may improve absorption and decrease the incidence of diarrhea.[83] Adding taurine at 1000–2000 mg/day will enhance the antihypertensive effects of magnesium.[83] Magnesium supplements should be avoided or used with caution in patients with known renal insufficiency or in those taking medications that induce magnesium retention.[83]

Calcium (Ca⁺⁺)

Population studies show a link between hypertension and calcium,[89] but clinical trials that administered calcium supplements to patients have shown inconsistent effects on BP.[73,89] The heterogeneous responses to calcium supplementation have been explained by Resnick.[90] This is the "ionic hypothesis"[90] of hypertension; CVD; and associated metabolic, functional, and structural disorders. Calcium supplementation is not recommended at this time as an effective means to reduce BP.

Zinc (Zn⁺⁺)

Low serum zinc levels in observational studies correlate with hypertension as well as CHD, T2DM, hyperlipidemia, elevated lipoprotein a (Lp(a)), and increased 2-hour postprandial plasma insulin levels and insulin resistance.[91,92] Zinc is transported into cardiac and vascular muscle and other tissues by metallothionein.[93] Genetic deficiencies of metallothionein with intramuscular zinc deficiencies may lead to increased oxidative stress, mitochondrial dysfunction, cardiomyocyte dysfunction, and apoptosis with subsequent myocardial fibrosis, abnormal cardiac remodeling, heart disease, heart failure, or hypertension.[93] Intracellular calcium increases oxidative stress, which is reduced by zinc.[93]

Bergomi et al.[94] evaluated Zn⁺⁺ status in 60 hypertensive subjects compared to 60 normotensive control subjects. An inverse correlation of BP and serum Zn⁺⁺ was observed. The BP was also inversely correlated to a Zn⁺⁺-dependent enzyme-lysyl oxidase activity. Zn⁺⁺ inhibits gene expression and transcription through NFκB and activated protein-1 (AP-1) and is an important cofactor for SOD.[91,93] These effects plus those on insulin resistance, membrane ion exchange, and renin-angiotensin-aldosterone system (RAAS) and SNS effects may account for Zn⁺⁺ antihypertensive effects.[91,93] Zinc intake should be 50 mg/day.[1]

PROTEIN

Observational and epidemiological studies demonstrate a consistent association between a high protein intake and a reduction in BP and incident BP.[95,96] The protein source is an important factor in the BP effect, animal protein being less effective than nonanimal or plant protein, especially almonds.[95–98] In the Inter-Salt Study of over 10,000 subjects, those with a dietary protein intake 30% above the mean had a lower BP by 3.0/2.5 mmHg compared to those who were 30%

below the mean (81 vs. 44 g/day).[95] However, lean or wild animal protein with less saturated fat and more essential ω-3 fatty acids may reduce BP, lipids, and CHD risk.[95,98] A meta-analysis confirmed these findings and also suggested that hypertensive patients and the elderly have the greatest BP reduction with protein intake.[96] Another meta-analysis of 40 trials with 3277 patients found reductions in BP of 1.76/1.15 mmHg compared to carbohydrate intake ($p < .001$).[99] Both vegetable and animal protein significantly and equally reduced BP at 2.27/1.26 mmHg and 2.54/.95 mmHg, respectively.[99] Increased dietary protein intake is inversely associated with risk for stroke in women with hypertension.[100] A randomized crossover study in 352 adults with prehypertension and stage I hypertension found a significant reduction in SBP of 2.0 mmHg with soy protein and 2.3 mmHg with milk protein compared to a high glycemic index diet over each of the 8-week treatment periods.[101] There was a nonsignificant reduction in DBP. Another parallel study over 4 weeks of 94 subjects with prehypertension and stage I hypertension found significant reductions on office BP of 4.9/2.7 mmHg in those given a combination of 25% protein intake versus the control group given 15% protein in an isocaloric manner.[102] The protein consisted of 20% pea, 20% soy, 30% egg, and 30% milk protein isolate.[102] The daily recommended intake of protein from all sources is 1.0–1.5 g/kg body weight, varying with exercise level, age, renal function, and other factors.[1,70,71]

Fermented milk supplemented with whey protein concentrate significantly reduces BP in human studies.[103–107] Administration of 20 g/day of hydrolyzed whey protein supplement rich in bioactive peptides significantly reduced BP over 6 weeks by 8.0 ± 3.2 mmHg in SBP and 5.5 ± 2.1 mm in DBP.[104] Milk peptides, which contain both caseins and whey proteins, are a rich source of ACEI peptides. Val-Pro-Pro and Ile-Pro-Pro given at 5–60 mg/day have variable reductions in BP with an average decrease in pooled studies of about 1.28–4.8/0.59–2.2 mmHg.[71,101,105–108] However, several recent meta-analyses did not show significant reductions in BP in humans.[107,109] Powdered fermented milk with *Lactobacillus helveticus* given at 12 g/day significantly lowered BP by 11.2/6.5 mmHg in 4 weeks in one study.[105] Milk peptides are beneficial in treating MS.[110] A dose–response study showed insignificant reductions in BP.[111] The clinical response is attributed to fermented milk's active peptides, which inhibit ACE.

Pins and Keenan[112] administered 20 g of hydrolyzed whey protein to 30 hypertensive subjects and noted a BP reduction of 11/7 mmHg compared to controls at 1 week, which was sustained throughout the study. Whey protein is effective in improving lipids, insulin resistance, glucose, arterial stiffness, and BP.[113] These data indicate that whey protein must be hydrolyzed to exhibit an antihypertensive effect, and the maximum BP response is dose dependent.

Bovine casein–derived peptides and whey protein–derived peptides exhibit ACEI activity.[103–112] These components include B-caseins, B-lg fractions, B2-microglobulin, and serum albumin.[103–105,112] The enzymatic hydrolysis of whey protein isolates releases ACEI peptides.

Marine collagen peptides (MCPs) from deep sea fish have antihypertensive activity.[114–116] A double-blind, placebo-controlled trial in 100 hypertensive subjects with diabetes who received MCPs twice a day for 3 months had significant reductions in DBP and mean arterial pressure.[114] Bonito protein (*Sarda orientalis*), from the tuna and mackerel family, has natural ACEI inhibitory peptides and reduces BP by 10.2/7 mmHg at 1.5 g/day.[115,117]

Sardine muscle protein, which contains valyl-tyrosine (Val-Tyr), significantly lowers BP in hypertensive subjects.[118] Kawasaki et al. treated 29 hypertensive subjects with 3 mg of Val-Tyr sardine muscle concentrated extract for 4 weeks and lowered BP by 9.7/5.3 mmHg ($p < .05$).[118] Levels of A-I increased as serum A-II and aldosterone decreased, indicating that Val-Tyr is a natural ACEI. A similar study with a vegetable drink with sardine protein hydrolysates significantly lowered BP by 8/5 mmHg in 13 weeks.[119]

Soy protein lowered BP in hypertensive patients in most studies[101,120–129] Soy protein intake was significantly and inversely associated with both SBP and DBP in 45,694 Chinese women consuming 25 g/day or more of soy protein over 3 years, and the association increased with age.[120] The SBP reduction was 1.9–4.9 mmHg lower and the DBP was 0.9–2.2 mmHg lower.[120] However, randomized clinical trials and meta-analyses have shown mixed results on BP with no change in BP to reductions of 7%–10% for SBP and DBP.[123–127] The recent meta-analysis of 27 trials found a significant reduction in BP of 2.21/1.44 mmHg.[122] Some studies suggest improvement in endothelial function, improved arterial compliance, reduction in HS-CRP and inflammation, ACEI activity, reduction in sympathetic tone, diuretic action, and reduction in both oxidative stress and aldosterone levels. [126,128,129] Fermented soy at about 25 g/day is recommended.

In addition to ACEI effects, protein intake may also alter catecholamine responses and induce a natriuretic effect.[118,119] Low protein intake coupled with low ω-3 fatty acid intake may contribute to hypertension in animal models.[130] The optimal protein intake, depending on level of activity, renal function, stress, and other factors, is about 1.0–1.5 g/kg/day.[1]

AMINO ACIDS AND RELATED COMPOUNDS

L-Arginine

L-arginine and endogenous methylarginines are the primary precursors for the production of nitric oxide (NO), which has numerous beneficial cardiovascular effects, mediated through conversion of L-arginine to NO by eNOS. Patients with hypertension, hyperlipidemia, DM, and atherosclerosis have increased levels of HS-CRP and inflammation; increased microalbumin; low levels of apelin (stimulates NO in the endothelium); increased levels of arginase (breaks down arginine); and elevated serum levels of ADMA, which inactivates NO.[131–135]

Under normal physiological conditions, intracellular arginine levels far exceed the Km (Michaelis–Menten constant [MMC]) of eNOS, which is less than 5 μmol.[136] However, endogenous NO formation is dependent on extracellular arginine concentration.[136] The intracellular concentrations of L-arginine are 0.1–3.8 mM in endothelial cells, whereas the plasma concentration of arginine is 80–120 μM, which is about 20–25 times greater than the MMC.[136,137] Despite this, cellular NO formation depends on exogenous L-arginine, and this is the arginine paradox. Renal arginine regulates BP and blocks the formation of endothelin, reduces renal sodium reabsorption, and is a potent antioxidant.[136] The NO production in endothelial cells is closely coupled to cellular arginine uptake, indicating that arginine transport mechanisms play a major role in the regulation of NO-dependent function. Exogenous arginine can increase renal vascular and tubular NO bioavailability and influence renal perfusion, function, and BP.[134] Molecular eNOS uncoupling may occur in the absence of tetrahydrobiopterin, which stabilizes eNOS, leading to the production of ROS.[137]

Human studies in hypertensive and normotensive subjects of parenteral and oral administrations of L-arginine demonstrate an antihypertensive effect as well as an improvement in coronary artery blood flow and peripheral blood flow in peripheral artery disease (PAD).[131,138–142] The BP was decreased by 6.2/6.8 mmHg on 10 g/day of L-arginine when provided as a supplement or though natural foods to a group of hypertensive subjects.[138] Arginine produces a statistically and biologically significant decrease in BP and improved metabolic effect in normotensive and hypertensive humans that is similar in magnitude to that seen in the DASH I diet.[138] Arginine given at 4 g/day also significantly lowered BP in women with gestational hypertension without proteinuria, reduced the need for antihypertensive therapy, decreased maternal and neonatal complications, and prolonged the pregnancy.[139,140] The combination of arginine (1200 mg/day) and N-acetyl cysteine (NAC) (600 mg bid) administered over 6 months to hypertensive patients with type 2 diabetes lowered SBP and DBP ($p < .05$), increased high-density lipoprotein (HDL)-C, decreased LDL-C and oxLDL, reduced HS-CRP, intercellular adhesion molecule (ICAM), vascular cell adhesion molecule (VCAM), PAI-I, fibrinogen, and IMT.[141] A study of 54 hypertensive subjects given arginine 4 g three times a day for 4 weeks had significant reductions in 24-hour ambulatory blood pressure monitoring (ABM).[142] A meta-analysis of 11 trials with 383 subjects administered arginine 4–24 g/day found average reduction in BP of 5.39/2.66 mmHg ($p < .001$) in 4 weeks.[143] Although these doses of L-arginine appear to be safe, no long-term studies in humans have been published at this time and there are concerns of a pro-oxidative effect or even an increase in mortality in patients who may have severely dysfunctional endothelium, advanced atherosclerosis, CHD, ACS, or MI.[144] In addition to the arginine–NO path, there exists a nitrate/nitrite pathway that is related to dietary nitrates from vegetables, beetroot juice, and the DASH diet that are converted to nitrites by symbiotic, salivary, gastrointestinal (GI), and oral bacteria.[145] Administration of beetroot juice or extract at 500 mg/day will increase nitrites and lower BP; improve endothelial function; and increase cerebral, coronary, and peripheral blood flow.[145]

L-Carnitine and Acetyl-L-Carnitine

L-carnitine is a nitrogenous constituent of muscle primarily involved in the oxidation of fatty acids in mammals. Animal studies indicate that carnitine has both systemic antihypertensive effects and antioxidant effects in the heart by upregulation of eNOS and PPARγ; inhibition of RAAS; modulation of NFkB; and downregulation of NOX2, NOX4, TGF-β, and CTGF, which reduces cardiac fibrosis.[146,147] Endothelial function, NO, and oxidative defense are improved, whereas oxidative stress and BP are reduced.[146–149]

Human studies on the effects of L-carnitine and acetyl-L-carnitine are limited, with minimal to no change in BP.[150–156] In patients with MS, acetyl-L-carnitine at 1 g bid over 8 weeks improved dysglycemia and reduced SBP by 7–9 mm Hg, but DBP was significantly decreased only in those with higher glucose.[153] Low carnitine levels are associated with a nondipping BP pattern in T2DM.[155] Carnitine has antioxidant and anti-inflammatory effects and may be useful in the treatment of essential hypertension, T2DM with hypertension, hyperlipidemia, cardiac arrhythmias, CHF, and cardiac ischemic syndromes.[1,150–152,154] Doses of 2–3 g twice a day are recommended.

Taurine

Taurine is a sulfonic β-amino acid that is considered a conditionally essential amino acid, which is not utilized in protein synthesis but is found free or in simple peptides with its highest concentration in the brain, retina, and myocardium.[156] In cardiomyocytes, it represents about 50% of the free amino acids and has the role of an osmoregulator, inotropic factor, and antihypertensive agent.[157]

Human studies have noted that essential hypertensive subjects have reduced urinary taurine as well as other sulfur amino acids.[1,156,157] Taurine lowers BP, systemic vascular resistance (SVR), and HR; decreases arrhythmias, CHF symptoms, and SNS activity; increases urinary sodium and water excretion; increases atrial natriuretic factor; improves insulin resistance; increases NO; and improves endothelial function. Taurine also decreases A-II, PRA, aldosterone, SNS activity, plasma norepinephrine, and plasma and urinary epinephrine; lowers homocysteine; improves insulin sensitivity, kinins, and acetyl choline responsiveness; decreases intracellular calcium and sodium; lowers response to β-receptors; has antioxidant, anti-atherosclerotic, and anti-inflammatory activities; decreases IMT and arterial stiffness; and may protect from risk of CHD.[1,156–162] A lower urinary taurine is associated with increased risk of hypertension and CVD.[162,163] A study of 31 Japanese males with essential hypertension placed on an exercise program for 10 weeks showed a 26% increase in taurine levels. The BP reduction of 14.8/6.6 mmHg was proportional to increases in serum taurine and reductions in plasma norepinephrine.[164] Fujita et al.[157] demonstrated a reduction in BP of 9/4.1 mmHg ($p < .05$) in 19 hypertension subjects given 6 g of taurine for 7 days. Taurine has numerous beneficial effects on the cardiovascular system and BP.[158] The recommended dose of taurine is 2–3 g/day at which no adverse effects are noted, but higher doses up to 6 g/day may be needed to reduce BP significantly.[1,70,71,156–164]

ω-3 Fats

The ω-3 fatty acids found in cold-water fish, fish oils, flax, flax seed, flax oil, and nuts lower BP in observational, epidemiological, and prospective clinical trials.[165–175] The findings are strengthened by a dose-related response in hypertension as well as a relationship to the specific concomitant diseases associated with hypertension.[165–175]

Studies indicate that docosahexaenoic acid (DHA) at 2 g/day reduces BP and heart rate.[165–175] The average reduction in BP is 8/5 mmHg and heart rate falls to about 6 beats per minute usually in about 6 weeks.[1,70,71,165,170–178] Fish oil at 4–9 g/day or in a combination of DHA and eicosapentaenoic acid (EPA) at 3–5 g/day will also reduce BP.[1,170–175] However, formation of EPA and ultimately DHA from α-lipoic acid (ALA) is decreased in the presence of high LA (the essential ω-6 fatty acid), saturated fats, trans fatty acids, alcohol, several nutrient deficiencies (magnesium and vitamin B 6), and aging, all of which inhibit the desaturase enzymes.[165] Eating cold-water fish three times per week may be as effective as high-dose fish oil in reducing BP in hypertensive patients, and the protein in the fish may also have antihypertensive effects.[1,165] In patients with chronic kidney disease, 4 g of ω-3 fatty acids reduced BP measured with 24-hour ABM over 8 weeks by 3.3/2.9 mmHg compared to placebo ($p < .0001$).[179]

The ideal ratio of ω-6 fatty acids to ω-3 fatty acids is between 1:1 and 1:4 with a polyunsaturated to saturated (P/S) fat ratio greater than 1.5 to 2.0.[2] ω-3 Fatty acids increase eNOS and nitric oxide, improve endothelial function, improve insulin sensitivity, reduce calcium influx, suppress ACE activity, and improve parasympathetic tone.[1,165–173] The ω-6 fatty acid family includes LA, GLA, dihomo-γ-linolenic acid (DGLA), and arachidonic acid (AA), which do not usually lower BP significantly but may prevent increases in BP induced by saturated fats.[180] GLA may block stress-induced hypertension by increasing PGE_1 and prostaglandin I_2 (PGI_2), reducing aldosterone levels, and reducing adrenal AT1R density and affinity.[177]

The ω-3 fatty acids have a multitude of other cardiovascular consequences that modulate BP such as increases in eNOS and nitric oxide, improvement in ED, reduction in plasma norepinephrine and increase in PNS tone, suppression of ACE activity, and improvement of insulin resistance.[180] The recommended daily dose is 3000–5000 mg/day of combined DHA and EPA in a ratio of 3 parts EPA to 2 parts DHA and about 50% of this dose as GLA combined with γ-/δ-tocopherol at 100 mg/g of DHA and EPA to get the ω-3 index to 8% or higher to reduce BP and provide optimal cardioprotection.[181] DHA is more effective than EPA for reducing BP and should be given at 2 g/day if administered alone.[165,175]

ω-9 FATS

Olive oil is rich in ω-9 monounsaturated fat (MUFA) oleic acid, which has been associated with BP and lipid reduction in Mediterranean and other diets.[182–185] Olive oil and MUFAs have shown consistent reductions in BP in most clinical studies in humans.[182–184,186–194] In one study, the SBP fell by 8 mmHg ($p ≤ .05$) and the DBP fell by 6 mmHg ($p ≤ .01$) in both clinic and 24-hour ambulatory BP monitoring in MUFA-treated subjects compared to PUFA-treated subjects.[182] In addition, the need for antihypertensive medications was reduced by 48% in the MUFA group versus 4% in the ω-6 PUFA group ($p < .005$). Extra virgin olive oil (EVOO) was more effective than sunflower oil in lowering SBP in a group of 31 elderly hypertensive patients in a double-blind randomized crossover study.[191] The SBP was 136 mmHg in the EVOO-treated subjects versus 150 mmHg in the sunflower-treated group ($p < .01$). Olive oil also reduces BP in hypertensive diabetic subjects.[192] It is the high oleic acid content in olive oil that reduces BP.[184] In stage I hypertensive patients, oleuropein-olive leaf (*Olea eurpoaea*) extract 500 mg bid for 8 weeks reduced BP by 11.5/4.8 mmHg, which was similar to captopril 25 mg bid.[193] *Olea europaea* L. aqueous extract administered to 12 patients with hypertension at 400 mg qid for 3 months significantly reduced BP ($p < .001$).[186] Olive oil intake in the EPIC study of 20,343 subjects was inversely associated with both SBP and DBP.[187] In the SUN study of 6863 subjects, BP was inversely associated with olive oil consumption, but only in men.[188] In a study of 40 hypertensive monozygotic twins, olive leaf extract demonstrated a dose–response reduction in BP at doses of 500–1000 mg/day in 8 weeks compared to placebo.[189] The low-dose groups decreased BP by 3/1 mmHg and the high-dose groups by 11/4 mmHg.[189] A double-blind, randomized crossover dietary intervention study over 4 months using polyphenol-rich olive oil 30 mg/day decreased BP in the study group by 7.91/6.65 mmHg and improved endothelial function.[190]

The ADMA levels, oxLDL, and HS-CRP were reduced in the olive oil group. Plasma nitrites and nitrates increased and hyperemic area after ischemia improved in the treated group. Olive oil inhibits the AT1R receptor, exerts L-type calcium channel antagonist effects, and improves wave reflections and augmentation index.[195–197]

EVOO also contains lipid-soluble phytonutrients such as polyphenols. Approximately 5 mg of phenols are found in 10 g of EVOO.[182,185] About 4 Tbsp of EVOO is equal to 40 g of EVOO, which is the amount required to get significant reductions in BP.

FIBER

Clinical trials with various types of fiber to reduce BP have been inconsistent.[198,199] Soluble fiber, guar gum, guava, psyllium, and oat bran may reduce BP and reduce the need for antihypertensive medications in hypertensive subjects, diabetic subjects, and hypertensive–diabetic subjects.[1,70,71,198,199] The average reduction in BP is about 7.5/5.5 mmHg on 40–50 g/day of a mixed fiber. There is improvement in insulin sensitivity, endothelial function, reduction in SNS activity, and increase in renal sodium loss.[1,70,71,198]

VITAMIN C

Vitamin C is a potent water-soluble electron donor. At physiological levels, it is an antioxidant, although at supraphysiological doses such as those achieved with intravenous vitamin C it donates electrons to different enzymes, which results in pro-oxidative effects. At physiological doses, vitamin C recycles vitamin E, improves ED, and produces a diuresis.[200] Dietary intake of vitamin C and plasma ascorbate concentration in humans is inversely correlated to SBP, DBP, and heart rate.[200–214]

An evaluation of published clinical trials indicates that vitamin C dosing at 250 mg twice daily will significantly lower SBP by 5–7 mmHg, and DBP by 2–4 mmHg over 8 weeks.[200–214] Vitamin C will induce a sodium water diuresis, improve arterial compliance, improve endothelial function, increase nitric oxide and PGI$_2$, decrease adrenal steroid production, improve sympathovagal balance, increase RBC Na/K ATPase, increase SOD, improve aortic elasticity and compliance, improve flow-mediated vasodilation, decrease pulse wave velocity and augmentation index, increase cyclic GMP, activate potassium channels, reduce cytosolic calcium, and reduce serum aldehydes.[212] Vitamin C prevents ED induced by an oral glucose load. Vitamin C enhances the efficacy of amlodipine, decreases the binding affinity of the AT1R for A-II by disrupting the ATR1 disulfide bridges, and enhances the antihypertensive effects of medications in the elderly with refractory hypertension.[1,70,71,204–209] In elderly patients with refractory hypertension already on maximum pharmacological therapy, 600 mg of vitamin C daily lowered the BP by 20/16 mmHg.[209] The lower the initial ascorbate serum level, the better the BP response. A serum level of 100 µmol/L is recommended.[1,70,71] The SBP and 24 ABM show the most significant reductions with chronic oral administration of vitamin C.[204–209] Block et al.[210] in an elegant depletion–repletion study of vitamin C demonstrated an inverse correlation of plasma ascorbate levels, SBP, and DBP. In a meta-analysis of 13 clinical trials with 284 patients, vitamin C at 500 mg/day over 6 weeks reduced SBP by 3.9 mmHg and DBP by 2.1 mmHg.[211] Hypertensive subjects were found to have significantly lower plasma ascorbate levels compared to normotensive subjects (40 vs. 57 µmol/L, respectively),[215] and plasma ascorbate is inversely correlated with BP even in healthy, normotensive individuals.[210]

VITAMIN E

Most studies have not shown reductions in BP with most forms of tocopherols or tocotrienols.[1,70,71] Patients with T2DM and controlled hypertension (130/76 mmHg) on prescription medications with an average BP of 136/76 mmHg were administered mixed tocopherols containing 60% γ-,

25% δ-, and 15% α-tocopherols.[216] The BP actually increased by 6.8/3.6 mmHg in the study patients ($p < .0001$) but was less compared to the increase with α-tocopherol of 7/5.3 mmHg ($p < .0001$). This may be a reflection of drug interactions with tocopherols via cytochrome P 450 (3A4 and 4F2) and reduction in the serum levels of the pharmacological treatments that were simultaneously being given.[216] γ-Tocopherol may have natriuretic effects by inhibition of the 70pS potassium channel in the thick ascending limb of the loop of Henle and lower BP.[217] Both α-tocopherol and γ-tocopherol improve insulin sensitivity and enhance adiponectin expression via PPARγ-dependent processes, which have the potential to lower BP and serum glucose.[218] If vitamin E has an antihypertensive effect, it is probably small and may be limited to untreated hypertensive patients or those with known vascular disease or other concomitant problems such as diabetes or hyperlipidemia.

Vitamin D

Vitamin D3 may have an independent and direct role in the regulation of BP and insulin metabolism.[219–229] Vitamin D influences BP by its effects on calcium phosphate metabolism, RAAS, immune system, control of endocrine glands, and ED.[220] If the vitamin D level is below 30 ng/mL, the circulating PRA levels are higher, which increases A-II, increases BP, and blunts plasma renal blood flow.[225] The lower the level of vitamin D, the greater the risk of hypertension, with the lowest quartile of serum vitamin D having a 52% incidence of hypertension and the highest quartile having a 20% incidence.[225] Vitamin D3 markedly suppresses renin transcription by a VDR-mediated mechanism via the JGA apparatus. Its role in electrolytes, volume, and BP homeostasis indicates that vitamin D3 is important in the amelioration of hypertension. Vitamin D lowers ADMA, suppresses proinflammatory cytokines such as TNF-α, increases nitric oxide, improves endothelial function and arterial elasticity, decreases vascular smooth muscle hypertrophy, regulates electrolytes and blood volume, increases insulin sensitivity, reduces free fatty acid concentration, regulates the expression of the natriuretic peptide receptor, and lowers HS-CRP.[221–225]

The hypotensive effect of vitamin D was inversely related to the pretreatment serum levels of 1,25 (OH)2 D3. Pfeifer et al. showed that short-term supplementation with vitamin D3 and calcium is more effective in reducing SBP than calcium alone.[229] In a group of 148 women with low 25 (OH)$_2$ D$_3$ levels, the administration of 1200 mg calcium plus 800 IU of vitamin D3 reduced SBP 9.3% more ($p < .02$) compared to 1200 mg of calcium alone. The HR fell by 5.4% ($p = .02$), but DBP was not changed. The range in BP reduction was 3.6/3.1 to 13.1/7.2 mmHg. The reduction in BP is related to the pretreatment level of vitamin D3, dose of vitamin D3, and serum level of vitamin D3, but BP is reduced only in hypertensive patients. Although vitamin D deficiency is associated with hypertension in observational studies, randomized clinical trials and their meta-analyses have yielded inconclusive results.[227] In addition, vitamin D receptor gene polymorphisms may effect the risk of hypertension in men.[228] A 25 hydroxyvitamin D level of 60 ng/mL is recommended.

Vitamin B6 (Pyridoxine)

Low serum vitamin B6 (pyridoxine) levels are associated with hypertension in humans.[230] One human study by Aybak et al.[231] proved that high-dose vitamin B6 at 5 mg/kg/day for 4 weeks significantly lowered BP by 14/10 mmHg. Pyridoxine (vitamin B6) is a cofactor in neurotransmitter and hormone synthesis in the CNS (norepinephrine, epinephrine, serotonin, GABA, and kynurenine), increases cysteine synthesis to neutralize aldehydes, enhances the production of glutathione, blocks calcium channels, improves insulin resistance, decreases central sympathetic tone, and reduces end organ responsiveness to glucocorticoids and mineralocorticoids.[1,70,71,232,233] Vitamin B6 is reduced with chronic diuretic therapy and heme pyrollactams (HPU). Vitamin B6 thus has a similar action to central α-agonists, diuretics, and CCBs. The recommended dose is 20 mg/day orally.

FLAVONOIDS

Over 4000 naturally occurring flavonoids have been identified in such diverse substances as fruits, vegetables, red wine, tea, soy, and licorice.[234] Flavonoids (flavonols, flavones, and isoflavones) are potent free radical scavengers that inhibit lipid peroxidation, prevent atherosclerosis, promote vascular relaxation, and have antihypertensive properties.[234] In addition, they reduce stroke and provide cardioprotective effects that reduce CHD morbidity and mortality.[235]

Resveratrol is a potent antioxidant and antihypertensive found in the skin of red grapes and in red wine. Resveratrol administration to humans reduces augmentation index, improves arterial compliance, and lowers central arterial pressure when administered as 250 mL of either regular or dealcoholized red wine.[236] There was a significant reduction in the aortic augmentation index of 6.1% with the dealcoholized red wine and of 10.5% with regular red wine. The central arterial pressure was significantly reduced by dealcoholized red wine at 7.4 mmHg and by regular red wine at 5.4 mmHg. Resveratrol increases flow-mediated vasodilation in a dose-related manner, improves ED, prevents uncoupling of eNOS, increases adiponectin, lowers HS-CRP, and blocks the effects of A-II.[237–240] The recommended dose is 250 mg/day of trans resveratrol.[142]

LYCOPENE

Lycopene is a fat-soluble phytonutrient in the carotenoid family. Dietary sources include tomatoes, guava, pink grapefruit, watermelon, apricots, and papaya in high concentrations.[241–245] Lycopene produces a significant reduction in BP, serum lipids, and oxidative stress markers.[241–245] Paran et al.[245] evaluated 30 subjects with grade I hypertension, age 40–65 years, taking no antihypertensive or antilipid medications and treated them with a tomato lycopene extract (10 mg lycopene) for 8 weeks. The SBP was reduced from 144 to 135 mmHg (9 mmHg reduction, $p < .01$), and the DBP fell from 91 to 84 mmHg (7 mmHg reduction, $p < .01$). Another study of 35 subjects with grade I hypertension showed similar results on SBP but not DBP.[241] Englehard gave a tomato extract to 31 hypertensive subjects over 12 weeks, demonstrating a significant BP reduction of 10/4 mmHg.[242] Patients on various antihypertensive agents including ACEI, CCB, and diuretics had a significant BP reduction of 5.4/3 mmHg over 6 weeks when administered a standardized tomato extract.[243] Other studies have not shown changes in BP with lycopene.[244] Lycopene and tomato extract improve ED and reduce plasma total oxidative stress.[246] The recommended daily intake of lycopene is 10–20 mg in food or in the supplement form.

PYCNOGENOL

Pycnogenol, a bark extract from the French maritime pine, at doses of 200 mg/day resulted in a significant reduction in SBP from 139.9 to 132.7 mmHg ($p < .05$) in 11 patients with mild hypertension over 8 weeks in a double-blind randomized placebo crossover trial. The DBP fell from 93.8 to 92.0 mmHg. Pycnogenol acts as a natural ACEI, protects cell membranes from oxidative stress, increases NO and improves endothelial function, reduces serum thromboxane concentrations, decreases myeloperoxidase activity, improves renal cortical blood flow, reduces urinary albumin excretion, and decreases HS-CRP.[247–251] Other studies have shown reductions in BP and a decreased need for ACEI and CCB and reductions in endothelin-1, HgA1C, fasting glucose, LDL-C, and myeloperoxidase.[248,249,251]

GARLIC

Clinical trials utilizing the correct dose, type of garlic, and well-absorbed long-acting preparations have shown consistent reductions in BP in hypertensive patients with an average reduction in BP of 8.4/7.3 mmHg.[252–253] Not all garlic preparations are processed similarly and are comparable in antihypertensive potency.[1] In addition, cultivated garlic (*Allium sativum*), wild uncultivated garlic or bear garlic (*Allium urisinum*), as well as the effects of aged, fresh, and long-acting garlic preparations differ.[1,70,71,253] Garlic is also effective in reducing BP in patients with uncontrolled hypertension already on antihypertensive medication.[254] A garlic homogenate-based supplement was administered to 34 prehypertensive and stage I hypertensive patients at 300 mg/day over 12 weeks with a reduction in BP of 6.6–7.5/4.6–5.2 mmHg. Aged garlic at doses of 240–960 mg/day given to 79 hypertensive subjects over 12 weeks significantly lowered SBP 11.8 ± 5.4mmHg in the high-dose garlic group. A longer acting garlic may reduce BP better than a shorter acting garlic. A Cochrane Database review indicated a net reduction in BP of 10–12/6–9 mmHg in all clinical trials with garlic. In a double-blind, parallel, and randomized placebo-controlled trial of 50 patients, 900 mg of aged garlic extract with 2.4 mg of *S*-allylcysteine was administered daily for 12 weeks and reduced SBP, 10.2 mmHg ($p = .03$), more than the control group.[254]

Approximately 10,000 mcg of allicin (one of the active ingredients in garlic) per day, the amount contained in four cloves of garlic (5 g), is required to achieve a significant BP-lowering effect.[1,70,71,253,254] Garlic has ACEI activity and calcium channel-blocking activity; reduces catecholamine sensitivity; improves arterial compliance; increases bradykinin and nitric oxide; and contains adenosine, magnesium, flavonoids, sulfur, allicin, phosphorous, and ajoenes that reduce BP.[1,70,71]

Seaweed

Wakame seaweed (*Undaria pinnatifida*) is the most popular, edible seaweed in Japan.[255] In humans, 3.3 g of dried wakame for 4 weeks significantly reduced both SBP, 14 ± 3 mmHg, and DBP, 5 ± 2 mmHg ($p < .01$).[256] In a study of 62 middle-aged, male subjects with mild hypertension given a potassium-loaded, ion-exchanging, sodium-adsorbing, and potassium-releasing seaweed preparation, significant BP reductions occurred at 4 weeks on 12 and 24 g/day of the seaweed preparation ($p < .01$).[257] The MAP fell by 11.2 mmHg ($p < .001$) in the sodium-sensitive subjects and 5.7 mmHg ($p < .05$) in the sodium-insensitive subjects, which correlated with PRA.

Seaweed and sea vegetables contain almost all of the seawater's 771 minerals and rare earth elements, fiber, and alginate in a colloidal form.[255–257] The primary effect of wakame appears to be through its ACEI activity from at least four parent tetrapeptides and possibly their dipeptide and tripeptide metabolites, especially those containing the amino acid sequence Val-Tyr, Ile-Tyr, Phe-Tyr, and Ile-Try in some combination.[255,258,259] Its long-term use in Japan has demonstrated its safety. Other varieties of seaweed may reduce BP by reducing intestinal sodium absorption and increasing intestinal potassium absorption.[257]

Sesame

Sesame has been shown to reduce BP in several small randomized, placebo-controlled human studies over 30–60 days.[260–268] Sesame lowers BP either alone[261–265] or in combination with nifedipine,[260,264] diuretics, and β-blockers.[261,265] In a group of 13 mild hypertensive subjects, 60 mg of sesamin for 4 weeks lowered SBP, 3.5 mmHg ($p < .044$), and DBP, 1.9 mmHg ($p < .045$).[262] Black sesame meal at 2.52 g/day over 4 weeks in 15 subjects reduced SBP by 8.3 mmHg ($p < .05$), but there was a nonsignificant reduction in DBP of 4.2 mmHg.[263] Sesame oil at 35 g/day significantly lowered central BP within 1 hour and also maintained BP reduction chronically in 30 hypertensive subjects, reduced heart rate, reduced arterial stiffness, decreased augmentation index and pulse wave velocity, decreased HS-CRP, improved NO, decreased endothelin-I, and improved antioxidant capacity.[268] In addition, sesame lowers serum glucose, HgbAIC, and LDL-C; increases HDL; reduces oxidative stress markers; and increases glutathione, SOD, GPx, CAT, vitamin C, vitamin E, and vitamin A.[260,261,263–265] The active ingredients are natural ACEIs such as sesamin, sesamolin, sesaminol glucosides, and furofuran lignans, which are also suppressors of NFkB.[266,267] All of these effects lower inflammation and oxidative stress, improve oxidative defense, and reduce BP.[266,267]

BEVERAGES: TEA, COFFEE, AND COCOA

Green tea, black tea, and extracts of active components in both have demonstrated reduction in BP in humans.[269–275] In a double-blind, placebo-controlled trial of 379 hypertensive subjects given green tea extract 370 mg/day for 3 months, BP was reduced significantly at 4/4 mmHg with simultaneous decreases in HS-CRP, TNF-α, glucose, and insulin levels.[272]

Dark chocolate (100 g) and *cocoa* with a high content of polyphenols (30 mg or more) have been shown to significantly reduce BP in humans.[276–287] A meta-analysis of 173 hypertensive subjects given cocoa for a mean duration of 2 weeks had a significant reduction in BP, 4.7/2.8 mmHg ($p = .002$ for SBP, and $p = .006$ for DBP).[276] Fifteen subjects given 100 g of dark chocolate with 500 mg of polyphenols for 15 days had a 6.4-mmHg reduction in SBP ($p < .05$) with a nonsignificant change in DBP.[277] Cocoa at 30 mg of polyphenols reduced BP in prehypertensive and stage I hypertensive patients by 2.9/1.9 mmHg at 18 weeks ($p < .001$).[278] Two more recent meta-analyses of 13 trials and 10 trials with 297 patients found a significant reduction in BP of 3.2/2.0 and 4.5/3.2 mmHg, respectively.[280,283] The BP reduction is the greatest in those with the highest baseline BP and those with at least 50%–70% cocoa at doses of 6–100 g/day.[280,282] Cocoa may also improve insulin resistance and endothelial function.[277,284,285]

Polyphenols, chlorogenic acids (CGAs), the ferulic acid metabolite of CGAs, and dihydrocaffeic acids decrease BP in a dose-dependent manner, increase eNOS, and improve endothelial function in humans.[288–290] CGAs in green coffee bean extract at doses of 140 mg/day significantly reduced SBP and DBP in 28 subjects in a placebo-controlled randomized clinical trial. A study of 122 male subjects demonstrated a dose–response in SBP and DBP with doses of CGA from 46 to 185 mg/day. The group that received the 185-mg dose had a significant reduction in BP of 5.6/3.9 mmHg ($p < .01$) over 28 days. Hydroxyhydroquinone is another component of coffee beans that reduces the efficacy of CGAs in a dose-dependent manner, which partially explains the conflicting results of coffee ingestion on BP.[288,290] Furthermore, there is genetic variation in the enzyme responsible for the metabolism of caffeine that modifies the association between coffee intake, amount of coffee ingested and the risk of hypertension, heart rate, MI, arterial stiffness, arterial wave reflections, and urinary catecholamine levels.[291] Fifty-nine percent of the population has the IF/IA allele of the *CYP1A2* genotype, which confers slow metabolism of caffeine. Heavy coffee drinkers who are slow metabolizers had a 3.00 hazard ratio for developing hypertension. In contrast, fast metabolizers with the IA/IA allele have a 0.36 hazard ratio for incident hypertension.[291]

ADDITIONAL COMPOUNDS

Melatonin demonstrates significant antihypertensive effects in humans in numerous double-blind, randomized, and placebo-controlled clinical trials at 3–5 mg/day.[292–302] The average reduction in BP is 6/3 mmHg. Melatonin stimulates GABA receptors in the CNS and vascular melatonin receptors, inhibits plasma A-II levels, improves endothelial function, increases NO, vasodilates, improves nocturnal dipping, lowers cortisol, and is additive with ARBs. β-Blockers reduce melatonin secretion.[303]

Hesperidin significantly lowered DBP 3 to 4 mmHg ($p < .02$) and improved microvascular endothelial reactivity in 24 obese hypertensive male subjects in a randomized, controlled crossover study over 4 weeks for each of three treatment groups consuming 500 mL of orange juice, hesperidin, or placebo.[304]

Pomegranate juice is rich in tannins and has numerous other properties that improve vascular health and reduces SBP by 5%–12%.[305,306] A study of 51 healthy subjects given 330 mg/day of pomegranate juice showed reduction in BP of 3.14/2.33 mmHg ($p < .001$).[306] Pomegranate juice also suppresses the postprandial increase in SBP following a high-fat meal.[306] Pomegranate juice reduces serum ACE activity by 36% and has antiatherogenic, antioxidant, and anti-inflammatory effects.[305,306] Pomegranate juice at 50 mL/day reduced carotid IMT by 30% over 1 year; increased PON by 83%; decreased oxLDL by 59%–90%; decreased antibodies to oxLDL by 19%; increased total antioxidant status by 130%; reduced TGF-β; increased catalase, SOD, and GPx; increased eNOS and NO; and improved endothelial function.[305–306] Pomegranate juice works like an ACEI.

Grape seed extract (GSE) was administered to subjects in a meta-analysis of randomized trials and demonstrated a significant reduction in SBP of 1.54 mmHg ($p < .02$).[307,308] A significant reduction in BP of 11/8 mmHg ($p < .05$) was seen in another dose–response study with 150–300 mg/day of GSE over 4 weeks.[309] GSE has a high phenolic content, which activates the PI3K/Akt signaling pathway that phosphorylates eNOS and increases NO.[309,310]

COENZYME Q10 (UBIQUINONE)

Coenzyme Q10 has consistent and significant antihypertensive effects in patients with essential hypertension.[1,311–320] The literature is summarized as follows:

- Compared to normotensive patients, essential hypertensive patients have a higher incidence (sixfold) of coenzyme Q10 deficiency documented by serum levels.[1]
- Doses of 120–225 mg/day of coenzyme Q10, depending on the delivery method or the concomitant ingestion with a fatty meal, are necessary to achieve a therapeutic level of 3 μg/mL.[1,316,317] This dose is usually 3–5 mg/kg/day of coenzyme Q10. Oral dosing levels may become lower with nanoparticle and emulsion delivery systems intended to facilitate absorption.[318] Adverse effects have not been characterized in the literature.
- Patients with the lowest coenzyme Q10 serum levels may have the best antihypertensive response to supplementation.
- The average reduction in BP is about 15/10 mmHg and heart rate falls to 5 beats per minute based on reported studies and meta-analysis.
- The antihypertensive effect takes time to reach its peak level at 4 weeks. Then the BP remains stable during long-term treatment. The antihypertensive effect is gone within 2 weeks after discontinuation of coenzyme Q10. The reductions in BP and SVR are correlated with the pretreatment and posttreatment serum levels of CoQ10. About 50% of patients respond to oral CoQ10 supplementation for BP.[312]
- Approximately 50% of patients on antihypertensive drugs may be able to stop between one and three agents. Both total dose and frequency of administration may be reduced.
- Patients administered CoQ10 with enalapril improved the 24-hour ABM better than enalapril monotherapy and also normalized endothelial function.[313]
- CoQ10 is a lipid-phase antioxidant and free radical scavenger, increases eNOS and NO, reduces inflammation and NFκB, and improves endothelial function and vascular elasticity.[1,314,315]

Other favorable effects on cardiovascular risk factors include improvement in the serum lipid profile and carbohydrate metabolism with reduced glucose and improved insulin sensitivity, reduced oxidative stress, reduced heart rate, improved myocardial left ventricular function and oxygen delivery, and decreased catecholamine levels.[1,314,315]

α-LIPOIC ACID

ALA is known as thioctic acid in Europe, where it is a prescription medication. It is a sulfur-containing compound with antioxidant activity in both water and lipid phases.[1,70,71] Its use is well established in the treatment of certain forms of liver disease and in the delay of onset of peripheral neuropathy in patients with diabetes. Recent research has evaluated its potential role in the treatment of hypertension, especially as part of the MS.[321–324] In a double-blind crossover study of 36 patients over 8 weeks with CHD and hypertension, 200 mg of lipoic acid with 500 mg of acetyl-L-carnitine significantly reduced BP by 7/3 mmHg and increased brachial artery diameter.[321] The

QUALITY study of 40 patients with DM and stage I hypertension showed significant improvements in BP, urinary albumin excretion, FMD, and insulin sensitivity over 8 weeks with a combination of quinapril (40 mg/day) and lipoic acid (600 mg/day), which was greater than either alone.[323] Lipoic acid increases levels of glutathione, cysteine, vitamin C, and vitamin E; inhibits NFκB; reduces endothelin -1, tissue factor, and VCAM-1; increases cAMP; downregulates CD4 immune expression on mononuclear cells; reduces oxidative stress and inflammation; reduces atherosclerosis in animal models; decreases serum aldehydes; and closes calcium channels, which improves vasodilation, increases NO and nitrosothiols, improves endothelial function, and lowers BP.[1,321–324] Lipoic acid normalizes membrane calcium channels by providing sulfhydryl groups, decreasing cytosolic free calcium, and lowering SVR. In addition, lipoic acid improves insulin sensitivity, lowering glucose and advanced glycosylation end products (AGEs), which improves BP control and lowers serum triglycerides. Morcos et al.[324] showed stabilization of urinary albumin excretion in DM subjects given 600 mg of ALA compared to placebo for 18 months ($p < .05$).

The recommended dose is 100–200 mg/day of R-lipoic acid with biotin 2–4 mg/day to prevent biotin depletion with long-term use of lipoic acid. R-lipoic acid is preferred to the L isomer because of its preferred use by the mitochondria.[1,70,71]

N-Acetyl Cysteine

NAC and L-arginine (ARG) in combination reduce endothelial activation and BP in hypertensive patients with T2DM.[325] Over 6 months, 24 subjects given placebo or NAC with ARG significantly reduced both SBP and DBP ($p = .05$).[325] In addition, oxLDL, HS-CRP, ICAM, VCAM, fibrinogen, and PAI-1 were decreased, whereas HDL, NO, and endothelial postischemic vasodilation were increased.[325] NAC increases NO via IL-1B and increases iNOS mRNA, increases glutathione by increasing cysteine levels, reduces the affinity for the AT1 receptor by disrupting disulfide groups, blocks the L-type calcium channel, lowers homocysteine, and improves IMT.[325–328] The recommended dose is 500–1000 mg bid.

Hawthorn

Hawthorn extract has been used for centuries for the treatment of hypertension, CHF, and other CVDs.[329–333] A recent four-period crossover design, dose–response study in 21 subjects with prehypertension or mild hypertension over 3½ days did not show changes in FMD or BP on standardized extract with 50 mg of oligomeric procyanidin per 250 mg extract with 1000 mg, 1500 mg, or 2500 mg of the extract.[329] Hawthorn showed noninferiority of ACEI and diuretics in the treatment of 102 patients with NYHC II CHF over 8 weeks.[331] Patients with hypertension and T2DM on medications for BP and DM were randomized to 1200 mg of hawthorn extract for 16 weeks; they showed significant reductions in DBP of 2.6 mmHg ($p = .035$).[332] Thirty-six mildly hypertensive patients were administered 500 mg of hawthorn extract for 10 weeks, and they showed a nonsignificant trend in DBP reduction ($p = .081$) compared to placebo.[333] Hawthorn acts like an ACEI, a beta blocker (BB), a CCB, and a diuretic. More studies are needed to determine the efficacy, long-term effects, and dose of hawthorn for the treatment of hypertension.

Quercetin

Quercetin is an antioxidant flavonol found in apples, berries, and onions that reduces BP in hypertensive individuals.[334–336] But the hypotensive effects do not appear to be mediated by changes in HS-CRP, TNF-α, ACE activity, ET-1, NO, vascular reactivity, or FMD.[334] Quercetin is metabolized by CYP 3A4. Quercetin was administered to 12 hypertensive men at an oral dose of 1095 mg, with reduction in mean BP by 5 mmHg, SBP by 7 mmHg, and DBP by 3 mmHg.[304] The maximal plasma level at 10 hours was 2.3 ± 1.8 μmol/L, with return to baseline levels at 17 hours.

Forty-one prehypertensive and stage I hypertensive subjects were enrolled in a randomized, double-blind, and placebo-controlled crossover study with 730 mg of quercetin per day versus placebo.[335] In the stage I hypertensive patients, the BP was reduced by 7/5 mmHg ($p < .05$), but there were no changes in oxidative stress markers.[335] Quercetin administered to 93 overweight or obese subjects at 150 mg/day (plasma levels of 269 nmol/L) over 6 weeks lowered SBP to 2.9 mmHg in the hypertensive group and up to 3.7 mmHg in SBP in the patients 25–50 years of age.[336] The recommended dose of quercetin is 500 mg bid.

CLINICAL CONSIDERATIONS

COMBINING FOOD AND NUTRIENTS WITH MEDICATIONS

Several of the strategic combinations of nutraceutical supplements together or with antihypertensive drugs have been shown to lower BP more than medications alone:

- Sesame with β-blockers, diuretics, and nifedipine
- Pycnogenol with ACEI and CCB
- Lycopene with ACEI, CCB, and diuretics
- ALA with ACEI or acetyl-L-carnitine
- Vitamin C with CCBs
- N-acetyl cysteine with arginine
- Garlic with ACEI, diuretics, and β-blockers
- Coenzyme Q10 with ACEI and CCB
- Taurine with magnesium
- Potassium with all antihypertensive agents
- Magnesium with all antihypertensive agents

Many antihypertensive drugs may cause nutrient depletions that can actually interfere with their antihypertensive action or cause other metabolic adverse effects manifest through the laboratory or with clinical symptoms.[337-339] Diuretics decrease potassium, magnesium, phosphorous, sodium, chloride, folate, vitamin B6, zinc, iodine, and coenzyme Q10; increase homocysteine, calcium, and creatinine; and elevate serum glucose by inducing insulin resistance. β-Blockers reduce coenzyme Q10. ACEIs and ARBs reduce zinc.

SUMMARY

- Vascular biology such as ED and VSMD plays a primary role in the initiation and perpetuation of hypertension, CVD, and TOD.
- Nutrient–gene interactions and epigenetics are a predominant factor in promoting beneficial or detrimental effects in cardiovascular health and hypertension.
- Food and nutrients can prevent, control, and treat hypertension through numerous vascular biology mechanisms.
- Oxidative stress, inflammation, and autoimmune dysfunction initiate and propagate hypertension and CVD.
- There is a role for the selected use of single and component nutraceutical supplements vitamins, antioxidants, and minerals in the treatment of hypertension based on scientifically controlled studies as a complement to optimal nutritional, dietary intake from food and other lifestyle modifications.[339]
- A clinical approach that incorporates diet, foods, nutrients, exercise, weight reduction, smoking cessation, alcohol and caffeine restriction, and other lifestyle strategies can be systematically and successfully incorporated into clinical practice (Table 9.3).

TABLE 9.3

An Integrative Approach to the Treatment of Hypertension

Intervention Category	Therapeutic Intervention	Daily Intake
Diet characteristics	DASH I, DASH II-Na$^+$ or PREMIER diet	Diet type
	Sodium restriction	1500 mg
	Potassium	5000 mg
	Potassium/sodium ratio	>3:1
	Magnesium	1000 mg
	Zinc	50 mg
Macronutrients	Protein: total intake from nonanimal sources, organic lean or wild animal protein, or cold-water fish	30% of total calories, which 1.5–1.8 g/kg body weight
	Whey protein	30 g
	Soy protein (fermented sources are preferred)	30 g
	Sardine muscle concentrate extract	3 g
	Milk peptides (VPP and IPP)	30–60 mg
	Fat:	30% of total calories
	ω-3 fatty acids	2 to 3 g
	ω-6 fatty acids	1 g
	ω-9 fatty acids	2–4 Tablespoons of olive or nut oil or 10–20 olives
	Saturated fatty acids from wild game, bison, or other lean meat	<10% total calories
	P/S fat ratio	>2.0
	ω-3 to ω-6 ratio	1.1–1.2
	Synthetic trans fatty acids	None (completely remove from diet)
	Nuts in variety	Ad libitum
	Carbohydrates as primarily complex carbohydrates and fiber	40% of total calories
	Oatmeal or	60 g
	Oat bran or	40 g
	β-Glucan or	3 g
	Psyllium	7 g
Specific foods	Garlic as fresh cloves or aged Kyolic garlic	4 Fresh cloves (4 g) or 600 mg aged garlic taken twice daily
	Sea vegetables, specifically dried wakame	3.0–3.5 g
	Lycopene as tomato products, guava, watermelon, apricots, pink grapefruit, papaya, or supplements	10–20 mg
	Dark chocolate	100 g
	Pomegranate juice or seeds	8 oz. or one cup
	Sesame	60 mg sesamin or 2.5 g sesame meal
Exercise	Aerobic	20 minutes daily at 4200 KJ/week
	Resistance	40 minutes per day
Weight reduction	Body mass index < 25	Lose 1 to 2 lb/week and increase the proportion of lean muscle
	Waist circumference:	
	<35 in. for women	
	<40 in. for men	
	Total body fat:	
	<22% for women	
	<16% for men	

(Continued)

TABLE 9.3   (*Continued*)

An Integrative Approach to the Treatment of Hypertension

Intervention Category	Therapeutic Intervention	Daily Intake
Other lifestyle recommendations	Alcohol restriction: Among the choice of alcohol, red wine is preferred due to its vasoactive phytonutrients	<20 g/day Wine <10 oz. Beer <24 oz. Liquor <2 oz.
	Caffeine restriction or elimination depending on CYP450 type	<100 mg/day
	Tobacco and smoking	Stop
Medical considerations	Medications that may increase blood pressure	Minimize use when possible, such as by using disease-specific nutritional interventions
Supplemental foods and nutrients	ALA with biotin	100–200 mg twice daily
	Amino acids:	
	Arginine	5 g twice daily
	Carnitine	1 to 2 g twice daily
	Taurine	1–3 g twice daily
	CGAs	150–200 mg
	Coenzyme Q10	100 mg once to twice daily
	Grape seed extract	300 mg
	Hawthorn extract	500 mg twice a day
	Melatonin	2.5 mg
	NAC	500 mg twice a day
	Olive leaf extract (oleuropein)	500 mg twice a day
	Pycnogenol	200 mg
	Quercetin	500 mg twice a day
	Resveratrol (trans)	250 mg
	Vitamin B6	100 mg once to twice daily
	Vitamin C	250–500 mg twice daily
	Vitamin D3	Dose to raise 25-hydroxyvitamin D serum level to 60 ng/mL
	Vitamin E as mixed tocopherols	400 IU

REFERENCES

1. Houston MC. Treatment of hypertension with nutraceuticals. Vitamins, antioxidants and minerals. *Exper Rev Cardiovasc Ther* 2007;5(4):681–691.
2. Eaton SB, Eaton SB III, Konner MJ. Paleolithic nutrition revisited: A twelve-year retrospective on its nature and implications. *Eur J Clin Nutr* 1997;51:207–216.
3. Houston MC, Harper KJ. Potassium, magnesium, and calcium: Their role in both the cause and treatment of hypertension. *J Clin Hypertens* 2008;10(7 suppl 2):3–11.
4. Layne J, Majkova Z, Smart EJ, Toborek M, Hennig B. Caveolae: A regulatory platform for nutritional modulation of inflammatory diseases. *J Nutr Biochem* 2011;22:807–811.
5. Dandona P, Ghanim H, Chaudhuri A, Dhindsa S, Kim SS. Macronutrient intake induces oxidative and inflammatory stress: Potential relevance to atherosclerosis and insulin resistance. *Exp Mol Med* 2010;42(4):245–253.
6. Berdanier CD. Nutrient-gene interactions. In: Ziegler EE, Filer LJ Jr, editors. *Present Knowledge in Nutrition*, 7th Ed. Washington, DC: ILSI Press; 1996, pp 574–580.

7. Talmud PJ, Waterworth DM. In-vivo and in-vitro nutrient-gene interactions. *Curr Opin Lipidol* 2000;11:31–36.
8. Lundberg AM, Yan ZQ. Innate immune recognition receptors and damage-associated molecular patterns in plaque inflammation. *Curr Opin Lipidol* 2011;22(5):343–349.
9. Zhao L, Lee JY, Hwang DH. Inhibition of pattern recognition receptor-mediated inflammation by bioactive phytochemicals. *Nutr Rev* 2011;69(6):310–320.
10. Houston MC. The importance of potassium in managing hypertension. *Curr Hypertens Rep* 2011; 13(4):309–317.
11. Broadhurst CL. Balanced intakes of natural triglycerides for optimum nutrition: An evolutionary and phytochemical perspective. *Med Hypotheses* 1997;49:247–261.
12. Eftekhari A, Mathiassen ON, Buus NH, Gotzsche O, Mulvany MJ, Christensen KL. Disproportionally impaired microvascular structure in essential hypertension. *J Hypertens* 2011;29(5):896–905.
13. Touyz RM. New insights into mechanisms of hypertension. *Curr Opin Nephrol Hypertens* 2012;21(2):119–121.
14. Xing T, Wang F, Li J, Wang N. Hypertension: An immunologic disease? *J Hypertens* 2012; 30(12):2440–2441.
15. Giannattasio C, Cattaneo BM, Mangoni AA et al. Cardiac and vascular structural changes in normotensive subjects with parental hypertension. *J Hypertens* 1995;13(2):259–264.
16. Goncharov A, Bloom M, Pavuk M, Birman I, Carpenter DO. Blood pressure and hypertension in relation to levels of serum polychlorinated biphenyls in residents of Anniston, Alabama. *J Hypertens* 2010;28(10):2053–2060.
17. Houston MC. Role of mercury toxicity in hypertension, cardiovascular disease, and stroke. *J Clin Hypertens (Greenwich)* 2011;13(8):621–627.
18. Al-Ghamdi A. Role of herpes simplex virus-1, cytomegalovirus and Epstein-Barr virus in atherosclerosis. *Pak J Pharm Sci* 2012;25(1):89–97.
19. Kotronias D, Kapranos N. Herpes simplex virus as a determinant risk factor for coronary artery atherosclerosis and myocardial infarction. *In Vivo* 2005;19(2):351–357.
20. Grahame-Clarke C, Chan NN, Andrew D et al. Human cytomegalovirus seropositivity is associated with impaired vascular function. *Circulation* 2003;108(6):678–683.
21. Nayak DU, Karmen C, Frishman WH, Vakili BA. Antioxidant vitamins and enzymatic and synthetic oxygen-derived free radical scavengers in the prevention and treatment of cardiovascular disease. *Heart Disease* 2001;3:28–45.
22. Kizhakekuttu TJ, Widlansky ME. Natural antioxidants and hypertension: Promise and challenges. *Cardiovasc Ther* 2010;28(4):e20–e32.
23. Kitiyakara C, Wilcox C. Antioxidants for hypertension. *Curr Opin Nephrol Hypertens* 1998;7:531–538.
24. Russo C, Olivieri O, Girelli D et al. Antioxidant status and lipid peroxidation in patients with essential hypertension. *J Hypertens* 1998;16:1267–1271.
25. Tse WY, Maxwell SR, Thomason H et al. Antioxidant status in controlled and uncontrolled hypertension and its relationship to endothelial damage. *J Hum Hypertens* 1994;8:843–849.
26. Mansego ML, Solar Gde M, Alonso MP et al. Polymorphisms of antioxidant enzymes, blood pressure and risk of hypertension. *J Hypertens* 2011;29(3):492–500.
27. Galley HF, Thornton J, Howdle PD, Walker BE, Webster NR. Combination oral antioxidant supplementation reduces blood pressure. *Clin Sci* 1997;92:361–365.
28. Dhalla NS, Temsah RM, Netticadam T. The role of oxidative stress in cardiovascular diseases. *J Hypertens* 2000;18:655–673.
29. Saez G, Tormos MC, Giner V, Lorano JV, Chaves FJ. Oxidative stress and enzymatic antioxidant mechanisms in essential hypertension. *Am J Hypertens* 2001;14:248A. Abstract P-653.
30. Nishihara M, Hirooka Y, Matsukawa R, Kishi T, Sunagawa K. Oxidative stress in the rostral ventrolateral medulla modulates excitatory and inhibitory inputs in spontaneously hypertensive rats. *J Hypertens* 2012;30(1):97–106.
31. Konno S, Hirooka Y, Kishi T, Sunagawa K. Sympathoinhibitory effects of telmisartan through the reduction of oxidative stress in the rostral ventrolateral medulla of obesity-induced hypertensive rats *J Hypertens* 2012;30(10):1992–1999.
32. Ghanem FA, Movahed A. Inflammation in high blood pressure: A clinician perspective. *J Am Soc Hypertens* 2007;1(2):113–119.
33. Amer MS, Elawam AE, Khater MS et al. Association of high–sensitivity C reactive protein with carotid artery intima-media thickness in hypertensive older adults. *J Am Soc Hypertens* 2011;5:395–400.

34. Vongpatanasin W, Thomas GD, Schwartz R et al. C-reactive protein causes downregulation of vascular angiotensin subtype 2 receptors and systolic hypertension in mice. *Circulation* 2007;115(8): 1020–1028.

35. Razzouk, Munter P, Bansilal S et al. C reactive protein predicts long-term mortality independently of low-density lipoprotein cholesterol in patients undergoing percutaneous coronary intervention. *Am Heart J* 2009;158(2):277–283.

36. Kvakan H, Luft FC, Muller DN. Role of the immune system in hypertensive target organ damage. *Trends Cardiovasc Med* 2009;19(7):242–246.

37. Rodriquez-Iturbe B, Franco M, Tapia E, Quiroz Y, Johnson RJ. Renal inflammation, autoimmunity and salt-sensitive hypertension. *Clin Exp Pharmacol Physiol* 2012;39(1):96–103.

38. Tian N, Penman AD, Mawson AR, Manning RD Jr, Flessner MF. Association between circulating specific leukocyte types and blood pressure. The Atherosclerosis Risk in Communities (ARIC) study. *J Am Soc Hypertens* 2010;4(6):272–283.

39. Muller DN, Kvakan H, Luft FC. Immune-related effects in hypertension on and target-organ damage. *Curr Opin Nephrol Hypertens* 2011;20(2):113–117.

40. Marketou ME, Kontaraki JE, Zacharis EA et al. TLR2 and TLR4 gene expression in peripheral monocytes in nondiabetic hypertensive patients: The effect of intensive blood pressure-lowering. *J Clin Hypertens (Greenwich)* 2012;14(5):330–335.

41. Luft FC. Neural regulation of the immune system modulates hypertension-induced target-organ damage. *J Am Soc Hypertens* 2012;6(1):23–26.

42. Herrada AA, Campino C, Amador CA, Michea LF, Fardella CE, Kalergis AM. Aldosterone as a modulator of immunity: Implications in the organ damage. *J Hypertens* 2011;29(9):1684–1692.

43. Colussi G, Catena C, Sechi LA. Spironolactone, eplerenone and the new aldosterone blockers in endocrine and primary hypertension. *J Hypertens* 2013;31(1):3–15.

44. Appel LJ, Moore TJ, Obarzanek E et al. A clinical trial of the effects of dietary patterns on blood pressure. DASH Collaborative *N Engl J Med* 1997;336(16):1117–1124.

45. Sacks FM, Svetkey LP, Vollmer WM et al. Effects on blood pressure of reduced dietary sodium and the Dietary Approaches to Stop Hypertension (DASH) diet. DASH-Sodium Collaborative Research Group. *N Engl J Med* 2001;344(1):3–10.

46. Sun B, Williams JS, Svetkey LP, Kolatkar NS, Conlin PR. Beta2-adrenergic receptor genotype affects the renin-angiotensin-aldosterone system response to the Dietary Approaches to Stop Hypertension (DASH) dietary pattern. *Am J Clin Nutr* 2010;92(2):444–449.

47. Chen Q, Turban S, Miller ER, Appel LJ. The effects of dietary patterns on plasma renin activity: Results from the Dietary Approaches to Stop Hypertension trial. *J Hum Hypertens* 2012;26(11):664–669.

48. Al-Solaiman Y, Jesri A, Zhao Y, Morrow JD, Egan BM. Low-sodium DASH reduces oxidative stress and improves vascular function in salt-sensitive humans. *J Hum Hypertens* 2009;23(12):826–835.

49. Lin PH, Allen JD, Li Y J, Yu M, Lien LF, Svetkey LP. Blood pressure-lowering mechanisms of the DASH dietary pattern. *J Nutr Metab* 2012;2012:472396.

50. Kotchen TA, McCarron DA. AHA Science Advisory. Dietary electrolytes and blood pressure. *Circulation* 1998;98:613–617.

51. Cutler JA, Follmann, Allender PS. Randomized trials of sodium reduction: An overview. *Am J Clin Nutr* 1997;65:643S–651S.

52. Svetkey LP, Sacks FM, Obarzanek E et al. The DASH diet, sodium intake and blood pressure (the DASH-Sodium Study): Rationale and design. *JADA* 1999;99:S96–S104.

53. Kawada T, Suzuki S. Attention of salt awareness to prevent hypertension in the young. *J Clin Hypertens (Greenwich)* 2011;13(12):933–934.

54. Weinberger MH. Salt sensitivity of blood pressure in humans. *Hypertension* 1996;27:481–490.

55. Morimoto A, Usu T, Fujii T et al. Sodium sensitivity and cardiovascular events in patients with essential hypertension. *Lancet* 1997;350:1734–1737.

56. Tomonari T, Fukuda M, Miura T et al. Is salt intake an independent risk factor of stroke mortality? Demographic analysis by regions in Japan. *J Am Soc Hypertens* 2011;5(6):456–462.

57. Kanbay M, Chen Y, Solak Y, Sanders PW. Mechanisms and consequences of salt sensitivity and dietary salt intake. *Curr Opin Nephrol Hypertens* 2011;20(1):37–43.

58. Dubach JM, Das S, Rosenzweig A, Clark HA. Visualizing sodium dynamics in isolated cardiomyocytes using fluorescent nanosensors. *Proc Natl Acad Sci USA* 2009;106(38):16145–16150.

59. Oberleithner H, Callies C, Kusche-Vihrog K et al. Potassium softens vascular endothelium and increases nitric oxide release. *Proc Natl Acad Sci USA* 2009;106(8):2829–2834.

60. Oberleithner H, Riethmüller C, Schillers H et al. Plasma sodium stiffens vascular endothelium and reduces nitric oxide. *Proc Natl Acad Sci USA* 2007;104(41):16281–16286.
61. Fels J, Oberleithner H, Kusche-Vihrog K. Ménageàtrois: Aldosterone, sodium and nitric oxide in vascular endothelium. *Biochim Biophys Acta* 2010;1802(12):1193–1202.
62. Oberleithner H, Kusche-Vihrog K, Schillers H. Endothelial cells as vascular salt sensors. *Kidney Int* 2010;77(6):490–494.
63. Kusche-Vihrog K, Callies C, Fels J, Oberleithner H. The epithelial sodium channel (ENaC): Mediator of the aldosterone response in the vascular endothelium? *Steroids* 2010;75(8–9):544–549.
64. Fels J, Callies C, Kusche-Vihrog K, Oberleithner H. Nitric oxide release follows endothelial nanomechanics and not vice versa. *Pflugers Arch* 2010;460(5):915–923.
65. Callies C, Fels J, Liashkovich I et al. Membrane potential depolarization decreases the stiffness of vascular endothelial cells. *J Cell Sci* 2011;124(Pt 11):1936–1942.
66. Kusche-Vihrog K, Urbanova K, Blanqué A et al. C-reactive protein makes human endothelium stiff and tight. *Hypertension* 2011;57(2):231–237.
67. Foulquier S, Dupuis F, Perrin-Sarrado C et al. High salt intake abolishes AT (2)-mediated vasodilation of pial arterioles in rats. *J Hypertens* 2011;29(7):1392–1399.
68. Kusche-Vihrog K, Oberleithner H. An emerging concept of vascular salt sensitivity. *F1000 Biol Rep* 2012;4:20.
69. Popov S, Silveira A, Wågsäter D et al. Salt-inducible kinase 1 influences Na (+),K (+)-ATPase activity in vascular smooth muscle cells and associates with variations in blood pressure. *J Hypertens* 2011;29(12):2395–2403.
70. Houston MC. Nutraceuticals, vitamins, antioxidants and mineral in the prevention and treatment of hypertension. *Prog Cardiovasc Dis* 2005;47(6):396–449.
71. Houston MC. Nutrition and nutraceutical supplements in the treatment of hypertension. *Exper Rev Cardiovasc Ther* 2010;8(6):821–833.
72. Messerli FH, Schmieder RE, Weir MR. Salt: A perpetrator of hypertensive target organ disease? *Arch Intern Med* 1997;157:2449–2452.
73. Kawasaki T, Delea CS, Bartter FC, Smith H. The effect of high-sodium and low-sodium intakes on blood pressure and other related variables in human subjects with idiopathic hypertension. *Am J Med* 1978;64:193–198.
74. Toda N, Arakawa K. Salt-induced hemodynamic regulation mediated by nitric oxide. *J Hypertens* 2011;29(3):415–424.
75. Oliver WJ, Cohen EL, Neel JV. Blood pressure, sodium intake, and sodium related hormones in the Yanomamo Indians, a "no-salt" culture. *Circulation* 1975;52(1):146–151.
76. Whelton PK, He J. Potassium in preventing and treating high blood pressure. *Semin Nephrol* 1999;19:494–499.
77. Gu D, He J, Xigui W, Duan X, Whelton PK. Effect of potassium supplementation on blood pressure in Chinese: A randomized, placebo-controlled trial. *J Hypertens* 2001;19:1325–1331.
78. Houston MC. The importance of potassium in managing hypertension. *Curr Hypertens Rep* 2011;13(4):309–317.
79. He J, Gu D, Kelly TN etal. Genetic variants in the renin-angiotensin-aldosterone system and blood pressure responses to potassium intake. *J Hypertens* 2011;29(9):1719–1730.
80. O'Donnell MJ, Yusuf S, Mente A et al. Urinary sodium and potassium excretion and risk of cardiovascular events. *JAMA* 2011;306(20):2229–2238.
81. Widman L, Wester PO, Stegmayr BG, Wirell MP. The dose dependent reduction in blood pressure through administration of magnesium: A double blind placebo controlled cross-over trial. *Am J Hypertens* 1993;6:41–45.
82. Laurant P, Touyz RM. Physiological and pathophysiological role of magnesium in the cardiovascular system: Implications in hypertension. *J Hypertens* 2000;18:1177–1191.
83. Houston M. The role of magnesium in hypertension and cardiovascular disease. *J Clin Hypertens (Greenwich)* 2011;13(11):843–847.
84. Rosanoff A, Weaver CM, Rude RK. Suboptimal magnesium status in theUnited States: Are the health consequences underestimated? *Nutr Rev* 2012;70(3):153–164.
85. Song Y, Liu S. Magnesium for cardiovascular health: Time for intervention. *Am J Clin Nutr* 2012;95(2):269–270.
86. Kupetsky-Rincon EA, Uitto J. Magnesium: Novel applications in cardiovascular disease—A review of the literature. *Ann Nutr Metab* 2012;61(2):102–110.

87. Cunha AR, Umbelino B, Correia ML, Neves MF. Magnesium and vascular changes in hypertension. *Int J Hypertens* 2012;2012:754250.

88. Kass L, Weekes J, Carpenter L. Effect of magnesium supplementation on blood pressure: A meta-analysis. *Eur J Clin Nutr* 2012;66(4):411–418.

89. McCarron DA. Role of adequate dietary calcium intake in the prevention and management of salt sensitive hypertensive. *Am J Clin Nutr* 1997;65:712S–716S.

90. Resnick LM. Calcium metabolism in hypertension and allied metabolic disorders. *Diabetes Care* 1991;14:505–520.

91. Garcia Zozaya JL, Padilla Viloria M. Alterations of calcium, magnesium, and zinc in essential hypertension: Their relation to the renin-angiotensin-aldosterone system. *Invest Clin* 1997;38:27–40.

92. Carpenter WE, Lam D, Toney GM, Weintraub NL, Qin Z. Zinc, copper, and blood pressure: Human population studies. *Med Sci Monit* 2013;19:1–8.

93. Shahbaz AU, Sun Y, Bhattacharya SK et al. Fibrosis in hypertensive heart disease: Molecular pathways and cardioprotective strategies. *J Hypertens* 2010;28:S25–S32.

94. Bergomi M, Rovesti S, Vinceti M, Vivoli R, Caselgrandi E, Vivoli G. Zinc and copper status and blood pressure. *J Trace Elem Med Biol* 1997;11:166–169.

95. Stamler J, Elliott P, Kesteloot H et al. Inverse relation of dietary protein markers with blood pressure. Findings for 10,020 men and women in the Intersalt Study. Intersalt Cooperative Research Group. International study of salt and blood pressure. *Circulation* 1996;94:1629–1634.

96. Altorf-van der Kuil W, Engberink MF, Brink EJ et al. Dietary protein and blood pressure: A systematic review. *PLoS One* 2010;5(8);e12102–e12117.

97. Jenkins DJ, Kendall CW, Faulkner DA et al. Long-term effects of a plant-based dietary portfolio of cholesterol-lowering foods on blood pressure. *Eur J Clin Nutr* 2008;62(6):781–788.

98. Elliott P, Dennis B, Dyer AR et al. Relation of Dietary Protein (Total, Vegetable, Animal) to Blood Pressure: INTERMAP Epidemiologic Study. Presented at the 18th Scientific Meeting of the International Society of Hypertension, Chicago, IL, August 20–24, 2000.

99. Rebholz CM, Friedman EE, Powers LJ, Arroyave WD, He J, Kelly TN. Dietary protein intake and blood pressure: A meta-analysis of randomized controlled trials. *Am J Epidemiol* 2012;176(suppl 7):S27–S43.

100. Larsson SC, Virtamo J, Wolk A. Dietary protein intake and risk of stroke in women. *Atherosclerosis* 2012;224(1):247–251.

101. He J, Wofford MR, Reynolds K et al. Effect of dietary protein supplementation on blood pressure: A randomized controlled trial. *Circulation* 2011;124(5):589–595.

102. Teunissen-Beekman KF, Dopheide J, Geleijnse JM et al. Protein supplementation lowers blood pressure in overweight adults: Effect of dietary proteins on blood pressure (PROPRES), a randomized trial. *Am J Clin Nutr* 2012;95(4):966–971.

103. FitzGerald RJ, Murray BA, Walsh DJ. Hypotensive peptides from milk proteins. *J Nutr* 2004;134(4):980S–988S.

104. Pins JJ, Keenan JM. Effects of whey peptides on cardiovascular disease risk factors. *J Clin Hypertens* 2006;8(11):775–782.

105. Aihara K, Kajimoto O, Takahashi R, Nakamura Y. Effect of powdered fermented milk with *Lactobacillus helveticus* on subjects with high-normal blood pressure or mild hypertension. *J Am Coll Nutr* 2005;24(4):257–265.

106. Gemino FW, Neutel J, Nonaka M, Hendler SS. The impact of lactotripeptides on blood pressure response in stage 1 and stage 2 hypertensives. *J Clin Hypertens* 2010;12(3):153–159.

107. Geleijnse JM, Engberink MF. Lactopeptides and human blood pressure. *Curr Opin Lipidol* 2010;21(1):58–63.

108. Cicero AF, Aubin F, Azais-Braesco V, Borghi C. Do the lactotripeptides isoleucine-proline-proline and valine-proline-proline reduce systolic blood pressure in European subjects? A meta-analysis of randomized controlled trials. *Am J Hypertens* 2013;26(3):442–449.

109. Usinger L, Reimer C, Ibsen H. Fermented milk for hypertension. *Cochrane Database Syst Rev* 2012;4.

110. Ricci-Cabello I, Herrera MO, Artacho R. Possible role of milk-derived bioactive peptides in the treatment and prevention of metabolic syndrome. *Nutr Rev* 2012;70(4):241–255.

111. Jauhiainen T, Niittynen L, Orešič M et al. Effects of long-term intake of lactotripeptides on cardiovascular risk factors in hypertensive subjects. *Eur J Clin Nutr* 2012;66(7):843–849.

112. Pins J, Keenan J. The antihypertensive effects of a hydrolyzed whey protein supplement. *Cardiovasc Drugs Ther* 2002;16(suppl):68.

113. Pal S, Radavelli-Bagatini S. The effects of whey protein on cardiometabolic risk factors. *Obes Rev* 2013;14(4):324–343.

114. Zhu CF, Li GZ, Peng HB, Zhang F, Chen Y, Li Y. Therapeutic effects of marine collagen peptides on Chinese patients with type 2 diabetes mellitus and primary hypertension. *Am J Med Sci* 2010;340(5):360–366.
115. De Leo F, Panarese S, Gallerani R, Ceci LR. Angiotensin converting enzyme (ACE) inhibitory peptides: Production and implementation of functional food. *Curr Pharm Des* 2009;15(31):3622–3643.
116. Lordan S, Ross P, Stanton C. Marine bioactives as functional food ingredients: Potential to reduce the incidence of chronic disease. *Drugs* 2011;9(6):1056–1100.
117. Fujita H, Yoshikawa M. LKPNM: A prodrug-type ACE-inhibitory peptide derived from fish protein. *Immunopharmacology* 1999;44(1–2):123–127.
118. Kawasaki T, Seki E, Osajima K et al. Antihypertensive effect of valyl-tyrosine, a short chain peptide derived from sardine muscle hydrolyzate, on mild hypertensive subjects. *J Hum Hypertens* 2000;14:519–523.
119. Kawasaki T, Jun CJ, Fukushima Y, Seki E. Antihypertensive effect and safety evaluation of vegetable drink with peptides derived from sardine protein hydrolysates on mild hypertensive, high-normal and normal blood pressure subjects. *Fukuoka Igaku Zasshi* 2002;93(10):208–218.
120. Yang G, Shu XO, Jin F et al. Longitudinal study of soy food intake and blood pressure among middle-aged and elderly Chinese women. *Am J Clin Nutr* 2005;81(5):1012–1017.
121. Teunissen-Beekman KF, Dopheide J, Geleijnse JM et al. Protein supplementation lowers blood pressure in overweight adults: Effect of dietary proteins on blood pressure (PROPRES), a randomized trial. *Am J Clin Nutr* 2012;95(4):966–971.
122. Dong JY, Tong X, Wu ZW, Xun PC, He K, Qin LQ. Effect of soya protein on blood pressure: A meta-analysis of randomised controlled trials. *Br J Nutr* 2011;106(3):317–326.
123. Teede HJ, Giannopoulos D, Dalais FS, Hodgson J, McGrath BP. Randomised, controlled, cross-over trial of soy protein with isoflavones on blood pressure and arterial function in hypertensive patients. *J Am Coll Nutr* 2006;25(6):533–540.
124. Welty FK, Lee KS, Lew NS, Zhou JR. Effect of soy nuts on blood pressure and lipid levels in hypertensive, prehypertensive and normotensive postmenopausl women. *Arch Inter Med* 2007;167(10):1060–1067.
125. Rosero Arenas MA, Roser Arenas E, Portaceli Arminana MA, Garcia MA. Usefulness of phyto-oestrogens in reduction of blood pressure. Systematic review and meta-analysis. *Aten Primaria* 2008;40(4):177–186.
126. Nasca MM, Zhou JR, Welty FK. Effect of soy nuts on adhesion molecules and markers of inflammation in hypertensive and normotensive postmenopausal women. *Am J Cardiol* 2008;102(1):84–86.
127. He J, Gu D, Wu X et al. Effect of soybean protein on blood pressure: A randomized, controlled trial. *Ann Intern Med* 2005;143(1):1–9.
128. Hasler CM, Kundrat S, Wool D. Functional foods and cardiovascular disease. *Curr Atheroscler Rep* 2000;2(6):467–475.
129. Tikkanen MJ, Adlercreutz H. Dietary soy-derived isoflavone phytoestrogens. Could they have a role in coronary heart disease prevention? *Biochem Pharmacol* 2000;60(1):1–5.
130. Begg DP, Sinclari AJ, Stahl LA, Garg ML, Jois M, Weisinger RS. Dietary proteins level interacts with omega-3 polyunsaturated fatty acid deficiency to induce hypertension. *Am J Hypertens* 2010;23(2):125–128.
131. Vallance P, Leone A, Calver A, Collier J, Moncada S. Endogenous dimethyl-arginine as an inhibitor of nitric oxide synthesis. *J Cardiovasc Pharmacol* 1992;20:S60–S62.
132. Sonmez A, Celebi G, Erdem G et al. Plasma apelin and ADMA levels in patients with essential hypertension. *Clin Exp Hypertens* 2010;32(3):179–183.
133. Michell DL, Andrews KL, Chin-Dusting JP. Endothelial dysfunction in hypertension: The role of arginase. *Front Biosci (Schol Ed)* 2011;3:946–960.
134. Rajapakse NW, Mattson DL. Role of L-arginine in nitric oxide production in health and hypertension. *Clin Exp Pharmacol Physiol* 2009;36(3):249–255.
135. Tsioufis C, Dimitriadis K, Andrikou E et al. ADMA, C-reactive protein and albuminuria in untreated essential hypertension: A cross-sectional study. *Am J Kidney Dis* 2010;55(6):1050–1059.
136. Rajapakse NW, Mattson DL. Role of cellular L-arginine uptake and nitric oxide production on renal blood flow and arterial pressure regulation. *Curr Opin Nephrol Hypertens* 2013;22(1):45–50.
137. Ruiz-Hurtado G, Delgado C. Nitric oxide pathway in hypertrophied heart: New therapeutic uses of nitric oxide donors. *J Hypertens* 2010;28(suppl 1):S56–S61.
138. Siani A, Pagano E, Iacone R, Iacoviell L, Scopacasa F, Strazzullo P. Blood pressure and metabolic changes during dietary L-arginine supplementation in humans. *Am J Hypertens* 2000;13:547–551.
139. Facchinetti F, Saade GR, Neri I, Pizzi C, Longo M, Volpe A. L-arginine supplementation in patients with gestational hypertension: A pilot study. *Hypertens Pregnancy* 2007;26(1):121–130.

140. Neri I, Monari F, Sqarbi L, Berardi A, Masellis G, Facchinetti F. L-arginine supplementation in women with chronic hypertension: Impact on blood pressure and maternal and neonatal complications. *J Matern Fetal Neonatal Med* 2010;23(12):1456–1460.

141. Martina V, Masha A, Gigliardi VR et al. Long-term *N*-acetylcysteine and L-arginine administration reduces endothelial activation and systolic blood pressure in hypertensive patients with type 2 diabetes. *Diabetes Care* 2008;31(5):940–944.

142. Ast J, Jablecka A, Bogdanski I, Krauss H, Chmara E. Evaluation of the antihypertensive effect of L-arginine supplementation in patients with mild hypertension assessed with ambulatory blood pressure monitoring. *Med Sci Monit* 2010;16(5):CR266–CR271.

143. Dong JY, Qin LQ, Zhang Z et al. Effect of oral L-arginine supplementation on blood pressure: A meta-analysis of randomized, double-blind, placebo-controlled trials. *Am Heart J* 2011;162(6):959–965.

144. Schulman SP, Becker LC, Kass DA et al. L-arginine therapy in acute myocardial infarction: The vascular interaction with age in myocardial infarction (VINTAGE MI) randomized clinical trial. *JAMA* 2006;295(1):58–64.

145. Miller GD, Marsh AP, Dove RW et al. Plasma nitrate and nitrite are increased by a high-nitrate supplement but not by high-nitrate foods in older adults. *Nutr Res* 2012;32(3):160–168.

146. Miguel-Carrasco JL, Monserrat MT, Mate A, Vázquez CM. Comparative effects of captopril and L-carnitine on blood pressure and antioxidant enzyme gene expression in the heart of spontaneously hypertensive rats. *Eur J Pharmacol* 2010;632(1–3):65–72.

147. Zambrano S, Blanca AJ, Ruiz-Armenta MV et al. L-carnitine protects against arterial hypertension-related cardiac fibrosis through modulation of PPAR-γ expression. *Biochem Pharmacol* 2013;85(7): 937–934.

148. Vilskersts R, Kuka J, Svalbe B et al. Administration of L-carnitine and mildronate improves endothelial function and decreases mortality in hypertensive Dahl rats. *Pharmacol Rep* 2011;63(3):752–762.

149. Mate A, Miguel-Carrasco JL, Monserrat MT, Vázquez CM. Systemic antioxidant properties of L-carnitine in two different models of arterial hypertension. *J Physiol Biochem* 2010;66(2):127–136.

150. Digiesi V, Cantini F, Bisi G, Guarino G, Brodbeck B. L-carnitine adjuvant therapy in essential hypertension. *Clin Ter* 1994;144:391–395.

151. Ghidini O, Azzurro M, Vita G, Sartori G. Evaluation of the therapeutic efficacy of L-carnitine in congestive heart failure. *Int J Clin Pharmacol Ther Toxicol* 1988;26(4):217–220.

152. Digiesi V, Palchetti R, Cantini F. The benefits of L-carnitine therapy in essential arterial hypertension with diabetes mellitus type II. *Minerva Med* 1989;80(3):227–231.

153. Ruggenenti P, Cattaneo D, Loriga G et al. Ameliorating hypertension and insulin resistance in subjects at increased cardiovascular risk: Effects of acetyl-L-carnitine therapy. *Hypertension* 2009;54(3):567–574.

154. Mate A, Miguel-Carrasco JL, Vázquez CM. The therapeutic prospects of using L-carnitine to manage hypertension-related organ damage. *Drug Discov Today* 2010;15(11–12):484–492.

155. Korkmaz S, Yıldız G, Kılıçlı F et al. Low L-carnitine levels: Can it be a cause of nocturnal blood pressure changes in patients with type 2 diabetes mellitus? *Anadolu Kardiyol Derg* 2011;11(1):57–63.

156. Huxtable RJ. Physiologic actions of taurine. *Physiol Rev* 1992;72:101–163.

157. Fujita T, Ando K, Noda H, Ito Y, Sato Y. Effects of increased adrenomedullary activity and taurine in young patients with borderline hypertension. *Circulation* 1987;75:525–532.

158. Huxtable RJ, Sebring LA. Cardiovascular actions of taurine. *Prog Clin Biol Res* 1983;125:5–37.

159. Feng Y, Li J, Yang J, Yang Q, Lv Q, Gao Y, Hu J. Synergistic effects of taurine and L-arginine on attenuating insulin resistance hypertension. *Adv Exp Med Biol* 2013;775:427–435.

160. Wójcik OP, Koenig KL, Zeleniuch-Jacquotte A, Pearte C, Costa M, Chen Y. Serum taurine and risk of coronary heart disease: A prospective, nested case-control study. *Eur J Nutr* 2013;52(1):169–178.

161. Abebe W, Mozaffari MS. Role of taurine in the vasculature: An overview of experimental and human studies. *Am J Cardiovasc Dis* 2011;1(3):293–311.

162. Yamori Y, Taguchi T, Hamada A et al. Taurine in health and diseases: Consistent evidence from experimental and epidemiological studies. *J Biomed Sci* 2010;17(suppl 1):S6.

163. Yamori Y, Taguchi T, Mori H, Mori M. Low cardiovascular risks in the middle aged males and females excreting greater 24-hour urinary taurine and magnesium in 41WHO-CARDIAC study populations in the world. *J Biomed Sci* 2010;17(suppl 1):S21.

164. Tanabe Y, Urata H, Kiyonaga A et al. Changes in serum concentrations of taurine and other amino acids in clinical antihypertensive exercise therapy. *Clin Exp Hypertens* 1989;11:149–165.

165. Mori TA, Bao DQ, Burke V, Puddey IB, Beilin LJ. Docosahexaenoic acid but not eicosapentaenoic acid lowers ambulatory blood pressure and heart rate in humans. *Hypertension* 1999;34:253–260.

166. Bønaa KH, Bjerve KS, Straume B, Gram IT, Thelle D. Effect of eicosapentaenoic and docosahexanoic acids on blood pressure in hypertension: A population-based intervention trial from the Tromso study. *N Engl J Med* 1990;322:795–801.
167. Mori TA, Burke V, Puddey I, Irish A. The effects of omega 3 fatty acids and coenzyme Q 10 on blood pressure and heart rate in chronic kidney disease: A randomized controlled trial. *J Hypertens* 2009;27(9):1863–1872.
168. Ueshima H, Stamler J, Elliot B, Brown CQ. Food omega 3 fatty acid intake of individuals (total, linolenic acid, long chain) and their blood pressure: INTERMAP study. *Hypertension* 2007;50 (20):313–319.
169. Mon TA. Omega 3 fatty acids and hypertension in humans. *Clin Exp Pharmacol Physiol* 2006;33(9):842–846.
170. Noreen EE, Brandauer J. The effects of supplemental fish oil on blood pressure and morning cortisol in normotensive adults: A pilot study. *J Complement Integr Med* 2012;9.
171. BhiseA, Krishnan PV, Aggarwal R, Gaiha M, Bhattacharjee J. Effect of low-dose omega-3 fatty acids substitution on blood pressure, hyperinsulinemia and dyslipidemia in Indians with essential hypertension: A pilot study. *Indian J Clin Biochem* 2005;20(2):4–9.
172. Cabo J, Alonso R, Mata P. Omega-3 fatty acids and blood pressure. *Br J Nutr* 2012;107(suppl 2): S195–S200.
173. Huang T, Shou T, Cai N, Wahlqvist ML, Li D. Associations of plasma n-3 polyunsaturated fatty acids with blood pressure and cardiovascular risk factors among Chinese. *Int J Food Sci Nutr* 2012;63(6):667–673.
174. Sagara M, Njelekela M, Teramoto T et al. Effects of docosahexaenoic acid supplementation on blood pressure, heart rate, and serum lipids in Scottish men with hypertension and hypercholesterolemia. *Int J Hypertens* 2011;2011:809198.
175. Passfall J, Philipp T, Woermann F, Quass P, Thiede M, Haller H. Different effects of eicosapentaenoic acid and olive oil on blood pressure, intracellular free platelet calcium, and plasma lipids in patients with essential hypertension. *Clin Investig* 1993;71(8):628–633.
176. Liu JC, Conklin SM, Manuck SB, Yao JK, Muldoon MF. Long-chain omega-3 fatty acids and blood pressure. *Am J Hypertens* 2011;24(10):1121–1126.
177. Engler MM, Schambelan M, Engler MB, Goodfriend TL. Effects of dietary gamma-linolenic acid on blood pressure and adrenal angiotensin receptors in hypertensive rats. *Proc Soc Exp Biol Med* 1998;218(3):234–237.
178. Sagara M, Njelekela M, Teramoto T et al. Effect of docosahexaenoic acid supplementation on blood pressure, heart rate, and serum lipid in Scottish men with hypertension and hypercholesterolemia. *Int J Hypertens* 2011;8:8091–8098.
179. Mori TA, Burke V, Puddey I et al. The effects of omega 3 fatty acids and coenzyme Q 10 on blood pressure and heart rate in chronic kidney disease: A randomized controlled trial *J Hypertens* 2009;27:1863–1872.
180. Chin JP. Marine oils and cardiovascular reactivity. *Prostaglandins Leukot Essent Fatty Acids* 1994;50:211–222.
181. Saravanan P, Davidson NC, Schmidt EB, Calder PC. Cardiovascular effects of marine omega-3 fatty acids. *Lancet* 2010;376(9740):540–550.
182. Ferrara LA, RaimondiS, d'Episcopa I. Olive oil and reduced need for antihypertensive medications. *Arch Intern Med* 2000;160:837–842.
183. Alonso A, Ruiz-Gutierrez V, Martínez-González MA. Monounsaturated fatty acids, olive oil and blood pressure: Epidemiological, clinical and experimental evidence. *Public Health Nutr* 2006;9(2):251–257.
184. Terés S, Barceló-Coblijn G, Benet M, Alvarez R, Bressani R, Halver JE, Escribá PV. Oleic acid content is responsible for the reduction in blood pressure induced by olive oil. *Proc Natl Acad Sci USA* 2008;105(37):13811–13816.
185. Thomsen C, Rasmussen OW, Hansen KW, Vesterlund M, Hermansen K. Comparison of the effects on the diurnal blood pressure, glucose, and lipid levels of a diet rich in monounsaturated fatty acids with a diet rich in polyunsaturated fatty acids in type 2 diabetic subjects. *Diabet Med* 1995;12:600–606.
186. Cherif S, Rahal N, Haouala M et al. A clinical trial of a titrated Olea extract in the treatment of essential arterial hypertension. *J Pharm Belg* 1996;51(2):69–71.
187. Psaltopoulou T,Naska A, Orfanos P, Trichopoulos D, Mountokalakis T, Trichopoulou A. Olive oil, the Mediterranean diet, and arterial blood pressure: The Greek European Prospective Investigation into Cancer and Nutrition (EPIC) study. *Am J Clin Nutr* 2004;80(4):1012–1018.
188. Alonso A, Martínez-González MA. Olive oil consumption and reduced incidence of hypertension: The SUN study. *Lipids* 2004;39(12):1233–1238.

189. Perrinjaquet-Moccetti T, Busjahn A, Schmidlin C, Schmidt A, Bradl B, Aydogan C. Food supplementation with an olive (*Olea europaea* L.) leaf extract reduces blood pressure in borderline hypertensive monozygotic twins. *Phytother Res* 2008;22(9):1239–1242.

190. Moreno-Luna R, Muñoz-Hernandez R, Miranda ML et al. Olive oil polyphenols decrease blood pressure and improve endothelial function in young women with mild hypertension. *Am J Hypertens* 2012;25(12):1299–1304.

191. Perona JS, Canizares J, Montero E, Sanchez-Dominquez JM, Catala A, Ruiz-Gutierrez V. Virgin olive oil reduces blood pressure in hypertensive elderly patients. *Clin Nutr* 2004;23(5):1113–1121.

192. Perona JS, Montero E, Sanchez-Dominquez JM, Canizares J, Garcia M, Ruiz-Gutierrez V. Evaluation of the effect of dietary virgin olive oil on blood pressure and lipid composition of serum and low-density lipoprotein in elderly type 2 subjects. *J Agric Food Chem* 2009;57(23):11427–11433.

193. Susalit E, Agus N, Effendi I et al. Olive (*Olea europaea*) leaf extract effective in patients with stage-1 hypertension: Comparison with captopril. *Phytomedicine* 2011;18(4):251–258.

194. Lopez-Miranda J, Perez-Jimenez F, Ros E et al. Olive oil and health: Summary of the II international conference on olive oil and health consensus report, Jaen and Cordoba (Spain) 2008. *Nutr Metab Cardiovasc Dis* 2010;20(4):284–294.

195. Zhang J, Villacorta L, Chang L et al. Nitro-oleic acid inhibits angiotensin II-induced hypertension. *Circ Res* 2010;107(4):540–548.

196. Scheffler A, Rauwald HW, Kampa B, Mann U, Mohr FW, Dhein SJ. *Olea europaea* leaf extract exerts L-type Ca (2+) channel antagonistic effects. *Ethnopharmacol* 2008;120(2):233–240.

197. Papamichael CM, Karatzi KN, Papaioannou TG et al. Acute combined effects of olive oil and wine on pressure wave reflections: Another beneficial influence of the Mediterranean diet antioxidants? *J Hypertens* 2008;26(2):223–229.

198. He J, Whelton PK. Effect of dietary fiber and protein intake on blood pressure: A review of epidemiologic evidence. *Clin Exp Hypertens* 1999;21:785–796.

199. Pruijm M, Wuerzer G, Forni V, Bochud M, Pechere-Bertschi A, Burnier M. Nutrition and hypertension: More than table salt. *Rev Med Suisse* 2010;6(282):1715–1720.

200. Sherman DL, Keaney JF, Biegelsen ES et al. Pharmacological concentrations of ascorbic acid are required for the beneficial effect on endothelial vasomotor function in hypertension. *Hypertension* 2000;35:936–941.

201. Ness AR, Khaw K-T, Bingham S, Day NE. Vitamin C status and blood pressure. *J Hypertens* 1996;14:503–508.

202. Duffy SJ, Bokce N, Holbrook. Treatment of hypertension with ascorbic acid. *Lancet* 1999;354:2048–2049.

203. Enstrom JE, Kanim LE, Klein M. Vitamin C intake and mortality among a sample of the United States population. *Epidemiology* 1992;3:194–202.

204. Block G, Jensen, CD, Norkus EP, Hudes M, Crawford PB. Vitamin C in plasma is inversely related to blood pressure and change in blood pressure during the previous year in young black and white women. *Nutr J* 2008;17(7):35–46.

205. Hatzitolios A, Iliadis F, Katsiki N, Baltatzi M. Is the antihypertensive effect of dietary supplements via aldehydes reduction evidence based: A systemic review. *Clin Exp Hypertens* 2008;30(7):628–639.

206. Mahajan AS, Babbar R, Kansai N, Agarwai, SK, Ray PC. Antihypertensive and antioxidant action of amlodipine and vitamin C in patients of essential hypertension. *J Clin Biochem Nutr* 2007;40(2):141–147.

207. Ledlerc PC, Proulx, CD, Arquin G, Belanger S. Ascorbic acid decreases the binding affinity of the AT! Receptor for angiotensin II. *Am J Hypertens* 2008;21(1):67–71.

208. Plantinga Y, Ghiadone L, Magagna, A, Biannarelli C. Supplementation with vitamins C and E improves arterial stiffness and endothelial function in essential hypertensive patients. *Am J Hypertens* 2007;20(4):392–397.

209. Sato K, Dohi Y, Kojima M, Miyagawa K. Effects of ascorbic acid on ambulatory blood pressure in elderly patients with refractory hypertension. *Arzneimittelforschung* 2006;56(7):535–540.

210. Block G, Mangels AR, Norkus EP, Patterson BH, Levander OA, Taylor PR. Ascorbic acid status and subsequent diastolic and systolic blood pressure. *Hypertension* 2001;37:261–267.

211. McRae MP. Is vitamin C an effective antihypertensive supplement? A review and analysis of the literature. *J Chiropr Med* 2006;5(2):60–64.

212. Simon JA. Vitamin C and cardiovascular disease: A review. *J Am Coll Nutr* 1992;11(2):107–125.

213. Ness AR, Chee D, Elliott P. Vitamin C and blood pressure—An overview. *J Hum Hypertens* 1997;11(6):343–350.

214. Trout DL. Vitamin C and cardiovascular risk factors. *Am J Clin Nutr* 1991;53(suppl 1):322S–325S.

215. National Center for Health Statistics, Fulwood R, Johnson CL, Bryner JD. Hematological and Nutritional Biochemistry Reference Data for Persons 6 Months-74 Years of Age: United States, 1976–1980. Washington, DC; U.S. Public Health Service; 1982 Vital and Health Statistics series 11, No. 232, DHHS publication No. (PHS) 83–1682.

216. Ward NC, Wu JH, Clarke MW, Buddy IB. Vitamin E effects on the treatment of hypertension in type 2 diabetics. *J Hypertension* 2007;227:227–234.

217. Murray ED, Wechter WJ, Kantoci D et al. Endogenous natriuretic factors 7: Biospecificity of a natriuretic gamma-tocopherol metabolite LLU alpha. *J Pharmacol Exp Ther* 1997;282(2):657–662.

218. Gray B, Swick J, Ronnenberg AG. Vitamin E and adiponectin: Proposed mechanism for vitamin E-induced improvement in insulin sensitivity. *Nutr Rev* 2011;69(3):155–161.

219. Hanni LL, Huarfner LH, Sorensen OH, Ljunghall S. Vitamin D is related to blood pressure and other cardiovascular risk factors in middle-aged men. *Am J Hypertens* 1995;8:894–901.

220. Bednarski R, Donderski R, Manitius L. Role of vitamin D in arterial blood pressure control. *Pol Merkur Lekarski* 2007;136:307–310.

221. Ngo DT, Sverdlov AL, McNeil JJ, Horowitz JD. Does vitamin D modulate asymmetric dimethylargine and C-reactive protein concentrations? *Am J Med* 2010;123(4):335–341.

222. Rosen CJ. Clinical practice. Vitamin D insufficiency. *N Engl J Med* 2011;364(3):248–254.

223. Pittas AG, Chung M, Trikalinos T et al. Systematic review: Vitamin D and cardiometabolic outcomes. *Ann Intern Med* 2010;152(5):307–314.

224. Motiwala Sr, Want TJ. Vitamin D and cardiovascular disease. *Curr Opin Nephrol Hypertens* 2011;20(4):345–353.

225. Bhandari SK, Pashayan S, Liu IL et al. 25-hydroxyvitamin D levels and hypertension rates. *J Clin Hypertens* 2011;13(3):170–177.

226. Kienreich K, Tomaschitz A, Verheyen N, Pieber TR, Pilz S. Vitamin D and arterial hypertension: Treat the deficiency! *Am J Hypertens* 2013;26(2):158.

227. Tamez H, Kalim S, Thadhani RI. Does vitamin D modulate blood pressure? *Curr Opin Nephrol Hypertens* 2013;22(2):204–209.

228. Wang L, Ma J, Manson JE, Buring JE, Gaziano JM, Sesso HD. A prospective study of plasma vitamin D metabolites, vitamin D receptor gene polymorphisms, and risk of hypertension in men. *Eur J Nutr* 2012 Dec 21. [Epub ahead of print].

229. Pfeifer M, Begerow B, Minne HW, Nachtigall D, Hansen C. Effects of a short-term vitamin D (3) and calcium supplementation on blood pressure and parathyroid hormone levels in elderly women. *J Clin Endocrinol Metab* 2001;86:1633–1637.

230. Keniston R, Enriquez JI Sr. Relationship between blood pressure and plasma vitamin B6 levels in healthy middle-aged adults. *Ann N Y Acad Sci* 1990;585:499–501.

231. Aybak M, Sermet A, Ayyildiz MO, Karakilcik AZ. Effect of oral pyridoxine hydrochloride supplementation on arterial blood pressure in patients with essential hypertension. *Arzneimittelforschung* 1995;45:1271–1273.

232. Paulose CS, Dakshinamurti K, Packer S, Stephens NL. Sympathetic stimulation and hypertension in the pyridoxine-deficient adult rat. *Hypertension* 1988;11(4):387–391.

233. Dakshinamurti K, Lal KJ, Ganguly PK. Hypertension, calcium channel and pyridoxine (vitamin B6). *Mol Cell Biochem* 1998;188(1–2):137–148.

234. Moline J, Bukharovich IF, Wolff MS, Phillips R. Dietary flavonoids and hypertension: Is there a link? *Med Hypotheses* 2000;55:306–309.

235. Knekt P, Reunanen A, Järvinen R, Seppänen R, Heliövaara M, Aromaa A. Antioxidant vitamin intake and coronary mortality in a longitudinal population study. *Am J Epidemiol* 1994;139:1180–1189.

236. Karatzi KN, Papamichael CM, Karatizis EN et al. Red wine acutely induces favorable effects on wave reflections and central pressures in coronary artery disease patients. *Am J Hypertension* 2005;18(9):1161–1167.

237. Biala A, Tauriainen E, Siltanen A et al. Resveratrol induces mitochondrial biogenesis and ameliorates Ang II-induced cardiac remodeling in transgenic rats harboring human renin and angiotensinogen genes. *Blood Press* 2010;19(3):196–205.

238. Wong RH, Howe PR, Buckley JD, Coates AM, Kunz, Berry NM. Acute resveratrol supplementation improves flow-mediated dilatation in overweight obese individuals with mildly elevated blood pressure. *Nutr Metab Cardiovasc Dis* 2011;21(11):851–856.

239. Bhatt SR, Lokhandwala MF, Banday AA. Resveratrol prevents endothelial nitric oxide synthase uncoupling and attenuates development of hypertension in spontaneously hypertensive rats. *Eur J Pharmacol* 2011;667(1–3):258–264.

240. Rivera L, Moron R, Zarzuelo A, Galisteo M. Long-term resveratrol administration reduces metabolic disturbances and lowers blood pressure in obese Zucker rats. *Biochem Pharmacol* 2009;77(6):1053–1063.

241. Paran E, Engelhard YN. Effect of lycopene, an oral natural antioxidant on blood pressure. *J Hypertens* 2001;19:S74. Abstract P 1.204.

242. Engelhard YN, Gazer B, Paran E. Natural antioxidants from tomato extract reduce blood pressure in patients with grade-1 hypertension: A double blind placebo controlled pilot study. *Am Heart J* 2006;151(1):100.

243. Paran E, Novac C, Engelhard YN, Hazan-Halevy I. The effects of natural antioxidants form tomato extract in treated but uncontrolled hypertensive patients. *Cardiovasc Drugs Ther* 2009;23(2):145–151.

244. Reid K, Frank OR, Stocks NP. Dark Chocolate or tomato extract for prehypertension: A randomized controlled trial. *BMC Complement Altern Med* 2009;9:22.

245. Paran E, Engelhard Y. Effect of tomato's lycopene on blood pressure, serum lipoproteins, plasma homocysteine and oxidative stress markers in grade I hypertensive patients. *Am J Hypertens* 2001;14:141A. Abstract P-333.

246. Xaplanteris P, Vlachopoulos C, Pietri P et al. Tomato paste supplementation improves endothelial dynamics and reduces plasma total oxidative status in healthy subjects. *Nutr Res* 2012;32(5):390–394.

247. Hosseini S, Lee J, Sepulveda RT et al. A randomized, double-blind, placebo-controlled, prospective 16 week crossover study to determine the role of pycnogenol in modifying blood pressure in mildly hypertensive patients. *Nutr Res* 2001;21:1251–1260.

248. Zibadi S, Rohdewald PJ, Park D, Watson RR. Reduction of cardiovascular risk factors in subjects with type 2 diabetes by pycnogenol supplementation. *Nutr Res* 2008;28(5):315–320.

249. Liu X, Wei J, Tan F, Zhou S, Wurthwein G, Rohdewald P. Pycnogenol French maritime pine bark extract improves endothelial function of hypertensive patients. *Lif Sci* 2004;74(7):855–862.

250. Van der Zwan LP, Scheffer PG, Teerlink T. Reduction of myeloperoxidase activity by melatonin and pycnogenol may contribute to their blood pressure lowering effect. *Hypertension* 2010;56(3):e35.

251. Cesarone MR, Belcaro G, Stuard S et al. Kidney low and function in hypertension: Protective effects of pycnogenol in hypertensive participants—a controlled study. *J Cardiovasc Pharmacol Ther* 2010;15(1):41–46.

252. Simons S, Wollersheim H, Thien T. A systematic review on the influence of trial quality on the effects of garlic on blood pressure. *Neth J Med* 2009;67(6):212–219.

253. Reinhard KM, Coleman CI, Teevan C, Vacchani P. Effects of garlic on blood pressure in patients with and without systolic hypertension: A meta-analysis. *Ann Pharmacother* 2008:42(12):1766–1771.

254. Reid K, Frank OR, Stocks NP. Aged garlic extract lowers blood pressure in patients with treated but uncontrolled hypertension: A randomized controlled trial. *Maturitas* 2010;67(2):144–150.

255. Suetsuna K, Nakano T. Identification of an antihypertensive peptide from peptic digest of wakame (*Undaria pinnatifida*). *J Nutr Biochem* 2000;11:450–454.

256. Nakano T, Hidaka H, Uchida J, Nakajima K, Hata Y. Hypotensive effects of wakame. *J Jpn Soc Clin Nutr* 1998;20:92.

257. Krotkiewski M, Aurell M, Holm G, Grimby G, Szckepanik J. Effects of a sodium-potassium ion-exchanging seaweed preparation in mild hypertension. *Am J Hypertens* 1991;4:483–488.

258. Sato M, Oba T, Yamaguchi T et al. Antihypertensive effects of hydrolysates of wakame (*Undaria pinnatifida*) and their angiotensin-1-converting inhibitory activity. *Ann Nutr Metab* 2002;46(6):259–267.

259. Sato M, Hosokawa T, Yamaguchi T et al. Angiotensin I converting enzyme inhibitory peptide derived from wakame (*Undaria pinnatifida*) and their antihypertensive effect in spontaneously hypertensive rats. *J Agric Food Chem* 2002;50(21):6245–6252.

260. Sankar D, Sambandam G, Ramskrishna Rao M, Pugalendi KV. Modulation of blood pressure, lipid profiles and redox status in hypertensive patients taking different edible oils. *Clin Chim Acta* 2005;355(1–2):97–104.

261. Sankar D, Rao MR, Sambandam G, Pugalendi KV. Effect of sesame oil on diuretics or beta-blockers in the modulation of blood pressure, athropometry, lipid profile and redox status. *Yale J Biol Med* 2006;79(1):19–26.

262. Miyawaki T, Aono H, Toyoda-Ono Y, Maeda H, Kiso Y, Moriyama K. Anti-hypertensive effects of sesamin in humans. *J Nutr Sci Vitaminol (Toyko)* 2009;55(1):87–91.

263. Wichitsranoi J, Weerapreeyakui N, Boonsiri P et al. Antihypertensive and antioxidant effects of dietary black sesame meal in pre-hypertensive humans. *Nutr J* 2011;10(1):82–88.

264. Sudhakar B, Kalaiarasi P, Al-Numair KS, Chandramohan G, Rao RK, Pugalendi KV. Effect of combination of edible oils on blood pressure, lipid profile, lipid peroxidative markers, antioxidant status, and electrolytes in patients with hypertension on nifedipine treatment. *Saudi Med J* 2011;32(4):379–385.

265. Sankar D, Rao MR, Sambandam G, Pugalendi KV. A pilot study of open label sesame oil in hypertensive diabetics. *J Med Food* 2006;9(3):408–412.

266. Harikumar KB, Sung B, Tharakan ST et al. Sesamin manifests chemopreventive effects through the suppression of NF-kappa-B-regulated cell survival, proliferation, invasion and angiogenic gene products. *Mol Cancer Res* 2010;8(5):751–761.

267. Nakano D, Ogura K, Miyakoshi M et al. Antihypertensive effect of angiotensin-I-converting enzyme inhibitory peptides from a sesame protein hydrolysate in spontaneously hypertensive rats. *Biosci Biotechnol Biochem* 206;70(5):1118–1126.

268. Karatzi K, Stamatelopoulos K, Lykka M et al. Acute and long-term hemodynamic effects of sesame oil consumption in hypertensive men. *J Clin Hypertens (Greenwich)* 2012;14(9):630–636.

269. Hodgson JM, Puddey IB, Burke V, Beilin LJ, Jordan N. Effects on blood pressure of drinking green and black tea. *J Hypertens* 1999;17:457–463.

270. Kurita I, Maeda-Yamamoto M, Tachibana H, Kamei M. Anti-hypertensive effect of Benifuuki tea containing *O*-methylated EGCG. *J Agric Food Chem* 2010;58(3):1903–1908.

271. McKay DL, Chen CY, Saltzman E, Blumberg JB. *Hibiscus sabdariffa* L. tea (tisane) lowers blood pressure in pre-hypertensive and mildly hypertensive adults. *J Nutr* 2010;140(2):298–303.

272. Bogdanski P, Suliburska J, Szulinska M, Stepien M, Pupek-Musialik D, Jablecka A. Green tea extract reduces blood pressure, inflammatory biomarkers, and oxidative stress and improves parameters associated with insulin resistance in obese, hypertensive patients. *Nutr Res* 2012;32(6):421–427.

273. Hodgson JM, Woodman RJ, Puddey IB, Mulder T, Fuchs D, Croft KD. Short-term effects of polyphenol-rich black tea on blood pressure in men and women. *Food Funct* 2013;4(1):111–115.

274. Medina-Remón A, Estruch R, Tresserra-Rimbau A, Vallverdú-Queralt A, Lamuela-Raventos RM. The effect of polyphenol consumption on blood pressure. *Mini Rev Med Chem* 2012 August 27. [Epub ahead of print].

275. Jiménez R, Duarte J, Perez-Vizcaino F. Epicatechin: Endothelial function and blood pressure. *J Agric Food Chem* 2012;60(36):8823–8830.

276. Taubert D, Roesen R, Schomig E. Effect of cocoa and tea intake on blood pressure: A meta-analysis. *Arch Intern Med* 2007;167(7):626–634.

277. Grassi D, Lippi C, Necozione S, Desideri G, Ferri C. Short-term administration of dark chocolate is followed by a significant increase in insulin sensitivity and a decrease in blood pressure in health persons. *Am J Clin Nutr* 2005;81(3):611–614.

278. Taubert D, Roesen R, Lehmann C, Jung N, Schomig E. Effects of low habitual cocoa intake on blood pressure and bioactive nitric oxide: A randomized controlled trial. *JAMA* 2007;298(1):49–60.

279. Cohen DL, Townsend RR. Cocoa ingestion and hypertension-another cup please? *J Clin Hypertens* 2007;9(8):647–648.

280. Reid I, Sullivan T, Fakler P, Frank OR, Stocks NP. Does chocolate reduce blood pressure? A meta-analysis. *BMC Med* 2010;8:39–46.

281. Egan BM, Laken MA, Donovan J, Woolson RF. Does dark chocolate have a role in the prevention and management of hypertension?: Commentary on the evidence. *Hypertension* 2010;55(6):1289–1295.

282. Desch S, Kobler D, Schmidt J et al. Low vs higher-dose dark chocolate and blood pressure in cardiovascular high-risk patients. *Am J Hypertens* 2010;23(6):694–700.

283. Desch S, Schmidt J, Sonnabend M et al. Effect of cocoa products on blood pressure: Systematic review and meta-analysis. *Am J Hypertens* 2010;23(1):97–103.

284. Grassi D, Desideri G, Necozione S et al. Blood pressure is reduced and insulin sensitivity increased in glucose intolerant hypertensive subjects after 15 days of consuming high-polyphenol dark chocolate. *J Nutr* 2008;138(9):1671–1676.

285. Grassi D, Necozione S, Lippi C et al. Cocoa reduces blood pressure and insulin resistance and improved endothelium-dependent vasodilation in hypertensives. *Hypertension* 2005;46(2):398–405.

286. Ellinger S, Reusch A, Stehle P, Helfrich HP. Epicatechin ingested via cocoa products reduces blood pressure in humans: A nonlinear regression model with a Bayesian approach. *Am J Clin Nutr* 2012;95(6):1365–1377.

287. Hooper L, Kay C, Abdelhamid A et al. Effects of chocolate, cocoa, and flavan-3-ols on cardiovascular health: A systematic review and meta-analysis of randomized trials. *Am J Clin Nutr* 2012;95(3): 740–751.

288. Yamaguchi T, Chikama A, Mori K et al. Hydroxyhydroquinone-free coffee: A double-blind, randomized controlled dose-response study of blood pressure. *Nutr Metab Cardiovasc Dis* 2008;18(6):408–414.

289. Chen ZY, Peng C, Jiao R, Wong YM, Yang N, Huang Y. Anti-hypertensive nutraceuticals and functional foods. *J Agric Food Chem* 2009;57(11):4485–4499.

290. Ochiai R, Chikama A, Kataoka K et al. Effects of hydroxyhydroquinone-reduced coffee on vasoreactivity and blood pressure. *Hypertens Res* 2009;32(11):969–974.

291. Kozuma K, Tsuchiya S, Kohori J, Hase T, Tokimitsu I. Anti-hypertensive effect of green coffee bean extract on mildly hypertensive subjects. *Hypertens Res* 2005;28(9):711–718.

292. Scheer FA, Van Montfrans GA, van Someren EJ, Mairuhu G, Buijs RM. Daily nighttime melatonin reduces blood pressure in male patients with essential hypertension. *Hypertension* 2004;43(2):192–197.

293. Cavallo A, Daniels SR, Dolan LM, Khoury JC, Bean JA. Blood pressure response to melatonin in type I diabetes. *Pediatr Diabetes* 2004;5(1):26–31.

294. Cavallo A, Daniels SR, Dolan LM, Bean JA, Khoury JC. Blood pressure-lowering effect of melatonin in type 1 diabetes. *J Pineal Res* 2004;36(4):262–266.

295. Cagnacci A, Cannoletta M, Renzi A, Baldassari F, Arangino S, Volpe A. Prolonged melatonin administration decreases nocturnal blood pressure in women. *Am J Hypertens* 2005;18(12 Pt 1):1614–1618.

296. Grossman E, Laudon M, Yalcin R et al. Melatonin reduces night blood pressure in patients with nocturnal hypertension. *Am J Med* 2006;119(10):898–902.

297. Rechcinski T, Kurpese M, Trzoa E, Krzeminska-Pakula M. The influence of melatonin supplementation on circadian pattern of blood pressure in patients with coronary artery disease-preliminary report. *Pol Arch Med Wewn* 2006;115(6):520–528.

298. Merkureva GA, Ryzhak GA. Effect of the pineal gland peptide preparation on the diurnal profile of arterial pressure in middle-aged and elderly women with ischemic heart disease and arterial hypertension. *Adv Gerontol* 2008;21(1):132–142.

299. Zaslavskaia RM, Scherban EA, Logvinenki SI. Melatonin in combined therapy of patients with stable angina and arterial hypertension. *Klin Med (Mosk)* 2009;86:64–67.

300. Zamotaev IuN, Enikeev AKh, Kolomets NM. The use of melaxen in combined therapy of arterial hypertension in subjects occupied in assembly line production. *Klin Med (Mosk)* 2009;87(6):46–49.

301. Rechcinski T, Trzos E, Wierzbowski-Drabik K, Krzeminska-Pakute M, Kurpesea M. Melatonin for non-dippers with coronary artery disease: Assessment of blood pressure profile and heart rate variability. *Hypertens Res* 2002;33(1):56–61.

302. Kozirog M, Poliwczak AR, Duchnowicz P, Koter-Michalak M, Sikora J, Broncel M. Melatonin treatment improves blood pressure, lipid profile and parameters of oxidative stress in patients with metabolic syndrome. *J Pineal Res* 2011;50(3):261–266.

303. De-Leersnyder H, de Biois MC, Vekemans M et al. Beta (1) adrenergic antagonists improve sleep and behavioural disturbances in a circadian disorder, Smith-Magenis syndrome. *J Med Genet* 2110;38(9):586–590.

304. Morand C, Dubray C, Milenkovic D et al. Hesperidin contributes to the vascular protective effects of orange juice: A randomized crossover study in healthy volunteers. *Am J Clin Nutr* 2011;93(1):73–80.

305. Basu A, Penugonda K. Pomegranate juice: A heart-healthy fruit juice. *Nutr Rev* 2009;67(1):49–56.

306. Aviram M, Rosenblat M, Gaitine D et al. Pomegranate juice consumption for 3 years by patients with carotid artery stenosis reduces common carotid intima-media thickness, blood pressure and LDL oxidation. *Clin Nutr* 2004;23(3):423–433.

307. Aviram M, Dornfeld L. Pomegranate juice inhibits serum angiotensin converting enzyme activity and reduces systolic blood pressure. *Atherosclerosis* 2001;18(1):195–198.

308. Feringa HH, Laskey DA, Dickson JE, Coleman CI. The effect of grape seed extract on cardiovascular risk markers: A meta-analysis of randomized controlled trials. *J Am Diet Assoc* 2011;111(8):1173–1181.

309. Sivaprakasapillai B, Edirisinghe K, Randolph J, Steinberg F, Kappagoda T. Effect of grape seed extract on blood pressure in subjects with the metabolic syndrome. *Metabolism* 2009;58(12):1743–1746.

310. Edirisinghe I, Burton-Freeman B, Tissa Kappagoda C. Mechanism of the endothelium-dependent relaxation evoked by grape seed extract. *Clin Sci (Lond)* 2008;114(4): 331–337.

311. Rosenfeldt FL, Haas Sj, Krum H, Hadu A. Coenzyme Q 10 in the treatment of hypertension: A meta-analysis of the clinical trials. *J Hum Hypertens* 2007;21(4):297–306.

312. Burke BE, Neuenschwander R, Olson RD. Randomized, double-blind, placebo-controlled trial of coenzyme Q10 in isolated systolic hypertension. *South Med J* 2001;94(11):1112–1117.

313. Mikhin VP, Kharchenko AV, Rosliakova EA, Cherniatina MA. Application of coenzyme Q (10) in combination therapy of arterial hypertension. *Kardiologiia* 2011;51(6):26–31.

314. Tsai KL, Huang YH, Kao CL et al. A novel mechanism of coenzyme Q10 protects against human endothelial cells from oxidative stress-induced injury by modulating NO-related pathways. *J Nutr Biochem* 2012;23(5):458–468.

315. Sohet FM, Delzenne NM. Is there a place for coenzyme Q in the management of metabolic disorders associated with obesity? *Nutr Rev* 2012;70(11):631–641.

316. Digiesi V, Cantini F, Oradei A et al. Coenzyme Q10 in essential hypertension. *Mol Aspects Med* 1994;15(suppl):S257–S263.

317. Langsjoen P, Langsjoen P, Willis R, Folkers K. Treatment of essential hypertension with coenzyme Q10. *Mol Aspects Med* 1994;15(suppl):S265–S272.
318. Ankola DD, Viswanad B, Bhardwaj V, Ramarao P, Kumar MN. Development of potent oral nanoparticulate formulation of coenzyme Q10 for treatment of hypertension: Can the simple nutritional supplements be used as first line therapeutic agents for prophylaxis/therapy? *Eur J Pharm Biopharm* 2007;67(2):361–369.
319. Trimarco V, Cimmino CS, Santoro M et al. Nutraceuticals for blood pressure control in patients with high-normal or grade1 hypertension. *High Blood Press Cardiovasc Prev* 2012;19(3):117–122.
320. Young JM, Florkowski CM, Molyneux SL et al. A randomized, double-blind, placebo-controlled crossover study of coenzyme Q10 therapy in hypertensive patients with the metabolic syndrome. *Am J Hypertens* 2012;25(2): 261–270.
321. McMackin CJ. Widlansky ME, Hambury NM, Haung AL. Effect of combined treatment with alpha lipoic acid and acetyl carnitine on vascular function and blood pressure in patients with coronary artery disease. *J Clin Hypertens* 2007;9:249–255.
322. Salinthone S, Schillace RV, Tsang C, Regan JW, Burdette DN, Carr DW. Lipoic acid stimulates cAMP production via G protein-coupled receptor-dependent and -independent mechanisms. *J Nutr Biochem* 2011;22(7):681–690.
323. Rahman ST, Merchant N, Haque T et al. The impact of lipoic acid on endothelial function and protein-uria in quinapril-treated diabetic patients with stage I hypertension: Results from the QUALITY study. *J Cardiovasc Pharmacol Ther* 2012;17(2):139–145.
324. Morcos M, Borcea V, Isermann B et al. Effect of alpha-lipoic acid on the progression of endothelial cell damage and albuminuria in patients with diabetes mellitus: An exploratory study. *Diabetes Res Clin Prac* 2001;52(3):175–183.
325. MartinaV, Masha A, Gigliardi VR et al. Long-term *N*-acetylcysteine and L-arginine administration reduces endothelial activation and systolic blood pressure in hypertensive patients with type 2 diabetes. *Diabetes Care* 2008;31(5):940–944.
326. Jiang B, Haverty M, Brecher P. *N*-acetyl-L-cysteine enhances interleukin-1beta-induced nitric oxide synthase expression. *Hypertension* 1999;34(4 Pt 1):574–579.
327. Vasdev S, Singal P, Gill V. The antihypertensive effect of cysteine. *Int J Angiol* 2009;18(1):7–21.
328. Meister A, Anderson ME, Hwang O. Intracellular cysteine and glutathione delivery systems. *J Am Coll Nutr* 1986;5(2):137–151.
329. Asher GN, Viera AJ, Weaver MA, Dominik R, Caughey M, Hinderliter AL. Effect of hawthorn standardized extract on flow mediated dilation in prehypertensive and mildly hypertensive adults: A randomized, controlled cross-over trial. *BMC Complement Altern Med* 2012;12:26.
330. Koçyildiz ZC, Birman H, Olgaç V, Akgün-Dar K, Melikoğlu G, Meriçli AH. *Crataegus tanacetifolia* leaf extract prevents L-NAME-induced hypertension in rats: A morphological study. *Phytother Res* 2006;20(1):66–70.
331. Schröder D, Weiser M, Klein P. Efficacy of a homeopathic Crataegus preparation compared with usual therapy for mild (NYHA II) cardiac insufficiency: Results of an observational cohort study. *Eur J Heart Fail* 2003;5(3):319–326.
332. Walker AF, Marakis G, Simpson E et al. Hypotensive effects of hawthorn for patients with diabetes taking prescription drugs: A randomised controlled trial. *Br J Gen Pract* 2006;56(527):437–443.
333. Walker AF, Marakis G, Morris AP, Robinson PA. Promising hypotensive effect of hawthorn extract: A randomized double-blind pilot study of mild, essential hypertension. *Phytother Res* 2002;16(1):48–54.
334. Larson A, Witman MA, Guo Y et al. Acute, quercetin-induced reductions in blood pressure in hypertensive individuals are not secondary to lower plasma angiotensin-converting enzyme activity or endothelin-1: Nitric oxide. *Nutr Res* 2012;32(8):557–564.
335. Edwards RL, Lyon T, Litwin SE, Rabovsky A, Symons JD, Jalili T. Quercetin reduces blood pressure in hypertensive subjects. *J Nutr* 2007;137(11):2405–2411.
336. Egert S, Bosy-Westphal A, Seiberl J et al. Quercetin reduces systolic blood pressure and plasma oxidised low-density lipoprotein concentrations in overweight subjects with a high-cardiovascular disease risk phenotype: A double-blinded, placebo-controlled cross-over study. *Br J Nutr* 2009;102(7):1065–1074.
337. Trovato A, Nuhlicek DN, Midtling JE. Drug-nutrient interactions. *Am Fam Physician* 1991;44(5):1651–1658.
338. McCabe BJ, Frankel EH, Wolfe JJ. Eds. *Handbook of Food-Drug Interactions*. CRC Press, Boca Raton, FL; 2003.
339. Houston MC. The role of cellular micronutrient analysis and minerals in the prevention and treatment of hypertension and cardiovascular disease. *Ther Adv Cardiovasc Dis* 2010;4:v165–v183.

10 The Role of Dentistry in Cardiovascular Health and General Well-Being

Mark A. Breiner

CONTENTS

If a person has cardiovascular disease, will a change in diet and supplements be sufficient to bring down inflammation? If the inflammatory markers are normal, is inflammation gone? What role does dentistry play in cardiovascular health and in health in general? Is there a level beyond inflammation that needs to be addressed?

I believe that cardiovascular problems and other health problems exist on two levels. The first of these is the physical level; this is the level of poor nutrition, mineral and vitamin deficiencies, and environmental toxins. This is also the level at which dentistry has a large impact. Impacted wisdom teeth, bite problems, mercury fillings, root canals, cavitations, and periodontal disease can have a major negative impact on a patient's health. At this level, the problems are addressed physically; supplements can be given, diets can be changed, and toxins can be eliminated. Dentally, for example, mercury fillings may be removed, bite problems can be corrected, and, sometimes, root-canaled teeth may be extracted. Medically, a bad heart valve may need to be replaced or a pacemaker needs to be placed.

The second level on which health problems exist involves a patient's core or "vital force." Addressing deep energetic imbalances can have a profound effect on a patient's emotions and health. Some of these imbalances have been passed down generationally. Other imbalances can be more recent, as, for example, from an accident or another traumatic experience, which leave an energetic imprint in the cellular matrix. These signals that disrupt normal function cause disharmony in the symphony of "cellular song." When these aberrant notes are removed, the melody of life will be harmonious and a high level of health will result. I believe this level plays a role in "susceptibility." For example, why would a 50-year-old who eats right, exercises, has low levels of toxins, has ideal blood work, and is *seemingly* healthy, suddenly drop dead of a heart attack? I have observed that when both the outer physical level and the inner energetic level have been addressed, patients have attained a level of health that had eluded them for years.

As you read through this chapter, it is important to remember that these two levels—the "physical" level and the "energetic" level—are intertwined.

PHYSICAL LEVEL

The topics of nutrition, diet, and supplementation are covered elsewhere in this book. I will focus on the major dental issues that affect the patient's cardiovascular and general health.

An obvious, but often overlooked, biological fact is that the blood that nourishes our lips, gums, tongue, teeth, and oral cavity is the same blood that courses throughout our body. Unfortunately, there is a serious lack of training about the systemic effects that dental procedures can have on overall body functioning. Dentists have been taught to make treatment decisions without recognizing the full impact of those decisions and with little appreciation for the relationship between the mouth and the rest of the body. The truth is that every dental procedure is an invasion of the human system, and that invasion may generate an adverse response elsewhere in the body.

As you read this chapter, you will discover that one cannot treat the mouth without having an impact on the entire body. You will also learn that health, or lack of health, will impact the oral cavity. Essentially, optimum health for the mouth necessitates optimum systemic health. Therefore, as a dentist striving to help a patient achieve maximum oral health, I have found it essential to treat the patient globally. With this philosophy in mind, I coined the term "Whole-Body Dentistry®."

When writing an article, I find it necessary to compartmentalize and categorize topics. However, this is not the way things work in real life. For example, I can discuss magnesium and its various functions and the problems associated with this deficiency. However, magnesium does not do its work in a vacuum; it is part of a greater whole. It is important to keep this concept in mind. Similarly, the mouth cannot be evaluated without considering what is occurring in the rest of the body and vice versa.

In general, a person's overall resistance is intimately tied to his or her genetic background, stress levels, toxins, pH, diet, and nutrition. Recent studies support this point of view, as they have demonstrated a correlation between periodontal disease and an increased incidence of heart disease. The resulting recommendation is that periodontal disease be treated to help prevent heart problems. It is now thought that the underlying factor in both periodontal disease and heart disease is inflammation. I will address inflammation, especially as it relates to dentistry and heart disease; however, that is not sufficient, it is also critical to address that which precedes inflammation to achieve optimal health.

Inflammation is a complex biological response of vascular tissues to irritants like oxidants, and bacterial and fungal infections. Food allergies and sensitivities, psychological or emotional stress, low-grade infection, dehydration, lack of sleep, environmental toxins, and a poor diet (too many trans fats or sugars) can also cause inflammation. Inflammation is, on the other hand, necessary, or wounds and infections would never heal. Acute inflammation is essential for life; however, as pointed out in other areas of this book, chronic inflammation is not good. Inflammation is the body's attempt at self-protection. It is the body's biological response to harmful or irritating substances. Inflammation does not mean infection; rather it is the response to the infection. Chronic inflammation, something that lasts for several months or longer, results from a chronic low-grade irritant, or an autoimmune response to a self-antigen.

Toxicity of the inner environment of the mouth is of great concern particularly because of the inflammation process that can be triggered by dental toxins. Metals in the mouth (mercury, nickel, tin, beryllium, etc.), toxins from root-canaled teeth, cavitations, and periodontal disease can cause chronic inflammation. Given that each of these can promote inflammation, and that inflammation is the underlying cause of heart disease, taking proper care of the mouth is very important in preventing and treating heart disease.

PERIODONTAL DISEASE AND THE INFLAMMATORY PROCESS

Periodontal disease is the most common infectious disease in the world. Periodontal disease involves multiple issues ranging from gingivitis, which is a simple inflammation of the gums, to periodontitis, which involves the loss of bone around the teeth as a result of chronic inflammation.

Gingivitis, the early stage of gum disease, involves only the gum tissue. The gums are often red and swollen and tend to bleed easily. In a healthy situation, there is a slight trough or sulcus between the tooth and the gum tissue. If gingivitis is present, the sulcus may deepen and form shallow pockets of 1–3 mm. This stage of periodontal diseases is easily reversible. Debridement of the pocket by the hygienist or dentist, good nutrition, supplementation with co-enzyme Q10 (CoQ10) and vitamin C, brushing, flossing, and often irrigation with an antimicrobial solution will ameliorate the problem. Hormonal changes (as in pregnancy) can also cause gingivitis.

When the inflammatory problem has progressed into the bone, it is called periodontitis. Pockets accompanied by bone loss are now present. Initially, these pockets will be 3–5 mm deep, but, if the process is not halted, they will become much deeper, reaching 5–10 mm or more. Keeping these pockets clean becomes more and more difficult and, as a result, patients' teeth may loosen. If this condition is left unchecked, and if enough bone is lost around the teeth, the teeth may need to be removed.

Patients are often unaware that they have periodontal disease. Therefore, to detect a problem at the earliest stage, it is very important to maintain regular dental visits. As part of an initial examination, I do a periodontal probing around every tooth. If I find a pocket of more than 3 mm deep, I suspect that bone has been lost; however, this is just historical information. How do I know if the pocket is actively infected and if the infectious process is ongoing? Bleeding on probing is one indication that this may be occurring. However, I find that the best way to make this determination is by viewing a plaque sample. Plaque is the sticky substance that you feel on your teeth at the end of the day. A sample can be gathered or taken from under the gum as well as from a pocket. This sample is then placed on a glass slide in a solution similar to saliva, and a coverslip is placed over it. Using a phase-contrast microscope, I can view the sample at a magnification of 400×. A healthy slide will have certain types of bacteria, but not a lot of "activity," whereas an unhealthy slide will be characterized by a lot of activity, lots of white blood cells, spirochetes, and, usually, amoebas. An amoeba is a parasite, and a spirochete is a snake-like bacteria. The spirochete associated with periodontal disease is called *Treponema denticola*. The specific amoeba associated with periodontal disease is called *Entamoeba gingivalis*. *T. denticola* and *E. gingivalis* are not seen in a healthy mouth. An unhealthy slide sample taken from a pocket would indicate an ongoing infection in that pocket. A healthy slide sample taken from a pocket would indicate that there had previously been a problem, but that it was presently quiescent. No pockets, but a microladen slide, tells me that a person may be at risk, at some point in the future, for periodontal disease and possibly other problems. As you can see, the use of a phase-contrast microscope in the dental office is very important.

The Heart Foundation reports that heart disease is the number one cause of death for both men and women in the United States, with more people dying of heart disease than of AIDS and all cancers combined.[1] With this alarming, but not surprising, statistic, it certainly is not in the best interest of a heart patient to have a high bacterial level in their plaque.

Also on the rise for the baby-boomer generation are replacements of various joints, e.g., hips, knees, and shoulders. It is important for the dentist to know if these patients (as well as heart patients) have a "poor" slide, before their hygiene visit, so steps can be taken to prevent a bacteremia. Subgingival irrigation with an antimicrobial agent both before and after a dental hygiene visit, for these patients, or even for a "healthy" patient with a bad slide will help prevent a problem. Bacteria are a major cause of inflammation, and as we are finding out, inflammation is an underlying cause of many diseases, not only periodontal disease.

TREATMENT OF PERIODONTITIS

The traditional method of treating periodontitis is debridement of the pocket and, often, surgery to decrease the depth of the pocket by moving the gums closer to where the bone currently is. The goal is to have a shallow pocket that can be easily cleaned by the patient. Some dentists send a sample from the pocket to a lab to be cultured. The lab identifies the specific bacteria present so that an appropriate antibiotic can be administered. There are small antibiotic-laden chips that can be placed in a pocket. These chips slowly release minute amounts of antibiotic, until, eventually, the chip resorbs. Recently, lasers have been used in place of scalpel surgery. The laser can sterilize the pocket and encourage the regeneration of bone. As opposed to surgery to move the tissue to where the bone is, laser treatment allows the bone to regrow to meet the tissue. In addition to having more tooth-stabilizing bone, the result of laser treatment is a more aesthetically pleasing appearance.

In treating periodontal disease, I find that it is important to take a whole-body approach; ultimately, this approach leads to improved host resistance. Assessment of a patient's nutritional status is beneficial. Important information can be obtained by blood and/or hair analysis. Supplementation with natural vitamin C, CoQ10, magnesium, calcium, homeopathic tissue salts, and immune enhancers such as thymus and the herb cat's claw can be advantageous. Bleeding gums and loose teeth, which are common indications of periodontal disease, are also among the symptoms of mercury toxicity; thus, removal of mercury (silver) fillings is beneficial. Addressing not just the "physical" level, but also the "energetic" level of imbalances is also important. In short, anything that can be done to enhance the immune system is valuable.

PERIODONTAL DISEASE AND YOUR HEART

Interestingly, research on the relationship of periodontal disease to heart disease goes back over 150 years. The book, *Death and Dentistry*, by Dr. Martin Fisher, published in 1940, chronicles the role of mouth bacteria in many diseases.[2] The impact of germs in the mouth on systemic disease was also shown in other research conducted many years ago; however, because that research is not "modern" research, it tends to be ignored. But the truth does not vary with time. In fact, the connection was even clearer before the introduction of antibiotics and the overwhelming number of pharmaceuticals used today.

Numerous studies have shown that those with periodontal disease have a higher incidence of heart disease. The same bacteria, which are specific to the mouth, have been isolated from heart tissue and arterial plaque.[3,4] Studies also show increased risk of stroke for those with periodontal disease.[5,6]

Elevated C-reactive protein (CRP) levels are a marker for increased stroke and heart attack risk. CRP is a key marker of inflammation and is produced in response to infection and injury. CRP also causes clotting, which can lead to heart attack, stroke, and pulmonary emboli. Many people with periodontal disease have elevated levels of CRP.[7] One study showed that prescribing 20 mg of the antibiotic doxycycline twice a day (normally 1000 mg/day is given) to patients with periodontal disease lowered CRP by 50%.[8] Doxycycline is specific for spirochetes. I have often observed that CRP decreases when a whole body approach is taken to reduce periodontal inflammation and/or infection.

Joyce, a 43-year-old woman, came to see me as a new patient. In discussing her medical history, she related that she had a high CRP level and that her physician had run extensive tests to uncover the source. All tests were negative. I viewed a sample of her plaque under a phase-contrast microscope and saw a multitude of spirochetes and amoebae. After Joyce's periodontal infection was treated and cleared, her slide normalized and her CRP dropped to a normal level; it has remained normal for the past 9 years.

METALS IN THE MOUTH

When amalgam fillings, which are an alloy of mercury and other metals, were first introduced into the United States in 1833, many dentists were outraged at the suggestion of placing such a highly toxic metal in their patients' mouths. The amalgam filling is an alloy of mercury with copper, tin, zinc, and silver. Because mercury is the main component of an amalgam, representing about 50% of the alloy, it is more accurate to call these fillings "mercury fillings"; however, for marketing purposes, they came to be called, "silver fillings." The controversy over the use of mercury in dental fillings continues to this very day, with the proponents saying there is no scientific evidence that mercury from fillings causes any harm. Today, everyone agrees that mercury does come out of the amalgam fillings. It comes off as a vapor (its most toxic form), which is easily absorbed. All the components of an amalgam filling are potentially toxic; however, mercury is by far the most toxic. Its effects are well documented. Mercury is mercury no matter where it comes from. Mercury causes psychological, neurological, immunological, endocrine, gastrointestinal, and oral disturbances.

MERCURY AND CARDIOVASCULAR PROBLEMS

Because mercury is so toxic, it will cause problems in any tissue or organ in which it resides, including the heart and the arteries. Studies have shown an affinity for accumulation in the cardiovascular system. In a 1983 study, animals were exposed to radioactively labeled mercury vapor by inhalation. A significant uptake of mercury was found in various organs, including the heart muscle.[9] Studies done on rats, mice, and monkeys have shown that exposure to inhaled mercury vapor results in a larger accumulation of mercury in the heart than does exposure to inorganic mercury.[10] In a study of idiopathic dilated cardiomyopathy (IDCM) patients, the mean mercury concentration was 22,000 times higher than that in control subjects.[11] In one study where animals were exposed to grinding of amalgam fillings, it was shown that mercury vapor from dental amalgam rapidly, and dramatically, accumulated in the heart tissue.[12] In another study radioactively labeled amalgam fillings were placed in the teeth of pregnant sheep. Within days after placement of the amalgam fillings, the radioactively labeled mercury was found in the heart tissue of the mother sheep and unborn fetuses.[13] A human study comparing subjects with and without amalgam fillings, showed that amalgam-bearing subjects had significantly higher blood pressure, lower heart rates, and lower hemoglobin and hematocrit levels. The subjects with the amalgam fillings had a greater incidence of chest pains, tachycardia, anemia, and fatigue.[14] Mercury also targets the pituitary, thyroid, and adrenal glands as well as the brain; all of these influence heart function.[15]

Numerous studies show that mercury damages the heart and blood vessels. Mercury has an effect on blood pressure and interferes with the electrical conduction pattern of the heart. It damages heart muscle tissue, blood vessels, and heart valves. I have had some patients with a reversal of their mitral valve prolapse after having mercury removed from their mouth and having mercury detoxed from their body. In addition, numerous cases of tachycardia and blood pressure problems have resolved with mercury removal. Mercury also causes blood to clot faster and easier.[16]

As previously mentioned, mercury causes oxidative stress and, therefore, inflammation. In fact, all the components of amalgam fillings cause oxidative stress. Not only for heart health but also for health in general, it is not a good idea to have mercury implanted in the mouth.

REMOVAL OF MERCURY "SILVER" FILLINGS

Because any stimulation of the fillings, such as with a dental drill, increases the amount of mercury vapor released, removal of mercury fillings should be done in a manner that protects the patient, the dentist, and the assistant. Patient safety precautions during amalgam removal include having the patient breathe oxygen, using large amounts of water and high-speed suction, use of a rubber dam to isolate teeth from the rest of the mouth, and coating the patient's mouth with a powder that has a strong affinity for mercury.

An equally important aspect of protecting the patient relates to preparation prior to mercury removal. It is essential to ascertain that the patient's organs of detoxification are functioning properly. In this regard, it is critical that the mesenchyme, which is the tissue that surrounds every cell of the body, be functioning optimally. Too often I see patients who have had their mercury fillings removed without proper preparation become extremely ill. It is beyond the scope of this chapter to go into depth as to what is needed to determine if the patient is at a point where they can have their mercury fillings removed. Suffice it to say that removal of mercury fillings is not to be taken lightly, and a patient should seek out a dentist trained in how to do this safely.

Some facts about mercury are as follows:

1. Amalgam fillings are approximately 40%–50% mercury.
2. Mercury continuously comes out of the fillings in the lethal vapor form.
3. Any stimulation to the fillings, e.g., chewing, grinding, and drinking hot liquids, increases the amount of vapor coming from the fillings.
4. Mercury from the fillings enters the body and builds up over time.
5. Mercury passes the placental barrier and accumulates in the fetus.
6. Mercury passes from the mother's milk to the infant.
7. There is no safe level of mercury in the human body.

ROOT CANALS AND THE INFLAMMATORY PROCESS

When a tooth dies as evidenced by pain, abscess, or radiographic evidence, a patient is confronted with a choice of extraction of the offending tooth or saving the tooth by having a root canal. Dentists are taught that it is usually best to keep a tooth in place by performing a root canal. If the tooth is at a point where it is beyond saving, dentists will usually recommend an extraction followed by an implant. Unfortunately, dentists are not taught about the possible systemic effects of either the root canal or the implant. However, the possible negative systemic effects are real and can have a devastating effect on the health of the patient. It is not just cardiovascular disease that has been related to the bacteria and toxins from root canals. Research has also shown these bacteria and toxins to be related to arthritis, breast tumors, gallbladder disease, eczema, torticollis, nephritis, cystitis, pernicious anemia, colitis, neuritis, sinusitis, hypertension, thyroid disease, atherosclerosis, heart valve problems, myocarditis, and more.[17–20] Notice how many of these are inflammatory in nature ("itis" denotes inflammation).

According to the American Dental Association, about 15 million root canals are being performed annually. This common procedure, however, is not without risk; root-canaled teeth are often the source of systemic toxins and are often the underlying cause of inflammation.

To appreciate why root-canaled teeth can be so dangerous, it is important to understand the process. A root canal is the removal of the pulpal tissue from the hollow tube within the root(s) of the tooth. This pulp is composed of nerves, blood, and lymphatic tissue. Dentists are taught to medicate the canal of the tooth during the root canal procedure to minimize the amount of bacteria left behind. The canal is usually packed with a latex material called gutta-percha, which supposedly seals off the canal. The underlying assumption is that the body will be able to tolerate a tooth that now contains a minimal amount of bacteria. The criteria for success are that a tooth does not hurt and that it appears normal on an x-ray. If it were just the pulp that was infected, a better outcome could be expected. However, the tooth's dentin, the tooth material that surrounds the pulp, is composed of literally millions of tiny tubules. These tubules exist to transport nutrients to the entire tooth. Although we think of tooth enamel as a hard and impenetrable material, it is actually made up of thousands of microscopic tubules. In fact, the dentin comprises so many tubules that if the tubules in your small lower front tooth were laid out end to end, it is estimated that they would form a line approximately 3 miles long.

During the root-canal procedure, the canal is partially sealed with the gutta-percha or other sealing materials, so the tooth no longer experiences the benefits from the constant cleansing oxygenating effect of the blood supply flowing through the tooth. When the bacteria left behind in the dental tubules are cut off from the normal oxygen and blood supply in this manner, they begin to metabolize differently. They change from an aerobic to an anaerobic form and begin to give off potent toxins. If your immune system is strong, your body may be able to quarantine the toxins by "walling" off the area. Sometimes, this may appear on an x-ray as a more radiolucent area indicating an abscess. Dr. Weston Price, a world-renowned researcher and dentist, did 25 years of research on the root canal issue in the 1920s and 1930s. He had been taught, as is still taught in dental schools today, that a radiolucent area is a bad sign. However, Dr. Price's research showed that a radiolucent area might indicate a positive reaction by a healthy well-functioning immune system to the toxins coming from a root-canaled tooth. Sometimes the reaction is so good that a drain, called a fistula, will open into the mouth through the gum. This is nature's way of expelling the toxins. Dr. Price considered a tooth with a radiolucent area on an x-ray less problematic than one without a radiolucent area. If your immune system cannot react effectively enough to quarantine these bacteria and their toxins, then these toxins enter into your body as negative agents, which then attack your genetically weak systems or your areas of stress. These bacteria are most often a form of a streptococcus.

Most people in the dental profession ignored the work of Dr. Price because it was done so long ago. However, as previously stated, the truth always remains the truth. Because his work was done before the advent of antibiotics, I would argue that the role of root canals in disease is much clearer. Dr. Price did hundreds of experiments. In one experiment, he took extracted root-canaled teeth from heart patients and implanted them under the skin of healthy rabbits. The rabbits immediately developed heart disease and died. Rabbits have an immune system similar to that of humans. When healthy teeth were implanted under the skin of rabbits for up to a year, nothing of consequence occurred. In additional studies, Dr. Price further demonstrated how potent and insidious root-canaled teeth could be. Root-canaled teeth taken from patients with heart disease were ground into a powder, which he sterilized and put through a filter to remove all bacteria. When a miniscule amount of that powder was injected into rabbits, they also died of heart disease. How could it be that root-canaled teeth seemed to cause heart disease in rabbits? What was it in the root-canaled teeth that caused this effect? The answer to these questions lies in the virtually indestructible toxins produced by the bacteria in root-canaled teeth. It was not only heart disease that was caused by the implanted root-canaled teeth. Dr. Price found that if a root-canaled tooth was removed from someone with, for example, arthritis, and that tooth was implanted under the skin of the rabbit, the rabbit would come down with arthritis. Whatever disease the host had, would be the disease that would manifest in the rabbit almost 100% of the time!

ROOT CANAL DECISIONS

To save a tooth, should a patient elect to do a root canal? If a patient has a root-canaled tooth, should it be removed? Some holistic dentists believe that all root-canaled teeth should be removed. However, I feel that the human body is too complex to look at this question in black and white. If a person has a strong immune system, he or she may be able to tolerate a root canal. Another factor to be considered is that every tooth is on an acupuncture meridian and thus each tooth relates to specific organs, tissues, joints, muscles, and vertebrae. This is an important factor in making the decision as to whether or not to have a root canal performed or as to whether or not to extract an existing root-canaled tooth. For example, if the patient has a weak liver, a root canal on the canine tooth, which is on the liver meridian, would be less likely to be tolerated than if that patient's liver were strong. On the other hand, balancing the patient's body chemistry and improving the function of his or her liver, may allow the person to tolerate a root-canaled tooth on this meridian.

Dr. Price showed that inoculating rabbits with an extract of root-canaled teeth from asymptomatic individuals usually did not produce any symptoms. Human beings have many compensatory mechanisms, and I feel that to say that all root-canaled teeth must be removed in everyone is too extreme. I have found that energetic testing via an electrodermal device (known as electroacupuncture according to Voll [EAV] testing, which is discussed below) is the best way to evaluate the current status of root canals and their effect on different parts of the body. I also use EAV testing to periodically monitor root-canaled teeth, especially if a person's health has changed.

Let me be clear, the safest thing is to never have a root canal. A root canal, which is being tolerated today, may not be tolerated at some point in the future. However, for some people the psychological impact of removing a tooth may have more of a negative impact on their health, than the root canal itself. For example, telling a 20-year-old female to remove her front tooth may be too much, psychologically, for her to handle.

It is important that the patient be educated about the possible negative effects of root canals, so that he or she can make an informed decision. For example, a patient of mine presented in pain with an abscess on her upper left first molar. She was 30 years old and had a broad smile that showed her upper teeth all the way back to the molars. Traditional treatment for a case like this would be a root canal. When I asked if anyone in her family had had breast cancer, I could see the shock in her eyes. Her mother had died at the age of 47 of breast cancer, and her mother's mother had died at the age of 55 of breast cancer. I then discussed the pros and cons of root canals and the fact that her infected molar was on the breast meridian. It was important that the patient be aware of this critical information before making her decision. It is also important that all patients be informed that a root-canaled tooth that is currently being tolerated may, at some future time, not be tolerated as a result of age, accident, illness, or mental trauma.

Dr. Price demonstrated that there was a greater risk of root canals creating a problem for individuals with a family history of degenerative diseases. In many of these otherwise healthy patients, the root canals actually trigger the onset of those diseases. Your family's health history is definitely one of the considerations that must be factored in when deciding whether or not to have a root canal. Also, you must consider the state of your own health at the time of making the decision. If you are chronically ill at the time you need the root canal, the wiser choice might be to have the tooth extracted.

Donald, a physician who worked for a pharmaceutical company, had high cholesterol and high blood pressure. The drugs he was taking for these conditions were causing side effects. While researching alternative methods for resolving his problems, Donald learned that dental issues could be contributing to his medical problems. Donald came to see me and I noted that he had mercury fillings and several root-canaled teeth. His mercury fillings and root-canaled teeth did not test well. After I removed his fillings, his cholesterol normalized. And, after I removed his three root-canaled teeth, Donald's blood pressure also returned to normal.

IMPLANTS AND INFLAMMATION

Just like natural teeth, implants can carry a risk with respect to inflammation. Similar to periodontitis, bone loss, called peri-implantitis, has been associated with a significant number of implants. However, given that there are no dental tubules present in an implant, the bacterial load may be less than that of a root-canaled tooth (see the section on "Root Canals and the Inflammatory Process"). However, implants are still a potential problem.[21,22]

Most implants are titanium, and even though titanium is considered a very biocompatible material, approximately 4% of those tested with the MELISA® test are allergic. Memory lymphocyte immunostimulation assay (MELISA) is a blood test that detects Type-IV allergy to metals, chemicals, environmental toxins, and molds from one single blood sample.

Studies have shown that titanium, through a process of corrosion, goes into the cells of the body and binds to proteins; this can produce an autoimmune reaction that can manifest as a skin rash, chronic fatigue, muscle pain, and a host of variable symptoms. In dentistry, if there are other metals present in the mouth from crowns or mercury fillings, corrosion increases.[23,24] Therefore, if a patient is going to have a titanium implant, it is preferable that there be no dissimilar metals present in the mouth. Often, the superstructure placed into the implant and the crown that is placed on top of that are composed of metals other than titanium. This creates galvanic currents, which in turn, have the potential to create health problems. Thus, it is best if the superstructure and crown are ceramic. Ceramic implants are beginning to be used in the United States, and these will decrease the problem of corrosion.

As stated before, every tooth and its corresponding area of the jaw are on acupuncture meridian, which relates to specific organs, tissues, joints, muscles, and vertebrae. Thus, one has to consider the potential effects of placing an implant onto that meridian. This relationship is one of the reasons galvanic currents can have a negative effect on a person's health.

CAVITATIONS AND INFLAMMATION

A cavitation is a hole in the bone, usually in an area where a tooth had been previously extracted and the bone has not filled in properly. Cavitations can occur in any bone in the body, but they are most frequently found in the jawbones. The most common site is the wisdom tooth area. When a tooth is extracted, the dentist typically leaves behind the periodontal membrane. The periodontal membrane is the ligamentous attachment between the tooth and the bone. In a normal healing process, the body fills in the space in the bone where the tooth was once located. Some experts speculate that if the periodontal membrane is not removed, incomplete healing occurs because the bone cells on either side of the space "sense" the presence of the periodontal membrane and "think" that the tooth is still there, thus not filling in the area with new bone. This results in a hole or spongy area of bone known as a cavitation. However, even if an excellent surgeon performed the extraction, and even if the membrane was removed, the patient may not heal properly. This is especially true in the case of individuals that are not in good health.

Recognized as far back as the 1800s, jawbone cavitations go by a number of names, such as ischemic osteonecrosis, neuralgia-inducing cavitational osteonecrosis (NICO), osteomyelitis of the jawbone, jaw osteitis, and others. These lesions characteristically are not painful or tender. They are silent and thus often go undetected. These jawbone lesions are like cesspools; they become filled with inflammatory bacteria and toxins. If your body can quarantine these toxins, the effects will be minimal. However, if the toxins go out into your system, they can cause a myriad of symptoms similar to root canals.

When looking at an x-ray of an extracted tooth site, one might see that the periodontal membrane left behind forms an image that appears to be a shadow of a tooth. When such an image is evident, it is often an indication of the presence of a cavitation. Most dentists are aware of this phantom tooth image; however, they do not recognize it as a source of potential health problems. How does one know if this phantom image, or any suspected area, is a cavitation and if it is, what is its effect on the person?

If a patient is having facial pain such as trigeminal neuralgia, injecting a couple of drops of anesthetic directly into the suspected area will almost immediately relieve the pain (if it is indeed caused by the cavitation). The relief will be temporary, but will become permanent, once the cavitation is treated.

Because most cavitations are silent, do not cause facial pain, and may not be obvious on an x-ray, it is difficult to determine if they exist. I find that the best way to check for cavitations is energetically.

Twenty years ago I developed a heart arrhythmia (PVCs). While I tried natural methods like vitamin and mineral supplementation, IV minerals, herbs and homeopathy, I did not succeed in reversing the arrhythmia. EAV evaluation (see the section on "Electroacupuncture According to Voll") revealed a cavitation in my lower left wisdom tooth area. That wisdom tooth had been extracted 25 years earlier. Given that the wisdom teeth area is located on the heart meridian, Dr. Voll observed in his patients a relationship between this area and heart problems. Surgical debridement (cleaning out) of the cavitation resolved the PVCs in a few days. I have had no further problem since that time. Up until the point of symptoms, my body had been able to compensate for the toxins and for the blockage of my energy flow through this meridian.

ELECTROACUPUNCTURE ACCORDING TO VOLL: HELPING TO TRACK DOWN INFLAMMATION AND CAUSES OF INFLAMMATION ENERGETICALLY

EAV was developed out of the research of Dr. Reinhold Voll, a practicing medical doctor, anatomy professor, acupuncturist, and homeopath. Dr. Voll began his clinical analysis in the late 1940s. Melding his various interests, Dr. Voll was able to scientifically document something that Chinese acupuncturists had known for centuries—that there are, in the human body, points on the skin having high levels of electrical conduction (less resistance), and that these points are known as acupuncture points. Fascinated by his confirmation of the existence of these energy pathways, Dr. Voll developed a simple metering device to measure the skin resistance over acupuncture points. This important component of the EAV device is basically an ohmmeter, which measures electron flow in a circuit. The meter has a metal cylinder attached at one end and a stylus attached at the other end. A small amount of current enters through the cylinder. Thus, if the stylus is touched to the cylinder, the reading on the meter will go to 100. This means that there is no resistance and there is a completed circuit.

Dr. Voll had his patients hold a small brass cylinder in one hand. Then he would touch the tip of the stylus to a specific acupuncture point. The stylus would introduce a minute amount of electrical current that would travel through the body to reach the cylinder thus forming a complete electrical circuit. The amount of skin resistance at the acupuncture site would then be recorded. Dr. Voll found normal skin resistance over a healthy acupuncture point to be 100,000 Ω. This equals 50 on the Voll galvanic skin response scale.

As previously mentioned, the human body is not just a physical being; it simultaneously operates via a series of electrical impulses that have been shown to follow certain pathways. These pathways can be accessed at various points on the skin, where there are changes in the electrical resistance or the ability of the tissue to conduct electricity. During 40 years of research Dr. Voll documented, throughout the body, an entire network of these energetic pathways, better known as energy meridians. Many correspond to traditional acupuncture meridians; many are new. He was also able to establish that each meridian acted like a "highway" for energy, connecting specific teeth, organs, tissues, and in fact, everything in the body.

A healthy pathway can sustain a certain level of electron flow. Inflammation tends to foster increased activity in the cells, thereby creating a more active environment through which electrons flow at a greater rate. Thus, if inflammation exists anywhere along the meridian pathway, the EAV testing will show a higher-than-average flow of electrons, as indicated by a reading of greater than 50.

Degenerative states cause cellular activity to slow and stagnate, making it more difficult for electrons to flow through the circuit. In such a state, the EAV testing would reveal a reading less than 50. Dr. Voll found that the most significant information he derived from EAV testing was revealed when the electron flow dropped from an initial reading to a lower reading. For example, a situation wherein the initial reading may be 55, but then drops to 35; this pattern indicates that a circuit, which was formerly capable of sustaining electron flow, is no longer able to do so. This type of drop evidences a disturbance in the circuit. Dr. Voll called this fall in reading an Indicator Drop.

Because the body consists of an energetic "web" of relationships, the major circuits have secondary and tertiary circuits connecting virtually all parts of the body. A highly skilled practitioner of EAV testing can establish a cause–effect relationship between any two points on the body. The use of EAV testing provides critical information that assists the practitioner in choosing the correct treatments to help a patient heal.

Because every major organ and, in fact, nearly everything in the human body is linked via meridians to a specific tooth and tooth area, the implications of EAV testing in a whole body approach to dentistry is exciting. For instance, EAV test results may indicate a hypothyroid condition, which might be caused by a cavitation in the upper first molar area, which is on the thyroid meridian. This type of early warning should be followed by traditional thyroid function testing to see if the condition has reached a physical point, where blood tests indicate a problem. However, it is important to remember that energetic changes always precede physical changes. Truly, preventive treatment would always begin as energy imbalances manifest; in this case, treatment would start before the problem shows up at a physical level in a blood test.

The fact that every tooth is on an acupuncture meridian, which relates to specific organs and tissues, is very important in helping to diagnose a problem with an individual tooth. Sometimes teeth are treated with a root canal or with an extraction (because the patient has pain), with the result being no resolution of the pain. For example, a patient presented with terrible pain in an upper canine (eye) tooth. At first it seemed obvious that a root canal or extraction was necessary. However, EAV testing revealed that a problem in the gallbladder was the underlying cause of the pain. Treatment of the gallbladder issue relieved the tooth pain.

EAV testing provides a phenomenal amount of information about the nature of what is happening in the body. It is an exceptional tool for helping to identify the type of traditional diagnostic testing that might be appropriate to confirm one's own suspicions as to what is occurring.

EAV equipment has also been used for allergy testing, and one study has actually shown EAV to be as accurate, or more accurate, than other forms of allergy testing.[25] EAV testing allows the practitioner to learn whether two seemingly unrelated symptoms in the body are indeed connected to one another.

EAV screening provides invaluable information about the patient's energetic "web" or currents and helps the practitioner determine the location of "energetic stressors" that are creating blockages or disturbances in the natural flow of energy. The stressors themselves can be anything alien to or out of balance in the body. They may include any foreign material implanted in the body, like fillings, crowns, implants, or root-canaled teeth. They may also emanate from issues involving sinuses, tonsils, impacted teeth, periodontal disease, cavitations, or various toxins. Even scars located on different parts of the body can act as stressors, affecting import meridians.

Stressors create a field of disturbance in the energetic web of the body. These fields of disturbance are most often in the head, because the mouth is where we most frequently have procedures performed. The results of such disturbances can be felt anywhere in the body and can actually block the effectiveness of any treatment.

Each individual has his or her own tolerance level for stressors. The range of responses to stressors is truly incredible. Certainly, factors such as diet, exercise, state of mind, genetics, and general well-being play an important role in how well a person's system can tolerate the stressors.

Ironically, a mishap at a presentation of EAV technology by Dr. Voll resulted in the discovery of one of EAV's most powerful abilities. Dr. Voll was giving a demonstration on a patient who had a large indicator drop on his prostate point. During a break, a helpful homeopath from the audience approached the patient and offered him a homeopathic remedy. The patient gratefully put the vial of medication in his pocket. After the break Dr. Voll resumed his demonstration with the same patient, but now found that the readings on the prostate point were normal.

After several confusing and somewhat embarrassing minutes of questioning his subject, Dr. Voll discovered the homeopath's remedy. Although the remedy was in a container in the patient's pocket, it was able to influence the readings. In fact, he discovered that the remedy influenced the readings even when it was simply held near enough to be in the patient's energy field. When the remedy was removed beyond the patient's energy field, the reading again indicated an energetic imbalance of the prostate.

This event ultimately led to one of the most interesting discoveries relating to meridians. It also provided a spectacular demonstration of how the human energy field does indeed extend beyond the boundaries of the physical body. In the following years, Dr. Voll developed a sophisticated means of selecting proper homeopathic remedies and various other substances based on EAV readings. He would place homeopathic remedies, vitamins, foods, and so on on a tray, which was in the circuit, to test their effects on the meridian readings. This method was very laborious but effective.

Modern EAV units are computerized, and the testing that Dr. Voll did manually is now much faster and more simplified. Although Dr. Voll needed the physical remedy or supplement, we now only need the frequency of what is being tested. Everything has its own unique energy signal or "energetic fingerprint," such as homeopathic remedies, foods, drugs, chemicals, and pesticides. Just as one can take one's voice frequency, digitalize it, and place it on a CD, one can take the energetic signal of anything and place it on a disk. Over the years, the energetic signals of countless substances have been entered into various EAV software programs, resulting in thousands of "virtual" bottles, so that the actual physical matter being tested is no longer necessary.

EAV is a wonderful instrument to help track down inflammation and causes of inflammation. Various toxins, such as pesticides or chemicals to which people are generally exposed, are often associated with inflammation. EAV testing allows one to evaluate whether or not particular substances present a problem, quantify the level of the problem, and track progress while removing those toxins from the body. Many practitioners are very skeptical of this type of testing because these concepts are based on the principles of energy rather than on the mechanical model, with which we are more familiar. However, for more than 20 years, I have clinically observed the successful results of this type of testing.

Therapy localization can be used to determine if a tooth, or if a cavitation, relates to a specific problem. For example, to discover whether or not a root canaled tooth on a lower right second molar is related to a chronic sinus problem, the following will be done. Using the hand holding the brass rod, the patient will place the index finger of this hand onto the root-canaled tooth. The tester will then place the stylus on various acupuncture points on the free hand, including the sinus point. If the root-canaled tooth is a problem for this patient, readings will change from the baseline readings (what they are without touching the root-canaled tooth). As an example, let us say there was an indicator drop on the sinus point when getting a baseline reading. This indicator drop signifies a problem in the sinus. If the patient therapy localizes to the root-canaled tooth and now we have no indicator drop on the sinus point, this indicates a cause-and-effect relationship; the root canal is having an effect on the sinus. One can then even output signals to see if bacteria from the root-canaled tooth are a problem and/or if other types of toxins (such as thioethers) are emanating from the dead tooth. This same method can be used to determine if the root-canaled tooth relates to a heart valve problem.

The use of EAV is also helpful in nutritional assessment. Supplements can be tested separately to see if each is compatible with the patient. Also, groupings of supplements can be tested at the same time, to see if they test well for the patient when taken together. It is not uncommon for supplements that test well individually, to not test well, when taken together as a particular grouping. Thus, various permutations of the prescribed supplements can be tested so that they are taken in optimal combinations.

BEYOND THE PHYSICAL: THE ENERGETIC LEVEL

The things that I have discussed thus far all have an inflammatory effect. It is important to manage these and to rid the body of these dental stressors. There are many other stressors; these include chemicals or pesticides, mold, parasites, and so on. It is important to address all of them. These can all be handled at a physical level, in other words, by doing things physically to remove them from the body. For instance, we can remove the mercury fillings, we can treat the periodontal disease and we can detoxify the body. However, is this enough? What is there beyond this?

I have observed that just a few mercury fillings or one root canal can have devastating effects on some people, while others are seemingly unaffected. Some people can be bitten by a tick, known to be carrying the Lyme bacteria, and remain Lyme free, even without antibiotics, while other people's health is forever changed, even with antibiotics. It all comes down to the resistance of the host. That resistance is composed of many different factors. I liken it to a balance scale. On one side of the scale is optimal health, on the other side are all those things opposing optimal health, both the physical and nonphysical. Many things will weigh down the bad side of the scale. The physical negatives include chemicals, pesticides, heavy metals, a bad structural relationship between the mandible and maxilla, impacted teeth, dead teeth, cavitations, infected tonsils, scars, poor nutrition, an out-of-balance acid–base level, a bad heart valve, or a bad hip. As we have discussed, these can be addressed at a physical level, and it is important that this be done. Unloading the physical stressors is straightforward and can substantially improve a person's health. A person may feel so much better that it seems as if nothing more needs to be done. Yet, if we look closely, there may still remain symptoms of grief or anxiety, digestive complaints, and so on. Then there are those people that have always felt well. We all know people who exercise, eat nutritiously, do not have a particularly stressful job or home life, feel well, and yet develop heart disease, cancer, or some other debilitating problem such as, for example, arthritis. If you question them, they will say that they were perfectly healthy up to this point of illness. However, if one looks more deeply, this is not the case. They all had symptoms. Often there were small problems that did not interfere with their lifestyle and tended to be ignored. These symptoms are the "voice of nature. They call out to us. These are the keys to unlocking a path to a much higher level of health. In such instances, we are at an energetic or vibrational level, the world of frequencies. There are different ways to access this level. One can approach it by dealing with the individual symptoms, as if one tuned only the violins in a symphony orchestra. As the violins are tuned, the sound of the instruments will become harmonious, with each note resonating with the universal note it is tuned to. There are a number of ways to tune into these aberrant frequencies. Different holistic modalities such as color therapy, music therapy, Rife machines, and homeopathic remedies are among a group of treatment modalities that can change frequencies and alleviate symptoms. However, other instruments in the orchestra may also be out of tune. If we could magically tune all the instruments in an orchestra with a master frequency, we could then create a beautiful symphony of sound. This is where I find homeopathy to be invaluable. Homeopathy can tune many instruments at one time. When that is done, many of the patient's symptoms will fall by the wayside. To better understand how homeopathy works, we need to understand its underlying principles. What are the foundational principles?

First is the law of "like cures like." The substance that will cause symptoms in a healthy person will take away those same symptoms in a sick person. Allergy shots are based on this concept of "like cures like." Unlike homeopathy, the shots actually give you a small amount of the allergen to which you are allergic, to desensitize you.

Second is the law of "potentization," which relates to the releasing of the inner energy of a substance. Unlike an allergy shot, a homeopathic remedy has no physical substance; it is an energetic signal or energetic vibration.

Another foundational principle of homeopathy is that symptoms are a manifestation between what Dr. Samuel Hahnemann called the "vital force" and something external such as a toxin or chronic infection.

Inherited traits or what Dr. Hahnemann called miasms, today we would refer to them as our genetic predispositions. Dr. Hahnemann found miasms to be the underlying cause of all chronic diseases. These miasms represent the core from which various symptoms emerge. The symptoms are given names like eczema, herpes, arthritis, heart disease, colitis, and so on. Looking at a patient's list of external symptoms (nature's voice), along with an understanding of the underlying miasms, the physician can find a specific homeopathic remedy, which can begin the process of true cure.

It is also extremely important to understand the fundamental truth about suppression of symptoms. Suppressing symptoms does not cure the underlying disease. Instead, the illness is driven deeper into the body until it manifests in another way. By the time a person exhibits pathology (an identifiable physical change), that person has probably been suffering for a long time. By "suffering" I mean that there have been symptoms, which were subtly or nonsubtly, crying out for treatment. Those symptoms may have been nagging and persistent, or they may have been symptoms that deal with the senses (ones for which modern medicine has no answers). For instance, a person may be affected by the phases of the moon. Another may catch cold whenever his or her chest is exposed to a draft. Others may have an altered sense of taste or be sensitive to smells. A child may have difficulty controlling his temper. These are the beginnings of what will follow. If not addressed in their early stages, these seemingly innocuous symptoms will eventually manifest themselves as external symptoms that modern medicine will now name and treat with a drug, which will suppress those symptoms. From a homeopathic perspective, these beginning changes are vibrational in nature; therefore, homeopathic remedies, which themselves are vibrational, should be used to treat them. The homeopathic remedy chosen should be based on the totality of symptoms, both physical and emotional.

Dr. Hahnemann also talked about "exciting" causes of the underlying miasms. Exciting causes are external stressors that can bring latent miasms to the surface or prevent a cure. Given that emotional stress, poor diet, toxins, drugs, and so on, can all be exciting causes, it is particularly important to treat both the physical and the nonphysical.

In summary, I feel that symptoms are nature's voice calling out to us. We need to answer nature's call. To do this, we must view dentistry in a global manner and address not only the problems in the mouth but also everything related to the mouth. It is not enough to treat inflammation. We need to address what is present even before inflammation. In other words, we need to treat the whole body. This approach leads not only to better oral health but also to better cardiovascular and general health.

REFERENCES

1. The Heart Foundation. Heart Disease Statitics, http://www.theheartfoundation.org/heart-disease-facts/heart-disease-statistics (accessed 2014).
2. Fischer MH. *Death and Dentistry*. Chicago, IL: Charles C. Thomas, 1940.
3. Leishman SJ, Do HL, Ford PJ. Cardiovascular disease and the role of oral bacteria. *J Oral Microbiol* 2010;2.
4. Demmer RT, Desvarieux M. Periodontal infections and cardiovascular disease: The heart of the matter. *J Am Dent Assoc* 2006;137(suppl):14S–20S.
5. Grau AJ, Becher H, Ziegler CM et al. Periodontal disease as a risk factor for ischemic stroke. *Stroke* 2004;35(2):496–501.
6. Wu T, Trevisan M, Genco RJ, Dorn JP, Falkner KL, Sempos CT. Periodontal disease and risk of cerebrovascular disease: The first national health and nutrition examination survey and its follow-up study. *Arch Intern Med* 2000;18:2749–2755.
7. Slade GD, Ghezzi EM, Heiss G, Beck JD, Riche E, Offenbacher S. Relationship between periodontal disease and C-reactive protein among adults in the Atherosclerosis Risk in Communities study. *Arch Intern Med* 2003;163:1172–1179.
8. Brown DL. MIDAS: Effects on inflammatory markers with low dose doxycycline versus placebo. American Heart Association's Scientific Sessions, 2002 http://www.theheart.org/article/198883.do (accessed 2009).
9. Placidi GF, Dell'Osso L, Viola PL, Bertelli A. Distribution of inhaled mercury (203Hg) in various organs. *Int J Tiss React* 1983;5:193–200.
10. Khayat A, Denker L. Whole body and liver distribution of inhaled mercury vapor in the mouse: Influence of ethanol and aminothiozole pretreatment. *J Appl Toxicol* 1983;3(2):66–73.
11. Frustace A, Magnavita N, Chimenti C. Marked elevation of myocardial trace elements in idiopathic dilated cardiomyopathy compared with secondary cardiac dysfunction. *J Am Coll Cardiol* 1999;33(6):1578–1583.
12. Cutright DE, Miller RA, Battistone GC, Milikan LJ. Systemic mercury levels caused by inhaling mist during high speed amalgam grinding. *J Oral Med* 1973;28(4):100–104.
13. Vimy MJ, Takahash Y, Lorscheider FL. Maternal-fetal distribution of mercury (203 Hg) released from dental amalgam fillings. *Am J Physiol* 1990;258:R939–R945.
14. Siberlund RI. Relationship between mercury and dental amalgam and the cardiovascular system. *Sci Total Environ* 1990;99(1–2):22–35.
15. Hahn LJ, Kloiber R, Leininger RW, Vimy MJ, Lorscheider FL. Whole-body imaging of the distribution of mercury released from dental fillings in monkey tissues. *FASEB J* 1990;4:3256–3260.

16. Kostka B, Michalska M, Krajewska U, Wierzbicki R. Blood coagulation changes in rats poisoned with methylmercuric chloride (MeHg). *Pol J Pharm* 1989;41(2):183–189.

17. Price WA. *Dental Infections Oral and Systemic.* The following volumes listed in footnotes 17–20 cover the many years of research by Dr. Weston Price* and are available from Price-Pottenger Nutrition Foundation http://www.ppnf.org (*Dr. Weston A. Price was a dentist and one of the foremost researchers of his time. Dr. Price did 25 years of research on the root canal issue at the beginning of the twentieth century).

18. Price WA. *Researches on Fundamentals of Oral and Systemic Expressions of Dental Infections.* Available from the Price-Pottenger Nutrition Foundation, http://www.ppnf.org.

19. Price WA. *Researches on Clinical Expressions of Dental Infections.* Available from the Price-Pottenger Nutrition Foundation, http://www.ppnf.org.

20. Price WA. *Dental Infections and the Degenerative Disease.* Available from the Price-Pottenger Nutrition Foundation, http://www.ppnf.org.

21. Serino G, Turri A. Extent and location of bone loss at dental implants in patients with peri-implantits. *J Biomech* 2011;44(2):267–271.

22. Khammissa RA, Feller L, Meyerov R, Lemmer J. Peri-implant mucositis and peri-implantitis: Bacterial infection. *SADJ* 2012;67(2):70, 72–74.

23. Reclaru L, Meyer JM. Study of corrosion between a titanium implant and dental alloys. *J Dent* 1994;22:159–168.

24. Ravnholt G, Jensen J. Corrosion investigation of two materials for implant: Supraconstructions coupled to a titanium implant. *Scand J Dent Res* 1991;99:181–186.

25. Tsui J, Lehman CW, Lam FM, Zhu DA. A food allergy study utilizing the EAV acupuncture technique. *Am J Acupuncture* 1984;12(2):105–116.

11 Lyme Disease and the Heart

William Lee Cowden

CONTENTS

BRIEF LYME DISEASE HISTORY

Lyme disease was first described as an outbreak of predominantly juvenile rheumatoid arthritis in Old Lyme, Connecticut, in the 1970s.[1] It was later shown to be an infectious illness transmitted to humans by the bite of a deer tick. Dr. Willy Burgdorfer identified the spirochete (spiral-shaped bacteria) *Borrelia burgdorferi* as the infectious agent.[2] It is now known that there are about a dozen other genetically related species in addition to the *B. burgdorferi* spirochete that can cause Lyme disease symptoms, especially *Borrelia afzelii* and *Borrelia garinii*. These species of spirochetes are collectively referred to as *Borrelia burgdorferi sensu lato*, and they can be transmitted to humans from various animals by various species of ticks.[3] There are also a variety of microbial coinfections carried by the same ticks that transmit *B. burgdorferi sensu lato* to humans and, often, these coinfections are transmitted to humans at the same time as the *Borrelia*. These coinfections include *Anaplasma phagocytophilum*, *Ehrlichia chaffeensis*, and *Coxiella burnetii*, as well as a variety of other *Rickettsia* (bacteria-like microbes); some *Bartonella* bacterial species; some *Babesia* protozoa species; various *Mycoplasma* bacterial species; certain worms (such as *Varestrongylus klapowi*) and, according to one European *Borrelia* researcher, also some *Chlamydia* species, *Yersinia enterocolitica*, *Campylobacter jejuni*, and human parvovirus B19.[4] When a person has coinfections along with *Borrelia*, it becomes much more complicated to make a proper, comprehensive diagnosis and to treat the person. Officials from the U.S. government's Center for Disease Control and Prevention recently announced that there are likely 300,000 new cases of Lyme disease in the United States each year because of a 10-fold underreporting of Lyme disease by physicians.[5]

DIAGNOSING LYME DISEASE AND COINFECTIONS

Standards for diagnosing and treating borreliosis and some of its coinfections have been published by the Infectious Diseases Society of America (IDSA).[6] Diagnosing *Borrelia* and all of the coinfections can be very challenging. The physical diagnostic hallmark of borreliosis is an erythema migrans (EM) skin rash (Figure 11.1) in a patient who has been bitten by a tick. However, a medical literature search revealed that at least 19% of U.S. *Borrelia* patients did not have an EM rash and many could not recall having been bitten by a tick.[7] Two practitioners in Houston, Texas (which is not considered an endemic area for Lyme disease), reported in 2003 that most of their 455 chronically ill patients who had symptoms in multiple systems of their bodies tested positive for *B. burgdorferi* after repeat Western blot or polymerase chain reaction (PCR) testing, even though two-thirds of them tested negative on the first test.[8] On the Centers for Disease Control and Prevention website,[9] there is a helpful diagram to aid physicians in diagnosing *Borrelia*. If the patient's symptoms suggest the possibility of borreliosis, the first test that they should do is a blood enzyme immunoassay (EIA) or a blood immunofluorescence assay (IFA). Only if one of those first tests is positive should a more specific blood test be done: a Western blot. If the initial EIA/IFA is negative and the signs/symptoms have persisted for greater than 30 days, an unspecified alternative diagnosis should be considered.

The incidence of false-negative blood tests in patients with the most advanced stage of *Borrelia* (called neuroborreliosis, meaning brain and/or spinal cord involvement) may be as high as 15%[10] because only *B. burgdorferi* is usually tested, rather than testing as well for the other species of *Borrelia* that can also commonly cause neuroborreliosis. Another reason for false-negative blood tests in Lyme patients is the presence or absence of certain human leukocyte antigens (the white blood cell proteins HLA-DR1 and HLA-DR7).[11] Furthermore, Lyme patients who have active live spirochetes in their joints and cerebrospinal fluid tend to have low or negative *Borrelia* antibodies in their serum,[12] which suggests that an excess of microbial antigens, resulting from rapidly growing microbes, might be overwhelming the immune system, forming immune complexes (which are not tested by most tests) and thus creating a negative antibody test. If Lyme disease test results are

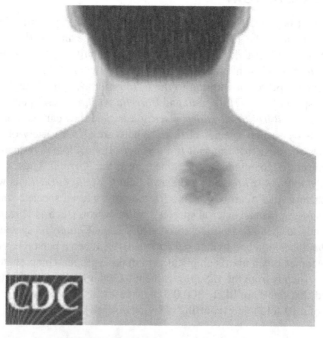

FIGURE 11.1   (See color insert.) Typical erythema migrans (EM) rash of Lyme borreliosis. (Courtesy of Centers for Disease Control and Prevention website.)

suspected to be false negative, it is a good idea to do a repeat test after a few weeks and also possibly test for *B. afzelii* and *B. garinii* or even some of the other less common *Borrelia* species in addition to *B. burgdorferi*. Testing for HLA-DR1 and HLA-DR7 may also be useful.

HOW LYME BORRELIOSIS AND COINFECTIONS CREATE MULTISYSTEM ILLNESS

Borreliosis often causes illness in many systems of the body, and several or all of the following conditions/symptoms can be found in the same patient: fatigue, fever, headaches, neuropathy, spinal nerve pain, inflammation in the eye, muscle pains, joint pains, skin rashes, lymph node swelling, various heart problems, gastrointestinal complaints, urinary symptoms, and even Guillain-Bare syndrome (a body-wide paralysis).[4] *Borrelia* is known as a great imitator, meaning that it imitates many different conditions. In fact, there are over 300 medical conditions linked to borreliosis by cause or by association.[13] Unfortunately, several of the common Lyme coinfections can cause many of the same conditions as *Borrelia*,[4,14–18] making it difficult to know whether *Borrelia* or other coinfections (or both *Borrelia* and the coinfections) are causing the ongoing symptoms after a usual treatment course for the microbes that were identified on the initial testing. In some cases, one or more of the coinfections are initially present without *Borrelia* and are not suspected by the treating practitioner because the patient did not have an EM rash. Blood testing for all of the possible coinfections is almost impossible because there are so many species that could be causing the symptoms and tests for some of the species are not readily available.

One solution to this dilemma is to do electrodermal screening (EDS) for the various suspected microbes. EDS, developed in Germany in the 1950s by Dr. Voll,[19] is like a lie-detector test, measuring galvanic skin response to a stressor[20]; but instead of the voice of a policeman being the stressor, the vibrational frequency of a microbe, toxin, or some other substance (generated by the EDS device) is the potential stressor. The frequency of a microbe that has never affected the patient will not create an abnormal galvanic skin response, but the frequency of a microbe recently affecting the patient will almost always produce an abnormal galvanic skin response. So, EDS is a useful data-gathering device used by many integrative medicine practitioners, but EDS does not make a diagnosis. It provides additional useful data, which a skilled integrative practitioner can factor into the patient's history, physical examination, laboratory tests, and imaging procedures to make a diagnosis. The EDS can also be used with fairly good accuracy to help predict which therapies might be helpful to consider for a specific patient and which therapies would likely produce an undesirable response in the patient. Some integrative practitioners also use some form of muscle testing to gather additional data that might assist in the diagnosis of Lyme disease and coinfections and to determine which therapies might be effective and which ones might be ineffective or potentially harmful for the patient.

OVERVIEW OF LYME EFFECTS ON THE HEART

Borrelia and all of the aforementioned coinfections (other than possibly *Anaplasma* and *Ehrlichia*) can cause heart disease. The most recent review of Lyme disease and the heart in peer-reviewed medical literature[21] failed to mention that coinfections and even other *Borrelia* species (besides *B. burgdorferi sensu stricto*) can cause heart disease. For this reason, physicians who are trying to offer the most help possible to their patients should educate themselves thoroughly about the effects that these microbes have on the heart and not rely on just one article for information. Studies published about 30 years ago revealed that carditis (inflammation of the heart) occurred in 4%–10% of untreated U.S. Lyme disease patients and even more than that if asymptomatic carditis was included[22] but that it occurred in only 0.3%–4% of European Lyme patients.[23] With more physicians recognizing Lyme disease and starting antibiotic therapy at earlier stages of the disease, Lyme carditis, which is a late-stage manifestation of Lyme, has become less common in endemic areas of the United States. But because many physicians still believe that Lyme disease can only occur near Lyme, Connecticut with an associated EM rash, there are still people with unrecognized/undiagnosed Lyme disease who have carditis, especially in nonendemic areas.

The most common cardiac indication that someone has Lyme carditis is atrioventricular (AV) block. The AV block is a condition in which there is impaired electrical conduction in the heart from the upper chambers (atria) to the lower chambers (ventricles) through the AV node (specialized electrical conducting cells between the heart chambers). Because severe AV block often results in a heart rate so slow that passing out can occur, this sometimes requires the patient to wear a temporary pacemaker for a few days while the carditis that caused the AV block is resolved with a course of appropriate antibiotics.[24,25] A permanent pacemaker is very rarely ever needed for Lyme carditis as the antibiotics usually resolve the AV block.

There are various other heart conditions/problems that may also be caused by Lyme disease. Junctional tachycardia[26] and fascicular tachycardia[27] are fast, abnormal heart rhythms that originate from the Lyme-induced inflammation in the electrical conducting tissue between the two lower (ventricular) chambers of the heart. Lyme can also cause mild left ventricular dysfunction and even rare cardiomegaly (heart chamber enlargement often with insufficient blood being pumped out of the heart with each beat).[28] Acute myopericarditis is an inflammation in the heart muscle and in the sac around the entire heart (the pericardium) that can be caused by Lyme.[28] This pericardial inflammation often results in fluid accumulation in the pericardial sac, which can then put such severe pressure on the heart chambers that they cannot adequately fill with blood during each beat of the heart and this can even be fatal.[28] Much less common ways in which Lyme affects the heart are endocarditis (an inflammation of one or more of the heart valves and inner lining of the heart)[29] and sick sinus syndrome (a disease process in the primary heart rhythm regulating center that causes the heart to beat much too fast at times and much too slowly at other times).[30] Also, supraventricular tachycardia (a very fast abnormal heart rhythm from the upper heart chambers) and even ventricular tachycardia (a very fast abnormal heart rhythm from the lower heart chambers) are other heart conditions rarely seen with Lyme carditis.[31] So patients with arrhythmias are often evaluated for coronary artery disease as a cause of the arrhythmia, but very rarely does a cardiologist think to look for Lyme disease as a cause. And if a blood test is done to look for Lyme disease, there is probably less than a 50% chance that the blood test will find *Borrelia*, even if it is the cause of the arrhythmia. It is important to remember that no tick bite or EM rash is necessary for Lyme disease to be the cause of an arrhythmia or other cardiac condition. And it is also important to understand the difficulties in diagnosing Lyme disease so that a person's cardiac condition is not attributed to something else.

When Lyme carditis has persisted for many weeks to months before diagnosis and treatment, a cardiomyopathy can develop. Cardiomyopathy is a generalized weakening of the heart muscle commonly associated with enlargement (dilation) of the heart chambers and with shortness of breath on minimal exertion and sometimes even at rest (especially when lying flat in bed at night). Advanced cardiomyopathy can easily result in congestive heart failure, which usually necessitates hospitalization. An Austrian study found that 26% of cardiomyopathy patients tested positive for *B. burgdorferi*, whereas only 8% of healthy blood donors tested positive.[32] In one research study in Prague, Czech Republic, heart muscle biopsies were done on patients with and without dilated cardiomyopathy (DCM).[33] In the DCM group, 24% of the heart biopsies were positive for *B. burgdorferi*, *B. afzelii*, or *B. garinii* but none in the control group (those with no DCM). In Warsaw, Poland, diseased hearts that were removed during heart transplantation were analyzed and found to have the DNA of *Borrelia* species, as well as some Lyme coinfections: *Coxiella* and *Bartonella*.[34] There are case reports of DCM in patients with known, or strongly suspected, *B. burgdorferi* infection whose DCM resolved after treatment with high-dose penicillin or ceftriaxone antibiotic.[35,36] This strongly suggests *B. burgdorferi* as the cause of the DCM in those cases. There is one fascinating case report of a 47-year-old woman who was given ceftriaxone antibiotic for fever, EM rash, shortness of breath, and passing out from complete AV heart block.[37] She had such a severe Herxheimer reaction (rapid toxin buildup from rapid microbe die-off) in her heart that she developed a life-threatening, very rapid heart rhythm and cardiogenic shock (very low blood pressure from heart failure). This required aggressive life support in the hospital to keep her alive. With 28 days of antibiotic therapy for Lyme disease, she recovered fully and the pumping function of her left ventricle (main heart pumping chamber) rose from 10% to 61% (normal is 55%–65%).

THERAPY FOR LYME CARDITIS IN GENERAL

If a patient has apparent Lyme carditis and chest pain, shortness of breath, passing out, or AV block, they should be hospitalized and continually monitored.[6] A temporary pacemaker may be required for advanced AV block, but a permanent pacemaker is very rarely ever needed. For Lyme carditis conditions that are severe enough to require hospitalization, an intravenous antibiotic, such as ceftriaxone, is recommended as an initial treatment; then once the patient's condition has improved sufficiently, the remainder of a 14- to 21-day treatment course can be completed with an oral antibiotic.[6] As seen in the cardiogenic shock case previously described, very aggressive and invasive therapies must be used occasionally to save a patient's life, but fortunately such therapies are rarely needed for people with Lyme carditis. And the various Lyme carditis conditions usually resolve fully with appropriate antibiotic therapy.

PHARMACEUTICAL ANTIBIOTIC RESEARCH IN LYME

A research study that was done on patients with Lyme disease, in which the patients were given trial treatments of antibiotics, revealed that tetracycline was more effective than penicillin and erythromycin for treating the EM rash, which occurs in early-stage Lyme disease. The patients who were treated with tetracycline had no major late-stage manifestations or complications from the illness, such as carditis, encephalitis (brain inflammation), or recurrent attacks of arthritis, but late-stage complications occurred in 7%–14% of the patients in the other two groups.[38] In 1990, patients who were given the combination of amoxicillin and probenecid for treating the EM Lyme rash had just as favorable results as those patients who were given doxycycline (a long-acting tetracycline antibiotic). This combination of antibiotics was also just as effective for preventing late-stage complications of Lyme disease.[39] Cephalexin was ineffective in treating early Lyme,[40] but cefuroxime was found to be as effective as doxycycline in treating early (EM rash) Lyme patients.[41] In treating early Lyme patients, however, azithromycin was less effective than amoxicillin.[42] Cefuroxime and amoxicillin were both found to be safe and effective for treating children 6 months to 12 years old with early Lyme disease[43] as tetracycline and doxycycline cause dental abnormalities and cannot be used in children. A study in 1997 found intravenous or intramuscular ceftriaxone equivalent to doxycycline in treating acute disseminated Lyme disease.[44] One study[45] found that for early Lyme there was no better 30-month outcome in those treated with 20 days of doxycycline, or 2 g of intravenous ceftriaxone followed by 10 days of doxycycline, compared to only 10 days of doxycycline (100 mg twice daily), but there was a four times greater risk of diarrhea in those given ceftriaxone. So, in summary, 10 days of doxycycline twice daily by mouth, or intravenous/intramuscular ceftriaxone, is the preferred treatment for adult Lyme patients and oral amoxicillin or cefuroxime is the preferred treatment for children.

LYME TREATMENT GUIDELINES FROM THE INFECTIOUS DISEASES SOCIETY OF AMERICA

The Lyme treatment guidelines were published by the IDSA in 2006.[6] The IDSA recommended only 14–28 days of pharmaceutical antibiotics for treatment whether the Lyme disease presented as acute EM or as late-stage disease with central nervous system involvement or very-late-stage arthritis or skin involvement (acrodermatitis chronica atrophicans [ACA]). Intravenous antibiotics were reserved for involvement of the heart, central nervous system, or peripheral nerves. The IDSA article[6] also said that "because of a lack of biologic plausibility, lack of efficacy, absence of supporting data, or the potential for harm to the patient" several therapies were not recommended for the treatment of Lyme disease, including various specific pharmaceutical antibiotics, "pulsed-dosing … , long-term antibiotic therapy, anti-*Bartonella* therapies, hyperbaric oxygen, ozone, fever therapy, intravenous immunoglobulin, cholestyramine, intravenous hydrogen peroxide, specific nutritional supplements, and others … ." It may be logical to avoid a few of these strategies/treatments, such as the antibiotics that are unproved in studies, like first-generation cephalosporins (the first antibiotics ever developed in this class of drugs), but recommendations to avoid other treatments/therapies are not logical or reasonable. For example, if a patient with advanced cardiomyopathy is proved, by appropriate testing, to have *Bartonella* myocarditis or endocarditis (with or without *Borrelia*), then the *Bartonella* should be treated with some of these other "forbidden" antibiotics to reduce the risk of the patient having to have a valve replacement or heart transplant.[34] Also, if objective testing proves that a patient with Lyme disease has a nutritional deficiency, it could be considered malpractice to withhold the needed nutrients from him or her. Certain nutrients are harmless and have a low risk of side effects, but they are likely to improve the patient's immune function or the production of adenosine triphosphate (ATP), which provides energy to the body so that it can heal. For example, 57% of the U.S. population ingests less magnesium than what is recommended by the U.S. Department of Agriculture.[46] Therefore, more than half of the population should be taking a magnesium nutritional supplement to maintain their health. This contradicts the aforementioned IDSA guidelines, which recommend avoiding such nutrients.

PHARMACEUTICAL TREATMENT FOR LATE-STAGE LYME DISEASE

The most common late-stage manifestations of Lyme disease are Lyme arthritis, Lyme DCM, ACA (a chronic inflammatory skin condition predominantly in the hands and feet), Lyme encephalomyelitis (an inflammation in the brain and spinal cord), and Lyme peripheral neuropathy (a loss of sensation in the feet, legs, and sometimes hands caused by *Borrelia*). The ACA and DCM are both rare in the United States but a bit more common in Europe. A study has shown that Lyme arthritis can be healed by 28–30 days of oral doxycycline or amoxicillin. Lyme arthritis that is resistant to 28–30 days of oral therapy may be treated with intravenous or intramuscular ceftriaxone 2 g/day for 14 days.[47] Intravenous or intramuscular ceftriaxone 2 g daily for 14–28 days is reported to be the best treatment for neurological Lyme disease[48] and usually helps to resolve other chronic manifestations of Lyme disease at the same time. Research by Judith Miklossy[49] has demonstrated that 25% of all Alzheimer's dementia cases are likely caused by *B. burgdorferi* infections and most of the remainder of the cases by other spirochetal bacteria that are commonly found in the human mouth. A prospective study has not yet been done though to determine if Alzheimer's dementia can be reversed by antimicrobial treatment.

INEFFECTIVENESS OF ANTIBIOTICS TO RESOLVE LATE-STAGE LYME SYMPTOMS

A fairly recent study was done on 63 Lyme patients who 6 months prior had been treated with antibiotics by following the IDSA guidelines[6] for short-term antibiotic treatment. After finishing treatment, 36% of these patients reported new-onset fatigue; 20% widespread pain; and 45% new difficulties with memory, focus, and concentration.[50] According to the IDSA guidelines, these patients should be labeled as having "posttreatment Lyme disease syndrome" (PTLDS). Interestingly, less than 10% of these patients reported greater than minimal depression across the entire testing period. The IDSA would say that their symptoms are a result of delayed immune reactions to the *Borrelia* antigens and that they do not have any active ongoing infections, but there may be another explanation. After *B. burgdorferi* is exposed for a few hours to antibiotics that are commonly used to treat Lyme disease, the spiral-shaped *B. burgdorferi* microbe forms several tiny blebs or granules along its length (Figure 11.2).[51] When spiral-shaped *B. burgdorferi* are placed into cerebrospinal fluid for a few hours, they also transform into these same small spherical forms (bleb, granule, or cystic form) and when those spherical bleb forms are moved from the cerebrospinal fluid to a BSK-H culture medium it takes more than 9 days for the *B. burgdorferi* to transform back into the spiral-shaped invasive form.[52] These *B. burgdorferi* blebs appear to contain all the DNA materials necessary to form an entirely new spiral-shaped bacteria when the noxious conditions resolve. These *B. burgdorferi* blebs also appear to be very resistant to any effect from standard antibiotics used to treat *Borrelia* according to IDSA guidelines. *B. burgdorferi* can also form biofilms (a matrix of complex sugar chains and other substances much like the thick, sticky human nasal secretions), which can envelope and shield the microbes hiding inside the biofilm from immune attack or antibiotic penetration.[53] When five different antibiotics were tested against *Borrelia* in bacterial culture tubes in the laboratory at the University of New Haven, Connecticut, it was found that many of the *Borrelia* blebs survived all five of the tested antibiotics and that the antibiotics also only reduced the *Borrelia* biofilm forms by 30%–55%.[54] The same research group found that a combination of Banderol and Samento (two Peruvian rain forest herbs) was able to significantly reduce the number of *B. burgdorferi* bleb forms and essentially eliminate all *B. burgdorferi* biofilms, much more effectively than the doxycycline antibiotic.[55] These same types of bleb forms of *B. burgdorferi* were found in the cerebrospinal fluid of all 10 multiple sclerosis (MS) patients in a study in Norway[56] but in only 1 of the 5 control patients without MS (and that 1 control patient had suffered from EM rash typical of *Borrelia* infection). When the cerebrospinal fluid samples from the MS patients were cultured, 2 out of the 10 grew spiral-shaped, rodlike microbes resembling *Borrelia*.

In a study with *B. burgdorferi*–infected mice, 3 months after treating with ceftriaxone antibiotic the mice's infection status was assessed by culture.[57] Joint tissue and heart tissue from these antibiotic-treated mice were transplanted under the skin (subcutaneously) into immune-deficient (SCID) mice who had no *Borrelia*. Even though the cultures were negative for *Borrelia* in the antibiotic-treated mice, various tissue samples that were collected from the SCID mice who had received the subcutaneously transplanted joint and heart tissue taken from the antibiotic-treated mice were positive for *Borrelia* DNA. This demonstrated that the *Borrelia* microbes remained alive and infectious after antibiotic treatment, but apparently they were more slowly reproducing than *Borrelia* that had never been treated with antibiotics. In addition, another research showed that *Borrelia* can survive for more than 14 days inside human fibroblasts exposed to concentrations of ceftriaxone antibiotic 10 times that recommended by the IDSA.[58] So, can something be done to try to help the so-called PTLDS patients?

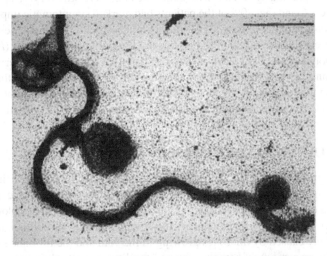

FIGURE 11.2 (See color insert.) *Borrelia* spirochete–forming granules soon after antibiotic exposure. (From Kersten A et al., *Antimicrob Agents Chemother*, 39, 5, 1127–1133, 1995. With permission.)

AN HERBAL PROGRAM MAY HELP MANY LYME PATIENTS

In 2003, I asked the question, "Can natural (non-pharmaceutical) therapies make a difference in chronically-ill Lyme patients with co-infections who have already been treated with antibiotics but who are given no hope of improvement by conventional Lyme-literate medical doctors?" Some other practitioners worked with me that year on a study in Dallas, Texas, to answer that question. Thirteen gravely ill Lyme patients with coinfections were treated for 18 weeks with a combination of natural remedies (predominantly herbal and nutritional). The 14 comparably ill Lyme patients with coinfections who served as controls in the study were treated during those 18 weeks with the best standard medical care possible from a Lyme-literate neurologist. All 13 of the natural treatment Lyme patients and the 14 other control Lyme patients had been previously treated with several courses of antibiotics for enzyme-linked immunosorbent assay (ELISA)-positive and Western blot-positive neuroborreliosis (*Borrelia* in the brain) but had not improved. Every 2 weeks, every patient filled out a 0 to 10 symptom-severity questionnaire and a Short-Form-8, a functionality and quality-of-life survey that had been used to evaluate patients in similar research studies over the previous 20 years. By the 10th week, all 13 patients receiving only natural therapies had a 75%–100% improvement in each of their symptoms. The 14 patients in the control group had minimal improvement in only some of their symptoms. By the 18th week of treatment, those who had received natural remedies had further improvement, but those in the control group did not. The natural treatment program was used on many other Lyme patients after the 18-week study was completed. It was modified to make it simpler (for better patient compliance) and more effective. For instance, additional antimicrobial herbals such as Banderol were added to Samento, which had been used in the initial study.

In early 2007, Richard Horowitz, MD, placed dozens of his PTLDS patients on the natural program developed in Dallas and reported at the International Lyme and Associated Diseases (ILADS) conference that 70% of his most ill patients had markedly improved within 6 months. Dr. Horowitz and others even used this program with fairly good results on Lyme patients who had never taken, and refused to take, pharmaceutical antibiotics. The "Microbial Defense" herbs in the natural program appeared to have good antimicrobial effects against not only *Borrelia* but also most coinfections, most fungal infections, many viruses, and even several parasites. Based on feedback from some of the patients who had failed Dr. Horowitz's treatment regimens, the CSP or Cowden Support Program (as the herbal regimen was then called by Dr. Horowitz) was modified a bit more to the way it has been used from 2008 through 2014.[59] The Borreliose Centrum (Borreliosis Center) in Germany in 2011 did a 9-month pilot study with 20 Lyme patients, using the revised CSP. These patients had all been previously treated with antibiotics but were still very symptomatic. After the study, the researchers found that 80% of the patients had marked symptomatic improvement in many areas, such as chronic fatigue, fibromyalgia, joint pain, chest pain, headache, fever, chills, sweats, insomnia, and anxiety. Furthermore, 90% had improved laboratory test results (*Borrelia* IgM, IgG by EIA and blot, polymerase chain reaction [PCR], Elispot-LTT, and CD57). Herxheimer reactions, or the detoxification reactions from rapid microbe die-off, occurred in 45% of the patients, but the CSP was otherwise tolerated well. The conclusion of all these unpublished pilot studies is that the natural products in CSP can make a marked difference in so-called PTLDS patients.

VENOUS VASCULITIS IN LYME DISEASE

Figure 11.3 is the infrared-imaging thermography (a picture from a camera that measures heat coming off the skin) of a woman with borreliosis and chronic headaches. You can see a red streak that extends up and down her neck over her jugular vein (the vein that carries blood from her brain back down into her chest). This image appears to represent venous vasculitis (an inflammation in the jugular vein likely caused by microbes growing in the vein and the immune system response to those microbes). Thermography of patients with no borreliosis usually shows no red streaking in the neck over the jugular vein.

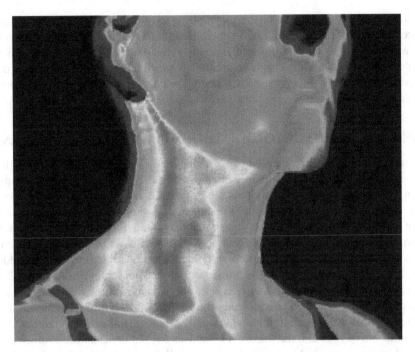

FIGURE 11.3 **(See color insert.)** Probable jugular venous vasculitis seen on infrared-imaging thermography of a woman with borreliosis and chronic headaches. (Courtesy of D. Hickey, unpublished data. With permission.)

The first description of inflammation near veins in patients with MS was in 1863.[60] More recently, Dr. Zamboni described a stenosis (narrowing) of the jugular veins in the neck (and certain other veins that drain blood from the brain) in every patient with MS that he evaluated but in none of his control patients without MS.[61] Dr. Zamboni named this condition chronic cerebrospinal venous insufficiency (CCSVI). When Dr. Zamboni did venous angioplasty (balloon dilation) of the narrowed neck veins of the patients with MS, several of the patients had marked improvement in their weakness and other MS symptoms. However, many of those who initially improved later worsened again and the jugular vein narrowing redeveloped. Dietrich Klinghardt, MD, PhD (pers. comm.), found that most of his MS patients had previously unrecognized Lyme borreliosis by blood tests. Those Lyme-positive MS patients had ultrasound testing of their neck veins using Dr. Zamboni's published procedures and were positive for CCSVI. Dr. Klinghardt did muscle testing on those Lyme-positive MS patients with CCSVI, which showed that *Borrelia* and some of the Lyme coinfections were present in high concentrations in the narrowed jugular veins of the MS patients. Dr. Klinghardt treated these MS patients with natural Lyme-eradicating therapies until no *Borrelia* or coinfections could be identified by muscle testing in their jugular veins. When these MS patients then had vein angioplasty for the CCSVI, their neurological symptoms markedly improved and did not recur later. Dr. Klinghardt also noted the CCSVI condition (by Zamboni's ultrasound) in a variety of other patients who were Lyme positive by blood tests but did not have MS (especially in children with autism and adult Lyme patients with neuroborreliosis symptoms). Recently, David Hickey, MD (pers. comm.), did ultrasound imaging for CCSVI (with Zamboni's technique) on a group of more than 25 Lyme-positive patients and did infrared imaging thermography on the same Lyme patients. If the ultrasound test was positive for CCSVI, then the thermography showed an obvious red streak over the jugular vein in almost every patient. A few of those Lyme patients have now been treated with sufficient herbal antimicrobial therapies (and no venous angioplasty) so that they are no longer positive for CCSVI by Dr. Zamboni's criteria.

A red streak over the jugular vein on thermography is a sign of inflammation in the jugular vein. Doctors are taught in formal training how much the inflammation in the arteries contributes to strokes, heart attacks, and other cardiovascular diseases, but much less is known about how inflammation in the veins affects health. This is an area where much research still needs to be done, but it is important for the reader to be aware that Lyme disease may be playing a large, previously unrecognized role in vascular diseases, especially venous diseases.

FOCUSING ON THE PHYSIOLOGY RATHER THAN THE LYME MICROBES

Too often, medical doctors are so focused on removing the microbes from the Lyme patient's body that they overlook the patient in whom these microbes dwell. There are a variety of conditions that can exist in a Lyme patient's body that could predispose the patient to becoming ill from a Lyme microbe or cause him or her to remain ill once infected. Immune weakness from various causes can make it easier for a microbial process to start and to continue. Toxicity, nutritional deficiencies, dehydration, hypoxia, gastrointestinal dysfunction with dysbiosis, and so on can create an environment that is more conducive to microbial growth. Sometimes, the microbial growth adds to these conditions. For example, as a result of the immune system response to viruses, fungi, *Borrelia*, or other microbes, thrombin (a clotting factor) is released, which, in turn, stimulates the production of fibrin (a clot-forming substance) and impairs the breakdown of fibrin.[62] The fibrin that attaches itself to the inner lining of the smallest blood vessels (capillaries) and prevents red blood cells from delivering sufficient oxygen into the tissues. This causes oxygen-deficient metabolism and buildup of lactic acid in the tissues.[63] Most microbes grow well in an oxygen-deficient, acidic environment. Human cells, however, do not function well in an acidic environment with low oxygen levels because human metabolic enzymes cannot make enough ATP (the essential energy molecule for the cell) under these conditions. Low ATP in the heart muscle of a Lyme patient can thus contribute to cardiomyopathy, congestive heart failure, and arrhythmias. In addition, many Lyme microbes produce biotoxins that are very toxic to human tissues, especially the electrical conducting tissues of the heart, and can further predispose to tissue dysfunction, heart block, cardiomyopathy, arrhythmias, and other illness. Therefore, comprehensive treatment for a patient with Lyme disease should not end after picking an appropriate antimicrobial agent, but it should also address issues of hydration, nutrition, sleep, tissue oxygenation, detoxification, gut function, excessive blood clotting, and other health issues.

The CSP was designed with these issues in mind. Patients on the CSP are encouraged to drink two to three quarts, or liters, of water per day spread out through the day so that tissues will have sufficient hydration to spontaneously detoxify. Patients on the CSP are also given Pinella, Burbur, and Parsley Detox tinctures to assist the detoxification of the brain, nervous tissue, liver, gall bladder, kidneys, and lymph vessels. Magnesium malate capsules in the CSP are given to address one of the most common nutritional deficiencies in chronically ill patients: magnesium deficiency. The Zeolite and Zeolite HP in the CSP are capsules of volcanic clay powder imprinted with energies to help detoxify heavy metals from the body. Sparga tincture in the CSP helps to detoxify the residuals of pharmaceutical sulfa drugs, which if present would impair production in the body of glutathione (a primary detoxification agent made by the body to bind and clear heavy metals and various man-made chemicals). Serrapeptase capsules in the CSP prevent excessive microbe-induced blood clotting, strip fibrin from the blood vessel linings so that oxygen can get into the tissues more easily, and also strip fibrin off microbes hiding in the body so that immune cells can identify and remove those microbes. Nutramedix Amantilla, Babuna, and Melatonin tinctures are used as needed in the CSP to improve sleep and reduce stress. Samento, Banderol, Cumanda, Houttuynia, Enula, and Mora are the herb tinctures used in the CSP on a cycling basis to reduce the microbial load in patients with *Borrelia* and coinfections. Several of these herbs are effective antifungals as well as being antibacterial, antiparasitic, and even antiviral. Because they are in alcoholic tinctures, they appear to be absorbed in the stomach and upper small intestine, so it is unlikely that they damage the healthy microbes in the gut like pharmaceutical antibiotic pills would.

Considerable evidence has accumulated that Lyme disease is quite capable of evading the patient's immune system, especially when treated with pharmaceutical antibiotics.[64] Because *B. burgdorferi* can invade and remain alive inside the white blood cells called macrophages[65] and lymphocytes[66] and even suppress the numbers of natural killer lymphocytes called CD57+ NK cells,[67] the immune system is often hard hit by *Borrelia* and therefore not very effective in eliminating *Borrelia* from the body. Further, chronic Lyme disease can even produce persistent inflammation from an autoimmune-like reaction induced by the *Borrelia*.[68]

Clinical experience is now mounting that the CSP is superior to doxycycline and other pharmaceutical antibiotics in dealing with these various Lyme-induced immune system problems and in treating advanced Lyme disease, especially if the symptoms have been present for more than a few weeks when the diagnosis is made and treatment is started. One of the best studied of the Nutramedix Microbial Defense herbs is Samento. It is an extract of the inner bark of *Uncaria tomentosa* (commonly called cat's claw), which is a vine that climbs up to 100 ft into the top of the Amazonian rain forest trees. Samento contains pentacyclic oxindole alkaloids (POAs), which stimulate the formation of new B and T lymphocytes (white blood cells responsible for antibody production and cellular immunity)[69]; but Samento, unlike most other forms of cat's claw on the market, contains no tetracyclic oxindole alkaloids (TOAs). Because TOAs block the immune stimulating effect of POAs, Samento may have better immune stimulating effect than most other cat's claw products, which means theoretically better effects against Lyme microbes as well as against cancers.[70] Samento also contains quinovic acid glycosides, which appear to have antiviral effects,[71] and Samento is anti-inflammatory,[72] just to name a few of its beneficial properties.

Dysbiosis: A Common Comorbid Condition in Lyme Carditis Patients

Some patients have intestinal dysbiosis (overgrowth of abnormal, disease-causing microbes in the gut) before they ever acquire Lyme disease.[73] This is most commonly caused by pharmaceutical antibiotic use, or by consuming antibiotic-tainted meats, dairy products, or eggs. Dysbiosis can also be caused by psychological stress, especially when protracted; physical stress (such as injuries); other prescription drugs and over-the-counter drugs (especially corticosteroids and nonsteroidal anti-inflammatory drugs like aspirin and ibuprofen); certain dietary factors (such as food preservatives, excessive dietary sugar, and genetically modified foods); as well as other causes. There should be nearly 1000 different species of friendly bacteria in the healthy human intestine,[74] but there are far fewer species in patients who have been exposed to antibiotics, either intentionally for Lyme treatment or unintentionally by eating certain antibiotic-contaminated meats, dairy, or eggs. Most Lyme patients who have been treated with antibiotics have dysbiosis because most antibiotics indiscriminately kill many of the friendly bacteria in the intestine and allow the overgrowth of disease-causing fungi or antibiotic-resistant bacteria.

Fungi in the gut can extend their tiny fingerlike projections (hyphae) through intestinal walls, which creates "leaky gut." Intestinal parasites can also burrow tiny holes in the intestinal wall. If incompletely digested, dietary proteins pass through these microscopic holes in the intestinal wall and food allergies can develop. Random food allergy reactions put additional stress on the immune system and the cardiovascular system. In addition, food allergy reactions can cause allergic gastroenteritis and/or celiac disease.[75] During allergic gastroenteritis, there can be swelling of the intestinal lining, which can impair the absorption of nutrients from the intestinal tract. Some of these nutrients, like magnesium, may be very important for heart function. In addition, allergic gastritis can damage parietal cells that line the stomach to the point where production and release of hydrochloric acid in the stomach is impaired. There can then be insufficient hydrochloric acid to make the protein-digesting enzyme in the stomach called pepsin, with a resultant impairment of dietary protein breakdown into its constituent amino acids. Also, hydrochloric acid, which is dumped by the stomach into the duodenum, is the primary stimulus for the body to release a hormone called cholecystokinin (CCK). If CCK production is deficient due to insufficient hydrochloric acid, then the gall bladder and bile ducts will not contract properly. This results in a deficiency of bile salts in the intestine, which are necessary to solubilize and absorb from the intestine fat-soluble vitamins (A, D, E, and K) and other essential fats (especially the ω-3 fats eicosapentaenoic acid [EPA] and docosahexaenoic acid [DHA]). Vitamin E is a very important antioxidant for the heart and blood vessels, and the ω-3 fats are protective against inflammation of the heart and blood vessels caused by excessive ω-6 fats in the diet. The EPA, and to a lesser extent DHA, have anti-inflammatory and antithrombotic actions in the body, which is very important in an inflammatory, excessive blood clot-forming condition like Lyme disease, especially Lyme carditis. In addition, deficiency of CCK results in insufficient release of pancreatic enzymes (proteases, lipases, etc.), which are involved in the digestion and absorption of amino acids and other essential nutrients. Therefore, restoring gastrointestinal health (and normal gut biosis) is paramount to the recovery of chronically ill patients, especially Lyme carditis patients.

Stress reduction techniques can also aid in gastrointestinal health, immune health, and cardiovascular health. When stress reduction is done before meals, gastrointestinal function improves. These techniques are important because most chronically ill patients are under tremendous stress. This stress often causes excessive cortisol production, which then weakens the immune system and causes stress-induced damage of the hydrochloric acid–producing cells of the stomach. Therefore, avoiding as many food allergens as possible; treating the gut dysbiosis with natural, herbal, antifungal, and antiparasitic remedies; and taking probiotics and prebiotic fibers (such as psyllium, slippery elm, or rice bran solubles) can often be quite helpful in the recovery of chronically ill Lyme patients. It can also be helpful to avoid nonsteroidal anti-inflammatory drugs, corticosteroid drugs, and pharmaceutical antibiotics and to take plant-derived digestive enzymes and possibly some ox-bile capsules with meals, until normal gut function is restored.

Man-Made Toxins: An Additional Comorbid Condition in Lyme Carditis

Toxins can impair immune function and the metabolic enzyme systems of cells, thereby making tissues and organs too "sick" to properly function. Toxicity in the heart definitely contributes to cardiomyopathy and probably contributes to cardiac arrhythmias and even AV heart block as well. Therefore, toxins can create a host of symptoms, some of which mimic Lyme disease, or can make Lyme disease more symptomatic, including from heart-related symptoms. When a patient is toxic, this predisposes the patient to becoming ill when exposed to *Borrelia* and coinfections and/or to remain ill after Lyme disease treatment. Toxins in the heart will increase the probability that *Borrelia* and other coinfections will concentrate enough in the heart to cause Lyme carditis symptoms. And when Lyme microbes infect the heart and cause inflammation there, the inflammation attracts more toxins, thus creating a self-sustaining cycle. Many of the toxins found in the body are absorbed from the enterohepatic circulation system (toxins absorbed from the intestines travel through the hepatic portal vein, poison the liver first, and then travel to, and poison, other vital organs thereafter). Some of the toxins in the body are produced in the gut by microbes that reside there. The toxins that these microbes produce are called biotoxins. Others are toxins that are ingested by the patient through food, water, and other fluids. Still others that the body harbors are toxins taken in through the skin, from such things as lotions and cosmetics and by bathing in unfiltered tap water, or that are breathed in through the lungs or taken in by other mucosal surfaces of the body. And some toxins result from patient exposure to dental restoration materials, implants, and other dental procedures.

Regardless of the route of initial exposure to a toxin, most toxins are metabolized to varying degrees in the liver and/or conjugated with carrier molecules and then dumped by the bile duct system of the liver into the upper intestine. Often, if a toxin "processed" in this manner is not passed into the toilet with feces quickly enough, gut microbes can cleave off the carrier molecules, thereby releasing the toxins to then be reabsorbed into the lymphatic system or the hepatic portal vein (thus retoxifying the body). Certain "toxin binders" can be taken by mouth to reduce the absorption (and reabsorption) of toxins. Some of the most common natural binders include fibers (dietary fibers, psyllium, slippery elm, rice bran, etc.), cracked chlorella, and clays (especially zeolite clay). One of the most effective pharmaceutical toxin binders is cholestyramine.[76] Because healthy people should have three bowel movements per day, most people with Lyme disease are considered to be constipated. If constipated people take too much fiber (especially if they are not drinking enough water every day), the constipation can become much more severe. In most cases, constipation can be avoided by drinking 2 oz. (60 mL) of pure water every 15 minutes throughout the day and by taking ascorbic acid (preferably unbuffered, non-corn-derived vitamin C) after most meals. In most Lyme patients, the dose of vitamin C should be gradually increased at every meal until the bowels are loose. The fiber can then be slowly increased in the diet so that the body will regain formed bowel movements. The ascorbic acid form of vitamin C taken on a full stomach at the end of a meal will usually not irritate the stomach, especially if taken with a supplemental fiber. Some practitioners have also found that if vitamin C is taken perfectly simultaneously with certain herbs, pharmaceuticals, and other supplements the absorption and/or tissue uptake of those herbs, pharmaceuticals, and supplements may be impaired by the vitamin C. Therefore, herbs, pharmaceuticals, and supplements should usually be taken before meals and vitamin C after those meals with fiber and/or clay supplements.

Common problematic toxins found in chronically ill Lyme patients include the following: heavy metals (especially mercury), pesticides, herbicides, solvents, most pharmaceuticals, and biotoxins (especially mycotoxins). Heavy metals can do all of the following: (1) bind to cellular enzymes in place of mineral cofactors and block cellular enzyme actions; (2) produce oxidant or free radical damage to tissues; or (3) bind to, and deactivate, other vital molecules in the body, such as glutathione. If heavy metals or other free radical substances (like *Borrelia* biotoxins, pesticides from foods, and chlorine from tap water) prevent cellular enzymes in the heart from producing enough ATP energy molecules, then the muscular contractions of the heart chambers are impaired, resulting in a cardiomyopathy. These are just a few mechanisms by which heavy metals create ill health. Sometimes, the body develops an immune reaction to the heavy metals whenever heavy metals become attached to healthy cells. This is regardless of whether the body becomes toxic from the metal or not. Immune reactions occur most commonly in response to nickel, palladium, gold, mercury, titanium, cadmium, and lead. Such reactions, which occur in the heart muscle and blood vessel linings as well as other tissues throughout the body, can be identified by blood tests through laboratories such as the MELISA laboratories (www.melisa.org). Immune reactions to metals can contribute to autoimmunity,[77] fatigue, and inflammation of the heart, blood vessels, and various other tissues (which can mimic Lyme-induced cardiovascular disease and make Lyme disease symptoms worse).

One of the most common and most problematic heavy metal toxins in chronically ill patients is mercury because it represents more than 50% of the composition of most dental amalgam fillings and is found in most fish that people eat. Mercury toxicity can cause hypertension, coronary heart disease, myocardial infarction, cardiac arrhythmias, reduced heart rate variability, increased carotid intima-media thickness and carotid artery obstruction, cerebrovascular accident, generalized atherosclerosis, proteinuria, and dysfunction or insufficiency of the kidneys,[78] as well as cardiomyopathy and various neurological and other conditions. As previously discussed, Lyme disease has been reported to cause cardiac arrhythmias, cardiomyopathy, and many other conditions also caused by mercury, so sometimes it is difficult to be sure whether Lyme disease or mercury or both are contributing to a specific condition, especially because a large percentage of Lyme patients have no history of tick bites or EM rash.

When heart muscle biopsies were analyzed for mercury content in patients with DCM compared to patients with coronary artery disease (controls), the mercury content of the heart was 22,000 times greater in DCM than in controls.[79] The first step in resolving toxicity from mercury, as with any other toxin, is to stop, or at least reduce, the ongoing uptake of that toxin into the body. If a patient has mercury-amalgam dental fillings, it may be important for him or her to cautiously have those amalgams removed by a dentist skilled in safe amalgam removal. The amalgams should be replaced with nonmetallic, biocompatible materials. Patients should also reduce their fish consumption, most of which is heavily contaminated with mercury. Instead, they should take distilled and/or chelated fish oils as supplements to provide their bodies with essential ω-3 oils, which are essential to the health of the heart, blood vessels, and most other tissues. After all amalgams are removed, gradual detoxification from mercury and other heavy metals can be done with zeolite, chlorella, dimercaptosuccinic acid (DMSA), dimercaptopropane-sulfonate (DMPS), ethylenediaminetetraacetic acid (EDTA), and other metal binders.

The primary sources of ongoing toxification of the body from other heavy metals must also be identified and avoided. All of the following heavy metals contribute, to varying degrees, to keeping people with advanced Lyme disease chronically ill and should be avoided whenever possible: aluminum is the first of these. It is found in antacids, aluminum cookware, aluminum foil, antiperspirants, and many toothpastes (as bauxite "inert" filler). Antimony is another toxic metal. It is often found in the textile industry (especially polyester clothing), some metal alloys, paints, glass and ceramics, solder, some batteries, bearing metals, semiconductors, some antiparasitic drugs, and in bedding/linens that are sprayed with antimony as a flame retardant. Antimony was found to be 12,000 times higher in concentration in heart muscle biopsies of patients with cardiomyopathy than in the heart muscle of patients without cardiomyopathy,[79] so antimony may also mimic Lyme carditis. Arsenic, another toxic metal, can be found in some soils (and the well water beneath those soils), fuel oils and coal, weed killers, pesticides, fungicides, pressure-treated lumber, rice, seafood, and commercially produced chicken. Cadmium is another toxic metal that can be found in batteries, cigarettes (and cigarette smoke), makeup (including lipstick, blush, foundation, and facial powders), various foods (including shellfish, coffee, tea, soft drinks, and some fruits), soldered water pipes, coal-burning furnaces, fungicides, pesticides, plastics, and hair-care products (including permanent solutions, hair dyes, bleaches, and hair sprays). Lead can be found in some hair color products, ceramic glazes, bullets, leaded paint, water from lead-soldered copper pipes, solder in food cans, soil, leaded gasoline, batteries, battery factories, lead smelters, cosmetics, and pesticides. Nickel can be found in stainless steel cookware, dental crowns and other dental metals, surgical prostheses, trace minerals, cigarette smoke, jewelry, industrial waste, hydrogenated fats, and fertilizers.

Radioactive metals (uranium, radium, plutonium, radioactive strontium, radioactive cesium, etc.) are found in ever-increasing amounts in the environment, as a result of the accumulation of over 300 nuclear weapons tests in the atmosphere since World War II, from nuclear power plants and from nuclear accidents (Chernobyl, Three Mile Island, and Fukushima). No one can avoid all of these toxic heavy metals, but once a serious effort has been made to avoid as many as feasible, a periodic detoxification can be undertaken with heavy metal binders. As stated before, these heavy metals and radioactive elements can accumulate in the heart, blood vessel linings, and other tissues of the body, causing free radical damage to tissues; impairment of metabolic enzyme function; and symptoms that mimic Lyme disease, including Lyme cardiovascular disease.

Accumulation of pesticides and herbicides in the body can be a large impediment to resolving chronic illnesses like Lyme disease because, like heavy metals, they create free radical damage in human tissues; disrupt normal function of metabolic enzymes; and alter the function of the autonomic nervous system, which is responsible for regulating heart rate, heart muscle contractility, and blood vessel tone. These and other man-made chemicals are taken into the body via skin contact and by breathing contaminated air, but pesticides and herbicides most commonly enter the body through the consumption of nonorganic food and drink. Because of the bioconcentration effect, nonorganic meats/dairy/eggs usually have several times more pesticides and herbicides than nonorganic vegetables. In a vegetarian diet, the sweetest nonorganic fruits have the most pesticides and herbicides, followed by other nonorganic fruits, then nonorganic root vegetables, and then other vegetables (with the least pesticides and herbicides). Therefore, when trying to reduce the intake of pesticides and herbicides it would be wise for people to always eat vegetarian when eating out so that they do not get the bioconcentration of food toxins in the animal-derived foods. They should also only eat organic meats and dairy products at home and try to make sure that most fruits (especially the sweetest ones) that they eat are organic and that the root vegetables are also organic. One type of bad oil that has found its way into foods is cottonseed oil. More pesticides and herbicides are sprayed on cotton plants than almost any other plant. Therefore, products with cottonseed oil should be avoided, because they are highly contaminated. People can reduce their exposure to other man-made chemicals by doing all of the following: (1) reading labels on all household products, (2) not putting anything on the skin or into the indoor air that could not be safely swallowed, (3) using low volatile organic compounds (low VOC) wall paints, (4) using only natural cleaning solutions in the house, (5) taking the outdoor shoes off at the door, and (6) opening several windows for ventilation of the house and office each day for several minutes (or even a few hours during better weather). It appears that various toxins (pesticides, herbicides, some heavy metals, solvents, other man-made chemicals, and possibly even biotoxins) are mobilized from the body, and associated symptoms are improved, when sitting in an infrared sauna at 110°F–160°F.[80] It is beneficial to take ginger, yarrow, or rapid-acting niacin at a dose of 100 mg (gradually building to 2000 mg) just before the sauna. This will cause a flushing and blood vessel dilation in the skin, which presumably then carries more of the heat-mobilized toxins into the sweat glands and sebaceous glands for excretion by the body. A cool shower, with a thorough soap lathering, immediately after the sauna helps to bind excreted toxins on the skin and to wash them down the drain. Because minerals are also lost in the sweat, people undergoing sauna should take supplemental minerals after the saunas.

MYCOTOXINS: YET ANOTHER COMORBID CONDITION IN LYME CARDITIS

Some people with Lyme disease have had mycotoxin exposure, which creates many of the same symptoms as Lyme disease. Animal research shows that some mycotoxins can cause various arrhythmias and even AV heart block, essentially indistinguishable from that seen with Lyme carditis.[81] Mycotoxins are chemicals produced by fungi that are immune disruptive, fat soluble, and usually not easily biodegradable. The fungal microbes that produce mycotoxins are sometimes found in the human body, in water-damaged buildings in which people live or work, or in food or fluids that people consume or sometimes come from a combination of all of the above. Some Lyme patients develop fungal overgrowth in their gut and/or sinuses after taking antibiotics and then become more ill because of the fungus and its mycotoxins. Other patients get mycotoxin exposure initially from a water-damaged building and then when they get a tick bite sometime after that they become much more ill from the *Borrelia* and coinfections than they might have been otherwise, due to the immune-damaging effects of the mycotoxins. If patients are affected by mycotoxins when they get infected with Lyme microbes, then *Borrelia* and/or coinfections are more likely to cause Lyme carditis and other more serious Lyme disease complications.

If mycotoxins are suspected to be affecting a patient, a reasonable quick and easy screening test to confirm this is the visual contrast sensitivity (VCS) test found on www.survivingmold.com. If a patient's vision is better than 20:50 and he or she fails the VCS test, then optic nerve toxicity is likely and mycotoxins are one of the most common causes of this toxicity. If a patient takes a repeat VCS test the following day, after a good night's sleep, and fails the test again, a reasonable next step is for that person to look carefully in every room in their home and workplace where water could be leaking: under every sink and toilet, around every shower and tub, behind every dishwasher, clothes washer, ice-maker, or any place where there could be a roof leak. If no moisture or fungal growth can be seen, then the person should also feel with their hands for moisture or unusual coolness in these areas. If there is coolness or moisture, this could indicate that subsurface moisture is also present. If no moisture, mold, or fungus can be found on inspection of these locations, then it is a good idea for that person to purchase from the plumbing department of one of the national chain hardware stores several petri dishes of culture medium used to culture mold from the air. One culture plate, with the lid off, should be placed on an outside window ledge, where there is no wind or sunlight, for the amount of time specified on the packaging. Other open culture plates should be placed in each interior room (also not in the sunlight) for the same length of time with no air purifiers running. The culture plates should then be collected after the specified length of time, the lids placed back on the culture plates, and a label placed on the bottom of each culture plate to indicate where it had been placed: for example, outside window ledge, master bathroom, master bedroom, kitchen, or laundry room, and so on. All of the closed and labeled culture plates should be placed in a single location inside the house where the temperature is comfortable and there is never any sunlight or fluorescent lights (a fireplace mantel or top of a piano are possible choices). The plates should then be examined daily and the number of mold colonies counted. If any plate has more fungal colonies than the "outside" plate, then that room is the likely source of the mycotoxins that are causing at least some of the patient's symptoms. Environmental specialists can then be contracted for further evaluation and/or mold remediation. It is very risky to a patient's health to try to remediate mold problems in their home on their own. Because mycotoxins, as well as other toxins previously discussed, can cause arrhythmias and other cardiac conditions similar to Lyme carditis, it is very important to evaluate cardiac disease patients for Lyme disease and for these various toxins.

CONCLUSION

Lyme disease is an underrecognized epidemic in the United States, with an estimated 300,000 new cases per year. Many doctors believe that Lyme disease is only found near Lyme; but in reality it is prevalent throughout the United States, as well as in many other countries. Lyme disease and its coinfections are difficult to diagnose because the blood tests are often falsely negative, but EDS and muscle testing may be helpful data-gathering tools to assist the practitioner in making a proper diagnosis when the blood tests fall short. Based on considerable research, it is likely that many people with Lyme disease are being inadequately treated with pharmaceutical antibiotics, in part, because of the limiting treatment standards published by the IDSA. As a result, many Lyme patients and their practitioners are resorting to natural, nonpharmaceutical treatment programs such as the CSP. The CSP successfully addresses *Borrelia*, other coinfections, as well as various comorbid conditions all at the same time.

Lyme disease can cause various cardiovascular effects such as AV heart block (and passing out), various other arrhythmias, cardiomyopathy, congestive heart failure, and even vasculitis (inflammation of the blood vessels). Because Lyme disease is known as a great imitator, the Lyme diagnosis should be considered irrespective of what symptoms are present, including arrhythmias and other predominantly cardiovascular symptoms. Fortunately, most cardiovascular effects of Lyme disease are short-lived once the diagnosis of Lyme disease is made and appropriate treatment is given. One underrecognized Lyme vascular disease, just recently noted on thermography, is jugular venous vasculitis, which appears to cause CCSVI. This is a blood vessel inflammation, presumably caused by *Borrelia* and other microbes, that results in a blood vessel narrowing, which then contributes to neurological diseases such as MS or autism.

A common treatment mistake that many conventional doctors make with Lyme patients is to be so focused on removing the microbes from the Lyme patient's body that they overlook the patient in whom those microbes dwell. Most Lyme patients, especially Lyme carditis patients, find much better success in recovering from illness if they address hydration, tissue oxygenation, nutrition, detoxification, gut function and sleep quality, as well as the microbial load. Natural therapies that address these other issues can help improve the Lyme patient markedly in many cases even without antibiotics, which may then resolve the cardiovascular condition caused by the Lyme.

REFERENCES

1. Steere AC, Malawista SE, Snydman DR et al. Lyme arthritis: An epidemic of oligoarticular arthritis in children and adults in three Connecticut communities. *Arthritis Rheum* 1977;20(1):7–17.
2. Burgdorfer W, Barbour AG, Hayes SF, Benach JL, Grunwaldt E, Davis JP. Lyme disease-a tick-borne spirochetosis. *Science* 1982;216(4552):1317–1319.

3. Masuzawa T. Terrestrial distribution of the Lyme Borreliosis agent *Borrelia burgdorferi sensu lato* in East Asia. *Jpn J Infect Dis* 2004;57(6):229–235.

4. Berghoff W. Chronic Lyme disease and coinfections: Differential diagnosis. *Open Neurol J* 2012;6:158–178.

5. New York Daily News: Associated Press. Lyme disease cases reach 300,000 per year in U.S. are under-reported: CDC http://www.nydailynews.com/life-style/health/lyme-disease-cases-reach-300-000-year-cdc-article-1.1431675#ixzz2ohUd29Ze (accessed November 19, 2014).

6. Wormser GP, Dattwyler RJ, Shapiro ED et al. The clinical assessment, treatment and prevention of Lyme disease, human granulocytic anaplasmosis and babesiosis: clinical practice guidelines by the Infectious Disease Society of America. *Clin Infect Dis* 2006;43:1089–1134.

7. Tibbles C, Edlow J. Does this patient have erythema migrans? *JAMA* 2007;297(23):2617–2627.

8. Harvey W, Salvato P. "Lyme disease": Ancient engine of an unrecognized borreliosis pandemic? *Med Hypotheses* 2003;60(5):742–759.

9. Centers for Disease Control and Prevention website. Lyme Disease, two-step laboratory testing process. http://www.cdc.gov/lyme/diagnosistesting/LabTest/TwoStep/index.html (accessed November 19, 2014).

10. Kaiser R. False-negative serology in patients with neuroborreliosis and the value of employing different borrelial strains in serologic assays. *J Med Microbiol* 2000;49(10):911–915.

11. Wang P, Hilton E. Contribution of HLA alleles in the regulation of antibody production in Lyme disease. *Front Biosci* 2001;6:B10–B16.

12. Tylewska-Wierzbanowska S, Chmielewski T. Limitation of serologic testing for Lyme borreliosis: evaluation of ELISA and Western blot in comparison to PCR and culture methods. *Wien Klin Wochenschr* 2002;114(13–14):601–605.

13. Bionatus website. 300+ medical conditions related to Lyme borreliosis. http://www.nutramedix.ec/ns/science-library/168-300-medical-conditions-related-to-lyme-borreliosis (accessed November 19, 2014).

14. Centers for Disease Control and Prevention website. Bartonella infection (cat scratch disease, trench Fever, and Carrión's disease) http://www.cdc.gov/bartonella/symptoms/index.html (accessed November 19, 2014).

15. Endresen GK. Mycoplasma blood infection in chronic fatigue and fibromyalgia syndromes. *Rheumatol Int* 2003;23(5):211–215.

16. Centers for Disease Control and Prevention website. Parasites—Babesiosis http://www.cdc.gov/parasites/babesiosis/disease.html (accessed November 19, 2014).

17. Center for Disease Control and Prevention website. Anaplasmosis http://www.cdc.gov/anaplasmosis/symptoms/index.html (accessed November 19, 2014).

18. Center for Disease Control and Prevention website. Ehrlichiosis http://www.cdc.gov/Ehrlichiosis/symptoms/index.html (accessed November 19, 2014).

19. Voll R. The phenomenon of medicine testing in EAV. *Amer J Acupunct* 1980;18(2):97–104.

20. Chen KG. The science of acupuncture—theory and practice: II. Electrical properties of meridians, with an overview of the electrodermal screening test. *IEEE Eng Med Biol Mag* 1996;15(3);58–63.

21. Krause P, Brockenstedt L. Lyme disease and the heart. *Circulation* 2013;127(7):e451–e454.

22. Steere A, Batsford WP, Weinberg M et al. Lyme carditis: Cardiac abnormalities of Lyme disease. *Ann Int Med* 1980;93(1):8–16.

23. Mayer W, Kleber FX, Wilske B et al. Persistent atrioventricular block in Lyme borreliosis. *Klin Wochenschr* 1990;68(8):431–435.

24. McAlister HF, Klementowicz PT, Andrews C, Fisher JD, Feld M, Furman S. Lyme carditis: An important cause of reversible heart block. *Ann Intern Med* 1989:110(5):339–345.

25. Bhattacharya IS, Dweck M, Francis M. Lyme carditis: a reversible cause of complete atrioventricular block. *J R Coll Physicians Edinb* 2010;40(2):121–122.

26. Frank DB, Patel AR, Sanchez GR, Shah MJ, Bonney WJ. Junctional tachycardia in a child with Lyme carditis. *Pediatr Cardiol* 2011;32(5):689–691.

27. Greenburg YJ, Brennan JJ, Rosenfeld LE. Lyme myocarditis presenting as fascicular tachycardia with underlying complete heart block. *J Cardiovasc Electrophysiol* 1997;8(3):323–324.

28. Lo R, Menzies DJ, Archer H, Cohen TJ. Complete heart block due to Lyme carditis. *J Invasive Cardiol* 2003;15(6):367–369.

29. Hidri N, Barraud O, de Martino S et al. Lyme endocarditis. *Clin Microbiol Infect* 2012;18(12):E531–E532.

30. Bartunek P, Němec J, Mrázek V et al. *Borrelia burgdorferi* as a cause of sick sinus syndrome? *Cas Lek Cesk* 1996;135(22):729–731.

31. Midttun M, Videbaek J. Serious arrhythmias in Borrelia infections. Ugeskr Laeger 1993;155(27):2147–2150.

32. Stanek G, Klein J, Bittner R, Glogar D. *Borrelia burgdorferi* as an etiologic agent in chronic heart failure? *Scand J Infect Dis Suppl* 1991;77:85–87.

33. Kubanek M, Šramko M, Berenová D et al. Detection of *Borrelia burgdorferi sensu lato* in endomyo-cardial biopsy specimens in individuals with recent-onset dilated cardiomyopathy. *Eur J Heart Fail* 2012;14(6):588–596.

34. Maczka I, Chmielewski T, Walczak E, Rózański J, Religa G, Tylewska-Wierzbanowska S. Tick-borne infections as a cause of heart transplantation. *Pol J Microbiol* 2011;60(4):341–343.

35. Wunderlich E, Graf A, Thess G, Foelske H. Dilated myocardial disease as sequel of chronic Lyme cardi-tis. *Z Cardiol* 1990;79(8):599–600.

36. Glasser R, Dusleag J, Reisinger E. Reversal by ceftriaxone of dilated cardiomyopathy *Borrelia burgdor-feri* infection. *Lancet* 1992;339(8802):1174–1175.

37. Koene R, Boulware DR, Kemperman M et al. Acute heart failure from lyme carditis. *Circ Heart Fail* 2012;5(2):e24–e26.

38. Steere AC, Hutchinson GJ, Rahn DW et al. Treatment of the early manifestations of Lyme disease. *Ann Intern Med* 1983;99(1):22–26.

39. Dattwyler RJ, Volkman DJ, Conaty SM, Platkin SP, Luft BJ. Amoxicillin plus probenecid versus doxy-cycline for treatment of erythema migrans borreliosis. *Lancet* 1990;336(8728):1404–1406.

40. Nowakowski J, McKenna D, Nadelman RB et al. Failure of treatment with cephalexin for Lyme disease. *Arch Fam Med* 2000;9:563–567.

41. Luger SW, Paparone P, Wormser GP et al. Comparison of cefuroxime axetil and doxycycline in treatment of patients with early Lyme disease associated with erythema migrans. *Antimicrob Agents Chemother* 1995;39:661–667.

42. Luft BJ, Dattwyler RJ, Johnson RC et al Azithromycin compared with amoxicillin in the treatment of erythema migrans: A double blind, randomized, controlled trial. *Ann Intern Med* 1996;124:785–791.

43. Eppes SC, Childs JA Comparative study of cefuroxime axetil versus amoxicillin in children with early Lyme disease. *Pediatrics* 2002;109:1173–1177.

44. Dattwyler RJ, Luft BJ, Kunkel MJ et al. Ceftriaxone compared with doxycycline for the treatment of acute disseminated Lyme disease*N Engl J Med* 1997;337:289–294.

45. Wormser GP, Ramanathan R, Nowakowski J et al. Duration of antibiotic therapy for early Lyme disease: A randomized, double-blind, placebo-controlled trial. *Ann Intern Med* 2003;138:697–704.

46. Agricultural Research Service of USDA. http://www.ars.usda.gov/Services/docs.htm?docid=15672 (accessed November 19, 2014).

47. Steere AC, Levin RE, Molloy PJ et al. Treatment of Lyme arthritis. *Arthritis Rheum* 1994;37:878–888.

48. Logigian EL, Kaplan RF, Steere AC. Chronic neurologic manifestations of Lyme disease. *N Engl J Med* 1990;323:1438–1444.

49. Miklossy J. Alzheimer's disease: A neurospirochetosis. Analysis of the evidence following Koch's and Hill's criteria. *J Neuroinflammation* 2011;8:90.

50. Aucott J, Rebman AW, Crowder LA, Kortte KB. Post-treatment Lyme disease syndrome symptomatol-ogy and the impact on life functioning: Is there something here? *Qual Life Res* 2013;22(1):75–84.

51. Kersten A, Poitschek C, Rauch S, Aberer E. Effects of penicillin, ceftriaxone, and doxycycline on mor-phology of *Borrelia burgdorferi*. *Antimicrob Agents Chemother* 1995;39(5):1127–1133.

52. Brorson O, Brorson SH. In vitro conversion of *Borrelia burgdorferi* to cystic forms in spinal fluid, and transformation to mobile spirochetes by incubation in BSK-H medium. *Infection* 1998;26(3):144–150.

53. Sapi E, Bastian SL, Mpoy CM et al. Characterization of biofilm formation by *Borrelia burgdorferi* in vitro. *PLoS One* 2012;7(10):e48277.

54. Sapi E, Kaur N, Anyanwu S et al. Evaluation of in-vitro antibiotic susceptibility of different morphologi-cal forms of *Borrelia burgdorferi*. *Infect Drug Resist* 2011;4:97–113.

55. Datar A, Kaur N, Patel S, Luecke DF, Sapi E. *In vitro* effectiveness of Samento and Banderol herbal extracts on the different morphological forms of *Borrelia burgdorferi*. *Townsend Lett* 2010;324:87–90.

56. Brorson O, Brorson SH, Henriksen TH, Skogen PR, Schøyen R. Association between multiple sclerosis and cystic structures in cerebrospinal fluid. *Infection* 2001;29(6):315–319.

57. Barthold SW, Hodzic E, Imai DM, Feng S, Yang X, Luft BJ. Ineffectiveness of tigecycline against persis-tent *Borrelia burgdorferi*. *Antimicrob Agents Chemother* 2010;54(2):643–651.

58. Klempner, MS, Noring R, Rogers RA. Invasion of human skin fibroblasts by the Lyme disease spiro-chetes, *Borrelia burgdorferi*. *J Infect Dis* 1993;167:1074–1081.

59. Bionatus website. Cowden support program http://www.nutramedix.ec/ns/lyme-protocol (accessed November 19, 2014).

60. Rindfleisch GE. Histologisches Detail zur grauen Degeneration von Gehirn und Ruckenmark. *Arch Pathol Anat Physiol Klin Med (Virchow)* 1863;26:474–483.

61. Zamboni P, Galeotti R, Menegatti E et al. Chronic cerebrospinal venous insufficiency in patients with multiple sclerosis. *J Neurol Neurosurg Psychiatry* 2009;80:392–399.
62. Berg D, Berg LH, Couvaras J, Harrison H. Chronic fatigue syndrome and/or fibromyalgia as a variation of antiphospholipid antibody syndrome (APS): an explanatory model and approach to laboratory diagnosis. *Blood Coagul Fibrinolysis* 1999;10(7):435–438.
63. Luft FC. Lactic acidosis update for critical care clinicians. *J Am Soc Nephrology* 2001;12 (suppl 1):S15–S19.
64. Berndtson K. Review of evidence for immune evasion and persistent infection in Lyme disease. *Int J Gen Med* 2013;6:291–306.
65. Montgomery RR, Nathanson MH, Malawista SE. The fate of *Borrelia burgdorferi*, the agent for Lyme disease, in mouse macrophages. Destruction, survival, recovery. *J Immunol* 1993;150(3):909–915.
66. Dorward DW, Fischer ER, Brooks DM. Invasion and cytopathic killing of human lymphocytes by spirochetes causing Lyme disease. *Clin Infect Dis* 1997; 25(suppl 1):S2–S8.
67. Stricker RB, Winger EE. Decreased CD57 lymphocyte subset in patients with chronic Lyme disease. *Immunol Lett* 2001;76(1):43–48.
68. Singh SK, Girschick HJ. Toll-like receptors in *Borrelia burgdorferi*-induced inflammation. *Clin Microbiol Infect* 2006;12(8):705–717.
69. Wurm M, Kacani L, Laus G, Keplinger K, Dierich MP. Pentacyclic oxindole alkaloids from *Uncaria tomentosa* induce human endothelial cells to release a lymphocyte-proliferation-regulating factor. *Planta Med* 1998;64(8):701–704.
70. Garcia Prado E, García Gimenez MD, De la Puerta Vázquez R, Espartero Sánchez JL, Sáenz Rodríguez MT. Antiproliferative effects of mitraphylline, a pentacyclic oxindole alkaloid of *Uncaria tomentosa* on human glioma and neuroblastoma cell lines. *Phytomed* 2007;14(4):280–284.
71. Aquino R, De Simone F, Pizza C, Conti C, Stein ML. Plant metabolites. Structure and in vitro antiviral activity of quinovic acid glycosides from *Uncaria tomentosa Guettarda platypoda*. *J Nat Prod* 1989;52:679–685.
72. Aquino R, De Feo V, De Simone F, Pizza C, Cirino G. Plant metabolites. New compounds and anti-inflammatory activity of *Uncaria tomentosa*. *J Nat Prod* 1991;54:453–459.
73. Hawrelak JA, Myers SP. The causes of intestinal dysbiosis: a review. *Altern Med Rev* 2004;9(2):180–197.
74. Sears CL. A dynamic partnership: Celebrating our gut flora. *Anaerobe* 2005;11(5):247–251.
75. Cingi C, Demirbas D, Songu M. Allergic rhinitis caused by food allergies. *Eur Arch Otorhinolaryngol* 2010;267:1327–1335.
76. Genuis SJ, Curtis L, Birkholz D. Gastrointestinal elimination of perfluorinated compounds using cholestyramine and *Chlorella pyrenoidosa*. *ISRN Toxicol* 2013;2013:657849.
77. Prochazkovw J, Sterzl I, Kucerova H, Bartova J, Stejskal VD. The beneficial effect of amalgam replacement on health in patients with autoimmunity. *Neuro Endocrinol Lett* 2004;25(3):211–218.
78. Houston MC. Role of mercury toxicity in hypertension, cardiovascular disease, and stroke. *J Clin Hypertens (Greenwich)* 2011;13:621–627.
79. Frustaci A, Magnavita N, Chimenti C et al. Marked elevation of myocardial trace elements in idiopathic dilated cardiomyopathy compared with secondary cardiac dysfunction. *J Am Coll Cardiol* 1999;33(6):1578–1583.
80. Crinnion W. Sauna as a valuable clinical tool for cardiovascular, autoimmune, toxicant-induced and other chronic health problems. *Alt Med Review* 2011;16(3):215–225.
81. Ngampongsa S, Ito K, Kuwahara M, Ando K, Tsubone H. Reevaluation of arrhythmias and alterations of the autonomic nervous activity induced by T-2 toxin through telemetric measurements in unrestrained rats. *Toxicol Mech Methods* 2012;22(9):662–673.

12 Metabolic Cardiology
The Missing Link in the Treatment and Management of Heart Failure

Stephen T. Sinatra

CONTENTS

Takeaways and key concepts:

1. Metabolic therapy involves the administration of a substance normally found in the body to enhance a metabolic reaction within the cell.
2. Such a therapy may be achieved in two ways. A substance can be given to correct a deficiency of a cellular component, or a substance can be given to achieve greater than normal levels in the body to drive an enzymatic reaction in a preferential direction.
3. Metabolic cardiology supports biochemical reactions that improve energy substrates in heart cells.
4. In this chapter, four metabolic substances that support cardiac metabolism are reviewed:

   a. Magnesium facilitates 300 enzymatic reactions.
   b. Coenzyme Q10, a lipid-soluble antioxidant, plays a vital role in oxidative phosphorylation.
   c. L-carnitine supports β-oxidation of fatty acids in mitochondria while removing toxic metabolic by-products at the same time.
   d. D-ribose is the energy-limiting substrate to support adenosine triphosphate (ATP) production in the myocyte.

5. Congestive heart failure (CHF) is literally an "energy-starved" heart, and compounds that enhance energy substrates must be given to positively impact heart function.
6. Diastolic dysfunction (DD) occurs when ATP levels fall and is the most important precursor of systolic dysfunction and, therefore, CHF.
7. Metabolic cardiology is a unique strategy to energize diastole and perhaps will be the standard of care for the treatment of heart failure as, in my opinion, it is the most effective therapy in the treatment of DD.

It seems like yesterday that I heard from my professors in medical school that the 5-year survival of CHF was worse than that of cancer. Several years later, after finishing a medical residency and a cardiovascular fellowship, I witnessed firsthand the sufferings and experienced the frustrations of managing patients with moderate to severe CHF. Unfortunately, that information over 40 years ago still rings true as most physicians managing heart failure on a day-to-day basis confront the same frustrations and difficulties in managing their patients.

Despite tremendous advances in technology, heart failure still remains the leading cause of hospitalization in the United States and its prevalence continues to increase as the population ages. The amount of human suffering associated with heart failure is enormous, and the financial burden placed on society is staggering. Although there has been considerable progress in the treatment of heart failure over the past 20 years with diuretics, ACE therapies,[1,2] β-receptor blockade,[3,4] and resynchronization therapy,[5–7] heart failure is still associated with an annual mortality of 10% and 30%–40%[8,9] of patients die within 1 year of diagnosis. The search for more effective treatments is one of the major challenges in clinical cardiology.

Recently, treating the heart at metabolic and cellular levels in heart failure has been acquiring increasing popularity. The preservation of mitochondrial function and the optimization of energy substrates in the heart has been gaining momentum as a new form of therapy.[10,11] Because the failing myocardium is "viable but dysfunctional,"[10] and not irreversibly damaged, treatment options that target the cardiomyocyte itself should be instituted as vulnerable and dysfunctional heart cells can still be rescued.[12] And if we consider the evidence for cardiomyocyte renewal in humans,[13] it makes even more sense to treat the myocardium at cellular and metabolic levels to help bolster progress in assisting the body's intrinsic stem cell wisdom for regenerative therapy.[14]

Although the genesis of heart failure includes multiple factors and many mechanisms, the essence of heart failure as an energy-starved heart running out of fuel identifies the myocardial energetics of the failing heart.[15,16] There is a definite energy disequilibrium between the work the heart has to perform and the available energy it has to fulfill its needs.

Thus, supporting energy substrates in heart cells will be a new cardiological approach that focuses on the biochemistry of cellular energy as "metabolic cardiology."[17] Many physicians are not trained to look at heart disease in terms of cellular biochemistry; therefore, the challenge in any metabolic cardiology discussion is in taking the conversation from "bench to bedside."[17]

Bioenergetics is the study of energy transformation in living organisms used in the field of biochemistry to reference cellular energy. Understanding the distinction between the concentration of adenosine triphosphate (ATP) in the cell and the efficiency of ATP turnover and recycling is central to our appreciation of cellular bioenergetics.

Once an understanding of how ATP repairs and restores heart cells is realized, targeted biochemical interventions to support ATP production and turnover will be strongly considered by physicians.

Metabolic therapies that help cardiomyocytes meet their absolute need for ATP fulfill a major clinical challenge of preserving pulsatile cardiac function while maintaining mitochondrial, cellular, and tissue viability. D-ribose, L-carnitine, and coenzyme Q10 work in synergy to help the ischemic or hypoxic heart preserve its energy charge.

In this chapter, we shall learn that the bottom line in the treatment of any form of cardiovascular disease, and especially in CHF, is the restoration of the heart's supply of ATP. Cardiac conditions like angina, CHF, silent ischemia, and DD all cause an ATP deficit. Metabolic cardiology is the missing link that has been eluding us for decades and is the major solution in improving quality of life for those struggling with CHF.

Although I struggled in my earlier career using conventional methodologies in heart failure, my new journey into metabolic cardiology commenced in 1982 when I successfully treated a 30-year-old female with congestive postpartum cardiomyopathy utilizing coenzyme Q10. For the next 30 plus years, I continued to use coenzyme Q10 while adding magnesium and later L-carnitine to the mix. Then, in 2004 the missing link I have been searching for suddenly materialized in a heartbeat.

I was attending a lecture at a symposium on antiaging medicine, when another like-minded, board-certified cardiologist started his sizzling presentation on a new nutrient, D-ribose. Jim Roberts, an integrative cardiologist like me, practices in Midwest, Ohio, to be specific. Within the first 15 minutes of his spellbinding lecture, I felt an enormous connection with him. I was inspired by his enthusiasm for treating people. Then, when I least expected it, I had an extraordinary epiphany—an "aha" moment. The metaphorical "lightbulb" went off in my head, as I listened to him describe how this new nutrient was working for his patients. Had I at last found the final puzzle piece for my metabolic approach to heart diseases? "Yes, this is it," I realized excitedly.

I had been combining traditional medical approaches to heart disease including pharmaceutical drugs, procedures, and surgeries with several targeted nutritional supplements to support and strengthen the heart. I'd say at least 85%–90% of my patients were improving, recovering, and maintaining those strides on my approach.

But at the end of the day, it's the other 10%–15% who still struggled in compromised bodies despite being faithful to my instructions that challenged me. I knew there must be another piece to the treatment puzzle in those cases, many of them with chronic CHF and/or hypertensive cardiovascular disease with significant mitral regurgitation. The final missing link had eluded me for decades.

It came as a flash in my mind as I sat there. There in my seat, my mental wheels were spinning wildly, adding Roberts' theory of how D-ribose contributed to the core program I had been using. I saw the heart as a busy network of vibrating cells and realized that it was all about treating the energy in each and every cardiac cell. The concept of metabolic cardiology is built on the premise that supporting cellular energy is the key to unlocking the heart's innate potential and it unfolded in my mind as if it had always been there, just waiting for me to get it.

Adding D-ribose to my basic foundation nutrient program started turning around that subgroup of people in my practice who needed something more, and even put new life into those who were doing well on other core nutrients like coenzyme Q10, L-carnitine, and magnesium. As my patients reported progress in their own words about having extraordinary symptom relief, it became clear that we needed to spread the news. In 2005, I wrote *The Sinatra Solution: Metabolic Cardiology*[18] with a fitting introduction by Dr. Jim Roberts. Later, we would coauthor a book together titled *Reverse Heart Disease Now*[19] and *The Sinatra Solution/Metabolic Cardiology* was updated and republished in April of 2008 and again in 2011.

The concept of metabolic cardiology is no fluke. Over the years, I've heard from hundreds of patients and physicians, even cardiovascular pediatric surgeons and electrophysiologists, who shared enough positive experiences with me that it's obvious that this approach in healing the heart absolutely works.

Once I understood how D-ribose would intertwine with the other key nutrients in my plan, it made perfect sense that this missing link could build and magnify the generation of energy within heart cells. Once I saw the heart muscle as "energy starved," how to promote energy recovery became clearer. It's all about supporting those energy-starved hearts and maintaining that support on a cellular level.

D-ribose is a building block of ATP—the energy of life. Remember, more than 30 years ago I first started my patients, and myself, on the vitamin-like antioxidant/nutrient called coenzyme Q10(CoQ10) or (ubiquinone). CoQ10 is effective on almost everything cardiac: blood pressure stabilization, oxygen utilization, angina, valvular problems, arrhythmias, and chronic heart failure. One of the first articles that caught my attention on coenzyme Q10 was an investigation in the *Annals of Thoracic Surgery* in 1982[20] in which Japanese researchers showed that patients come off heart–lung bypass machines more easily postoperatively when CoQ10 was taken for the month before needed heart surgery. It reduced pulmonary wedge pressure and increased cardiac index.[20] As an antioxidant and membrane stabilizer, it helps to prevent the oxidation of low-density lipoprotein. I even tracked some heart transplant candidates who were able to come off the transplant list as long as they maintained the higher CoQ10 blood levels that I monitored for them.

I learned enough about carnitines more than 20 years ago when I wrote *L-Carnitine and the Heart*. I then added them to my basic game plan, which of course always includes a solid multi-vitamin/multimineral at its base. The carnitines are effective in the β-oxidation of fats as well as transporting toxic metabolites safely out of the mitochondria, the powerhouses of the cells that generate ATP.

Eventually, I added magnesium supplementation because, like CoQ10, the nutrient does so many things right for the heart. An essential component for over 300 of the body's enzymatic reactions, magnesium helps to increase ATP turnover in the energy-starved heart.

Despite all my successes, there was still something sticking in my craw; something was amiss. I had doubts because not everyone with angina or heart failure got better on my program. Even though I was able to reduce suffering and pain for most, just one clinical failure could keep me up at night. Like most physicians and healthcare providers, it's that one case where all your best efforts just aren't good enough, or helped only a little, that gets you obsessing. One failure means more than nine successes. It was the failures that kept me going; they drove me, in fact. I kept reading, reread-ing, and trying multiple nutraceutical supports. So, the day I heard of D-ribose, the pivotal pentose sugar/nutrient that forms the basic molecule generating ATP, I knew in my own mind that we were onto something big in terms of helping more people get well.

In 2005, I coined the term metabolic cardiology, after I sent a letter to the editor to the journal *Clinical Cardiology*[21] commenting on the use of coenzyme Q10 for patients awaiting heart trans-plantation. In essence, metabolic cardiology describes the biochemical interventions we are learn-ing to employ to directly improve energy metabolism in heart cells.

Metabolic cardiology offers the greatest hope for the largest number of patients with cardiovas-cular disease. My 40 plus years as a cardiologist has afforded me time and experience to add what had been considered alternatives to the pharmaceutical and technical standard-of-care treatments that were basic to my studies in postgraduate training of cardiology. But this specialty that I hold so close to my heart still has considerable limitations that need to be addressed before any explaining or discussing how to implement metabolic cardiology into clinical practice.

Pharmaceutical drugs, bypass surgery, angioplasty, stent placements, pacemakers, and implant-able defibrillators all have their place, and many lives would be lost without these high-tech interventions. Cardiologists face a daily dilemma concerning the best diagnostic procedures to rec-ommend to their patients and then, based on those test results, which surgical and/or pharmaceutical interventions to select. To complicate the choice, the evaluations we order and the treatments we select may actually create unnecessary risks for patients, risks that are out of proportion to the ben-efits they will experience. For example, we consider angioplasty and stent procedures on too many patients who are asymptomatic. Continuing technological advances, although necessary, add to the complexity of the decision-making process.

Cardiologists have grown reliant on these sophisticated medical processes. But, somewhere along the way something has gone amiss. Recently, there has been much mistrust and skepticism among the public toward the conventional medical model. Starving for new information, massive numbers of patients are consulting alternative therapy practitioners, visiting bookstores and health food stores in record numbers, searching the Internet for advice and creating a multibillion-dollar industry outside the mainstream medical community.

What is driving even our most conservative patients to look at other forms of therapies? There are many reasons for the increased popularity of alternative medicine, including patient dissatisfaction with ineffective conventional treatments, pharmacological drug side effects, drug errors, and high price of medications.

Many patients are now questioning the need for potentially life-threatening drugs and invasive interventions that carry considerable side effects, complications, and even mortality.

Recent research reviews and an analysis of peer-reviewed medical journals, as well as government health statistics, demonstrate that our trusted medical model can cause more harm than good. Complications from standard-of-care interventions, medical errors, and overuse of antibiotics are increasing at an alarming rate. When we consider that the fourth leading cause of death in the United States is properly prescribed medications[22] in a hospital setting, something's got to give.

For some patients, traditional medicine and the use of prescription medication can be very helpful in alleviating symptoms. For others, the side effects of strong drugs can be almost as problematic as the initial symptoms. In other cases, the drugs simply aren't providing enough relief. You feel better but not up to par.

Natural therapies, which are virtually side effect free, can reduce our reliance on conventional medicines. They are being utilized, and even preferred, by more and more people. In many cases, alternative therapies can augment traditional medicines and provide the final measure of relief that is lacking with drug therapy alone. Many patients benefit greatly from blending conventional and alternative therapies—a strategy I call "smart medicine." But before discussing any therapeutic interventions, we must first focus on why we become ill.

I've spent decades analyzing the body's electrical potential in electrocardiograms (ECGs or EKGs), watching its ultrasonic synchronous vibrations on echocardiograms, and studying its pulsating structure in invasive procedures like angiography of the great vessels and heart chambers. I have come to appreciate the complexity and perfection of the human body and also the key importance of cellular and vibrational energy.

Every cell generates its own energy through enzymatic reactions in the mitochondria that generate ATP. But to understand pathology and illness, we need to focus on the damage that happens to the repair loops in each cell.

The health of the cell is negatively impacted by bodily trauma; emotional blocks; environmental toxins; pharmaceutical drugs; trans fats; and, most recently, electromagnetics. When the cells are bombarded with one or more of these agents, a departure from their healthy electrical potential and synchronous vibration occurs. For example, both atrial fibrillation and congestive cardiomyopathy may occur as a result of mercury toxicity, and disturbed heart rate variability may occur as result of chaotic electromagnetic fields (EMFs).

SECRETS OF THE CELL

It is my firm belief that the reason we become ill—whether it is heart disease or any other condition—is really more about the jeopardized integrity of the cellular membrane of each and every cell than anything else. Whatever the target organs, when the cell membrane is threatened normal functioning is impaired. Simply stated, a healthy, semipermeable cell wall (membrane) allows nutrients in and toxins out. To be healthy, the cell's membrane must be able to breathe as it ushers in the nutrients that support its metabolism and safely transports out the waste products of those chemical reactions to be excreted. In other words, the cellular membrane must be able to take in oxygen, water, glucose, nutrients, hormones, and so on, and excrete waste and toxic by-products.

When the integrity of the cell membrane is impaired, dysfunctional energetic relationships may manifest provoking degenerative processes that eventually cause insidious and relentless inflammation, a cycle that, if unchecked, continuously damages the cell.

In heart cells, decreased ATP concentrations in mitochondria may reflect defects in cellular metabolism.[23] In one small study investigating the relationship between left ventricular chamber dynamics and the pathophysiology of ventricular dysfunction, biochemical events are more relevant in cellular energy production.[23] The free energy of hydrolysis of ATP—or the amount of chemical energy available to fuel cellular function—is vitally important.[24,25] We shall soon see that in heart disease the bioenergetic property of cardiac cells is impaired because of the faulty metabolism of

ATP, especially in situations of coronary ischemia. To maintain the heart's pulsatory and vibratory energy levels, supporting the mitochondrial production of ATP is critical.

Every cell has the same basic structures, in addition to being specialized. Unlike well-armored nuclear DNA (the genetic material in the nucleus of the cell), mitochondrial DNA have no defense mechanisms. The mitochondria generate the chemical energy (ATP) that is transferred to mechanical energy. In the heart muscle cell, this means managing cellular respiration, calcium and sodium pumps, contracting and relaxing, conducting impulses, and so on.

In the process of mitochondrial respiration and the genesis of ATP, not all the oxygen is converted to carbon dioxide and water. About 3%–5% of the oxygen generated results in breakdown products known as free radicals. Because mitochondrial DNA has no defense mechanisms, it is vulnerable to these unstable, unpaired electrons typical of free radical oxidative stress. So, it is absolutely essential to repair and support vulnerable mitochondrial activity from the relentless free radical stress of mitochondrial respiration that can negatively impact tissue and organ function.

In cardiology, solving the heart's energy crisis is essential to optimizing cardiovascular function. For decades, heart disease prevention has inappropriately and inadvertently been focused on lowering lipids (cholesterol) in an effort to prevent or slow down coronary artery disease. Rather, it behooves us to shift the focus to mitochondria and employ nutritional strategies targeting improved ATP synthesis and, therefore, heart function. Metabolic cardiology, a form of metabolic medicine, highlights the importance of sustaining key enzymatic and biochemical reactions in a preferential direction to revitalize the life of the cells in the heart and body. It is now widely accepted that one characteristic of the failing heart is persistent and progressive loss of energy. The requirement for energy to support the systolic and diastolic work of the heart is absolute. Therefore, a disruption in cardiac energy metabolism, and the energy supply/demand mismatch that results, can be identified as the pivotal factor contributing to the inability of failing hearts to meet the hemodynamic requirements of the body. In her landmark book, *ATP and the Heart*, Joanne Ingwall, PhD,[26] describes the metabolic process associated with the progression of CHF and identifies the mechanisms that lead to a persistent loss of cardiac energy reserves as the disease process unfolds.

The heart contains approximately 700 mg of ATP, enough to fuel about 10 heartbeats. At a rate of 60 beats per minute, the heart will beat 86,400 times in the average day, forcing the heart to produce and consume an amazing 6,000 g of ATP daily and causing it to recycle its ATP pool 10,000 times every day. This process of energy recycling occurs primarily in the mitochondria of the myocyte. These organelles produce more than 90% of the energy consumed in the healthy heart. In the heart cell, 3,500–5,000 mitochondria fill about 35% of the cell volume. Disruption in mitochondrial function significantly restricts the energy-producing processes of the heart, causing a clinically relevant impact on heart function that translates to peripheral tissue involvement.

The heart consumes more energy per gram than any other organ, and the chemical energy that fuels the heart comes primarily from ATP (Figure 12.1). The chemical energy held in ATP is resident in the phosphoryl bonds, with the greatest amount of energy residing in the outermost bond holding the ultimate phosphoryl group to the penultimate group. When energy is required to provide the chemical driving force to a cell, this ultimate phosphoryl bond is broken and chemical energy is released. The cell then converts this chemical energy to mechanical energy to do work.

In the case of the heart, this energy is used to sustain stretching and contracting, drive ion pump function, synthesize large and small molecules, and perform other necessary activities of the cell. The consumption of ATP in the enzymatic reactions that release cellular energy yields the metabolic by-products adenosine diphosphate (ADP) and inorganic phosphate (Pi) (Figure 12.2). A variety of metabolic mechanisms have evolved within the cell to provide rapid rephosphorylation of ADP to restore ATP levels and maintain the cellular energy pool. But, these metabolic mechanisms

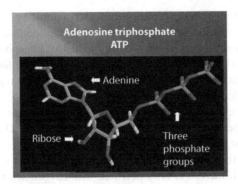

FIGURE 12.1 **(See color insert.)** Adenosine triphosphate (ATP) is composed of D-ribose, adenine, and three phosphate groups. Breaking the chemical bond attaching the last phosphate group to ATP releases the chemical energy that is converted to mechanical energy to perform cellular work.

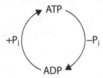

FIGURE 12.2 When ATP is used, the remaining by-products are adenosine diphosphate (ADP) and inorganic phosphate (P_i). ADP and P_i can then recombine to form ATP in the cellular processes of energy recycling. When oxygen and food (fuel) are available, energy recycling occurs unimpeded millions of times per second in every cell in the body. Lack of oxygen or mitochondrial dysfunction severely limits the cell's ability to recycle its energy supply.

are disrupted in CHF, tipping the balance in a manner that creates a chronic energy supply/demand mismatch that results in an energy deficit.

The normal nonischemic heart is capable of maintaining a stable ATP concentration despite large fluctuations in workload and energy demand. In a normal heart, the rate of cellular ATP synthesis via rephosphorylation of ADP closely matches ATP utilization. The primary site of cellular ATP rephosphorylation is the mitochondria, where fatty acid and carbohydrate metabolic products flush down the oxidative phosphorylation pathways. ATP recycling can also occur in the cytosol via the glycolytic pathway of glucose metabolism, but in normal hearts this pathway accounts for only about 10% of ATP turnover.

ATP levels are also maintained through the action of creatine kinase in a reaction that transfers a high-energy phosphate creatine phosphate (PCr) to ADP to yield ATP and free creatine. Because the creatine kinase reaction is approximately 10-fold faster than ATP synthesis via oxidative phosphorylation, creatine phosphate acts as a buffer to ensure consistent availability of ATP in times of acute high metabolic demand. Although there is approximately twice as much creatine phosphate in the cell as ATP, there is still only enough to supply energy to drive about 10 heartbeats, making the maintenance of high levels of ATP availability critical to cardiac function.

The content of ATP in heart cells progressively falls in CHF, frequently reaching and then stabilizing at levels that are 25%–30% lower than normal.[27] The fact that ATP falls in the failing heart means that the metabolic network responsible for maintaining the balance between energy supply and demand is no longer functioning normally in these hearts. It is well established that oxygen deprivation in ischemic hearts contributes to the depletion of myocardial energy pools, but the loss of energy substrates in the failing heart is a unique example of chronic metabolic failure in the well-oxygenated myocardium.

The mechanism explaining energy depletion in heart failure is the loss of energy substrates and the delay in their resynthesis. In conditions where energy demand outstrips supply, ATP is consumed at a rate faster than it can be restored via oxidative phosphorylation or the alternative pathways of ADP rephosphorylation. The cell has a continuing need for energy; so it will use all its ATP stores and then break down the by-product, ADP, to pull the remaining energy out of this compound as well. What's left is adenosine monophosphate (AMP).

Because a growing concentration of AMP is incompatible with sustained cellular function, it's quickly broken apart and the by-products are washed out of the cell. The net result of this process is a depletion of the cellular pool of energy substrates. When the by-products of AMP catabolism are washed out of the cell, they are lost forever (Figure 12.3). It takes a long time to replace these lost energy substrates even if the cell is fully perfused with oxygen again. This reduction in energy is like a depleted car battery struggling to start your engine. In diseased hearts, the energy pool depletion via this mechanism can be significant, reaching levels that exceed 40% in ischemic heart disease and 30% in heart failure.

Under high-workload conditions, even normal hearts display a minimal loss of energy substrates. These substrates must be restored via the de novo pathway of ATP synthesis. This pathway is slow and energy costly, requiring the consumption of six high-energy phosphates to yield one newly synthesized ATP molecule. The slow speed and high energy cost of de novo synthesis highlights the importance of cellular mechanisms designed to preserve energy pools. In normal hearts, the salvage pathways are the predominant means by which the ATP pool is maintained.

Whereas de novo synthesis of ATP proceeds at a rate of approximately 0.02 nM/min/g in the heart, the salvage pathways operate at a 10-fold higher rate.[28] The function of both the de novo and salvage pathways of ATP synthesis is limited by the cellular availability of 5-phosphoribosyl-1-pyrophosphate (PRPP) (Figure 12.4). PRPP initiates these synthetic reactions and is the sole compound capable of donating the D-ribose-5-phosphate moiety required to re-form ATP and preserve the energy pool. In muscle tissue, including that of the heart, formation of PRPP is slow and rate limited, impacting the rate of ATP restoration via the de novo and salvage pathways.

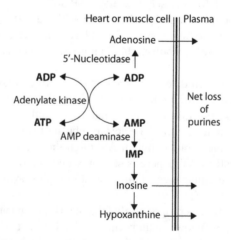

FIGURE 12.3   When the cellular concentration of ATP falls and ADP levels increase, two molecules of ADP can combine. This reaction provides one ATP, giving the cell additional energy, and one adenosine monophosphate (AMP). The enzyme adenylate kinase (also called myokinase) catalyzes this reaction. The AMP formed in this reaction is then degraded, and the by-products are washed out of the cell. The loss of these purines decreases the cellular energy pool and is a metabolic disaster to the cell.

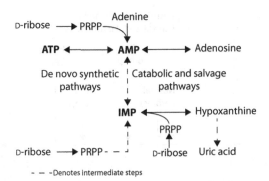

FIGURE 12.4 Replacing lost energy substrates through the de novo pathway of energy synthesis begins with D-ribose. D-ribose can also "salvage" AMP degradation products, capturing them before they can be washed out of the cell. Both the de novo and salvage pathways of energy synthesis are rate limited by the availability of D-ribose in the cell.

ENERGY STARVATION IN THE FAILING HEART

The chronic mechanism explaining the loss of ATP in CHF is decreased capacity for ATP synthesis relative to ATP demand. In part, the disparity between energy supply and demand in hypertrophied and failing hearts is associated with a shift in relative contribution of fatty acid versus glucose oxidation to ATP synthesis. The major consequence of the complex readjustment toward carbohydrate metabolism is that the total capacity for ATP synthesis decreases. At the same time, the demand for ATP continually increases as hearts work harder to circulate blood in the face of the increased filling pressures that are associated with CHF and hypertrophy.

The net result of this energy supply/demand mismatch is a decrease in the absolute concentration of ATP in the failing heart, and this decrease in absolute ATP level is reflected in a lower energy reserve in the failing and hypertrophied heart. A declining energy reserve is directly related to heart function, with diastolic function being the first to be affected, followed by systolic function, and finally global performance (Figure 12.5). In ischemic or hypoxic hearts, the cell's ability to match ATP supply and demand is disrupted leading to both depletion of the cardiac energy pool and dysfunction in mitochondrial ATP turnover mechanisms. When ATP levels drop, diastolic heart function deteriorates.

DD is an early sign of myocardial failure despite the presence of normal systolic function and preserved ejection fraction. Higher concentrations of ATP are required to activate calcium pumps necessary to facilitate cardiac relaxation and promote diastolic filling. This observation leads to the conclusion that, in absolute terms, more ATP is needed to fill the heart than to empty it, consistent with Starling's law that requires more energy in diastole than in systole. The absolute requirement for ATP in the context of cardiac conditions in which energy is depleted makes a metabolic therapeutic approach such a reasonable intervention.

Laplace's law confirms that pressure overload increases energy consumption in the face of abnormalities in energy supply. In failing hearts, these energetic changes become more profound as left ventricle remodeling proceeds,[29–31] but they are also evident in the early development of the disease.[32] It has additionally been found that similar adaptations occur in the atrium, with energetic abnormalities constituting a component of the substrate for atrial fibrillation in CHF.[33] Atrial fibrillation following coronary artery bypass surgery (CABS) has also been identified as a sequelae of DD.[34]

Left ventricular hypertrophy is initially an adaptive response to chronic pressure overload, but it is ultimately associated with a 10-fold greater likelihood of subsequent chronic CHF. While metabolic abnormalities are persistent in CHF and left ventricular hypertrophy, at least half of all patients with left ventricular hypertrophy-associated heart failure have preserved systolic function, with components of diastolic heart failure.

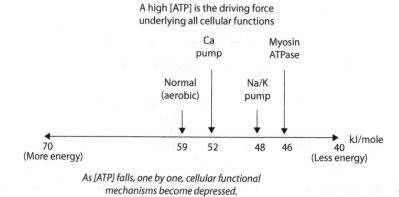

FIGURE 12.5   (See color insert.) Cellular energy levels can be measured as the free energy of hydrolysis of adenosine triphosphate, or the amount of chemical energy available to fuel cellular function. Healthy, normal hearts contain enough energy to fuel all the cellular functions with a contractile reserve for use in emergency. Cellular mechanisms used in calcium management and cardiac relaxation require the highest level of available energy. Sodium/potassium pumps needed to maintain ion balance are also significant energy consumers. The cellular mechanisms associated with contraction require the least amount of cellular energy. (Adapted from Braunwald E et al. *Mechanisms of Contraction of the Normal and Failing Heart.* 2nd ed. Boston: Little, Brown, 1976; Lewis BS and Gotsman MS, *Am Heart J* 99:101–13, 1980.)

Oxidative phosphorylation is directly related to oxygen consumption, which is not decreased in patients with pressure overload left ventricular hypertrophy. Metabolic energy defects, instead, relate to the absolute size of the energy pool and the kinetics of ATP turnover through oxidative phosphorylation and creatine kinase. Dysfunctional ATP kinetics is similar in both systolic and diastolic heart failure and may be both an initiating event and a consequence.

Inadequate ATP availability would be expected to initiate and accentuate the adverse consequences of abnormalities in energy-dependent pathways. Factors that increase energy demand, such as adrenergic stimulation and systolic overload, exaggerate the energetic deficit. Consequently, the hypertrophied heart is more metabolically susceptible to stressors such as increased chronotropic and inotropic demand, and ischemia.

In humans, this metabolic deficit is shown to be greater in compensated left ventricular hypertrophy (with or without concomitant CHF) than in dilated cardiomyopathy.[35,36] Hypertensive heart disease alone was not shown to contribute to alterations in high-energy phosphate metabolism, but it can contribute to left ventricular hypertrophy and DD that can later alter cardiac energetics.[37,38] Further, for a similar clinical degree of heart failure, volume overload hypertrophy does not, but pressure overload does, induce significant high-energy phosphate impairment.[38,40] This explains why hypertensive patients or patients with aortic valvular disease are so much more vulnerable in the setting of even mild CHF.

Type 2 diabetes has also been shown to contribute to altering myocardial energy metabolism early in the onset of diabetes, and these alterations in cardiac energetics may contribute to left ventricular functional changes.[41] The effect of age on progression of energetic altering has also been reviewed, with results of both human[42] and animal[43] studies suggesting that increasing age plays a moderate role in the progressive changes in cardiac energy metabolism that correlates to DD, left ventricular mass, and ejection fraction.

Cardiac energetics also provides important prognostic information in patients with heart failure, and determining the myocardial contractile reserve has been suggested as a method of differentiating which patients seeking to reverse left ventricular remodeling[44] would most likely respond to cardiac resynchronization therapy (CRT). Patients with a positive contractile reserve are more likely to respond to CRT and reverse remodeling of the left ventricle. Nonresponders show a negative contractile reserve, suggesting increased abnormality in cardiac energetics.

Taken together, results of clinical and laboratory studies confirm that energy metabolism in CHF and left ventricular hypertrophy is of vital clinical importance. Impaired diastolic filling and stroke volume limit the delivery of oxygen-rich blood to the periphery. This chronic oxygen deprivation forces peripheral muscles to adjust and downregulate energy turnover mechanisms, a contributing cause of symptoms of fatigue, dyspnea, and muscle discomfort associated with CHF.

Treatment options that include a metabolic intervention with therapies shown to preserve energy substrates or accelerate ATP turnover are indicated for at-risk populations or patients at any stage of disease. D-ribose, coenzyme Q10, L-carnitine, and magnesium provide critical energy support to the compromised heart.

ENERGY NUTRIENTS FOR CONGESTIVE HEART FAILURE

D-RIBOSE (RIBOSE)

The effect of the pentose monosaccharide D-ribose on cardiac energy metabolism has been studied since the 1970s, with clinical studies describing its value as an adjunctive therapy in ischemic heart disease first appearing in 1991. Ribose is a naturally occurring simple carbohydrate that is found in every living tissue, and natural synthesis is via the oxidative pentose phosphate pathway of glucose metabolism. But the poor expression of gatekeeper enzymes glucose-6-phosphate dehydrogenase and 6-phosphogluconate dehydrogenase limits its natural production in heart and muscle tissue. The primary metabolic fate of ribose is the formation of PRPP required for purine synthesis and salvage via the purine nucleotide pathway. PRPP is rate limiting in purine synthesis and salvage, and concentration in tissue defines the rate of flux down this pathway. In this way, ribose is rate limiting for preservation of the cellular adenine nucleotide pool.

As a pentose, ribose is not used by cells as a primary energy fuel. Unlike glucose, ribose is preserved for the important metabolic task of stimulating purine nucleotide synthesis and salvage for the production of ATP. Approximately 98% of consumed ribose is quickly absorbed into the bloodstream and is circulated to remote tissue with no first pass effect by the liver. As ribose passes through the cell membrane, it is phosphorylated by membrane-bound ribokinase before entering the pentose phosphate pathway downstream of the gatekeeper enzymes. In this way, administered ribose is able to increase intracellular PRPP concentration and initiate purine nucleotide synthesis and salvage.

The study of ribose in CHF was first reported in the *European Journal of Heart Failure* in 2003.[45] Until that time, the clinical benefit for ribose in cardiovascular disease was largely confined to its increasing role in treating coronary artery disease and other ischemic heart diseases, where its benefit has been well established. The reported double blind, placebo-controlled crossover study included patients with chronic coronary artery disease and New York Heart Association (NYHA) class II/III CHF. Patients underwent two treatment periods of 3 weeks each, during which either oral ribose (5 g t.i.d.) or placebo (glucose, 5 g t.i.d.) was administered. Following a 1-week washout period, the alternate test supplement was administered for a subsequent 3-week test period. Before and after each 3-week trial period, assessment of myocardial function was made by echocardiography and the patient's exercise capacity was determined using a stationary exercise cycle. Participants also completed a quality of life questionnaire. Ribose administration significantly enhanced all indices of diastolic heart function and exercise tolerance and was also associated with improved quality of life score. By comparison, none of these parameters were changed with glucose (placebo) treatment.

In addition to impaired pump function, CHF patients exhibited compromised ventilation and oxygen uptake efficiency that presents as dyspnea. Ventilation efficiency slope and oxygen uptake efficiency slope are highly sensitive predictors of CHF patient survival that can be measured using submaximal exercise protocols, which include pulmonary assessment of oxygen and carbon dioxide levels. In one study, ribose administration (5 g, t.i.d.) to NYHA class III/IV CHF patients significantly improved ventilation efficiency, oxygen uptake efficiency, and stroke volume, as measured by oxygen pulse.[46]

A second study[47] showed that in NYHA class II/III CHF patients ribose administration significantly maintained VO2max compared to placebo and improved ventilatory efficiency to the respiratory compensation point. A third,[48] similar, study involving patients with NYHA class III CHF investigated the effect of ribose on Doppler Tei Myocardial Performance Index (MPI), VO2max, and ventilatory efficiency, all powerful predictors of heart failure survival in a class III heart failure population. Results showed that ribose improved MPI and ventilatory efficiency while preserving VO2max. Results of these studies show that ribose stimulates energy metabolism along the cardiopulmonary axis, thereby improving gas exchange.

Increased cardiac load produces unfavorable energetics that depletes myocardial energy reserves. Because ribose is the rate limiting precursor for adenine nucleotide metabolism, its role in preserving energy substrates in remote myocardium following infarction was studied in a rat model.[49] In this study, male Lewis rats received continuous venous infusion of ribose or placebo via an osmotic minipump for 14 days. About 1 to 2 days after pump placement, animals underwent ligation of the left anterior descending coronary artery to produce an anterior wall myocardial infarction. Echocardiographic analysis performed preoperatively and at 2 and 4 weeks following infarction was used to assess functional changes as evidenced by ejection indices, chamber dimensions, and wall thickness.

By all three measured indices, ribose administration better maintained the myocardium. Contractility and wall thickness were increased, whereas less ventricular dilation occurred. This study showed that the remote myocardium exhibits a significant decrease in function within 4 weeks following myocardial infarction and that, to a significant degree, ribose administration attenuates this dysfunction.

This is an important clinical concept as I've seen many patients experience typical and atypical chest symptoms as well as generalized weakness following stent and angioplasty procedures. When temporary ischemia occurs in the myocardium, following balloon inflation, ATP levels drop. It may take the body several days to make up the deficit with de novo ATP synthesis[15,26]. In my experience, ribose is a significant factor in supporting energy substrate levels that enhance ATP production, thus alleviating symptoms in these patients. Temporary or prolonged ischemia results in lower myocardial energy levels. Increasing the cardiac energy level not only improves symptoms and function but also may delay vulnerable changes in a variety of CHF conditions. This therapeutic advantage ribose provides in improving cardiac index and left ventricular function suggests its value as an adjunct to traditional therapy for ischemia and CHF.

Because D-ribose administration creates favorable physiological parameters on cardiac function and has been shown to enhance the recovery of high-energy phosphates following myocardial ischemia, it was hypothesized that D-ribose could improve cardiological indices for off-pump coronary artery bypass procedures.[50] In a retrospective analysis of 366 patients undergoing off-pump CABS, 308 received D-ribose as a perioperative metabolic protocol. D-ribose patients had a greater improvement in cardiac index post revascularization compared with non-D-ribose patients (37% vs. 17%, $p < .0001$).[50] The research has suggested that a larger randomized placebo-controlled prospective trial be considered to further test the hypothesis that ribose should be considered standard management in myocardial ischemia.

Researchers and practitioners using ribose in cardiology practice recommend a dose range of 10–15 g/day as metabolic support for CHF or other heart diseases. In my practice, patients are placed on a regimen of 5 g/dose three times a day for any form of CHF and/or myocardial ischemia. Individual doses greater than 10 g are not recommended because high single doses of a hygroscopic carbohydrate may cause mild gastrointestinal discomfort or transient lightheadedness. As ribose has a lower glycemic index, it should be administered with meals or mixed in beverages containing a secondary carbohydrate source when administered to diabetic patients prone to hypoglycemia. I also frequently recommend ribose in fruit juices to these patients or in diabetic patients taking insulin.

COENZYME Q10 AND THE HEART

Coenzyme Q10 or ubiquinone, so named for its ubiquitous nature in cells, is a fat-soluble compound that functions as an antioxidant and coenzyme in the energy-producing pathways. As an antioxidant, the reduced form of CoQ10 inhibits lipid peroxidation in both cell membranes and serum low density lipoprotein and also protects proteins and DNA from oxidative damage. Coenzyme Q10 also has membrane-stabilizing activity. However, its bioenergetic activity and electron transport function for its role in oxidative phosphorylation is probably its most important function.

The electron transport chain is a series of oxidation–reduction (REDOX) chemical reactions that allow the mitochondria to transform the food you eat into energy (ATP). The electrons need CoQ10 to make their way down the electron transport chain or ATP production slows, causing a decrease in energy production, an increase in free radicals, and potentially disease or even death.

In CHF, oxidative phosphorylation slows due to a loss of mitochondrial protein and lack of expression of key enzymes involved in the cycle. Disruption of mitochondrial activity may lead to a loss of coenzyme Q10 that can further depress oxidative phosphorylation. In patients taking statin-like drugs, the mitochondrial loss of coenzyme Q10 may be exacerbated by restricted coenzyme Q10 synthesis resulting from 3-hydroxy-3-methylglutaryl coenzyme A (HMG-CoA) reductase inhibition (Figure 12.6). One study on this association was reported by Japanese researchers in the 2008 *International Heart Journal*.[51] In essence, long-term treatment with atorvastatin may increase plasma levels of brain natriuretic peptide (BNP) in coronary artery disease when associated with a greater reduction in plasma coenzyme Q10. Although statins and other pharmaceutical drugs appear to be the most significant source of CoQ10 deficiency in the general population, other sources of coenzyme Q10 decline appear in tissues that are highly metabolically active, such as those of the heart, immune system, inflamed gingival, and overactive thyroid gland. As we age, the levels of CoQ10 in our body decrease.[52] This may be due to decreased endogenous production, an insufficiency in the diet, or the cumulative effects of stress and free radicals. Although there is no evidence that healthy individuals need to supplement with CoQ10, tissues will benefit from coenzyme Q10 support during times of metabolic stress.

Although coenzyme Q10 is found in relatively high concentrations in the liver, kidney, and lung, the heart requires the highest levels of ATP activity because it is continually aerobic and contains more mitochondria per gram than any other tissue in the body. Cardiomyocytes, for example, contain more than 3500 mitochondria per cell compared to a biceps muscle cell that houses approximately 200 mitochondria per cell. Tissue deficiencies and low serum blood levels of coenzyme Q10 have been reported across a wide range of cardiovascular diseases, including DD, CHF, hypertension,

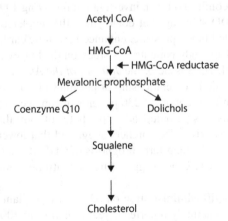

FIGURE 12.6   Statin drugs (HMG-CoA reductase inhibitors) can reduce natural coenzyme Q10 synthesis in the body.

aortic valvular disease, and coronary artery disease, and research suggests that coenzyme Q10 support may be indicated in these disease conditions.[53,54]

Although the medical literature generally supports the use of coenzyme Q10 in CHF, the evaluated dose–response relationships for this nutrient have been confined to a narrow dose range, with the majority of clinical studies having been conducted on subjects who were taking only 90–300 mg daily. At such doses, some patients have responded, whereas others have not. In more than two dozen controlled trials of supplemental CoQ10 in CHF, only three investigations,[55–57] which failed to show improvement in any significant cardiovascular function, had major limitations.

In the well-known study conducted by Permanetter et al.,[55] a 100-mg dose of coenzyme Q10 failed to show improvement. However, actual blood levels of CoQ10 were not obtained in this investigation; thus, it is impossible to know if a therapeutic blood level was ever achieved. In the second trial by Watson et al.,[56] a mean treatment plasma CoQ10 level of 1.7 µg/mL was obtained with only 2 of the 30 patients having a plasma level greater than 2.0 µg/mL.

The third study performed by Khatta and colleagues[57] demonstrated a mean treatment plasma CoQ10 level of 2.2 ± 1.1 µg/mL and indicated that approximately half the patients had treatment levels as low as 1.0 µg/mL. Unfortunately, these last two clinical trials are frequently quoted as CoQ10 failures despite the fact that a biosensitive result was not achieved.

In patients with CHF or dilated cardiomyopathy, I generally use higher doses of coenzyme Q10 in ranges of at least 300 mg or more to get a biosensitive result requiring a blood level at least greater than 2.5 µg/mL and preferably 3.5 µg/mL.[58] In a previous analysis in three patients with refractory CHF, higher doses of CoQ10 were required to get such a biosensitive or therapeutic result.[59]

In an investigation at the Lancisi Heart Institute in Italy, researchers studied 23 patients with a mean age of 59 years, using a double-blind, placebo-controlled, and crossover design. Patients were assigned to receive 100 mg of oral CoQ10 three times a day plus supervised exercise training. The study concluded that CoQ10 supplementation improved functional capacity, endothelial function, and left ventricular contractility in CHF without any side effects.[60]

In a previous long-term study of 424 patients with systolic dysfunction and/or DD in the presence of CHF, dilated cardiomyopathy, or hypertensive heart disease, a dose of 240 mg/day maintained blood levels of coenzyme Q10 above 2.0 µg/mL and allowed 43% of the participants to discontinue one to three conventional drugs over the course of the study.[61] Patients were followed for an average of 17.8 months, and during that time a mild case of nausea was the only reported side effect. This long-term study clearly shows coenzyme Q10 to be a safe and effective adjunctive treatment for patients with systolic and/or diastolic left ventricular dysfunction with or without CHF, dilated cardiomyopathy, and hypertensive heart disease.

These results are further confirmed by an investigation involving 109 patients with hypertensive heart disease and isolated DD showing that coenzyme Q10 supplementation resulted in clinical improvement, lowered elevated blood pressure, enhanced diastolic cardiac function, and decreased myocardial thickness in 53% of study patients.[62] A study on the longevity merits of CoQ10 in heart failure was published in a fall 2008 issue of the *Journal of the American College of Cardiology*.[63] New Zealand researchers studied the relationship of plasma CoQ10 levels and survival in patients with chronic heart failure. In their cohort of 236 patients (mean age 77 years), they concluded that plasma CoQ10 concentrations was an independent predictor of mortality. The higher blood levels were the best predictors for survival. Researchers suggested that lower concentrations of plasma CoQ10 might be detrimental in the long-term prognosis of CHF. Because CoQ10 depletion is associated with worse outcomes in CHF, they suggest further controlled intervention studies on CoQ10 supplementation.

This effect of coenzyme Q10 administration on 32 heart transplant candidates with end-stage CHF and cardiomyopathy was actually reported 4 years[64] earlier in 2004. The study was designed to determine if coenzyme Q10 could improve the pharmacological bridge to transplantation, and the results showed three significant findings. First, following 6 weeks of coenzyme Q10 therapy the study group showed elevated blood levels from an average of 0.22 mg/L to 0.83 mg/L, an increase of 277% (please note that different laboratories in other countries have different standardizations of CoQ10). By contrast, the placebo group measured 0.18 mg/L at the onset of the study and 0.178 mg/L at 6 weeks. Second, the study group showed significant improvement in 6-minute walk test distance, shortness of breath, NYHA functional classification, fatigue, and episodes of waking for nocturnal urination. No such changes were found in the placebo group. These results strongly show that coenzyme Q10 therapy may augment pharmaceutical treatment of patients with end-stage CHF and cardiomyopathy.

Very recently, three coenzyme Q10 studies were published, suggesting even more evidence for its consideration in left ventricular dysfunction. In one small study of 28 patients with ischemic left ventricular systolic dysfunction, taking 300 mg of coenzyme Q10 supplement per day versus 28 placebo controls, 8 weeks of supplementation improved mitochondrial functioning and brachial flow-mediated dilatation (FMD).[65] The researchers concluded that coQ10 improved endothelial function via reversal of mitochondrial dysfunction in patients with diminished ejection fraction. In another study (Q-Symbio)[66] presented in Lisbon, Portugal (2013), investigators studied 420 patients and reported not only a reduction in hospital admissions in the CoQ10 group but also a significant decrease in mortality with 18 patients in the CoQ10 group versus 36 placebo. The investigators concluded that CoQ10 should strongly be considered as part of the maintenance treatment of CHF.

Finally, in another double-blind, placebo-controlled trial[67] among elderly Swedish citizens, 443 patients aged 70–88 years, selenium and coQ10 were administered versus placebo. There was a significant reduction in mortality in the active group, 5.9% versus 12.6 controls. In addition, N-terminal pro-B-type natriuretic peptide (NT-Pro-BNP) and echocardiographic measurements were significantly improved.

To summarize, CoQ10 is one of the body's most important endogenous compounds as a powerful antioxidant and membrane stabilizer as well as a critical electron donor for mitochondrial cellular production. Multiple controlled studies have confirmed my observation in three decades of CoQ10 applications in thousands of patients. It is the most efficacious, bioenergetic, and therapeutic compound I've ever discovered in the treatment and management of CHF.

LEVOCARNITINE (L-CARNITINE OR CARNITINE)

Carnitine is derived naturally in the body from the amino acids lysine and methionine. Biosynthesis occurs in a series of metabolic reactions involving these amino acids, complemented with niacin, vitamin B_6, vitamin C, and iron. Although carnitine deficiency is rare in a healthy, well-nourished population consuming adequate protein, CHF, left ventricular hypertrophy, and other cardiac conditions causing renal insufficiency can lead to cellular depletion and conditions of carnitine deficiency.

The principal role of carnitine is to facilitate the transport of fatty acids across the inner mitochondrial membrane to initiate β-oxidation. The inner mitochondrial membrane is normally impermeable to activated coenzyme A (CoA) esters. To affect transfer of the extracellular metabolic by-product acyl-CoA across the cellular membrane, the mitochondria deliver its acyl unit to the carnitine residing in the inner mitochondrial membrane. Carnitine (as acetyl-carnitine) then transports the metabolic fragment across the membrane and delivers it to coenzyme A residing inside the mitochondria. This process of acetyl transfer is known as carnitine shuttle, and the shuttle also works in reverse to remove excess acetyl units from the inner mitochondria for disposal. Excess acetyl units that accumulate inside the mitochondria disturb the metabolic burning of fatty acids.

Nature created carnitine to serve as a freight train or ferryboat to carry fatty acids into the mitochondria. More importantly, it's not only the burning of fat in the mitochondria that fuels the energy for ATP, but as a high-energy organism, we humans produce a lot of toxic waste products. This is where the carnitines are so absolutely phenomenal and instrumental, especially in cardiac health.

Not only do these carnitines shuttle in the fatty acids to be burned in the mitochondria as fuel but they also shuttle out the toxic metabolites as well.

Other crucial functions of intracellular carnitine include the metabolism of branched-chain amino acids, ammonia detoxification, and lactic acid clearance from tissue. Carnitine also exhibits antioxidant and free radical scavenger properties.

Although the role of carnitine in the utilization of fatty acids and glucose in cardiac metabolism has been known for decades, the relationship between carnitine availability in heart tissue, carnitine metabolism in the heart, and carnitine's impact on left ventricular function has been elucidated only recently. Two independent studies have investigated the relationship between tissue carnitine levels and heart function and whether plasma or urinary carnitine levels might actually serve as markers for impaired left ventricular function in patients with CHF.

In the first study of carnitine tissue levels and CHF, the myocardial tissue from 25 cardiac transplant recipients with end-stage CHF and 21 control donor hearts was analyzed for concentrations of total carnitine, free carnitine, and carnitine derivatives. Compared to controls, the concentration of carnitines in the heart muscle of heart transplant recipients was significantly lower in patients, and the level of carnitine in the tissue was directly related to ejection fraction. This study concluded that carnitine deficiency in the heart tissue might be directly related to heart function.[68]

The second study measured plasma and urinary levels of L-carnitine in 30 patients with CHF and cardiomyopathy and compared them to 10 control subjects with no heart disease.[69] Results showed that patients with CHF had higher plasma and urinary levels of carnitine, suggesting that carnitine was being released from the challenged heart muscle cells. Similarly, the results showed that the level of plasma and urinary carnitine was related to the degree of left ventricular systolic dysfunction and ejection fraction, showing that elevated plasma and urinary carnitine levels—indices of carnitines being leached out of compromised cardiomyocytes—might represent measurable physiological markers for myocardial damage and impaired left ventricular function.

More recently, free L-carnitine levels and levels of its derivative palmitoyl-carnitine were increased in CHF patients and correlated with NT-Pro-BNP and NYHA functional class status. In this study of 183 heart failure patients and 111 healthy controls, higher levels of palmitoyl-carnitine were also associated with more adverse outcomes. The authors believed these findings suggested prognostic value and recommended additional investigational analysis of L-carnitine administration in heart failure candidates.[70]

A previous investigation examined the effect of long-term carnitine administration on mortality in patients with CHF and dilated cardiomyopathy. This study followed 80 patients with moderate to severe heart failure (NYHA class III/IV) for 3 years. After a 3-month period of stable cardiac function on normal medication, patients were randomly assigned to receive either 2 g of carnitine per day or a matched placebo. After an average of 33.7 months of follow-up 70 patients remained in the study (33 taking placebo and 37 supplementing with carnitine), and at the end of the study period 63 had survived (27 placebo and 36 carnitine). This study determined that carnitine provided a benefit to longer term survival in late-stage heart failure in dilated cardiomyopathy.[71]

A similar placebo-controlled study evaluated 160 myocardial infarction survivors for 12 months.[72] A total of 80 subjects were included in each group; the study group received a daily dose of 4 g of L-carnitine, and the controls received a placebo. Both the carnitine and control groups continued their conventional therapeutic regimen while on the test substance. Subjects in both groups showed improvement in arterial blood pressure, cholesterol levels, rhythm disorders, and signs and symptoms of CHF over the study period, but all-cause mortality was significantly lower in the carnitine group than the placebo group (1.2% and 12.5%, respectively). A further double blind, placebo-controlled trial by Singh and coworkers studied 100 patients with suspected myocardial infarction. Patients taking carnitine (2 g/day for 28 days) showed improvement in arrhythmia, angina, onset of heart failure, and mean infarct size, as well as a reduction in total cardiac events. There was a significant reduction in cardiac death and nonfatal infarction in the carnitine group versus the placebo group (15.6% vs. 26%, respectively).[73]

In a European study of 472 patients published in the *Journal of the American College of Cardiology*, 9 g/day of carnitine was administered intravenously for 5 days followed by 6 g/day orally for the next 12 months.[74] The study validated previous findings, demonstrating an improvement in ejection fraction and a reduction in left ventricular size in carnitine-treated patients. Although the European study was not designed to demonstrate outcome differences, the combined incidence of CHF death after discharge was lower in the carnitine group than the placebo group (6.0% vs. 9.6%, respectively), a reduction of more than 30%.

In a later study, only 1500 mg of L-carnitine in 29 patients with NYHA class II symptoms and preserved left ventricular function demonstrated not only an improvement in shortness of breath in the carnitine group but also improved diastolic relationships on echocardiographic analysis after only 3 months of treatment.[75]

The most recent review of the benefits of L-carnitine and cardiovascular function was reported as a meta-analysis in the Mayo Clinic's proceedings in 2013.[76] A total of 13 clinical trials involving 3629 patients post-myocardial infarction (MI) were evaluated. L-carnitine's benefits were attributed to the ability of L-carnitine to limit infarct size, stabilize membranes, and improve compromised cellular energy production. The major improvements in these vulnerable post-MI patients not only showed a reduction of angina symptoms by 40% and reduced arrhythmia by 60% but a striking reduction in all-cause death by 27%.[76]

A newer form of carnitine called glycine propionyl L-carnitine (GPLC) has demonstrated significant advantages in the production of nitric oxide and lower malondialdehyde (MDA), a marker of lipid peroxidation and oxidative damage. This form of carnitine has demonstrated the important property of vasodilation via a nitric oxide mechanism. GPLC also blocked key steps in the process of platelet aggregation and adhesion, as well as reducing levels of lipid peroxidation and oxidative damage.[77]

To summarize, without carnitine fats, which are a high-energy fuel for the heart, cannot be converted to ATP. The heart uses free fatty acids as its main energy source, and the only way for long-chain fatty acids to get to the inner mitochondrial membrane where energy is produced is via the carnitine shuttle. Thus, the addition of L-carnitine is very important in the synergy of metabolic cardiology.

MAGNESIUM: SWITCHING ON THE ENERGY ENZYMES

Magnesium is an essential mineral that is critical for energy-requiring processes, in protein synthesis, membrane integrity, nervous tissue conduction, neuromuscular excitation, muscle contraction, hormone secretion, maintenance of vascular tone, and intermediary metabolism. Deficiency may lead to changes in neuromuscular, cardiovascular, immune, and hormonal function; impaired energy metabolism; and reduced capacity for physical work. Magnesium deficiency is now considered to contribute to many diseases, and the role for magnesium as a therapeutic agent is expanding. A published German study[78] brings this point into focus.

Researchers in this study evaluated a random population of about 16,000 people, who were assigned to subgroups based on gender, age, and state of health. Low blood levels of magnesium, or hypomagnesemia, was identified in 14.5% of all persons examined, and suboptimal levels were found in yet another 33.7%—a total of 58.2%—more than half of those evaluated.[78] Thus, low magnesium situations are more common than we think.

Magnesium deficiency reduces the activity of important enzymes used in energy metabolism. Hypomagnesemia can result in progressive vasoconstriction, coronary spasm, and even sudden death.[79] In anginal episodes due to coronary artery spasm, treatment with magnesium has been shown to be efficacious.[80]

Magnesium deficiency, which is better detected by mononuclear blood cell magnesium than the standard serum level performed at most hospitals, predisposes to excessive mortality and morbidity in patients with acute MI.[81]

Unless we have adequate levels of magnesium in our cells, the cellular processes of energy metabolism cannot function. Small changes in magnesium levels can have a large effect on heart and blood vessel function. Although magnesium is found in most foods, particularly beans, figs, and vegetables, deficiencies are increasing. Softened water, depleted soils, and a trend toward lower vegetable consumption are the culprits contributing to these rising deficiencies.

SUMMARY

The energy-starved heart is often not considered by physicians who treat cardiac disease on a day-to-day basis. Angiotensin-converting enzyme inhibitors and angiotensin receptor II blockers improve survival in ischemic and nonischemic heart failure and should be considered as a conventional approach in any patient with heart failure. However, therapies that target the cardiomyocyte itself must also be employed[11] as it has been shown that the function of cardiomyocytes in the failing heart, although metabolically compromised, can be potentially improved and restored.[11] Therapies that go beyond symptomatic relief (diuretics), and the neurohormonal axis, must also be considered that target the cellular, mitochondrial, and metabolic defects. Metabolic support with D-ribose, coenzyme Q10, L-carnitine, and magnesium is critical for the maintenance of contractile reserve and energy charge in minimally oxidative ischemic or hypoxic hearts. Preservation of cellular energy charge provides the chemical driving force required to complete ATPase reactions needed to maintain cell and tissue viability and function. D-ribose, coenzyme Q_{10}, L-carnitine, and magnesium exert a physiological benefit that has a positive impact on cardiac function.

A metabolic cardiology approach using these components is suggested here: when taking the suggested amounts, it is recommended that the total dose be given in divided doses after breakfast and after dinner. For D-ribose, take 5-g (one scoop) dose, three times a day.

Mild to moderate CHF:

1. Multivitamin/mineral foundation program with 1 g of fish or calamarine oil
2. Coenzyme Q10: 300–400 mg
3. L-carnitine: 2000–2500 mg
4. D-ribose: 15 g
5. Magnesium: 400–800 mg

Severe CHF, dilated cardiomyopathy, and patients awaiting heart transplantation:

1. Multivitamin/mineral foundation program with 1 g of fish or calamarine oil
2. Coenzyme Q10: 360–600 mg
3. L-carnitine: 2500–3500 mg
4. D-ribose: 15 g
5. Magnesium: 400–800 mg

Note: If quality of life is still not satisfactory, add 1500 mg of Hawthorn berry and 2 to 3 g of taurine, as the addition of these two nutraceuticals has helped many of my patients with severe refractory CHF.

CONCLUSION

Cardiovascular function depends on the operational capacity of myocardial cells to generate the energy to expand and contract. Insufficient myocardial energy significantly contributes to CHF. Literally, heart failure occurs when a heart is energy starved.

Although there may be several causes of myocardial dysfunction, the energy deficiency in cardiac myocytes plays a significant role and is probably the major factor in CHF. It is no longer enough that physicians focus on the fluid retention aspects of "pump failure." For instance, diuretic therapies target the kidneys indirectly to relieve the sequelae of CHF without addressing the root cause. Inotropic agents attempt to increase contractility directly, yet fail to offer the extra energy necessary to assist the weakened heart muscle. Metabolic solutions, on the other hand, treat the heart muscle cells directly.

Physicians must consider the biochemistry of "pulsation." It is critically important to treat both the molecular and the cellular components of the heart when managing CHF. Remember, one characteristic of the failing heart is the persistent and progressive loss of cellular energy substrates and abnormalities in cardiac bioenergetics that directly compromise diastolic performance, with the capacity to impact global cardiac function. It took me 35 years of cardiology practice to learn that the heart is all about ATP, and the bottom line in the treatment of any form of cardiovascular disease, especially CHF and cardiomyopathy, is restoration of the heart's energy reserve. Metabolic cardiology addresses the biochemical interventions that directly improve energy substrates and therefore energy metabolism in heart cells. In simple terms, sick hearts leak out and lose vital ATP and the endogenous restoration of ATP cannot keep pace with the relentless depletion of energy substrates, especially in situations of ischemia. When ATP levels drop, diastolic function, the most important precursor of CHF, deteriorates. As epidemiological studies suggest that DD is present in more than half of patients admitted to hospitals with CHF,[82] it makes sense to target myocardial energetics with effective modalities that truly work.

D-ribose, coenzyme Q10, L-carnitine, and magnesium all act to promote cardiac energy metabolism and help normalize myocardial adenine nucleotide concentrations. These naturally occurring compounds exert a physiological benefit that positively impacts diastolic heart function. All are recommended as adjunctive metabolic therapies in the treatment of heart failure and cardiomyopathy.

Acknowledging this metabolic support for the heart provides the missing link that has been eluding cardiologists for decades and offers hope for the future treatment of cardiovascular disease. Energizing diastole and myocyte metabolism is the most effective therapy for diastolic heart failure and some day may become the standard of care for all forms of heart disease[82] and especially CHF.[17,18] Such potential treatment strategies are currently being modulated from the bench to the bedside.[17,83]

REFERENCES

1. The CONSENSUS Trial Study Group. Effects of enalapril on mortality on mortality in severe congestive heart failure: Results of the Cooperative North Scandinavian Enalapril Survival Study (CONSENSUS). *N Engl J Med* 1987;316:1429–1435.
2. Pfeffer MA, Braunwalk E, Moye LA et al. Effect of captopril on mortality and morbidity in patients with left ventricular dysfunction after myocardial infarction: Results of the Survival and Ventricular Enlargement Trial. *N Engl J Med* 1992;327:669–677.
3. CIBIS Investigators and Committees. A randomized trial of B-blockade in heart failure: The Cardiac Bisoprolol Insufficiency Study (CIBIS). *Circulation* 1994;90:1765–1773.
4. Packer M, Bristow MR, Cohn JN et al. The effect of carvedilol on morbidity and mortality in patients with chronic heart failure. *N Engl J Med* 1996;334:1349–1355.
5. Agnetti N, Kaludercic LA, Kane ST et al. Modulation of mitochondrial proteome and improved mitochondrial function by biventricular pacing of dyssynchronous failing hearts. *Circ Cardiovasc Genet* 2010;3:78–87.
6. Kitaizumi K, Yukiiri K, Masugata H et al. Positron emission tomographic demonstration of myocardial oxidative metabolism in a case of left ventricular restoration after cardiac resynchronization therapy. *Circ J* 2008;72:1900–1903.
7. Christenson SD, Chareonthaitawee P, Burnes JE et al. Effects of simultaneous and optimized sequential cardiac resynchronization therapy on myocardial oxidative metabolism and efficiency. *J Cardiovasc Electrophysiol* 2008;19:125–132.
8. McMurray JJ, Pfeffer MA. Heart failure. *Lancet* 2005;365:1877–1889.
9. Gheorghiade M, Peterson ED. Improving postdischarge outcomes in patients hospitalized for acute heart failure syndromes. *JAMA* 2011;305:2456–2457.

10. Stanley WC, Hoppel CL. Mitochondrial dysfunction in heart failure: Potential for therapeutic interventions? *Cardiovasc Res* 2000;45:805–806.
11. Bayeva M, Gheorghiade M, Ardehali H. Mitochondria as a therapeutic target in heart failure. *J Am Coll Cardiol* 2013;61(6):599–610.
12. Ardehali H, Sabbah HN, Burke MA et al. Targeting myocardial substrate metabolism in heart failure: Potential for new therapies. *Eur J Heart Fail* 2012;14:120–129.
13. Bergmann O, Bhardwaj RD, Bernard S et al. Evidence for cardiomyocyte renewal in humans. *Science* 2009;324:98–102.
14. Parmacek MS, Epstein JA. Cardiomyocyte renewal. *N Engl J Med* 2009;361;1:86–88.
15. Ingwall JS, Weiss RG. Is the failing heart energy starved? On using chemical energy to support cardiac function. *Circ Res* 2004;95:135–145.
16. Neubauer S. The failing heart: An engine out of fuel. *N Engl J Med* 2007;356(11):1140–1151.
17. Sinatra ST. Metabolic cardiology: The missing link in cardiovascular disease. *Altern Ther Health Med* 2009;15(2):48–50.
18. Sinatra ST. The Sinatra Solution/Metabolic Cardiology. Laguna Beach, CA: Basic Health Publications, 2005.
19. Sinatra ST, Roberts JC. *Reverse Heart Disease Now*. Hoboken, NJ: John Wiley, 2007.
20. Tanaka J, Tominaga R, Yoshitoshi et al. Coenzyme Q10: The prophylactic effect on low cardiac output following cardiac valve replacement. *Ann Thorac Surg* 1982;33:145–151.
21. Sinatra ST. Letter to the Editor: Coenzyme Q10 in patients with end-stage heart failure awaiting cardiac transplantation: A randomized, placebo-controlled study. *Clin Cardiol* 2004;27(10):A26.
22. Lazaron J, Pomeranz B, Corey P. Incidence of adverse drug reaction in hospitalized patients. *JAMA* 1998;279:1200–1205.
23. Bashore TM, Magorien DJ, Letterio J, et al. Histologic and biochemical correlates of left ventricular chamber dynamics in man. *J Am Coll Cardiol* 1987;9:734.42.
24. Braunwald E, Ross J Jr, Sonnenblick EH. *Mechanisms of Contraction of the Normal and Failing Heart*. 2nd ed. Boston: Little, Brown; 1976, p. 170.
25. Lewis BS, Gotsman MS. Current concepts of left ventricular relaxation and compliance. *Am Heart J* 1980;99:101–13.
26. Ingwall JS. *ATP and the Heart*. Boston, MA: Kluwer Academic Publishers, 2002.
27. Ingwall JS. On the hypothesis that the failing heart is energy starved: Lessons learned from the metabolism of ATP and creatine. *Cur Hypertens Rep* 2006;8:457–464.
28. Manfredi JP, Holmes EW. Purine salvage pathways in myocardium. *Ann Rev Physiol* 1985;47:691–705.
29. Gourine AV, Hu Q, Sander PR et al. Interstitial purine metabolites in hearts with LV remodeling. *Am J Physiol Heart Circ Physiol* 2004;286:H677–H684.
30. Hu Q, Wang Q, Lee J et al. Profound bioenergetics abnormalities in peri-infarct myocardial regions. *Am J Physiol Heart Circ Physiol* 2006;291:H648–H657.
31. Ye Y, Gong G, Ochiai K et al. High-energy phosphate metabolism and creatine kinase in failing hearts: A new porcine model. *Circ* 2001;103:1570–1576.
32. Maslov MY, Chacko VP, Stuber M et al. Altered high-energy phosphate metabolism predicts contractile dysfunction and subsequent ventricular remodeling in pressure-overload hypertrophy mice. *Am J Physiol Heart Circ Physiol* 2007;292:H387–H391.
33. Cha Y-M, Dzeja PP, Shen WK et al. Failing atrial myocardium: Energetic deficits accompany structural remodeling and electrical instability. *Am J Physiol Heart Circ Physiol* 2003;284:H1313–H1320.
34. Melduni R, Suri RM, Seward JB et al. Diastolic dysfunction in patients undergoing cardiac surgery: A pathophysiological mechanism underlying the initiation of new-onset post-operative atrial fibrillation. *J Am Coll Cardiol* 2011;58(9):953–961.
35. Bache RJ, Zang J, Murakami Y et al. Myocardial oxygenation at high workstates in hearts with left ventricular hypertrophy. *Cardiovasc Res* 1999;42(3):567–570.
36. Smith CS, Bottomley PA, Schulman SP et al. Altered creatine kinase adenosine triphosphate kinetics in failing hypertrophied human myocardium. *Circ* 2006;114:1151–1158.
37. Weiss RG, Gerstenblith G, Bottomley PA. ATP flux through creatine kinase in the normal, stressed, and failing human heart. *Proc Natl Acad Sci U S A* 2005;102(3):808–813.
38. Beer M, Seyfarth T, Sandstede J et al. Absolute concentrations of high-energy phosphate metabolites in normal, hypertrophied, and failing human myocardium measured noninvasively with (31) P-Sloop magnetic resonance spectroscopy. *JACC* 2002;40(7):1267–1274.
39. Lamb HJ, Beyerbacht HP, van der Laarse A et al. Diastolic dysfunction in hypertensive heart disease is associated with altered myocardial metabolism. *Circ* 1999;99(17):2261–2267.

40. Neubauer S, Horn M, Pabst T et al. Cardiac high-energy phosphate metabolism in patients with aortic valve disease assessed by 31P-magnetic resonance spectroscopy. *J Investig Med* 1997;45(8):453–462.
41. Diamant M, Lamb HJ, Groeneveld Y et al. Diastolic dysfunction is associated with altered myocardial metabolism in asymptomatic normotensive patients with well-controlled type 2 diabetes mellitus. *JACC* 2003;41(2):328–335.
42. Schocke MF, Metzler B, Wolf C et al. Impact of aging on cardiac high-energy phosphate metabolism determined by phosphorous-31 2-dimensional chemical shift imaging (31P 2D CSI). *Magn Reson Imaging* 2003;21(5):553–559.
43. Perings SM, Schulze K, Decking U et al. Age-related decline of PCr/ATP-ratio in progressively hypertrophied hearts of spontaneously hypertensive rats. *Heart Vessels* 2000;15(4):197–202.
44. Ypenburg C, Sieders A, Bleeker GB et al. Myocardial contractile reserve predicts improvement in left ventricular function after cardiac resynchronization therapy. *Am Heart J* 2007;154(6):1160–1165.
45. Omran H, Illien S, MacCarter D et al. D-ribose improves diastolic function and quality of life in congestive heart failure patients: A prospective feasibility study. *Eur J Heart Failure* 2003;5:615–619.
46. Vijay N, MacCarter D, Washam M et al. Ventilatory efficiency improves with d-ribose in congestive heart failure patients. *J Mol Cell Cardiol* 2005;38(5):820.
47. Carter O, MacCarter D, Manneback S et al. D-ribose improves peak exercise capacity and ventilatory efficiency in heart failure patients. *JACC* 2005;45(3 suppl A):185A.
48. Sharma R, Munger M, Litwin S et al. D-ribose improves Doppler TEI myocardial performance index and maximal exercise capacity in stage C heart failure. *J Mol Cell Cardiol* 2005;38(5):853.
49. Befera N, Rivard A, Gatlin G et al. Ribose treatment helps preserve function of the remote myocardium after myocardial infarction. *J Surg Res* 2007;137(2):156.
50. Perkowski DJ, Wagner S, Schneider JR. A targeted metabolic protocol with D-ribose for off-pump coronary artery bypass procedures: A retrospective analysis. *Ther Adv Cardiovasc Dis* 2011;5(4):185–192.
51. Suzuki T, Nozawa T, Sobajima M. Atorvastatin-induced changes in plasma coenzyme Q10 and brain natriuretic peptide in patients with coronary artery disease. *Int Heart J* 2008;49(4):423–433.
52. Lass A. Mitochondrial coenzyme Q content and aging. *Biofactors* 1999;9(2–4):199–205.
53. Langsjoen PH, Langsjoen AM. Overview of the use of CoQ10 in cardiovascular disease. *Biofactors* 1999;9(2–4):273–284.
54. Langsjoen PH, Littarru GP, Silver MA. Role of concomitant coenzyme Q10 with statins for patients with hyperlipidemia. *Curr Topics Nutr Res* 2005;3(3):149–158.
55. Permanetter B, Rossy W, Klein G et al. Ubiquinone (coenzyme Q10) in the long-term treatment of idiopathic dilated cardiomyopathy. *Eur Heart J* 1992;13(11):1528–1533.
56. Watson PS, Scalia GM, Gaibraith AJ et al. Is coenzyme Q10 helpful for patients with idiopathic cardiomyopathy? *Med J Aust* 2001;175(8):447, author reply 447–448.
57. Khatta M, Alexander BS, Krichten CM et al. The effect of coenzyme Q10 in patients with congestive heart failure. *Ann Intern Med* 2000;132(8):636–640.
58. Sinatra ST. Letter to the editor: Coenzyme Q10 and congestive heart failure. *Ann Intern Med* 2000;133(9):745–746.
59. Sinatra ST. Coenzyme Q10: A vital therapeutic nutrient for the heart with special application in congestive heart failure. *Conn Med Nov* 1997;61(11):707–711.
60. Belardinelli R, Mucaj A, Lacalaprice F et al. Coenzyme Q10 and exercise training in chronic heart failure. *Eur Heart J* 2006;27(22):2675–2681.
61. Langsjoen PH, Langsjoen P, Willis R et al. Usefulness of coenzyme Q10 in clinical cardiology: A long-term study. *Mol Aspects Med* 1994;15:S165–S175.
62. Langsjoen P, Willis R, Folkers K. Treatment of essential hypertension with coenzyme Q10. *Mol Aspects Med* 1994;15 (suppl):265–272.
63. Molyneux S, Florkowski C, George P et al. Coenzyme Q10: An independent predictor of mortality in chronic heart failure. *JACC* 2008;52(18):1435–1441.
64. Berman M, Erman A, Ben-Gal T et al. Coenzyme Q10 in patients with end-stage heart failure awaiting cardiac transplantation: A randomized, placebo-controlled study. *Clin Cardiol* 2004;27:295–299.
65. Dai YL, Luk TH, Yiu KH et al. Reversal of mitochondrial dysfunction by coenzyme Q10 supplement improves endothelial function in patients with ischaemic left ventricular systolic dysfunction: A randomized controlled trial. *Atherosclerosis* 2011;216(2):395–401.
66. Mortensen SA, Kumar A, Dolliner P et al. The Effect of Coenzyme Q10 on Morbidity and Mortality in Chronic Heart Failure. Results from Q-SYMBIO Study. Presented at Heart Failure Congress 2013 Final Programme Number 440, Coenzyme Q10 as Adjunctive Treatment of Chronic Heart Failure: A Randomized

Double Blind Multicenter Trial With Focus on Changes in Symptoms, Biomarker Status with BNP and Long Term Outcome. *JACC Heart Fail* 2014 Sep 25. p.ii: S2213-1779(14)00336-9.

67. Alehagen U, Johansson P, Bjornstedt M et al. Cardiovascular mortality and N-terminal-proBNP reduced after combined selenium and coenzyme Q10 supplementation: A 5-year prospective randomized double-blind placebo-controlled trial among elderly Swedish citizens. *Int J Cardiol* 2013;167(5):1860–1866.

68. El-Aroussy W, Rizk A, Mayhoub G et al. Plasma carnitine levels as a marker of impaired left ventricular functions. *Mol Cell Biochem* 2000;213(1–2):37–41.

69. Narin F, Narin N, Andac H et al. Carnitine levels in patients with chronic rheumatic heart disease. *Clin Biochem* 1997;30(8):643–645.

70. Ueland T, Svardal A, Oie E et al. Disturbed carnitine regulation in chronic heart failure: increased plasma levels of palmitoyl-carnitine are associated with poor prognosis. *Int J Cardiol* 2013;167(5):1892–1899.

71. Rizos I. Three-year survival of patients with heart failure caused by dilated cardiomyopathy. *Am Heart J* 2000;139(2 Pt 3):S120–S123.

72. Davini P, Bigalli A, Lamanna F et al. Controlled study on L-carnitine therapeutic efficacy in post-infarction. *Drugs Exp Clin Res* 1992;18:355–365.

73. Singh RB, Niaz MA, Agarwal P et al. A randomized, double-blind, placebo-controlled trial of L-carnitine in suspected acute myocardial infarction. *Postgrad Med* 1996;72:45–50.

74. Iliceto S, Scrutinio D, Bruzzi P et al. Effects of L-carnitine administration on left ventricular remodeling after acute anterior myocardial infarction: The L-carnitine Eocardiografia Digitalizzata Infarto Miocardioco (CEDIM) Trial. *JACC* 1995;26(2):380–387.

75. Serati AR, Motamedi MR, Emami S et al. L-carnitine treatment in patients with mild diastolic heart failure is associated with improvement in diastolic function and symptoms. *Cardiology* 2010;116:178–182.

76. DiNicolantonio JD. L-carnitine in the secondary prevention of cardiovascular disease: systemic review and meta-analysis. *Mayo Clinic Proceed* 2013;88(6):544–551.

77. Bloomer RJ, Smith WA, Fisher-Wellman KH. Glycine propionyl-L-carnitine increases plasma nitrate/nitrite in resistance trained men. *J International Society of Sports Nutr* 2007;4:22.

78. Schimatschek HF, Rempis R. Prevalence of hypomagnesemia in an unselected German population of 16,000 individuals. *Magnes Res* 2001;14(4):283–290.

79. Turlapaty PDMV, Altura BM. Magnesium deficiency produces spasms of coronary arteries: relationship to etiology of sudden death ischemic heart disease. *Science* 1980;208:198.

80. McLean RM. Magnesium and its therapeutic uses: A review. *Am J Med* 1994;96:63.

81. Elin RJ. Magnesium metabolism in health and disease. *Dis Mon* 1998;34:161.

82. Baliga RR, Young JB. Energizing diastole. *Heart Fail Clin* 2008;4(1):9–13.

83. Schwarz K, Siddiqi N, Singh S et al. The breathing heart: Mitochondrial respiratory chain dysfunction in cardiac disease. *Int J Cardiol* 2014;171(2):134–143.

13 Be the Willow
Stress, Resiliency, and Diseases of the Heart

Mimi Guarneri and Ryan Bradley

CONTENTS

Man should not try to avoid stress any more than he should shun food, love, or exercise.

Hans Selye, MD, endocrinologist (1907–1982)

Notice that the stiffest tree is most easily cracked,
while the bamboo or willow survives by bending with the wind.

Bruce Lee, American actor (1940–1973)

Willows never forget how it feels to be young.

William Stafford, American poet (1914–1993)

INTRODUCTION

Life is incomplete without stress. Stress creates the inflection points of our emotional experiences of life, i.e., the roller coaster of life itself. In the cognitive domain, stress creates motivation, vigilance, and stimulates productivity. Although many of us often wish for less stress, or maintain an ideal vision of complete relaxation, without stress the experience of life would be bland, boring, and blunted by a lack of emotional extremes. The inherent requirement of stress for having rich life experiences was recognized in the mid-1900s by physician and chemist, Dr. Hans Selye, during his research on the role glucocorticoids have in eliciting and maintaining the stress response. In his book, *The Stress of Life*,[1] Dr. Selye describes the connections between the brain and the adrenal glands, articulating what has come to be known as the hypothalamic–pituitary–adrenal (HPA) axis. In addition to describing the overall importance of stress, Dr. Selye also described stress—and reactions to stress—along a continuum of optimally balanced vigilance and engagement in life to exhaustion and chronic disease states, resulting from the long-term consequences of maladaptation to stress. Selye's recommendation for dynamic balance in relation to stress is closely related to the contemporary term "allostasis," which refers to the simultaneous regulation of multiple physiologic processes in response to physical, environmental and psychosocial challenges, i.e., stressors.[2,3] Optimal allostasis, therefore, requires flexibility and dynamism, balancing multiple systems for optimal performance. However, even though the numerous interconnections in human physiology provide checks and balances to maintain allostasis, all infrastructure has limitations (no matter how expertly designed) and "allostatic load" refers to the gradual "wear and tear" of the various physiologic mechanisms involved, i.e., long-term consequences of maladaptation.

The concept of "allostasis" is closely related to "resiliency." By definition, resiliency is the quality of an object (or individual!) to hold or return to their shape after being bent, compressed, or stretched (or stressed!). With stress, building resiliency for regaining allostasis becomes an important goal—and a much more sophisticated goal than simply prescribing antidepressants or herbal adaptogens (although each may help as an element of a broader therapeutic strategy). By recognizing the importance of stress for living a dynamic life filled with rich emotional experiences (vs. the scarier thought of living a bland life without stress), the goal changes from eliminating stress, to managing stress by training ourselves and our patients to differentiate significant stressors from background noise, and then choose when and how to react. Guiding patients toward practicing stress management and resiliency-building behaviors, e.g., meditation, socialization, and spirituality, can provide them with tools to quickly return to allostasis following even significant stressors. These cumulative skills build resiliency to stress, and retrain previously reflexive reactions.

In this chapter, we describe some of the known connections between stress and cardiovascular disease (CVD), including a discussion of emerging research on the genetic pathways triggered by stress and careful exploration of "significant" stress and its contribution to CVD risk. We then provide a brief summary of the clinical evidence on numerous therapeutic interventions, including personal behavioral practices, mind–body interventions, combined physical and breathe practices, and formal clinical programs, that can help patients build resilience to stress, regain allostasis, reduce allostatic load, all of which help reduce their risk of significant cardiovascular morbidity and mortality.

MECHANISMS OF STRESS

Our robust physiologic stress response, has provided us with numerous evolutionary advantages, and ensured the survival of our species for millions of years. The major hormones of stress—epinephrine, norepinephrine, and cortisol[4,5]—increased our blood pressure to deliver more oxygen and nutrients to our muscles when we needed to run from aggressors, and chase after our food. The same hormones in different ratios helped us survive famine by blunting our sensitivity to insulin and shifting our metabolism to generate fuel when needed using gluconeogenesis and adipolysis. However, whether for better or worse, the *stressors* of life have changed but our physiological response has remained conserved. When under chronic stress, the same hormones that once protected us from our harsh environments now threaten our physiology with prolonged maladaptive changes including the following:

- Impaired glucose metabolism via chronic cortisol elevations and aberrant gluconeogenesis
- Weight gain from disrupted diurnal cortisol rhythms
- Cardiac arrhythmia via skewed sympathetic to parasympathetic nervous tone
- Hypertension from elevated catecholamines
- Hyperlipidemia and excess circulated free fatty acids from lipolysis
- Increased inflammation, i.e., increased TNF-α, from elevated catecholamines
- Coronary spasm via skewed sympathetic to parasympathetic nervous tone
- Immune suppression from excess cortisol
- Increased anxiety from excess catecholamines
- Hypersensitivity to pain from increased inflammatory mediators[6]

Providing a genetically rooted explanation for the cellular dysfunction caused by stress, Bhasin et al. recently applied transcriptome analysis to identify the genes temporally affected by relaxation, and discovered relaxation response was associated with increased transcription of genes associated with cellular energy metabolism, mitochondrial APT production, insulin secretion, telomere maintenance, and reduced transcription of genes associated with chronic inflammation, i.e., NF-κB.[7,8] These findings led the authors to coin "mitochondrial resilience" to describe the adaptive changes that result from relaxation. Thus mitochondrial maladaptation, i.e., reduced ATP production, reduced energy metabolism, increased oxidative stress, and reduced telomere maintenance, can be considered underlying cellular consequences of chronic stress. This innovative concept provides mechanistic support for stress as a mitochondrial toxin that reduces its ability to respond dynamically to a changing metabolic environment, i.e., maintains allostasis. Is it not surprising chronic stress has negative consequences for the most densely mitochondrial-laden tissue of the body—the heart.

As described in detail by McEwen and Gianaros,[9] central to our perception of potentially stressful stimuli, and thus our response, are complex interactions of several brain centers, with reaction originating in the deep emotional limbic centers of the brain, i.e., the amygdala, and then interacting with our memory of life experiences, i.e., the hippocampus, and our rational, cognitive centers, i.e., the prefrontal cortex. Interestingly, our perceptions of stress and reactions to stressors are connected to our developmental environment, including the *in utero* environment and during early childhood, including variables like food availability, parental nurturing behaviors, self-esteem, and education.[9–11] Therefore, our final reaction to stress is a complex mixture of voluntary and involuntary limbic responses, blended with a myriad of influences from our past experiences (e.g., injury, reward, support, and isolation) and our cognitive beliefs.

On one hand, the many influences on our response to stress may seem overwhelming and uncontrollable, i.e., we are destined to overreact and we can blame our parents; however, understanding the neurobiology provides several opportunities for education and reprogramming. For example, educating patients on how their responses to stress are a combination of voluntary and involuntary responses creates less judgment, provides an opportunity to query patients on past life experiences, and provides an opportunity to focus on the voluntary elements of their stress reactions to stress reprograming using cognitive behavioral therapy, mindfulness-based stress reduction, or other techniques. Also, the overarching regulating properties of the hippocampus and the prefrontal cortex, suggest that stress response, and increased resiliency, can be re-trained through repetitive exposure to potential stressors that do not need to lead to deleterious consequences, i.e., re-training social interactions, forming healthy relationships, and so on. Supporting this concept, animal studies in rats suggest that with continued exposure to stressors without consequence, i.e., repeated immobilization and forced swim testing, led to loss of fear memory and increased resiliency.[4] Offering patients reassurance and support, while encouraging them to face their fears and re-engage, may be one effective approach to reprogramming a deeply wired response.

STRESS AND CARDIOVASCULAR DISEASE

Chronic maladaptation to stress leads to both increases in circulating stress hormones and disrupted circadian rhythms of the normal cycles of stress hormones. As described earlier, this chronic dysregulation has direct and indirect consequences to the cardiovascular system, i.e., increased heart rate, blood pressure, oxidative stress, circulating blood fat, circulating blood sugar, and so on. Yet, many of these risk factors are multifactorial, influenced by diet, physical activity, genetics, and general state of health, so what is the independent effect of stress on cardiovascular health?

Because of its robust design and wide-reaching international recruitment, the INTERHEART case–control study has done more to increase the cardiology community's appreciation for the impact of stress on CVD risk than any other research to date. INTERHEART was designed to determine risk factors for first myocardial infarction (MI) and was conducted in 52 countries around the world, accumulating over 15,000 events.[12,13] The findings related to psychosocial stress and MI risk were staggering, with increased psychosocial stress attributing over 30% of population attributable risk for first MI. To thoroughly assess the contribution of stress to MI in INTERHEART, it is important to learn how "stress" was defined in the study. In INTERHEART, psychosocial stress was measured as a composite index composed of scores from five domains of stress: stress at home or at work, financial stress, past significant trauma (e.g., loss of a spouse or child), presence of depression, and locus of control.[13] Not surprisingly, having higher degrees of stress at work and home, greater financial stress, having experienced major life stress (e.g., business failure, major intra-family conflict, job loss, death of a spouse, and subject of violence), having depression, and/ or experiencing a low locus of control were all associated with increased risk for MI. Each component of the index contributes differently to the population attributable risk (see Table 13.1). Of note, although experiencing two or more major stressful events in life increased risk, business failure and having a major intrafamily conflict lend the greatest increases in risk, whereas the frequency of life stresses such as divorce, loss of another family member, or injury were similar between cases and controls.

Of all psychosocial risk factors, depression has been the most studied in relation to its impact on CVD. The relationship between depression and CVD appears to be bidirectional,[14] with major depressive disorder being more common in CVD patients,[15] as well as depression occurring as a common sequelae to MI.[16] The accumulation of evidence for positive associations between depression and worsened CVD prognosis finally led to its recognition in 2014 as an independent risk factor by the American Heart Association.[17] Many studies suggest depression predisposes to cardiovascular events, and worsen prognosis once events occur.[18–24] Depression worsens outcomes in unstable angina, even after controlling for other prognostic factors, such as left

TABLE 13.1

Impact of Psychosocial Risk Factors and First MI: INTERHEART

Psychosocial Risk Factor	Population Attributable Risk (PAR) for MI[13](%)
Low locus on control	16
Financial stress	11
Major stressful life event	10
Depression	9
Chronic stress at home or work	8
Total with adjustment for demographic variables and smoking	29
Total with adjustment for demographic and all other risk variables	32.5

ventricular ejection fraction and number of diseased vessels.[25] Patients with depression after MI are even more vulnerable, and experience higher mortality rates during the 18 months postinfarction than their nondepressed counterparts.[22] Toward the end of one's life journey, the absence of depression may be more significant to chances of recovery from chronic illness and exhaustion than history of CVD.[26]

Other studies before and since INTERHEART have recognized domains of psychosocial stress, in addition to depression, to have an impact on CVD. Supporting the significance of workplace stress on CVD outcomes, the massive meta-cohort study by Kivimaki et al. combined individual-level data from 30 European cohorts studies, collecting a total of 197,473 participants, 15% of whom reported job strain. Job strain was associated with a significant independent risk factor for coronary disease, contributing a 3.4% population attributable risk.[27] In contrast to INTERHEART, the Coronary Artery Risk Development in Young Adults (CARDIA) study demonstrated that time, urgency/impatience, and hostility, but not depression or anxiety, were linked to increased MI risk.[28] Brackett et al.[29] were among the first investigators to demonstrate a relationship between a type "A"–driven personality and increased risk for adverse CVD outcome. In their prospective cohort study over 5 years, having a type "A" personality was an independent predictor of sudden cardiac death.

POTENTIAL MECHANISMS FOR STRESS-INDUCED CVD

One potential behavioral mechanism for the higher morbidity and mortality witnessed in depressed patients may be differential self-care, including reduced adherence to medications and other self-care practices. Ziegelstein et al. found patients with depression reported lower inherence to low-fat-diet, regular-exercise, and stress-management plans. Individuals with major depression also reported taking their medications less often than prescribed.[30] Individuals with depression are also more likely to use alcohol excessively, which may also contribute to worsened outcomes. However, behavioral differences only accounted for a small percentage (3%) of the differences in CVD mortality for people with depression included in the National Health Interview Study.[31] Numerous biochemical mechanisms have been proposed, including increased inflammatory cytokines, oxidative stress, reduced heart rate variability (HRV), and tendency for coagulation.[32] Cortisol reactivity has also been proposed as a potential mechanism of stress-induced CVD, which is supported by the findings of Hamer et al. who found salivary cortisol concentrations correlated with progression of coronary calcification in healthy men and women over 3 years.[33] Clearly, part of the difficulty in trying to find the mechanism is trying to separate the parts, rather than accepting depression as an individualized biobehavioral syndrome—and that patients caught in the cycle of depression need to be recognized, evaluated, and given help.

GENDER DIFFERENCES IN THE EFFECTS OF STRESS ON CVD

Fortunately, the effects of stress on CVD risk in women have been given special attention in CVD research recently and suggest stress may have greater negative effects on women compared to men.[34–36] Specifically, stress and job strain are more likely to impact angina symptoms in women,[36] and recurrent depression predicts worsening coronary artery calcification.[34] These differences are important to appreciate, as they correspond also with differences in the presentation of CVD symptoms in women,[37] including a higher contribution of C-reactive protein (CRP) to risk (associated with increased stress and depression)[38,39] and a greater contribution of arteriole spasm to angina symptoms (also associated with increased stress and depression).[40] Notably, research suggests CRP increased in women relative to men, and continues to increase in women beginning at puberty.[37] Estrogen may mediate the effects of stress in women (and likely in men, though not well studied) as clinical research suggests estrogen replacement therapy blunts the usual increases in both cortisol and catecholamines following mental stress.[41] Other potential mechanisms include increased sensitivity of women to oxytocin—a hormone released during social interactions—which is theorized to ameliorate the neuroendocrine and cardiovascular effects of stress.[42]

Not surprisingly, the concerns of women vary with age, with women over age 60 tending to be concerned more with functional capacity, physical resiliency, and memory changes, whereas women below 60 years of age tend to be more concerned with emotional issues regarding work and family.[35] The differences between men and women summarized here underscore the importance of including a holistic history in the clinical encounter, including queries about emotional health, home, and work stress, especially in women with symptoms of potential CVD and/or in women with increased traditional CVD risk. Thus, interventions, including cognitive behavior therapies and other stress management interventions, should be tailored to meet the current needs of patients based on their age, gender, and current risk, rather than relying on generalized recommendations.

THERAPEUTIC INTERVENTIONS

Once a patient is identified with significant stressor, conventional Western medicine offers few non-pharmacologic options, which may not be effective in the context of CVD. Fortunately, there are various nonpharmacological mind–body therapies that are effective treatments for stress. Table 13.2 provides a summary of mind–body and other interventions that can be recommended to patients to build intrinsic or extrinsic resiliency. These therapies can be used in both inpatient and outpatient care settings, and many of these techniques can be taught to the patient for self-treatment. Once patients learn stress reduction techniques, these techniques become tools they can use to reduce allostatic load whenever necessary, and increasing the number of tools in one's toolbox builds resiliency.

TABLE 13.2

Interventions to Help Patients Reduce Allostatic Load and Build Resiliency

Personal Behaviors	Mind–Body Practices	Breathing and Movement Practices	Clinical Programs and Interventions
• Socialization	• Breathing exercises	• Yoga	• Stress management programs
• Pet ownership	• Guided imagery	• Tai chi	• Anger management programs
• Prayer	• Hypnosis	• Qi gong	• Cognitive behavioral therapy
• Volunteering	• Progressive muscle relaxation		• Comprehensive lifestyle change programs
• Spirituality	• Meditation		
• Gratitude	• Biofeedback HeartMath MBSR		

One goal shared by many mind–body and stress management practices in reaching the "relax-ation response," alters the ratio of sympathetic to parasympathetic tone, and thus increases HRV. Lower HRV is an independent risk factor for sudden cardiac death, all-cause death, and the cardiac event recurrence.[43–46]

THE THERAPEUTIC ENCOUNTER

The stress of life is real, and can have a significant deleterious effect on the cardiovascular risk of our patients, and the outcomes of our patients with known CVD. Our duty as physicians is to identify, evaluate, and offer treatment for risk factors in an effort to prevent disease and reestablish health. The honor of being an integrative medicine provider is having a range of therapeutic options to patients, which will help them build resilience and reduce their allostatic load. However, neither fancy devices nor disciplined meditation practices are likely to be effective unless we create the space for a therapeutic encounter during which they can openly discuss their stress history and the current impact of stress on their lives.

PERSONAL BEHAVIORAL PRACTICES

One of the many benefits of being integrative medicine providers is being able to empower our patients to take control of their health, by directing them to personal and behavioral practices that do not require formal programs or intensive interventions to be effective. Many suggestions for lifestyle modifications can be made to patients, letting their preferences and philosophies guide the final choices for intervention. Behavioral changes, such as getting out more into the community, reconnecting with friends, and volunteering, are relatively simple ways to encourage patients to build resiliency to stress.

SOCIALIZATION AND SOCIAL SUPPORT

Life is stressful—share the (allostatic) load! Supporting the concept that resiliency can be improved by building community, social support may influence prognosis in CVD. In participants of the CAST-1 trial, perceived social support was a significant independent predictor of mortality from arrhythmia.[47] Although, Frasure-Smith et al. found elevated Beck depression scores were correlated to cardiac mortality, and the association between depression and mortality decreased with increasing social support.[22] Notably, social support was related to greater-than-expected improvement in depression symptoms for those survivors who were depressed at baseline, and those with higher baseline depres-sion scores . Therefore, although post-MI depression is a predictor of 18-month mortality, social sup-port can decrease the magnitude of depression, providing some evidence for a potential mechanism of social support in the improvement cardiovascular outcomes. Craig et al. demonstrated a significant relationship between increased social support and reduced cardiovascular reactivity in MI survivors.[48]

VOLUNTEERISM

One of the greatest lessons of life is learning the many benefits of generosity, "In giving, we receive." Again, suggesting the importance of service, social connection, and reaching out beyond one's self, vol-unteerism has been linked to less depression and pain, less anxiety, and a greater sense of life purpose.[49]

PET OWNERSHIP

Pet ownership can not only provide medical benefits associated with stress reduction but also convey a sense of companionship and purpose. A wide variety of research methods demonstrated support for both physical and psychological health benefits of pet ownership, including less depression, lower cardiovascular risk, fewer physician visits, and reduced mortality.[50–52] Pet ownership appears to be effective in building resiliency, reducing the impact of stress and perhaps mimicking the effects of social support.[53] Pet ownership may be particularly helpful after MI, a vulnerable time during which owning a pet appears to reduce depression and increase HRV.[50,54]

SPIRITUALITY

We define spirituality as any path that leads to the recognition of the Divine. Meta-analyses support the role of spirituality and spiritual practices to increase coping, and build resiliency to stress,[55] and multiple studies have been conducted linking religious practices and spirituality with improved health and lower rates of heart disease.[56–59] Supporting the concept that self-care behaviors are improved by improving coping strategies for stress, people who are religious tend to have greater adherence to medication, exercise more, eat healthier diets, drink less alcohol, quit smoking more readily and use more preventive services.[59] Some observational data supports that these behaviors translate into improved health outcomes:

- Secular Jewish persons had significantly higher odds for the first MI compared to Orthodox Jewish patients (odds ratio: 4.2 for men and 7.3 for women) after adjustments for age, ethnicity, education, smoking, physical activity, and body mass index (BMI).[58]
- A 23-year prospective study of more than 10,000 Israeli civil servants and municipal employees found that Orthodox Jewish men had a 20% decreased risk of fatal coronary heart disease compared with nonreligious men, after adjusting for age, blood pressure, lipids, smoking, diabetes, BMI, and baseline coronary heart disease.[57]
- A prospective study of 232 people (age, 55 years) undergoing elective heart surgery found that lack of participation in social groups and lack of strength or comfort from religion were the most consistent predictors of death, after adjusting for age, previous cardiac surgery, and preoperative functional status.[56]

PRAYER

Investigating a sample of caregivers under a moderate burden of stress, Wilks et al.[60] demonstrated the use of prayer increased with the magnitude of stress, but prayer was also associated with improved resiliency compared to those participants who did not pray. Therefore, prayer seemed to moderate the effects of caregiver burden on resiliency.

GRATITUDE

Although many of us were taught to express thanks to friends, family, and the Divine, how many of us truly remember every day to be thankful for our breath, and for the opportunity to follow the dynamic path of life? Although the science of gratitude is relatively new, gratitude as an element of positive outlook has been linked to reduced depression,[61] improved cardiac outcomes,[62] and recommended as a strategy to build resiliency and improve well-being.[63]

MIND–BODY PRACTICES

Mind–body practices help create mental calm, affect allostasis, and offer multiple strategies for developing resiliency in our patients. Once learned, mind–body practices can be practiced nearly anywhere, from home to an elevator during a busy workday. Both assisted (e.g., biofeedback) and unassisted (e.g., guided imagery) exercises are accessible to patients depending on their interests and preferences.

BREATHING EXERCISES

Breathing exercises, including the breath exercises inherent in meditation and yoga, have been part of spiritual traditions for thousands of years. One of our favorite mantras to use with patients in the clinic is: "The mind controls the body. The breath controls the mind." Followed by a breathing exercise, this mantra immediately redirects the focus to the breath, and away from the physical symptoms, and expands their shallow breathing. Breathing exercises can result in a 6- to 9-mmHg reduction in BP.[64] Practice inhaling for a count of two, then exhaling for a count of two, gradually lengthen the breathing to counts of three, four, or more for a target breathing rate of six to seven breaths per minute. It is important to note that as soon as it feels like a struggle or competition, you are no longer in the parasympathetic zone.

Other types of self-guided relaxation, including progressive muscle relaxation, are effective at eliciting a relaxation response.[65] Progressive muscle relaxation encourages relaxation through awareness of the sensations present in the main muscle groups. For example, first take a few quieting breaths and then focus on your feet, either simply bringing awareness to any muscle tension there or intentionally contracting the muscles, then, exhaling, relaxing, and releasing the tension. Next, move your attention to the lower leg and repeat the tensing and relaxing. This technique aims to elicit the relaxation response through this repetitive mental focus and intentional adoption of a relaxed state.

GUIDED IMAGERY AND HYPNOSIS

Guided imagery uses the power of thought to influence psychological states and physiological functions. Guided imagery is a therapeutic technique that allows an individual to use his or her own imagination to achieve a desirable outcome such as decreased pain perception and reduced anxiety. Guided imagery has been studied as a pre-and postsurgical intervention in cardiothoracic surgery patients, and it showed reductions in both pain and anxiety.[66] Reaching a state of hypnosis, or a state of heightened mental focus and awareness, often involves guided imagery. Hypnosis has been limitedly evaluated in CVD, but available results suggest hypnosis can increase HRV by reducing sympathetic tone, reduce blood pressure, and improve anxiety.[67,68]

MEDITATION

Interest in formal meditation practices was ignited in the United States with the introduction of Transcendental Meditation (TM) by Maharishi Mahesh Yogi in 1967. Instruction is offered in simple breathing techniques. TM is practiced for 20 minutes twice daily, and offers a simple, unique technique for meditation and relaxation. It is one of the most studied integrative medicine therapies with research dating back to 1970s.

Both observational research and clinical trials suggest benefits of TM, leading to its recent "Level B" evidence ranking for the treatment of hypertension by the American Heart Association in a recent scientific statement.[69] Research by Schneider et al.[70] in adults over age 55 with hypertension demonstrated those who practiced TM had improved blood pressure and reduced cardiovascular morbidity and mortality over 5 years. More recently, Schneider et al.[71] extended their observational findings to clinical trials and demonstrated a 48% reduction in risk for primary composite cardiovascular endpoints in black men and women who practiced TM compared to controls. Additional clinical trials have showed improved blood pressure, insulin sensitivity, and HRV from TM practice, suggesting TM activates a relaxation response.[72] Providing evidence of a potential effect of meditation on atherosclerotic disease regression, 9 months of TM practice reduced carotid intimal medial thickness (IMT) in black Americans with hypertension, compared to increased carotid IMT in controls.[73]

MINDFULNESS-BASED STRESS REDUCTION

Mindfulness-based stress reduction (MBSR) is a structured group program that teaches meditation focused on moment-to-moment awareness. MBSR utilizes the techniques of mindfulness meditation, gentle yoga, and coordinated deep breathing to decrease pain and anxiety. A meta-analysis investigating MBSR for a wide spectrum of clinical populations demonstrated MBSR was effective at alleviating stress and suffering associated with various diseases.[74] Numerous studies have shown perceived improvement in quality of life, reduced symptoms of stress, and improved sleep quality from MBSR practices.[75–77]

More specific to CVD, Hughes et al.[78] conducted a randomized controlled trial of MBSR, compared to progressive muscle relaxation (another mind–body practice for stress reduction), for high blood pressure. After 8 weeks, MBSR resulted in significant reductions in systolic (−4.8 mmHg) and diastolic blood pressure (−1.9 mmHg), greater than reductions achieved from progressive muscle relaxation. Similar benefits on blood pressure were measured by Parswani et al.[79] when they evaluated MBSR in men with coronary heart disease. In their 3-month trial, people randomized to MBSR had significant reductions in anxiety, depression, perceived stress, blood pressure (−2.8 mmHg systolic/−1.9 mmHg diastolic), and BMI. Although not a formal trial, we recently published a compelling case report describing a patient's experience in which MBSR training reduced her blood pressure from "stage 2" (>160/100) to the normal after 11 weeks.[80] MBSR also has established benefits in obesity, including reductions in risk factors relevant to CVD risk. Dalen et al.[81] evaluated a mindfulness intervention in a group of obese men and found after 3 months that mindfulness practice improved weight loss, binge eating, depression, and perceived stress while lowering CRP.

BIOFEEDBACK

Biofeedback involves monitoring and displaying physiological information directly to the patient, including heart rate, muscle tension, and skin temperature, allowing for instruction on methods to improve HRV and other risk factors. During monitoring, patients are taught relaxation techniques such as deep breathing and muscle relaxation. Lehrer et al.[82,83] demonstrated that training subjects to maximize peak heart rate differences, i.e., increase HRV, using biofeedback could increase homeostatic reflexes, lower blood pressure, and improve lung function. In cardiovascular patients, biofeedback can be used effectively to reduce stress, increase HRV, improve exercise tolerance, and lower blood pressure, including both systolic and diastolic blood pressure.[84–89] A recent American Heart Association scientific review committee assigned "Level B" evidence to biofeedback techniques for reducing blood pressure.[69]

There are many tools and techniques that can be used to provide biofeedback to patients including thermometers, heart rate monitors, and computer-assisted devices to measure breathing, pulse, and muscle tension. One of the best studied is the Resp-e-Rate (InterCure, New York) device. The device was approved by FDA for the treatment of hypertension, and generally consists of breathing monitor linked to headphones. The device then senses the breathing pattern and provides audio guidance about how to change your breathing patterns to optimize a parasympathetic respiratory pattern (longer, slower breaths). In clinical trials, Resp-E-Rate users have reduced their blood pressure at an average of 14 mmHg systolic (the top number) and 8 mmHg diastolic (the bottom number).[90] Another similar device is Healing Rhythms (Wild Divine, San Diego, California). Even better, each of these devices is covered by some insurers.

HEARTMATH

Similar to biofeedback, but anchored more on the emotional plane, is HeartMath. HeartMath is a series of techniques that helps people focus on their emotional responses to stress. We all know what it feels like to "get our blood pumping" when we are angry; that is an example of an emotional response to stress causing high blood pressure. In fact, it is thought that the expression "seeing red" relates to blood vessels dilating in the eyes in response to really high blood pressure.

HeartMath has nothing to do with arithmetic; it uses a concept called *rhythm coherence* based on the premise that modern life stressors influence the coherence of heart rhythms, and that the coherence itself can be influenced by intentionally and sincerely focusing on positive feelings. In general, the techniques help you focus on remembering positive experiences (and how the mind–body feel in those situations) and then cultivating the ability to "interrupt" yourself when negative feelings begin. There are many specific exercises used to teach participants to develop this pattern. HeartMath focuses attention on the heart, uses heart-centered breathing (described as extending the exhalation longer than the inhalation) and other mind–body exercises such as "freeze-frame."[91] People who practice HeartMath principles generally experience blood pressure reductions of about 10 mmHg.

MIXED-BREATHING AND PHYSICAL PRACTICES

YOGA

Although the asanas of yoga have sprung up in most gyms and strip malls, there is still a long way to go before the other elements of traditional yoga take root. From its beginning, yoga was neither a physical nor a breathing practice, but a way of being. The eight limbs of yoga foster changes in mental attitude, social practices, diet, the practice of asanas (postures), breathing practices (pranayamas), and meditation to reach a higher realm of being, closer to the Divine. When practiced completely, behavioral qualities of nonviolence, satisfaction, restraint, and honesty, combine with disciplined physical and mental practices, to create clarity, interconnection, and resilience.

Specific to CVD, yoga deserves mention in the context of several specific clinical conditions. Hypertension is probably the most studied, and most intuitive, application of yoga practice. However, research on yoga for hypertension show mixed results,[92–95] leading to its evidence ranking of "Level C" by the American Heart Association in their recent scientific statement on nondrug approaches to hypertension.[69] Cardiac arrhythmia may be more sensitive to effects of yoga, and clinical trial results suggest reductions in ectopic beats in people with palpitations,[96] and improvements in paroxysmal atrial fibrillation.[97] In the YOGA My Heart trial, yoga practice reduced heart rate, number of fibrillation episodes, and blood pressure in patients with paroxysmal atrial fibrillation while reducing depression and anxiety and improving all domains of health-related quality of life.[97]

Yoga has also demonstrated benefits in established coronary artery disease, including stabilization and improvement in angina symptoms, increased myocardial perfusion, and regression of atheroma volume.[98,99] Notably, adherence to the yoga-based stress management program in the famous Lifestyle Heart Trial, which demonstrated reversal of coronary disease by intensive lifestyle modification, was strongly associated with the degree of reduction in plaque volume during the course of the trial.[100,101]

Supported mechanisms for the beneficial effects of yoga on vascular health include improvement in endothelial function,[102] perhaps secondary to reduced lipid peroxidation.[103]

TAI CHI

Tai chi is an element of traditional Chinese medicine (TCM) that implements coordination of different breathing patterns with a variety of flowing postures and body motions. Supporting benefit of tai chi in patients with CVD, several small randomized trials in people with stable NYHA stage II chronic heart failure and preserved ejection fraction have evaluated tai chi training vs. usual care for changes in functional capacity and mood.[104–106] Improvements measured in patients receiving tai chi included improved mood, quality of life, 6-minute walk distance, exercise self-efficacy, and serum B-type natriuretic peptide levels.

Qi Gong

Qi gong is an element of TCM that implements coordination of different breathing patterns with a variety of physical postures and body motions. It is a very safe low-impact form of physical exercise and meditation, and can be performed by almost anyone including patients with exercise-limiting diseases. Qi gong practice can be implemented at home on a daily basis. Although Qi gong is often taught for general health maintenance, it can be used as a therapeutic intervention. Qi gong has demonstrated benefits for rehabilitation in congestive heart failure and reducing hypertension while reducing generalized stress and anxiety.[107–110] Although some controversy remains over the benefits of Qi gong on hypertension, it appears to be at least as effective as the positive controls used in the trials. Reductions in blood pressure during Qi gong practice were correlated with reduced concentrations of catecholamines, suggesting Qi gong can effectively induce a relaxation response.[111] Research by Sun et al. in people with type 2 diabetes demonstrated that daily Qi gong practice reduced blood sugar and decreased perceived stress, whereas students also trended toward lower rates of depression and reduced body weight.[112–114]

CLINICAL SERVICES FOR STRESS REDUCTION AND INCREASED RESILIENCY

Cognitive Behavioral Therapy

Recent trials indicate a cognitive behavioral therapy (CBT) intervention, consisting of twenty 2-hour sessions focused on stress management, reduced risk for composite CVD events, and reduced recurrent MI events in older adults with an event history.[115]

Comprehensive Stress Reduction Programs

Studies by Blumenthal et al. and Düsseldorp et al. demonstrate the positive impact stress reduction can have on cardiovascular endpoints. Blumenthal[116] demonstrated stress management significantly reduces the risk of events in patients with CVD. One hundred and thirty-six patients with CVD were randomized to usual care, physical activity training, or stress management. Stress management training consisted of sixteen 1½-hour sessions during which patients were instructed in biofeedback and progressive muscle relaxation. Both endothelial function and HRV improved in the stress management intervention. Previous observational research by Blumenthal et al.[117] suggested a 50% reduction in cardiac events for patients with coronary artery disease who attended their hospital-based stress management program.[117] Stress management programs appear to prolong life in women with CVD. Orth-Gomer et al.[118] reported that women randomized to a stress management program after MI (including 20 sessions over a year that provided education about risk factors, training on relaxation techniques, methods for self-monitoring, and cognitive restructuring, with an emphasis on coping with stress exposure from family and work, plus self-care and compliance with clinical advice) had a 67% reduction in cardiovascular mortality over 7 years of follow-up. However, not all research has demonstrated benefit of protocolized stress reduction interventions on cardiovascular risk factors. The Trials of Hypertension Prevention (THOP-I) tested whether a standardized stress management intervention, including group and individual sessions during training on four relaxation methods, techniques to reduce stress reactions, cognitive approaches, communication skills, time management, and anger management, would lower systolic blood pressure. Only minor changes in blood pressure resulted, including a small, but significant −1.36 mmHg reduction in the intervention subgroup who were higher adherent.[119] Despite some conflicting results, Düsseldorp et al. summarize the support for psychoeducational program for CVD risk reduction and improved outcomes in their meta-analysis demonstrating improvements in blood pressure, weight, and lipids following health education and stress management programs, plus improved smoking, physical activity, and eating behaviors, all leading to a 29% reduction in MI recurrence and a 34% reduction in overall cardiovascular mortality.[120] Sure sounds like stress management programs should be an element of best practices in care for CVD.

COMPREHENSIVE MULTI-BEHAVIORAL LIFESTYLE CHANGE PROGRAMS

Despite the inherent complexity in multifactorial interventions, several significant studies support the benefits of adherence to comprehensive lifestyle-change programs. The Lifestyle Heart Trial[100] led by Ornish et al., was the first clinical trial to definitively demonstrate the feasibility of reversing coronary artery disease through intensive lifestyle change. The Lifestyle Heart Trial intervention included the strict low-fat diet, aerobic physical activity training, group support, and a yoga-based stress reduction program. Adherence to the stress management program was associated with reduced stenosis diameter at both 1- and 5-year follow-up evaluations.[101] Daubenmier et al. also demonstrated additive and interrelated effects of stress reduction, improved diet, and increased physical activity on reduced cardiovascular risk.[121]

However, not all comprehensive lifestyle programs have demonstrated reversal of coronary artery calcification (CAC).[122] The SAFE-LIFE trial measured no change in CAC after a 3-year intervention consisting of stress management techniques, including mindfulness meditation, guided imagery, yoga breathing techniques, and body scan, plus CBT and training in coping.[123] SAFE-LIFE participants were also encouraged toward a Mediterranean diet, and encouraged (but not trained) to increase their physical activity. Despite not demonstrating reductions in CAC, SAFE-LIFE participant did experience reductions in blood pressure, heart rate, and doses of anti-ischemic medications. Notably, the SAFE-LIFE intervention was much less intensive then the intervention in the Lifestyle Heart Trial, i.e., Mediterranean vs. very low-fat diet, physical activity recommendations versus specific training, and individual vs. group stress management practice, which may explain the differential results.[100,123]

Supporting the concept that multibehavioral lifestyle change may be effective at the cellular level, only "multisystem resiliency"—defined by Puterman et al. as healthy emotion regulation, strong social connections, and health behaviors (sleep and exercise)—and not improvement in individual domains of resiliency, moderated the strong association between depression and reduced telomere length.[124] The biological importance of building multidimensional resiliency is supported by other findings by Ornish et al., who demonstrated that increased telomere length results from comprehensive lifestyle change—and that increases in telomere length were associated with reductions in psychological stress (and also reductions in low-density lipoproteins [LDL]).[125] However, to bring this discussion full circle, because telomere regulation and metabolic regulation are closely linked through the mitochondria,[126] this concept could be extended as multisystem resilience leading to increased mitochondrial resiliency.

CONCLUSION

Stress is inherent to a dynamic life, filled with diverse experiences and emotions. Therefore, the therapeutic goal becomes helping patients identify significant stressors, and adapt effectively by reaching allostasis, or a dynamic balance with stress. Chronic maladaptation to psychosocial stress is an important independent risk factor for developing primary CVD, and for worsened outcomes for those with CVD. Although pharmacological therapies can reduce the symptoms of anxiety and depression associated with financial stress, workplace stress, and past trauma, drugs do not provide patients with long-lasting approaches to build either extrinsic or intrinsic resiliency to stress. Numerous therapeutic strategies are available to the integrative medicine provider to help patients build resiliency including recommendations for socialization, spirituality, prayer, pet ownership, as well as personal practices like yoga and meditation. Finally, formal stress management programs and comprehensive lifestyle change programs, when available, offer structured and effective alternatives to home-based personal practices, and may lead to significant stabilization or reversal of CVD, including coronary disease. However, before teaching our patients to bend like the willow, rather than break under the load, we must first listen and learn about the impact of stress on their life and relationships. Helping our patients open their hearts to the experiences, pleasures, and disappointments of life, while helping them protect themselves by developing the skills to maintain dynamic balance through life's stressors, is a lofty, but achievable goal, through the practice of integrative medicine.

ACKNOWLEDGMENTS

This chapter was made possible by an educational grant from the Miraglo Foundation and The Taylor Endowment Fund For Holistic Medicine Education and Research.

REFERENCES

1. Selye H. *The Stress of Life*. New York, NY: McGraw-Hill, 1956.
2. Goldstein DS, McEwen B. Allostasis, homeostats, and the nature of stress. *Stress* 2002;5:55–58.
3. Logan JG, Barksdale DJ. Allostasis and allostatic load: Expanding the discourse on stress and cardiovascular disease. *J Clin Nurs* 2008;17:201–208.
4. Wong DL, Tai TC, Wong-Faull DC, et al. Epinephrine: A short- and long-term regulator of stress and development of illness: A potential new role for epinephrine in stress. *Cell Mol Neurobiol* 2012;32:737–748.
5. Chrousos GP, Kino T. Glucocorticoid signaling in the cell. Expanding clinical implications to complex human behavioral and somatic disorders. *Ann N Y Acad Sci* 2009;1179:153–166.
6. Crettaz B, Marziniak M, Willeke P et al. Stress-induced allodynia—evidence of increased pain sensitivity in healthy humans and patients with chronic pain after experimentally induced psychosocial stress. *PLoS One* 2013;8:e69460.
7. Bhasin MK, Dusek JA, Chang BH et al. Relaxation response induces temporal transcriptome changes in energy metabolism, insulin secretion and inflammatory pathways. *PLoS One* 2013;8:e62817.
8. Dusek JA, Otu HH, Wohlhueter AL et al. Genomic counter-stress changes induced by the relaxation response. *PLoS One* 2008;3:e2576.
9. McEwen BS, Gianaros PJ. Central role of the brain in stress and adaptation: Links to socioeconomic status, health, and disease. *Ann N Y Acad Sci* 2010;1186:190–222.
10. Mastorci F, Vicentini M, Viltart O et al. Long-term effects of prenatal stress: Changes in adult cardiovascular regulation and sensitivity to stress. *Neurosci Biobehav Rev* 2009;33:191–203.
11. Seery MD. Challenge or threat? Cardiovascular indexes of resilience and vulnerability to potential stress in humans. *Neurosci Biobehav Rev* 2011;35:1603–1610.
12. Anand SS, Islam S, Rosengren A et al. Risk factors for myocardial infarction in women and men: Insights from the INTERHEART study. *Eur Heart J* 2008;29:932–940.
13. Rosengren A, Hawken S, Ounpuu S, et al. Association of psychosocial risk factors with risk of acute myocardial infarction in 11119 cases and 13648 controls from 52 countries (the INTERHEART study): Case-control study. *Lancet* 2004;364:953–962.
14. Elderon L, Whooley MA. Depression and cardiovascular disease. *Prog Cardiovasc Dis* 2013;55:511–523.
15. O'Neil A, Williams ED, Stevenson CE et al. Co-morbid cardiovascular disease and depression: Sequence of disease onset is linked to mental but not physical self-rated health. Results from a cross-sectional, population-based study. *Soc Psychiatry Psychiatr Epidemiol* 2012;47:1145–1151.
16. Huffman JC. Review: Depression after myocardial infarction is associated with increased risk of all-cause mortality and cardiovascular events. *Evid Based Ment Health* 2013;16:110.
17. Lichtman JH, Froelicher ES, Blumenthal JA, et al. Depression as a risk factor for poor prognosis among patients with acute coronary syndrome: Systematic review and recommendations: A scientific statement from the american heart association. *Circulation* 2014;129(12):1350–1369.
18. Thombs BD, de Jonge P, Coyne JC et al. Depression screening and patient outcomes in cardiovascular care: A systematic review. *JAMA* 2008;300:2161–2171.
19. Frasure-Smith N, Lesperance F. Reflections on depression as a cardiac risk factor. *Psychosom Med* 2005;67(suppl 1):S19–25.
20. Frasure-Smith N, Lesperance F. Depression and coronary artery disease. *Herz* 2006;31(suppl 3):64–68.

21. Frasure-Smith N, Lesperance F. Depression and anxiety as predictors of 2-year cardiac events in patients with stable coronary artery disease. *Arch Gen Psychiatry* 2008;65:62–71.
22. Frasure-Smith N, Lesperance F, Talajic M. Depression and 18-month prognosis after myocardial infarction. *Circulation* 1995;91:999–1005.
23. Lesperance F, Frasure-Smith N, Talajic M, Bourassa MG. Five-year risk of cardiac mortality in relation to initial severity and one-year changes in depression symptoms after myocardial infarction. *Circulation* 2002;105:1049–1053.
24. Davidson KW, Burg MM, Kronish IM et al. Association of anhedonia with recurrent major adverse cardiac events and mortality 1 year after acute coronary syndrome. *Arch Gen Psychiatry* 2010;67:480–488.
25. Lesperance F, Frasure-Smith N, Juneau M, Theroux P. Depression and 1-year prognosis in unstable angina. *Arch Intern Med* 2000;160:1354–1360.
26. Whitson HE, Thielke S, Diehr P et al. Patterns and predictors of recovery from exhaustion in older adults: The cardiovascular health study. *J Am Geriatr Soc* 2011;59:207–213.
27. Kivimaki M, Nyberg ST, Batty GD et al. Job strain as a risk factor for coronary heart disease: A collaborative meta-analysis of individual participant data. *Lancet* 2012;380:1491–1497.
28. Yan LL, Liu K, Matthews KA et al. Psychosocial factors and risk of hypertension: The Coronary Artery Risk Development in Young Adults (CARDIA) study. *JAMA* 2003;290:2138–2148.
29. Brackett CD, Powell LH. Psychosocial and physiological predictors of sudden cardiac death after healing of acute myocardial infarction. *Am J Cardiol* 1988;61:979–983.
30. Ziegelstein RC, Fauerbach JA, Stevens SS et al. Patients with depression are less likely to follow recommendations to reduce cardiac risk during recovery from a myocardial infarction. *Arch Intern Med* 2000;160:1818–1823.
31. Saint Onge JM, Krueger PM, Rogers RG. The relationship between major depression and nonsuicide mortality for U.S. adults: The importance of health behaviors. *J Gerontol B Psychol Sci Soc Sci* 2014;69(4):622–632.
32. Lang UE, Borgwardt S. Molecular mechanisms of depression: Perspectives on new treatment strategies. *Cell Physiol Biochem* 2013;31:761–777.
33. Hamer M, Endrighi R, Venuraju SM, Lahiri A, Steptoe A. Cortisol responses to mental stress and the progression of coronary artery calcification in healthy men and women. *PLoS One* 2012;7:e31356.
34. Matthews KA, Chang YF, Sutton-Tyrrell K, Edmundowicz D, Bromberger JT. Recurrent major depression predicts progression of coronary calcification in healthy women: Study of Women's Health Across the Nation. *Psychosom Med* 2010;72:742–747.
35. Murray JC, O'Farrell P, Huston P. The experiences of women with heart disease: What are their needs? *Can J Public Health* 2000;91:98–102.
36. Billing E, Hjemdahl P, Rehnqvist N. Psychosocial variables in female vs male patients with stable angina pectoris and matched healthy controls. *Eur Heart J* 1997;18:911–918.
37. Shaw LJ, Bairey Merz CN, Pepine CJ et al. Insights from the NHLBI-Sponsored Women's Ischemia Syndrome Evaluation (WISE) Study: Part I: Gender differences in traditional and novel risk factors, symptom evaluation, and gender-optimized diagnostic strategies. *J Am Coll Cardiol* 2006;47:S4–S20.
38. Lopresti AL, Maker GL, Hood SD, Drummond PD. A review of peripheral biomarkers in major depression: The potential of inflammatory and oxidative stress biomarkers. *Prog Neuropsychopharmacol Biol Psychiatry* 2014;48:102–111.
39. Valkanova V, Ebmeier KP, Allan CL. CRP, IL-6 and depression: A systematic review and meta-analysis of longitudinal studies. *J Affect Disord* 2013;150:736–744.
40. Plourde A, Lavoie KL, Ouellet K et al. Hemodynamic, hemostatic, and endothelial reactions to acute psychological stress in depressed patients following coronary angiography. *Psychophysiology* 2013;50:790–798.
41. Komesaroff PA, Esler MD, Sudhir K. Estrogen supplementation attenuates glucocorticoid and catecholamine responses to mental stress in perimenopausal women. *J Clin Endocrinol Metab* 1999;84:606–610.
42. Kubzansky LD, Mendes WB, Appleton A, Block J, Adler GK. Protocol for an experimental investigation of the roles of oxytocin and social support in neuroendocrine, cardiovascular, and subjective responses to stress across age and gender. *BMC Public Health* 2009;9:481.
43. Bigger JT, Fleiss JL, Rolnitzky LM, Steinman RC. The ability of several short-term measures of RR variability to predict mortality after myocardial infarction. *Circulation* 1993;88:927–934.
44. Bigger JT Jr., Fleiss JL, Steinman RC et al. Frequency domain measures of heart period variability and mortality after myocardial infarction. *Circulation* 1992;85:164–171.

45. Bigger JT Jr., Fleiss JL, Steinman RC et al. RR variability in healthy, middle-aged persons compared with patients with chronic coronary heart disease or recent acute myocardial infarction. *Circulation* 1995;91:1936–1943.

46. Kleiger RE, Miller JP, Bigger JT Jr., Moss AJ. Decreased heart rate variability and its association with increased mortality after acute myocardial infarction. *Am J Cardiol* 1987;59:256–262.

47. Gorkin L, Schron EB, Brooks MM et al. Psychosocial predictors of mortality in the Cardiac Arrhythmia Suppression Trial-1 (CAST-1). *Am J Cardiol* 1993;71:263–267.

48. Craig FW, Lynch JJ, Quartner JL. The perception of available social support is related to reduced cardiovascular reactivity in Phase II cardiac rehabilitation patients. *Integr Physiol Behav Sci* 2000;35:272–283.

49. Depner CE, Ingersoll-Dayton B. Supportive relationships in later life. *Psychol Aging* 1988;3:348–357.

50. Friedmann E, Thomas SA, Son H. Pets, depression and long term survival in community living patients following myocardial infarction. *Anthrozoos* 2011;24:273–285.

51. Anderson WP, Reid CM, Jennings GL. Pet ownership and risk factors for cardiovascular disease. *Med J Aust* 1992;157:298–301.

52. Headey B. Pet ownership: Good for health? *Med J Aust* 2003;179:460–461.

53. Friedmann E, Thomas SA. Pet ownership, social support, and one-year survival after acute myocardial infarction in the Cardiac Arrhythmia Suppression Trial (CAST). *Am J Cardiol* 1995;76:1213–1217.

54. Friedmann E, Thomas SA, Stein PK, Kleiger RE. Relation between pet ownership and heart rate variability in patients with healed myocardial infarcts. *Am J Cardiol* 2003;91:718–721.

55. Boudreaux ED, O'Hea E, Chasuk R. Spiritual role in healing. An alternative way of thinking. *Prim Care* 2002;29:439–454, viii.

56. Oxman TE, Freeman DH Jr., Manheimer ED. Lack of social participation or religious strength and comfort as risk factors for death after cardiac surgery in the elderly. *Psychosom Med* 1995;57:5–15.

57. Goldbourt U, Yaari S, Medalie JH. Factors predictive of long-term coronary heart disease mortality among 10,059 male Israeli civil servants and municipal employees. A 23-year mortality follow-up in the Israeli Ischemic Heart Disease Study. *Cardiology* 1993;82:100–121.

58. Friedlander Y, Kark JD, Stein Y. Religious orthodoxy and myocardial infarction in Jerusalem—a case control study. *Int J Cardiol* 1986;10:33–41.

59. Mueller PS, Plevak DJ, Rummans TA. Religious involvement, spirituality, and medicine: Implications for clinical practice. *Mayo Clin Proc* 2001;76:1225–1235.

60. Wilks SE, Vonk ME. Private prayer among Alzheimer's caregivers: Mediating burden and resiliency. *J Gerontol Soc Work* 2008;50:113–131.

61. Lambert NM, Fincham FD, Stillman TF. Gratitude and depressive symptoms: The role of positive reframing and positive emotion. *Cogn Emot* 2012;26:615–633.

62. Dubois CM, Beach SR, Kashdan TB et al. Positive psychological attributes and cardiac outcomes: Associations, mechanisms, and interventions. *Psychosomatics* 2012;53:303–318.

63. Szloboda P. Gratitude practices: A key to resiliency, well-being & happiness. *Beginnings* 2008;28:6,7.

64. Mori H, Yamamoto H, Kuwashima M, et al. How does deep breathing affect office blood pressure and pulse rate? *Hypertens Res* 2005;28:499–504.

65. Mandle CL, Jacobs SC, Arcari PM, Domar AD. The efficacy of relaxation response interventions with adult patients: A review of the literature. *J Cardiovasc Nurs* 1996;10:4–26.

66. Kshettry VR, Carole LF, Henly SJ, Sendelbach S, Kummer B. Complementary alternative medical therapies for heart surgery patients: Feasibility, safety, and impact. *Ann Thorac Surg* 2006;81:201–205.

67. Gay MC. Effectiveness of hypnosis in reducing mild essential hypertension: A one-year follow-up. *Int J Clin Exp Hypn* 2007;55:67–83.

68. Hippel CV, Hole G, Kaschka WP. Autonomic profile under hypnosis as assessed by heart rate variability and spectral analysis. *Pharmacopsychiatry* 2001;34:111–113.

69. Brook RD, Appel LJ, Rubenfire M et al. Beyond medications and diet: Alternative approaches to lowering blood pressure: A scientific statement from the american heart association. *Hypertension* 2013;61:1360–1383.

70. Schneider RH, Alexander CN, Staggers F et al. Long-term effects of stress reduction on mortality in persons > or = 55 years of age with systemic hypertension. *Am J Cardiol* 2005;95:1060–1064.

71. Schneider RH, Grim CE, Rainforth MV et al. Stress reduction in the secondary prevention of cardiovascular disease: Randomized, controlled trial of Transcendental Meditation and health education in Blacks. *Circ Cardiovasc Qual Outcomes* 2012;5:750–758.

72. Paul-Labrador M, Polk D, Dwyer JH et al. Effects of a randomized controlled trial of Transcendental Meditation on components of the metabolic syndrome in subjects with coronary heart disease. *Arch Intern Med* 2006;166:1218–1224.

73. Castillo-Richmond A, Schneider RH, Alexander CN et al. Effects of stress reduction on carotid athero-sclerosis in hypertensive African Americans. *Stroke* 2000;31:568–573.

74. Grossman P, Niemann L, Schmidt S, Walach H. Mindfulness-based stress reduction and health benefits. A meta-analysis. *J Psychosom Res* 2004;57:35–43.

75. Carlson LE, Speca M, Patel KD, Goodey E. Mindfulness-based stress reduction in relation to quality of life, mood, symptoms of stress and levels of cortisol, dehydroepiandrosterone sulfate (DHEAS) and melatonin in breast and prostate cancer outpatients. *Psychoneuroendocrinology* 2004;29:448–474.

76. Tacon AM, McComb J, Caldera Y, Randolph P. Mindfulness meditation, anxiety reduction, and heart disease: A pilot study. *Fam Community Health* 2003;26:25–33.

77. Robert McComb JJ, Tacon A, Randolph P, Caldera Y. A pilot study to examine the effects of a mindfulness-based stress-reduction and relaxation program on levels of stress hormones, physical functioning, and submaximal exercise responses. *J Altern Complement Med* 2004;10:819–827.

78. Hughes JW, Fresco DM, Myerscough R et al. Randomized controlled trial of mindfulness-based stress reduction for prehypertension. *Psychosom Med* 2013;75:721–728.

79. Parswani MJ, Sharma MP, Iyengar S. Mindfulness-based stress reduction program in coronary heart disease: A randomized control trial. *Int J Yoga* 2013;6:111–117.

80. Oberg EB RM, Bradley R. Self-directed mindfulness training and improvement in blood pressure, migraine frequency, and quality of life. *Glob Adv Health Med* 2013;2:20–25.

81. Dalen J, Smith BW, Shelley BM et al. Pilot study: Mindful Eating and Living (MEAL): Weight, eating behavior, and psychological outcomes associated with a mindfulness-based intervention for people with obesity. *Complement Ther Med* 2010;18:260–264.

82. Lehrer P, Vaschillo E, Lu SE, et al. Heart rate variability biofeedback: Effects of age on heart rate variability, baroreflex gain, and asthma. *Chest* 2006;129:278–284.

83. Lehrer PM, Vaschillo E, Vaschillo B. Resonant frequency biofeedback training to increase cardiac variability: Rationale and manual for training. *Appl Psychophysiol Biofeedback* 2000;25:177–191.

84. Nakao M, Nomura S, Shimosawa T, Fujita T, Kuboki T. Blood pressure biofeedback treatment of white-coat hypertension. *J Psychosom Res* 2000;48:161–169.

85. Nakao M, Nomura S, Shimosawa T et al. Clinical effects of blood pressure biofeedback treatment on hypertension by auto-shaping. *Psychosom Med* 1997;59:331–338.

86. Nakao M, Yano E, Nomura S, Kuboki T. Blood pressure-lowering effects of biofeedback treatment in hypertension: A meta-analysis of randomized controlled trials. *Hypertens Res* 2003;26:37–46.

87. Kranitz L, Lehrer P. Biofeedback applications in the treatment of cardiovascular diseases. *Cardiol Rev* 2004;12:177–181.

88. Del Pozo JM, Gevirtz RN, Scher B, Guarneri E. Biofeedback treatment increases heart rate variability in patients with known coronary artery disease. *Am Heart J* 2004;147:E11.

89. Swanson KS, Gevirtz RN, Brown M et al. The effect of biofeedback on function in patients with heart failure. *Appl Psychophysiol Biofeedback* 2009;34:71–91.

90. Schein MH, Gavish B, Herz M et al. Treating hypertension with a device that slows and regularises breathing: A randomised, double-blind controlled study. *J Hum Hypertens* 2001;15:271–278.

91. McCraty R, Atkinson M, Tomasino D. Impact of a workplace stress reduction program on blood pressure and emotional health in hypertensive employees. *J Altern Complement Med* 2003;9:355–369.

92. Adhana R, Gupta R, Dvivedii J, Ahmad S. The influence of the 2:1 yogic breathing technique on essential hypertension. *Indian J Physiol Pharmacol* 2013;57:38–44.

93. Jayasinghe SR. Yoga in cardiac health (a review). *Eur J Cardiovasc Prev Rehabil* 2004;11:369–375.

94. Miles SC, Chun-Chung C, Hsin-Fu L et al. Arterial blood pressure and cardiovascular responses to yoga practice. *Altern Ther Health Med* 2013;19:38–45.

95. Bhavanani AB, Madanmohan, Sanjay Z, Basavaraddi IV. Immediate cardiovascular effects of pranava pranayama in hypertensive patients. *Indian J Physiol Pharmacol* 2012;56:273–278.

96. Ravindra PN, Madanmohan, Pavithran P. Effect of pranayam (yoga breathing) and shavasan (relaxation training) on the frequency of benign ventricular ectopics in two patients with palpitations. *Int J Cardiol* 2006;108:124–125.

97. Lakkireddy D, Atkins D, Pillarisetti J et al. Effect of yoga on arrhythmia burden, anxiety, depression, and quality of life in paroxysmal atrial fibrillation: The YOGA My Heart Study. *J Am Coll Cardiol* 2013;61:1177–1182.

98. Manchanda SC, Narang R, Reddy KS et al. Retardation of coronary atherosclerosis with yoga lifestyle intervention. *J Assoc Physicians India* 2000;48:687–694.

99. Yogendra J, Yogendra HJ, Ambardekar S et al. Beneficial effects of yoga lifestyle on reversibility of ischaemic heart disease: Caring heart project of International Board of Yoga. *J Assoc Physicians India* 2004;52:283–289.

100. Ornish D, Scherwitz LW, Billings JH et al. Intensive lifestyle changes for reversal of coronary heart disease. *JAMA* 1998;280:2001–2007.

101. Pischke CR, Scherwitz L, Weidner G, Ornish D. Long-term effects of lifestyle changes on well-being and cardiac variables among coronary heart disease patients. *Health Psychol* 2008;27:584–592.

102. Sivasankaran S, Pollard-Quintner S, Sachdeva R et al. The effect of a six-week program of yoga and meditation on brachial artery reactivity: Do psychosocial interventions affect vascular tone? *Clin Cardiol* 2006;29:393–398.

103. Yadav RK, Ray RB, Vempati R, Bijlani RL. Effect of a comprehensive yoga-based lifestyle modification program on lipid peroxidation. *Indian J Physiol Pharmacol* 2005;49:358–362.

104. Yeh GY, Wood MJ, Wayne PM et al. Tai chi in patients with heart failure with preserved ejection fraction. *Congest Heart Fail* 2013;19:77–84.

105. Yeh GY, McCarthy EP, Wayne PM et al. Tai chi exercise in patients with chronic heart failure: A randomized clinical trial. *Arch Intern Med* 2011;171:750–757.

106. Yeh GY, Wood MJ, Lorell BH et al. Effects of tai chi mind-body movement therapy on functional status and exercise capacity in patients with chronic heart failure: A randomized controlled trial. *Am J Med* 2004;117:541–548.

107. Chan CL, Wang CW, Ho RT et al. A systematic review of the effectiveness of qigong exercise in cardiac rehabilitation. *Am J Chin Med* 2012;40:255–267.

108. Guo X, Zhou B, Nishimura T, Teramukai S, Fukushima M. Clinical effect of qigong practice on essential hypertension: A meta-analysis of randomized controlled trials. *J Altern Complement Med* 2008;14:27–37.

109. Lee MS, Lim HJ, Lee MS. Impact of qigong exercise on self-efficacy and other cognitive perceptual variables in patients with essential hypertension. *J Altern Complement Med* 2004;10:675–680.

110. Lee MS, Pittler MH, Guo R, Ernst E. Qigong for hypertension: A systematic review of randomized clinical trials. *J Hypertens* 2007;25:1525–1532.

111. Lee MS, Lee MS, Kim HJ, Moon SR. Qigong reduced blood pressure and catecholamine levels of patients with essential hypertension. *Int J Neurosci* 2003;113:1691–1701.

112. Sun GC, Lovejoy JC, Gillham S et al. Effects of Qigong on glucose control in type 2 diabetes: A randomized controlled pilot study. *Diabetes Care* 2010;33:e8.

113. Putiri AL, Lovejoy JC, Gillham S et al. Psychological effects of Yi Ren Medical Qigong and progressive resistance training in adults with type 2 diabetes mellitus: A randomized controlled pilot study. *Altern Ther Health Med* 2012;18:30–34.

114. Sun GC DX, Andrew Zhou XH, Putiri A, Bradley R. Effects of Yi Ren Medical Qigong on body weight in people with type 2 diabetes mellitus: A secondary analysis of a randomized controlled pilot study. *J Integrative Med Ther* 2014;1:5.

115. Gulliksson M, Burell G, Vessby B et al. Randomized controlled trial of cognitive behavioral therapy vs standard treatment to prevent recurrent cardiovascular events in patients with coronary heart disease: Secondary prevention in Uppsala primary health care project (SUPRIM). *Arch Intern Med* 2011;171:134–140.

116. Blumenthal JA, Sherwood A, Babyak MA et al. Effects of exercise and stress management training on markers of cardiovascular risk in patients with ischemic heart disease: A randomized controlled trial. *JAMA* 2005;293:1626–1634.

117. Blumenthal JA, Babyak M, Wei J et al. Usefulness of psychosocial treatment of mental stress-induced myocardial ischemia in men. *Am J Cardiol* 2002;89:164–168.

118. Orth-Gomer K, Schneiderman N, Wang HX et al. Stress reduction prolongs life in women with coronary disease: The Stockholm Women's Intervention Trial for Coronary Heart Disease (SWITCHD). *Circ Cardiovasc Qual Outcomes* 2009;2:25–32.

119. Batey DM, Kaufmann PG, Raczynski JM et al. Stress management intervention for primary prevention of hypertension: Detailed results from Phase I of Trials of Hypertension Prevention (TOHP-I). *Ann Epidemiol* 2000;10:45–58.

120. Dusseldorp E, van Elderen T, Maes S, Meulman J, Kraaij V. A meta-analysis of psychoeduational programs for coronary heart disease patients. *Health Psychol* 1999;18:506–519.

121. Daubenmier JJ, Weidner G, Sumner MD et al. The contribution of changes in diet, exercise, and stress management to changes in coronary risk in women and men in the multisite cardiac lifestyle intervention program. *Ann Behav Med* 2007;33:57–68.

122. Lehmann N, Paul A, Moebus S et al. Effects of lifestyle modification on coronary artery calcium progression and prognostic factors in coronary patients—3-year results of the randomized SAFE-LIFE trial. *Atherosclerosis* 2011;219:630–636.

123. Michalsen A, Grossman P, Lehmann N et al. Psychological and quality-of-life outcomes from a comprehensive stress reduction and lifestyle program in patients with coronary artery disease: Results of a randomized trial. *Psychother Psychosom* 2005;74:344–352.

124. Puterman E, Epel ES, Lin J et al. Multisystem resiliency moderates the major depression-telomere length association: Findings from the Heart and Soul Study. *Brain Behav Immun* 2013;33:65–73.

125. Ornish D, Lin J, Daubenmier J et al. Increased telomerase activity and comprehensive lifestyle changes: A pilot study. *Lancet Oncol* 2008;9:1048–1057.

126. Chen LY, Zhang Y, Zhang Q et al. Mitochondrial localization of telomeric protein TIN2 links telomere regulation to metabolic control. *Mol Cell* 2012;47:839–850.

14 Women and Heart Disease
Special Considerations

Stephen T. Sinatra

CONTENTS

For decades, cardiovascular disease (CVD) has been the leading cause of death and disability for both men and women in the United States. In 2010 alone, it claimed almost 600,000 lives, the majority of which were people over the age of 64 years.[1] Cancer comes a close second, followed at a distance by chronic lower respiratory diseases, strokes, and accidents. One of the main reasons why CVD is such a deadly enemy may be lack of recognition of its more subtle signs and symptoms until it is too late. The good news is that you can help prevent or reverse CVD before it's too late.

"MODUS OPERANDI" OF CARDIOVASCULAR DISEASE

CVD is usually characterized by coronary artery disease, a condition of blood vessel damage due to a combination of silent inflammation, endothelial deterioration, and plaque buildup. When the integrity of blood vessels becomes compromised, a silent but deadly process unfolds over time. As arteries may start to calcify, continually pumping blood through the body becomes a more strenuous activity for the heart and blood pressure may rise. Chronic high blood pressure, or hypertension, is major risk factor for CVD. Additionally, as the immune system constantly repairs damage in blood vessels, blood vessel walls get more inflamed. As inflammation increases, so does the likelihood that plaques in arterial walls will become unstable and rupture. When unstable plaques break open, blood clots can enter the bloodstream, get lodged in blood vessels, and block blood flow. Three potentially devastating events can happen at this point due to lack of oxygen: a person may have an acute myocardial infarction (MI), may die from arrhythmia (chaotic and/or irregular pulsations of the heartbeat due to the sudden loss of oxygen from ischemia), or may have a central nervous system event.

Although heart disease is the number one cause of death among both women and men,[2,3] CVD is still often overlooked as a significant women's health issue. This may be due to a misunderstanding by the medical community about how heart disease manifests in women. CVD,[2,3] and not breast cancer, is the leading cause of death for women. For nearly three decades, in fact, more women than men have died each year from cardiovascular causes and nearly two-thirds of them who died suddenly had no previous symptoms. It is thus very important to identify at-risk women early so that effective prevention strategies can be started.

Over the year, in articles and lectures, and in working with my own patients, I have tried to educate women to be alert to the uniqueness of their gender when it comes to cardiovascular issues. Women have generally been lumped together and treated similarly as men. As I wrote in my 2000 book *Heart Sense for Women*[4] (Lifeline Press), men and women are definitely different when it comes to heart health factors and treatment.

Until recently, medical school training rarely prepared physicians to recognize symptoms of CVD that are specific to women. Instead, because for so many years the traditional prototype for diagnosing and treating heart disease had been the middle-aged man, physicians were taught to diagnose and treat what manifests as CVD in men. The diagnosis of heart disease in the female is a much more difficult process compared to men.

Although women generally are better in touch with their emotional pain and stress than men are, they tend to experience more subtle or vague physical symptoms of heart disease and cardiac events than men. Whereas men may experience a crushing pain in their chests (angina) when having a heart attack, women's symptoms may include the following:

- Discomfort, pressure, or pain in the chest and/or back
- Tingling or pain in the jaw, elbow, or arm (both men and women tend to feel pain in the left elbow or arm when having ischemia)
- Shortness of breath and/or light-headedness with exertion
- Sudden, profound fatigue
- Tightness in the throat
- Dizziness and/or vertigo
- Indigestion (women often feel that if they could "just burp," they would feel better)
- Nausea and/or vomiting
- Disproportionate sweating with activity

Sometimes, women's symptoms are mild enough for them to think they just have the flu and doctors may misdiagnose women's symptoms as other, less serious conditions such as hypoglycemia, indigestion, muscle strain, or simply just anxiety or stress. Myocardial ischemia may be manifested as both typical and atypical symptoms in women. In my experience, the diagnosis of angina in women is more complex and a poorly understood process.

Angina—chest pain often described as a "heart cramp"—is a symptom of ischemia, restricted blood flow that results in an insufficient supply of oxygen to heart and other vital tissues. Most often, ischemia is due to plaque buildup in coronary arteries (CVD), which causes a partial blockage; but it can also be caused by a blood clot, which completely blocks blood flow and may result in a heart attack. Without enough oxygen, the heart quickly becomes depleted of the energy it needs to continue circulating blood throughout the rest of the body; it begins to cramp, and the person feels numbness and/or pain.

As angina can be a sure sign of a heart issue, it's crucial for both women and health professionals alike to recognize women's symptoms. With men, angina is typically felt as a sharp, crushing pain in the middle of the chest or on either side. Women, on the other hand, tend to experience *dull* or *aching* pain, or even just a sense of heaviness, tightness, soreness, or pressure in the chest. Also, with men, angina pain usually comes on after exercise or exertion and generally improves with rest; women may experience it without any obvious cause or remedy, and rest may not help.

Women's angina symptoms might even be mistaken for heartburn (women commonly feel a need to just burp to feel better), and women may not know they have angina and are therefore at risk for a heart attack, until the condition is dire. Gastrointestinal distress is often one of the most commonly disregarded signs of CVD. Women also tend to feel pain or pressure radiating into their jaws or necks; they could easily seek help at the dentist's office instead of going to the hospital with such symptoms. I remember one woman who had a cardiac arrest in the emergency room as she was waiting to see an oral surgeon for jaw pain.

For men and women alike, shortness of breath and sudden fatigue are often early warning signs that the heart isn't getting enough oxygenated blood. However, whereas the onset of these symptoms is usually sudden in men, women tend to experience chronic breathlessness or may awaken in the middle of the night with difficulty catching their breath. Women's fatigue may be unexplained or generalized.

One possible explanation for these differences is that women may be more in tune with changes in their bodies that indicate heart disease. Unfortunately for men, a heart attack is all too often the initial symptom that is recognized. The other side of the coin is that women may also be more prone to dismiss their pain and discomfort, having learned to bear the physical effects of menstruation, pregnancy, and childbirth; they may not seek medical attention until the situation becomes dire.

Also, some women may incorrectly associate and write off menopausal discomforts, such as sweating, irregular heartbeat, insomnia, and irritability, as aging, when in fact they may be subtle symptoms of cardiac disease.

A woman's risk of having a cardiac event significantly increases after she goes through menopause. This is because of her gradual loss of heart-protective estrogen. As a woman ages, she tends to experience a greater increase in lipid levels, high blood pressure, weight gain, and hormonal imbalance.

Younger women, although less commonly, have heart attacks too. They are oftentimes "vitally exhausted," from working, caring for or raising children and/or other family members, or possibly enduring rough emotional situations like divorce or death of loved ones. Feeling burned out, overloaded, and stressed is an indication of potential cardiac problems, even for people who appear healthy on the surface. Excessive stress not only depletes the immune system and leads to the inflammation that causes CVD but also causes blood to thicken and blood pressure to rise. Although estrogen protects younger women, it will not, on its own, prevent heart attacks. Stress management is one key to preventing heart attacks in all ages of women, as well as men.

Statistically, men tend to experience cardiac events about a decade earlier than women. But, in general, they have a better chance at recovery. Also, men usually report symptoms that appear as "mechanical difficulties" or changes in physical function in their bodies, rather than as problems of the heart, or of their emotional lives. With women, cardiac complications may not present recognizable symptoms and may be mistaken for general malaise. Many coronary-related events in women are actually "silent" heart attacks, where symptoms remain unrecognized and treatment is delayed or neglected. Such a silent heart attack may be recognized only when an electrocardiogram (EKG) is routinely done sometime afterward.

Another factor that is more prevalent in women compared to men in my experience is the use of denial as a maladaptive coping mechanism.

According to the dictionary,[5] denial, psychologically speaking, means "a condition in which someone will not admit that something sad, painful, etc., is true or real." Denial in cardiology refers to a fairly common habit among patients to not admit that they have a heart problem. Such denial can be deadly. Too often, I have seen patients who even with severe chest or arm pain minimize their symptoms by calling them something else, anything other than heart pain. And all too often, I treated them afterward for serious heart attacks.

Individuals who deny they have a medical emergency are jeopardizing not only their health but also their very life. Over the years, many patients, even those experiencing severe chest and arm pain, would try to minimize their situation, saying that they had something other than a heart condition. Often, I would treat these deniers for serious heart attacks.

I remember one man many years ago who was a woodcutter. He had severe left arm pain for 4 days that practically brought him to tears. He was convinced it was bursitis. At one point, he went into heart failure and passed out. In the emergency room, he developed ventricular fibrillation and we shocked him back and he survived. Afterward, he was totally stunned by the realization that he'd had a heart attack.

You might think that such kind of denial is a "macho" or manly thing. But it's not. Both genders fall into the denial trap. I vividly recall the case of a woman in her fifties who developed chest pain while hosting a dinner party. The pain had risen up to her jaw. She postponed going to the emergency room until hours later at 1:00 a.m., after her final guest had departed. She had a massive heart attack and almost died in the emergency room. Later, she told me that she didn't think she could possibly have a heart problem. Women, research indicates, often delay seeking help because they think heart disease is an almost always male problem and they prefer to self-medicate. The fact is that more women than men die of heart attacks.

Whether you are a man or a woman, denial is absolutely a real cardiovascular risk factor. I have treated dozens of patients in total denial, not only of their symptoms of heart disease but also of heart damage itself.

In cardiology today, such denial is regarded seriously because when deniers delay or refuse to seek medical care they lose out on the benefits (including lower mortality rates) achieved by recent advances in treatment. The American Heart Association has waged public education campaigns for years emphasizing that about half of all heart attack deaths occur within 1 hour after symptoms appear and usually outside the hospital. Outcomes are clearly optimized when care is obtained during that first hour after symptom onset. Many deniers receive care significantly later.

In a 2010 study[6] involving over 100,000 people with a relatively mild form of heart attack in which a blood clot doesn't totally occlude a particular coronary artery, researchers found that the average patient came to the hospital about 2½ hours after first feeling the symptoms. It was note that 11% of the patients waited 12 or more hours before putting in a 9-1-1 call or getting to the hospital. Seniors, women, nonwhites, smokers, and diabetics tended to delay the most.

In a Swedish study of first-time heart attacks, involving 78 men and 29 women, researchers monitored whether the patients sought help within or beyond 4 hours and also whether they attended a follow-up rehabilitation program. The results are as follows: a total of 49 patients procrastinated, and 76 failed to participate in rehabilitation. The researchers interviewed all patients and found that "high deniers" were both delayers and nonattenders.[7]

Years ago, people were reluctant to come into the emergency room even with chest pain. Thanks to the advent of thrombolytic and stent therapy, there has been a huge advance in treatment and survival. The earlier you get in, the faster you get blood flow revived and the better the survival. Such early stenting in acute heart attack is the most important factor in surviving, and limiting infarct size. Although chest pain is the most common symptom of pre-infarction angina for both men and women, women were still more likely to present without chest pain than men in a cohort study of 1015 patients of which 30% were women.[8]

I try to closely follow cardiovascular research. My antenna is always alert to new revelations that can help women better understand their uniqueness and take appropriate and timely action. With that in mind, I want to share new details regarding four underreported areas of cardiovascular concern for women: hypertension, lower extremity peripheral artery disease (PAD), diastolic dysfunction (DD), and mitral valve prolapse (MVP).

Before my book, *Heart Sense for Women*,[4] I tended to treat men and women with hypertension in the same way. As I wrote the book, it became clear that there were real gender-specific issues that I needed to recognize as a clinician. More recently, a comprehensive review article in the journal *Hypertension Research*[9] made this point unequivocally clear.

Here are some conclusions from that article:

- Aside from smoking cessation, hypertension control is the single most important intervention to reduce the risk of future cardiovascular events in women.
- Total life expectancy is almost 5 years less for women of 50 years with high blood pressure compared to those without it. Early high blood pressure is considered if your level is

over 130 (systolic) or 84 (diastolic). More recent teaching suggests optimal blood pressure readings of 120/80 and lower.

- Among the elderly, high blood pressure actually affects more women than men and, in general, is underdiagnosed and undertreated.

The article, written by two Emory University researchers, covers various hormonal and menopause factors. For instance, there is a slight but significant increase in blood pressure among women taking the widely prescribed, but risky, pharmaceutical hormone replacement therapy of equine estrogen (Premarin) and medroxyprogesterone (Provera) to relieve menopausal symptoms.[9,10]

I vividly recall a patient in her late fifties who had developed a leaking mitral valve related to a sudden increase in blood pressure. She had no history of hypertension. Her doctor prescribed different medications to which she didn't respond. She then consulted a surgeon who wanted to operate on her valve. Looking for another opinion, she came to see me. I asked if she was on hormones. When she said "yes," I figured she was hypersensitive because of medroxyprogesterone, which is known to cause coronary artery constriction. The resulting blood pressure increase was likely affecting her mitral valve, resulting in significant mitral regurgitation. I took her off the hormonal drugs, and she normalized. It was a dramatic eye-opener for me. If a woman desires hormonal therapy, she should only consider natural, bioidentical estrogen and progesterone under the supervision of a knowledgeable doctor. In Chapter 13, Dr. Pam Smith discusses this subject in great detail.

In younger women, hypertension may be as much as three times more common among individuals taking oral contraceptives. For such a hypertensive person, stopping "the pill" may reduce systolic pressure by 15 points within 6 months.[9] When a woman does become pregnant, hypertension occurs in about 6%–8% of cases[11] and can increase the risk of maternal and fetal mortality. Many women with high blood pressure deliver healthy babies (high blood pressure during pregnancy is called eclampsia). But pregnancy—and the increased blood volume required to nurture a growing fetus—can potentially raise blood pressure to extremely high levels. For this reason, expectant mothers also should have blood pressure readings taken routinely. Hypertension can develop rapidly in the last 3 months of pregnancy. When this happens, a woman may need treatment, even after delivery.

Stress and hypertension have been traditionally associated with men, but that's clearly an obsolete concept. Just ask any working mom, as an example. In my book,[4] I reported on a 40-year-old attorney who had a heart attack after divorcing her husband and moving out of state with her two young children to be close to her parents, one of who had Alzheimer's disease. Clearly, that's a classic formula for stress, high blood pressure, and heart problems. With good medical care, the woman survived her MI and later came to see me about dealing with lifestyle and stress issues.

Summing up the situation, the authors of the journal article said that prevention of cardiovascular events by blood pressure control is "30–100 percent higher in women than in men" and that a 15-point increase in systolic blood pressure raises the risk of CVD by 56% in women compared with 32% in men.[10] Those two statistics make it quite clear that a woman needs to pay attention to her blood pressure and do something about it if it is higher; further, if a woman does have any blood pressure issues, she must be cautious about the routine use of over-the-counter analgesics.

A 2005 study looked at nonnarcotic analgesics and the risk of incident hypertension in U.S. women.[12] The study found that women aged 51–77 years who took an average daily dose of more than 500 mg of acetaminophen or one Extra Strength Tylenol had about double the risk of developing high blood pressure in 3 years. Women in the same age range who took more than 400 mg of nonsteroidal anti-inflammatory drugs (NSAIDs), equal to about two ibuprofen, had a 78% risk of developing high blood pressure over those who did not take any nonsteroidals. Younger women, aged 34–53 years, who took an average of 500 mg of acetaminophen a day had a twofold higher risk of developing high blood pressure. Similar aged women who took 400 mg of NSAIDs had a 60% risk increase over those who did not take the meds. The study also demonstrated that aspirin did not increase these risks. The study involved 5123 women participating in the Nurse's Health Study at Harvard Medical School and Brigham and Women's Hospital in Boston.[12] Although none of the women had high blood pressure when the study began, higher doses of acetaminophen and NSAIDs independently increased the risk of hypertension in these women. Although NSAIDs increase renal sodium absorption, both acetaminophen and NSAIDs may impair endothelial function, which may explain why blood pressure increases. Because the results of this study have confirmed previous investigations, it makes sense to educate women about the overzealous use of these analgesics.

If you take painkillers regularly, be sure to inform your doctor and find out about safer medications. I recommend Traumeel, a homeopathic remedy available in health food stores or online at www.traumeel.com. You can buy it as a topical cream or sublingual tablet, and it works great for various muscle aches and pains, without potentially devastating effects on blood pressure as optimal blood pressure control is essential for women in helping to prevent DD.

Women with high blood pressure are much more prone to DD, a condition involving progressive stiffening of the heart muscle that weakens the left ventricle's pumping ability. It can lead to the most common and serious form of heart failure that affects women. Shortness of breath in a hypertensive woman frequently suggests that she has DD and because standard medicine has no effective treatment over time DD may progress to diastolic heart failure.

DIASTOLIC HEART FAILURE

Diastolic heart failure is the accumulation of fluid in the body resulting from compliance issues of the left ventricle or a "stiffening of the heart muscle." When the myocardium does not relax fully, the cavity inside the heart remains compromised and is unable to fill properly. In essence, during diastole the filling cycle struggles. Therefore, patients may feel shortness of breath and may complain of chest pain, fatigue, and even leg swelling. Their symptoms and physical findings are similar with patients with systolic heart failure caused by a weakened heart[13] (often referred to as heart failure with impaired systolic function), and their prognosis in most cases is poor.[13,14] The morbidity and mortality caused by diastolic heart failure, again, often referred to as heart failure with well-preserved systolic function, is very similar to systolic heart failure. The estimated health-care cost is $30 billion dollars in the United States for 2010.[15] Thus, diastolic heart failure and systolic dysfunction places a great burden on the health-care system in the United States.

The identification of effective treatments for diastolic heart failure remains an important area of concern given the predominance of women with diastolic heart failure,[16] lack of specific therapies,[17,18] and high mortality and morbidity associated with this affliction.[13,14] The scope of this heart failure epidemic was projected for those over 40 years to be 20%, a level well in excess of many conditions associated with aging.[19]

The treatment for diastolic heart failure remains severely limited as pharmaceutical drugs have been shown to be of little benefit based on randomized clinical studies.[20] The Women's Health Coalition Report[20] also lamented on the lack of effective treatments for DD and indicated that the prognosis has not changed over the last 15 years. Clearly, an alternative to standard pharmaceutical intervention is needed.

We must, therefore, look to cardiac energetics and metabolic support with a focus on adenosine triphosphate (ATP) and energy substrates in mitochondria.[21] Because biopsies of heart tissue in heart failure patients reveal diminished quantities of ATP in the mitochondria,[22] investigating therapies that promote the basis of cellular metabolism must be utilized. Myocytes contain the highest concentrations of mitochondria cellular constituents necessary to generate the huge amounts of ATP required to fuel the high-energy demand of cardiac energetics.[21,23]

The energetic imbalance of heart failure is characterized by an increase in energy demand and a decrease in energy production, transfer, and substrate utilization resulting in an ATP deficit. DD is the result of the heart muscle's inability to relax sufficiently after contraction because it cannot maintain the higher concentrations of ATP required to effectively activate the calcium pumps necessary to facilitate cardiac relaxation and diastolic filling.[21,23,24] All patients with heart failure have DD to some degree. Similar energetic adaptations occur in the atrium, which may contribute to atrial fibrillation.[25]

Because the requirements of myocytes for ATP is absolute,[23] incorporating a metabolic approach with nutritional biochemical interventions that preserve and promote mitochondrial support and ATP production must be considered. For example, in a randomized controlled trial 300 mg of coenzyme Q10 reduced plasma pyruvate/lactate ratios and improved endothelial function via reversal of mitochondrial dysfunction in patients with ischemic left ventricular systolic dysfunction.[26] Such a metabolic cardiology approach does not create adverse effects and may be supportive in patients with DD. Patients prone to DD such as the aging population as described in a recent *Journal of the American Medical Association* study[27] may also need metabolic support.

An effective solution for failing ATP production involves nutraceutical support with coenzyme Q10, L-carnitine, magnesium, and D-ribose.[21,24] Supplied on a daily basis, they provide essential raw materials that support cellular energy substrates needed by mitochondria to rebuild feeble ATP levels. Such treatment options that incorporate metabolic interventions targeted to preserve ATP energy substrates (D-ribose) or accelerate ATP turnover (L-carnitine and coenzyme Q10) are indicated for at-risk populations and patients undergoing cardiovascular surgery. This metabolic cardiology approach does not create adverse effects and may be supportive in preventing atrial fibrillation often seen in patients with DD after undergoing cardiac surgery[28] as well as in patients with hypertension and MVP where DD is also frequently seen.

MITRAL VALVE PROLAPSE

MVP is a relatively benign condition of the mitral valve (which lies between the left atrium and the left ventricle and is shaped like a bishop's hat or miter). Sometimes, the mitral valve leaflets become thickened, voluminous, or stretched, which may cause a slight to severe leakage of the valve. Many times on physical examination, a mid to late systolic click may be heard followed by a murmur or leak. While most patients don't even know they have MVP, a few are particularly bothered by somatic symptoms (from chest discomforts to irregular heartbeats and even shortness of breath). In the rare cases, surgery may be considered if spontaneous rupture of the chordae tendinae occurs resulting in a severe left ventricular overload state with mitral regurgitation and left ventricular failure.

During my cardiovascular fellowship, I studied under Dr. Robert Jeresaty, the author of the book *Mitral Valve Prolapse*.[29] As his senior cardiovascular fellow, I participated in gathering data for him on over 300 patients in our MVP clinic. I did dozens of phonocardiograms in which a graphic display of mid and late systolic clicks followed by frequent late systolic murmurs was recorded. Recording the data and examining many patients, I realized that MVP, fortunately, was terribly symptomatic for only a very few patients. However, one especially bothersome symptom was shortness of breath, which was difficult to evaluate. Although arrhythmias and chest pain and documentation of clicks and murmurs were relatively straightforward, the shortness of breath was perplexing. Therefore, we decided to study 20 patients with MVP with pulmonary function studies.

All these patients were nonsmokers, and chest radiographs were obtained to document structural thoracic wall deformities, which were present in several of the patients. The lack of any significant correlation between shortness of breath and either pulmonary function abnormalities or chest wall deformity suggested that the symptoms of dyspnea may be nonpulmonary in origin.[30] Although decreased left ventricular compliance seen in the prolapse of the mitral valve was one possible mechanism,[31] none of the authors (myself included) were privy to the nature of DD, which has been a relatively new correlation in the last two decades. We published the paper in July of 1979.[30] Looking back, these patients most likely had DD, but we were not aware of this pathologic abnormality as it took about another 20 years to diagnose DD via echocardiographic analysis using tissue Doppler to assess mitral valve velocities.[32]

Unfortunately, the therapeutic treatment in these patients, and particularly in those with severe shortness of breath, was limited with β-blockers, which was the only treatment we had to offer. β-Blockers were particularly effective in the treatment of arrhythmia and atypical chest pain; however, it was fruitless in most of the cases with shortness of breath. After I understood the phenomenon of DD many years later, I realized why these patients experienced shortness of breath. Metabolic cardiology has been the most effective treatment in patients with MVP and especially in those with shortness of breath and fatigue. The conventional literature attests to the efficacy of magnesium.

Magnesium has shown efficacy in relieving symptoms of MVP. In a double-blind study of 181 participants,[33] 80 serum magnesium levels were assessed in 141 patients with symptomatic MVP and compared to those of 40 healthy control subjects. While decreased serum magnesium levels were found in more than half (60% to be exact) of the patients with MVP, only 5% of the control subjects showed similar decreases. The second phase of the study investigated response to treatment.

Participants with magnesium deficits were randomly assigned to receive magnesium supplement or placebo, and results for the magnesium group were dramatic. The mean (average) number of symptoms per patient was significantly reduced with magnesium supplementation; significant reductions were noted in weakness, chest pain, shortness of breath, palpitations, and even anxiety. Decreases in the amount of adrenalin-like substances in the urine were noted as well. The researchers made two conclusions.

First, many patients with MVP with severe symptoms do have low serum magnesium levels. Second, supplementation with the crucial mineral leads to an improvement in symptoms and a decrease in adrenalin-like hormones.[33] For these individuals, magnesium supplementation may be the solution for reducing symptomatology while improving quality of life at the same time.

In my experience, the combination of 400 mg of magnesium in a combined form of citrate, glycinate, turinate, and orotate and 100–200 mg of coenzyme Q10 has been extremely promising. I've seen that it alleviates 80%–90% of symptoms, including chest pain, shortness of breath, easy fatigability, and palpitations. The enhanced quality of life most likely was due to some improvement in DD, which is frequently seen on echocardiographic analysis in women with MVP. On occasion, a full metabolic prescription was required with the addition of 5 g of D-ribose and 1 g of L-carnitine twice a day in symptomatic patients with MVP with moderate to severe mitral regurgitation. This similar metabolic approach is also extremely therapeutic in PAD. PAD is another significant clinical problem for women.

PERIPHERAL ARTERY DISEASE

Peripheral artery disease (PAD) is the third leading cause of arteriosclerotic cardiovascular morbidity followed by coronary artery disease and stroke. In a broad-based review of the literature involving 34 studies worldwide,[34] PAD has become a global problem involving over 200 million people, with smoking, diabetes, and hypertension being the prevalent risk factors.[34]

Arterial disease (atherosclerosis) is never limited to the coronary arteries. If you have it in one place, you likely have it elsewhere. PAD refers to atherosclerotic disease in the arteries of your lower legs.

PAD has received scant public recognition and it has always been considered a man's disease. In my practice, I saw many more men than women with PAD symptoms, most typically cramping and pain in the calves when walking (called intermittent claudication). Women don't seem to develop those symptoms as often unless they are smokers. They usually complain more of fatigue and functional decline in the legs. But the following revelations from a recent American Heart Association "call to action" article published in the journal *Circulation*[35] clearly illustrates how prevalent and serious a problem of PAD appears to be for women.

PAD increases with age for both men and women, yet evidence suggests that over 40 years of age more women than men are affected.

PAD is so common that it has equal morbidity and mortality and perhaps even higher medical costs than coronary artery disease and ischemic stroke. The gender associations between PAD and cardiovascular events and mortality are not well defined; however, population-based studies suggest a higher trend among women.

The summary statements by the authors indicate the following[35]:

- Most women with PAD, like men, do not have classic symptoms of intermittent claudication.
- Women with PAD have greater functional impairment and a more rapid functional decline than women without PAD.
- Women (and particularly black females) are more likely than men to experience graft failure or limb loss.
- There is a need to identify women with or at risk for PAD, especially black women, to lower cardiovascular ischemic event rates, loss of independent functional capacity, and ischemic amputation rates.
- Women in the United States attend as many or more PAD physician visits as men, which confirms the very large burden of PAD in women.
- Women predominantly see doctors and other clinicians for PAD in the outpatient office setting.

The risks associated with PAD are not fully recognized by clinicians and governmental agencies and certainly not the public. The evaluation of PAD is tedious and complex, involving a meticulous evaluation of peripheral pulses, targeted blood pressure measurements involving brachial and tibial arteries, duplex ultrasound, as well as advanced imaging studies in some patients. Although many successful treatments frequently involve pharmaceutical and surgical procedures including arterial stents, many patients without major obstructions to blood vessels continue to be symptomatic despite conventional methodologies. Frequently, small vessel disease is present and a metabolic approach is warranted.

My metabolic cardiology recommendations for women include the following targeted nutritional supplement program for PAD support:

- A high-quality multimineral/vitamin formula.
- A total of 100–300 mg of coenzyme Q10 and 200–600 mg of magnesium, both of which help to lower blood pressure and support endothelial function.
- A total of 1–3 g of broad-spectrum L-carnitine or 2 g of glycine propionyl L-carnitine (GPLC), a proprietary form of L-carnitine. L-carnitine helps clear out metabolic wastes that aggravate vasoconstriction in small blood vessels generated by cellular energy production. Cellular efficiency and aerobic capacity are supported when toxic by-products or the β oxidation of fats are shuttled out of the mitochondria. GPLC does the same and also helps to improve blood flow by boosting nitric oxide, a biochemical that keeps blood vessels relaxed.
- A total of 5 g D-ribose, three times daily.
- A total of 1 to 2 g ω-3 fatty acid (fish or squid oil).

Another simple and therapeutic intervention for diffuse distal vessel disease is earthing. Earthing, where you reconnect with the Earth's healing energy by being barefoot outdoors or sleeping, working, or relaxing indoors on earthing sheets or mats, in my opinion, is yet another simple and therapeutic intervention for diffuse distal vessel disease. Earthing generates healing benefits such as improved blood viscosity and ζ potential,[36] reduced inflammation, decreased pain, lower blood pressure, a calming effect on the nervous system with a downregulation of heightened sympathetic tone with improved heart rate variability,[37] better sleep, and more energy—all positives for supporting vascular pathology.

To summarize, the recognition and treatment of PAD is a widespread problem that is frequently undiagnosed and mismanaged. Remember that arteriosclerotic CVD is a diffuse process and when plaquing shows up in one area of the body it is most likely present in other areas as well. So, the diagnosis of PAD could literally tip off the physician that other areas of the body such as the carotid and coronary arteries are most likely involved as well. Although PAD was not considered to be a major pathology in women, it clearly has become a major problem afflicting women and especially African-American women.

SUMMARY AND CONCLUSIONS

Women are vastly different than men. In the coronary circulation for example, their arteries are smaller and more difficult to navigate with stents and even bypass grafting and this is probably why they have an increased mortality following acute MI, stent, and coronary artery bypass surgery interventions. They are also exposed to a number of life circumstances that influence classical cardiovascular risk factors. For example, in younger women oral contraceptives may elevate blood pressure slightly. However, in women with a family history of hypertension oral contraceptives may be a most aggregating factor in raising the numbers. Pregnancy is also another consideration in which increased blood volume required to nurture a growing fetus can potentially raise blood pressure to high levels. Menopause with age-related hormonal declines can cause a woman's arteries to become less elastic and more constrictive, thus contributing to inflammation as well as higher blood pressure. Coronary artery disease goes up significantly when a woman approaches menopausal years.

Metabolic syndrome is another area where women need to be aggressively treated as women with type 2 diabetes or insulin resistance with higher triglyceride levels have more risk as opposed to men. DD, which is more prevalent in women with hypertension and occurring in MVP, frequently found in more women than men, is another area of marked concern given the fact that conventional medicine has very few options to offer.

Even painkillers in women can have a detrimental effect on their health. Acetaminophen, ibuprofen, and aspirin are three of the most frequently used drugs by both women and men. Prospective cohort studies among older women and even younger women demonstrate that higher doses of acetaminophen and NSAIDs independently increase the risk of hypertension in women. The high prevalence rate of hypertension in the United States may be related to the overzealous use of acetaminophen and NSAIDs.

In the final analysis, a gender-specific approach, although increasing in popularity, has not always been to the advantage of women. As previously mentioned, there are several considerations and concerns that are germane to women. Again, aside from smoking cessation, hypertension management is the single most important intervention to reduce the risk of future cardiovascular events. However, the diagnosis and management of hypertension and its relationship to DD warrants the need for a gender-specific focus as more aggressive diagnosis and treatment methodologies are required more for women. Another area of concern is the routine use of statin drugs in women, which was discussed in Chapter 3. Remember, women have more side effects as opposed to their male counterparts and the therapeutic efficacy in women is much weaker as opposed to men.

CVD is the major leading cause of death in women today. Conducting appropriate gender-specific differences research and analysis of CVD trials has been difficult due to insufficient recruitment of women. Although this has contributed to a lack of understanding of gender differences in CVD, improved participation rates of women in new cardiovascular trials would yield more information concerning appropriate prevention, detection, accurate diagnosis, as well as proper treatment of all women with heart disease. In the near future, gender-specific medicine will probably be able to stand on its own and physicians will have a better understanding in the diagnosis and treatment of women with CVD.

REFERENCES

1. Hoyert DL, Xu JX. Deaths: Preliminary data for 2011. *National Vital Statistics Reports* 2011;61(6):1–52.
2. Mosca L, Mochari-Greenberger H, Dolor RJ et al. Twelve-year follow-up of American women's awareness of cardiovascular disease risk and barriers to heart health. *Circulation: Cardiovascular Quality Outcomes* 2010;3:120–7.
3. Kochanek KD, Xu JQ, Murphy SL et al. Deaths: Final data for 2009. *National vital statistics reports* 2011;60(3).
4. Sinatra ST. *Heart Sense for Women*. Washington, DC: LifeLine Press; 2000.
5. Second Edition. *Encarta Webster's Dictionary of the English Language*. New York: Bloomsbury Publishing; 1999.
6. Ting HH, Chen AY, Roe MT et al. Delay from symptom onset to hospital presentation for patients with non-ST-segment elevation myocardial infarction. *Arch Intern Med* 2010;170(20):1834–1841. http://www.ncbi.nlm.nih.gov/pubmed/21059977.
7. Stenstrom U, Nilsson AK, Stridh C et al. Denial in patients with a first-time myocardial infarction: Relations to pre-hospital delay and attendance to a cardiac rehabilitation programme. *Eur J Cardiovasc Prev Rehabil* 2005;12(6):568–571. http://www.ncbi.nlm.nih.gov/pubmed/16319547.
8. Khan NA, Daskalopoulou SS, Karp I et al; GENESIS PRAXY Team. Sex differences in acute coronary syndrome symptom presentation in young patients. *JAMA Intern Med* 2013;173(20):1863–1871.
9. Engberding N, Wenger NK. Management of Hypertension in Women. *Hypertension Research* 2012;35;251–260. http://www.nature.com/hr/journal/v35/n3/full/hr2011210a.html.
10. Wassertheil-Smoller S, Anderson G, Psaty BM et al. Hypertension and its treatment in postmeno-pausal women: Baseline data from the Women's Health Initiative. *Hypertension* 2000;36:780–789.
11. "Medical researchers have found that birth control pills increase blood pressure in some women" and "According to the National Heart, Lung, and Blood Institute (NHLBI), high blood pressure affects 6–8 percent of all pregnancies in the United States." – The American Heart Association (AHA). High Blood Pressure and Women. *Heartorg* accessed June 24, 2014. http://www.heart.org/HEARTORG/Conditions/HighBloodPressure/UnderstandYourRiskforHighBloodPressure/High-Blood-Pressure-and-Women_UCM_301867_Article.jspc.
12. Forman JP, Stampfer MJ, Curhan GC. Non-narcotic analgesic dose and risk of incident hypertension in US women. *Hypertension* 2005;46(3):500–507.
13. Bhatia RS, Tu JV, Lee DS et al. Outcome of heart failure with preserved ejection fraction in a population-based study. *N Engl J Med* 2006;355:260–269.
14. Owan TE, Hodge DO, Herges RM et al. Trends in prevalence and outcome of heart failure with preserved ejection fraction. *N Engl J Med* 2006;355:251–259.
15. Roger VL, Go AS, Lloyd-Jones DM et al. Heart disease and stroke statistics-2011 update: A report from the American heart association. *Circulation* 2011 Feb 1;123(4):e18–e209.
16. Yancy CW, Lopatin M, Stevenson LW, De Marco T, Fonarow GC. Clinical presentation, management, and in-hospital outcomes of patients admitted with acute decompensated heart failure with preserved systolic function: A report from the acute decompensated heart failure national registry (adhere) database. *J Am Coll Cardiol* 2006;47:76–84.
17. Hunt SA, Abraham WT, Chin MH et al. 2009 focused update incorporated into the acc/aha 2005 guidelines for the diagnosis and management of heart failure in adults a report of the american college of cardiology foundation/American heart association task force on practice guidelines developed in collaboration with the international society for heart and lung transplantation. *J Am Coll Cardiol* 2009;53:el–e90.
18. Paulus WJ, van Ballegoij JJ. Treatment of heart failure with normal ejection fraction: An inconvenient truth! *J Am Coll Cardiol* 2010;55:526–537.
19. Redfield MM, Jacobsen SJ, Burnett JC Jr, Mahoney DW Bailey KR, Rodeheffer RJ. Burden of systolic and diastolic ventricular dysfunction in the community: Appreciating the scope of the heart failure epidemic. *JAMA* 2003;289(2):194–202.
20. Wenger NK, Hayes SN, Pepine CJ et al. Cardiovascular care for women: The 10-Q report and beyond. *Am J Cardiol* 2013 Aug 15;112(4):S2.
21. Sinatra ST. Metabolic cardiology: An integrative strategy in the treatment of congestive heart failure. *Altern Ther Health Med* 2009;15(3):44–52.
22. Bashore TM, Magorien DJ, Letterio J, Shaffer P, Unverferth DV. Histologic and biochemical correlates of left ventricular chamber dynamics in man. *J Am Coll Cardiol* 1987;9(4):734–42.

23. Ingwall JS, Weiss RG. Is the failing heart energy starved? On using chemical energy to support cardiac function. *Circ Res* 2004;95(2):135–145.
24. Sinatra ST. Metabolic cardiology: The missing link in cardiovascular disease. *Altern Ther Health Med* 2009;15(2):48–50.
25. Cha YM, Dzeja PP, Shen WK et al. Failing atrium myocardium: Energetic deficits accompany structural remodeling and electrical instability. *Am J Physiol* Heart *Circ Physiol* 2003;284(4): H1313–H1320.
26. Dai Y, Luk T, Yiu K et al. Reversal of mitochondrial dysfunction by coenzyme Q10 supplement improves endothelial function in patients with ischemic left ventricular systolic dysfunction: A randomized controlled trial. *Atherosclerosis* 2011;216:395–401.
27. Kane GC, Karon BL, Mahoney DW et al. Progression of left ventricular diastolic dysfunction and risk of heart failure. *JAMA* 2011;306(8):856–863.
28. Melduni RM, Suri RM, Seward JB et al. Diastolic dysfunction in patients undergoing cardiac surgery: A pathological mechanism underlying the initiation of new-onset post-operative atrial fibrillation. *J Am Coll Cardiol* 2011;58:953–961.
29. Jeresaty R. *Mitral Valve Prolapse.* New York, NY: Raven Press, 1979.
30. ZuWallack R, Sinatra S, Lahiri B et al. Pulmonary function studies in patients with prolapse of the mitral valve. *Chest* 1979;76(1):17–20.
31. Jeresaty RM. Mitral valve prolapse-click syndrome. *Prog Cardiovasc Dis* 1973;15:623–652.
32. Halley CM, Houghtaling PL, Khalil MK et al. Mortality rate in patients with diastolic dysfunction and normal systolic function. *Arch Intern Med* 2011;171(2):1082–1087.
33. Kitlinski M, Stepniewski M, Nessler J et al. Is magnesium deficit in lymphocytes a part of the mitral valve prolapse syndrome? *Magnes Res* 2004;17(1):39–45.
34. Fowkes FG, Rudan D, Rudan I et al. Comparison of global estimates of prevalence and risk factors for peripheral artery disease in 2000 and 2010: A systematic review and analysis. *Lancet* 2013;382(9901):1329–1340.
35. Hirsch AT, Allison MA, Gomes MS et al. A call to action: Women and peripheral artery disease: A scientific statement from the American Heart Association. *Circulation* 2012;125(11):1449–1472.
36. Chevalier G, Sinatra ST, Oschman JL, Delany RM. Earthing (grounding) the human body reduces blood viscosity: A major factor in cardiovascular disease. *J Altern Complement Med* 2013;19(2):102–10.
37. Chevalier G, Sinatra ST. Emotional stress, heart rate variability, grounding, and improved autonomic tone: Clinical applications. *Integr Med: A Clin J* 2011;10(3):16–21.

15 Hormones and Their Effects on the Cardiovascular System

Pamela Smith

CONTENTS

HORMONES AND THEIR EFFECT ON THE CARDIOVASCULAR SYSTEM IN WOMEN

Hormones in women have a major impact on the cardiovascular system. Much has been discussed in the medical literature concerning insulin and its effects on the cardiovascular system. There are other hormones, however, that also play a major role in women's heart health such as estrogen, progesterone, testosterone, dehydroepiandrosterone (DHEA), cortisol, thyroid hormone, melatonin, and pregnenolone. These hormones all interact with each other in the body. They are like a symphony. Consequently, if one hormone is playing out of tune all of the hormones will be affected.

Before menopause, women have a lower risk of developing cardiovascular disease than men of the same age.[1–3] After menopause, women start having an increased risk of developing heart disease.

ESTROGEN

Estrogen has 400 functions in a woman's body. Consequently, when estrogen levels start to decline women can develop many symptoms. The following are signs and symptoms of estrogen deficiency:[71]

- Acne/oily skin
- Anxiety
- Arthritis
- Brittle hair and nails
- Fatigue/low energy especially at the end of the day
- Cognitive decline
- Decreased breast size
- Decrease in dexterity
- Decrease in sexual interest and function
- Depression
- Stress incontinence
- Insulin resistance
- Difficulty losing weight even with diet and exercise
- Dry eyes
- Hypertension
- Hypercholesterolemia
- Hypertriglyceridemia
- Food cravings
- Increase in facial hair
- Increase in tension headaches/migraines
- Infertility
- Joint pain
- Increased risk of developing heart disease and strokes
- More wrinkles/aging skin
- Osteoporosis/osteopenia
- Panic attacks
- High testosterone levels
- Insomnia/restless sleep
- Thinning skin
- Thinning hair
- Urinary tract infections
- Vaginal dryness
- Vulvodynia
- Weight gain

Epidemiological studies have shown that estrogen replacement therapy may reduce the risk of heart disease by 50% in postmenopausal women.[4-6] Furthermore, studies have shown a 40%–50% reduction in cardiovascular morbidity and mortality with hormone replacement therapy.[7] Menopause, whether it is natural or surgical, is commonly associated with a change in lipid profile that is not desirous:

- Elevation of low-density lipoprotein (LDL).
- Higher total cholesterol.
- Triglyceride levels rise.
- Lower high-density lipoprotein (HDL).
- LDL to HDL ratio may move to a nonfavorable value even if the total cholesterol level does not change.

Estrogen replacement helps to normalize the lipid profile[8,9]:

- Decreases total cholesterol
- Lowers LDL
- Raises HDL
- Increases large very-low-density lipoprotein (VLDL) particles
- Lowers remnant VLDL levels

Furthermore, another study showed that triglycerides improved in women who used transdermal (applied to the skin) estrogen.[12] Estrogen replacement therapy also positively affects other cardiovascular risk factors. Research has shown that patients who have an elevated lipoprotein(a) have a 70% higher rate of developing heart disease over 10 years.[10,187,196,197] Lipoprotein(a) levels are decreased by estrogen replacement therapy by up to 15%.[11]

There are many mechanisms by which medical studies have shown that estrogen replacement therapy is cardioprotective, besides estrogen's positive effects on lipid studies. There are even estrogen and progesterone receptor sites on the atrial and ventricular fiber level of the heart.[25]

- Estrogen may improve arterial function independent of lipid effects.[13]
- Estrogen stimulates endothelial nitric oxide synthase (eNOS) in vascular endothelial cells.[14]
- Estrogen enhances endothelial dependent vasodilation mediated by nitric oxide.[15]
- Estrogen has effects on posttranscriptional and translation modulation of proteins and enzymes.[16–19]
- Estrogen has positive effects on the mitochondria.[20–22]
- Estrogen suppresses reactive oxygen species through other mechanisms than the mitochondria.[23,24]
- The most prominent effects of estrogen on vascular reactivity are through its ability to influence endothelial function.[26]
- Estrogen promotes vasodilation through an eNOS-dependent mechanism.
- Estrogen increases flow-mediated vasodilation.[27]
- Estrogen affects production of other endothelial factors.[28]
- Estrogen increases the release of endothelium-derived relaxing factors in postmenopausal women.[29]
- Estrogen stimulates muscarinic and β-adrenergic cardiac receptors.[30]
- Estradiol decreases arterial impedance in the carotid and uterine arteries in postmenopausal women.[31]
- Estrogen increases left ventricular systolic flow measurements, which increase stroke volume, and helps to preserve myocardial contractility.[32]
- Estrogen is a calcium channel blocker.
- Estrogen affects the regulation of intracellular calcium.
- Estrogen may limit the progression of fibro-fatty lesions.[33]
- Estrogen limits neointimal formation following arterial injury.[34,35]
- Estrogen may limit the progression of atherosclerotic plaque formation.[36,37]
- Estrogen helps with the rapid repair of vascular wounds.[38,39]
- Estriol replacement prevents coronary hyperreactivity in vascular smooth muscle.[40]
- Estrogen reduces carotid intima-media thickness (IMT) in postmenopausal women.[41,42]
- Estrogen positively modulates the quantity of arterial calcification and intimal hyperplasia.[43,44]
- Estrogen replacement has been shown to suppress the stress response to both physical and emotional stresses that can lead to high cholesterol, elevated blood sugar, high blood pressure, heart disease, and weight gain.[45]
- Estrogen regulates adrenergic neurotransmission through several mechanisms. It modulates neuronal activity through binding to estrogen receptors, thereby regulating

its effects on catecholamine reuptake at the synaptic cleft, has genomic regulation of α-adrenergic receptors, and competes with norepinephrine for adrenergic binding sites.[51,52]

- Women on estrogen replacement therapy have been shown to have coronary calcification scores lower than women not on estrogen replacement.[53–55]
- Estrogen applied transdermally has an anti-inflammatory effect.[56–58]
- Estradiol improves insulin sensitivity in women with coronary heart disease.[59]
- Estrogen lowers fibrinogen levels.[60]
- Estrogen reduces infiltration of leukocytes to arteries after endothelium denudation and cytokine-induced gene transcription in smooth muscle.[112,113]

There is much less information on estrogen's effects on veins than on arteries. Studies suggest that the presence of ovarian hormones affects endothelial production of inhibitory prostanoids in veins just as it does in arteries.[46]

Estrogen has been shown to also affect blood pressure. The depletion of estrogen with a rise in androgens in women at menopause reduces local inhibitory signals while elevating procontractile signals at the vascular wall. This leads to increased peripheral resistance and blood pressure in the absence of a decrease in sympathetic tone. In addition, estrogen depletion elevates sympathetic tone and circulating levels of norepinephrine, which result in an elevation of blood pressure especially if the person is under stress.[105] Estrogen depletion is also associated with withdrawal of inhibitory tone (such as imparted by the parasympathetic system), which increases peripheral resistance and lowers heart rate variability. Studies have shown that estrogen replacement has positive effects on blood pressure by several different mechanisms. Estrogen replacement has been shown to restore heart rate variability.[106] In addition, studies have shown that estrogen decreases serum angiotensin-converting enzyme (ACE) activity by 20%.[47,48] Furthermore, estrogen inhibits the renin–angiotensin system by reducing the transcription of ACE in endothelial cells.[49] Estrogen also upregulates endothelium-derived vasodilator factors with simultaneous downregulation of vasoconstrictor factors like endothelin-1.[50,114] Likewise, estrogen replacement ameliorates the problems with sympathetic tone.

In review of the studies presented here, estrogen replacement therapy has many beneficial effects on the cardiovascular system. The timing of estrogen replacement is important for both cardiovascular health and memory maintenance. The ability for estrogen replacement therapy to prevent or slow the progression of vascular remodeling or plaque formation may be somewhat limited if not begun at the time of menopause. This same concept holds true for the actions of estrogen on the mitochondria. It is still important to replace estrogen in menopausal women who have low levels; however, the more positive effects on cardiovascular disease occur if estrogen is replaced as soon as the patient becomes deficient.

Estrogen for hormone replacement therapy should always be prescribed transdermally and should include both estradiol and estriol because both hormones have a positive effect on the heart. This combination is called biest. Oral estrogen should not be considered as it is proinflammatory. This is due to the fact that hepatic metabolism of[17] β-estradiol produces proinflammatory metabolites in higher concentrations if given orally as opposed to the transdermal application of estrogen,[107] whereas transdermal application of estrogen has been shown to have an anti-inflammatory effect.[108–111] In addition, estrogen replacement transdermally has been shown to lower interleukin (IL)-6, tumor necrosis factor (TNF)-α, and IL-1.[114] There are other negative reasons why estrogen should not be prescribed orally as hormone replacement. Estrogen by mouth can cause any of the following[115]:

- Increases blood pressure
- Increases triglycerides

- Increases estrone (the estrogen that should not be replaced because it is the estrogen that is linked to breast cancer)
- Gallstones
- Elevates liver enzymes
- Increases sex hormone–binding globulin (SHBG) (which decreases bioavailable testosterone levels)
- Interrupts tryptophan metabolism and consequently serotonin metabolism
- May lower growth hormone
- Increases C-reactive protein (CRP)
- Increases carbohydrate cravings
- Increases prothrombic effects

Transdermally applied, estradiol has been shown not to increase the risk of developing a cardiovascular accident (CVA).[116] Other studies showed no risk with transdermal estradiol use in the development of thrombolism.[117,118] In the future, intravenous (IV) estrogen may be used to treat heart attacks and heart rhythms that are not regular.[61]

When prescribing estrogen, progesterone should also be given even in women who have had a total hysterectomy. Again, the hormones in the body are a symphony so that balance between the hormones is paramount. In addition, prescribed hormones should always be in the natural form, also called bioidentical form. In medicine, the word natural means that the hormone is of the same chemical structure that God gave the patient. The word synthetic denotes that the chemical structure is not the same one that the individual is born with. Furthermore, natural does not technically have to do with the derivation of the drug. In this case, however, natural hormones that are prescribed are derived from yams or soy.

PROGESTERONE

Progesterone levels can be low at any age. Women with premenstrual syndrome (PMS), postpartum depression, and women who are peri-and postmenopausal are all commonly low in progesterone. Other causes of low progesterone in women include high sugar intake; deficiency of vitamins A, B6, and C; deficiency of zinc; hypothyroidism; high intake of saturated fat; stress; antidepressant use; and high prolactin levels.[198–202] Signs and symptoms of progesterone loss include the following[71]:

- Anxiety
- Depression
- Irritability
- Mood swings
- Insomnia
- Pain and inflammation
- Osteoporosis/osteopenia
- Excessive menstruation
- Hypersensitivity
- Nervousness
- Migraine headaches related to menstrual cycle
- Weight gain
- Decreased libido
- Decreased HDL
- High LDL
- Incontinence
- Palpitations

Natural progesterone is very different from synthetic progestins. Progestins do not balance estrogen, and they interfere with the body's own production of progesterone. Progestins may also be associated with any of the following[203–205]:

- Increased appetite[203]
- Weight gain[203]
- Fluid retention
- Irritability
- Depression
- Headache
- Decreased energy
- Bloating
- Breast tenderness
- Decreased sexual interest
- Acne
- Hair loss
- Nausea
- Insomnia
- May increase the symptoms of progesterone loss
- Protects only the uterus and not the breast from cancer[173]
- Counteracts many of the positive effects of estrogen on serotonin[209]

Likewise, progesterone and progestins have different effects on smooth muscle cell proliferation and hence on the risk of developing heart disease. Progesterone inhibits smooth muscle cell proliferation, and progestins may increase proliferation of heart artery smooth muscle cells.[62] Furthermore, progesterone inhibits vascular cell adhesion molecule-1 expression, which helps to prevent heart disease, and progestins do not inhibit vascular cell adhesion molecule-1.[63] In addition, progestins can raise LDL and lower HDL. Lastly, progestins can cause spasm of the coronary arteries.[205] Likewise, in postmenopausal women progesterone, and not progestin, enhances the beneficial effect that estrogen has on exercise-induced myocardial ischemia.[64] Very importantly, progestins can stop the protective effects that estrogen has on the heart.[205–208] In contrast, natural progesterone increases the beneficial effects that estrogen has on blood vessels.[212–214]

Natural progesterone, unlike synthetic progestins, has the following other positive effects on a women's body[210]:

- Helps balance estrogen
- Lowers blood pressure[65]
- Leaves the body quickly[211]
- Improves sleep
- Has a natural calming affect
- Helps the body use and eliminate fats
- Lowers cholesterol
- May protect against breast cancer as it has an antiproliferative effect[215,216]
- Increases scalp hair
- Helps balance fluids in the cells
- Increases metabolic rate[217]
- Is a natural diuretic
- Is a natural antidepressant
- Is anti-inflammatory
- Stimulates the production of new bone
- Enhances the action of thyroid hormones

- Improves libido
- Helps restore proper cell oxygen levels
- Induces conversion of E1 to the inactive E1S form
- Promotes Th2 immunity
- Is neuroprotective/promotes myelination

For all of the aforementioned reasons, when prescribing progesterone the natural form progesterone and not the synthetic form progestin should be employed.

TESTOSTERONE

Testosterone in women is made in the adrenal glands and ovaries. Women can have low testosterone levels at any age due to stress, medications, chemotherapy, childbirth, depression, endometriosis, and menopause. Signs and symptoms of testosterone deficiency include the following[71]:

- Anxiety
- Decline in muscle tone/muscle wasting despite adequate calorie and protein intake
- Decreased HDL
- Decreased sex drive
- Droopy eyelids
- Dry, thin skin with poor elasticity
- Dry, thinning hair
- Fatigue
- Hypersensitive, hyperemotional states
- Less dreaming
- Loss of pubic hair
- Low self-esteem
- Mild depression
- Saggy cheeks
- Thin lips
- Weight gain

Testosterone replacement in women who are deficient has been shown to relax coronary arteries and allow more blood to flow to the heart. It has also been shown to decrease symptoms of angina.[66–68] In another medical trial, testosterone replacement in postmenopausal women was found to lower lipoprotein(a) levels by up to 65%.[69] Testosterone can be increased in other ways besides hormone replacement: exercise; decreasing calorie intake; getting enough sleep; increasing the amount of protein in the diet; weight loss if the patient is overweight; stress reduction; taking the amino acids arginine, leucine, or glutamine; and zinc supplementation (if the patient is deficient, as zinc aids in the metabolization of testosterone).

Testosterone is only replaced in women who have their own estrogen or who are already receiving estrogen replacement. If the estrogen level is low and testosterone is replaced, it increases the patient's risk of heart disease if estrogen is not also supplemented. As discussed earlier, if estrogen is being prescribed then progesterone is always given as well.

Just like any other hormone in the body, too high or too low levels of testosterone are not desirous. High testosterone levels can occur in women who have polycystic ovarian disease (polycystic ovary syndrome [PCOS]) or in some women after menopause.[70,71] Individuals with elevated testosterone levels have an increased risk for the following major diseases:

- Diabetes[77]
- Heart disease[78]

- Hypertension[79]
- Infertility[80]
- Hormonally related cancers (breast, ovarian, and uterine)[81,82]
- Obesity[83]

Women with PCOS have an increased risk of developing heart disease compared to women without PCOS.[119–121] Up to 70% of women in the United States with PCOS have dyslipidemias.[94,122–126] In addition, elevated testosterone levels in women can lower HDL.[127] Furthermore, homocysteine levels are commonly increased in patients with PCOS.[128] Women with PCOS tend to have a higher than usual rate of elevated CRP. Also, women with PCOS frequently have decreased total antioxidant status and increased oxidative stress. These patterns may be some of the contributing causes of an increased risk in the development of coronary artery disease in women with polycystic ovarian disease.[130] Women with PCOS also have four times the rate of hypertension than women who do not have PCOS.[131] Furthermore, because women with PCOS tend to have insulin resistance, their insulin resistance and hyperinsulinemia may be associated with elevated blood pressure.[132] In addition, studies have shown that women with PCOS store fat better and burn calories at a slower rate than women who do not have this disease process.[133–135]

PCOS affects almost 10% of women in the United States. The following are signs and symptoms of PCOS or high testosterone levels at menopause[72,86–88,93–98]:

- Obesity/inability to lose weight easily
- High testosterone
- Irregular or absent menstrual cycles
- Infertility or recurrent miscarriages
- Hirsutism
- Alopecia
- Oily skin and/or acne
- Acrochordons (skin tags)
- Depression/irritability/tension
- Acanthosis nigricans
- Gray–white breast discharge
- Sleep apnea
- Pelvic pain
- Thinning scalp hair
- Insulin resistance
- Hypertension
- Decreased SHBG
- High estrone
- Elevated DHEA levels
- Abnormal lipid levels
- Ovarian cysts
- Low progesterone levels

Some scientists believe that PCOS has a hereditary component.[73,74] It is noted that 40% of women with PCOS have a sister with PCOS. Further, 35% of women with PCOS have a mother with PCOS.[89] There is a suggestion in the medical literature that women with PCOS are born with a gene that triggers higher than normal levels of androgens or insulin.[90,91] Studies have also shown that the high levels of testosterone and insulin in patients with PCOS are lined by a gene called *follistatin*. *Follistatin* plays a role in the development of ovaries and is needed to make insulin.[92] Furthermore, phthalates, bisphenol A, cadmium, and mercury toxicities may be related to the development of PCOS because they are endocrine disrupters.[94]

Stress may be a contributing factor to PCOS.[75] Studies have shown that many women with PCOS cannot process cortisol effectively, which can lead to elevated cortisol levels in the body. High cortisol levels may increase the risk of weight gain, high cholesterol, and high blood sugar and blood pressure, thus increasing the individual's risk of development of heart disease.[76] Likewise, hypothyroidism may be a cause of PCOS. A study conducted on teenage women with hypothyroidism showed that on ultrasound the ovarian cysts resolved when their hypothyroidism was treated.[99]

The full range of treatment of PCOS conventionally and from a metabolic approach is beyond the scope of this chapter. In considering the lowering of testosterone levels, the following therapies have been proved to be successful: saw palmetto 240–260 mg twice a day or metformin 250–500 mg daily, or spironolactone 100 mg twice a day.

Dehydroepiandrosterone

The majority of DHEA is made by the adrenal glands, but a small amount is made in the brain and skin. DHEA production declines with age. A study of postmenopausal women with coronary risk factors undergoing coronary angiography for suspected myocardial ischemia showed that lower DHEA-S levels were linked with higher cardiovascular mortality and mortality due to any cause.[84] Likewise, DHEA replacement has been shown to lower triglycerides and increase insulin sensitivity.[71] DHEA supplementation should not be considered in patients with a hormonally related cancer.

Cortisol

Cortisol is the only hormone in the body that may rise with age. Cortisol has many functions in the body, one of which is to help the body deal with stress. When the body is stressed, cortisol levels elevate. This can increase the risk of development of heart disease because high cortisol levels are commonly associated with high blood sugar, hypertension, hypercholesterolemia, hypertriglyceridemia, insomnia, and weight gain. Furthermore, if cortisol levels are consistently high it may affect the conversion of T4 to T3, which may lead to hypothyroidism. In addition, stress can lead to perivascular coronary artery inflammation, endothelial dysfunction, and hypercoagulable states such as elevated fibrinogen; elevated von Willebrand factor; elevated homocysteine; and high activity of factors XII, XI, IX, VIII, plasminogen, 2-antiplasmin, and plasminogen-activating factor.[145] In a medical trial called the INTERHEART study, psychosocial factors like stress were shown to be more potent predictors of the incidence of heart attack than diabetes, smoking, hypertension, and obesity.[103]

Furthermore, when the body stays in a constant state of stress it depletes the body of important nutrients such as magnesium, potassium, B vitamins, vitamin C, and zinc, many of which are needed to help the adrenal glands function optimally.

Melatonin

Melatonin has many functions in the body. One of them is to be cardioprotective. Melatonin is a vasodilator and free radical scavenger and inhibits the oxidation of LDL-C.[140] Melatonin levels have been found to be lower in patients with coronary heart disease compared to healthy patients. One study showed that melatonin levels in patients with coronary heart disease were only one-fifth that of health controls.[85] Low levels of this important hormone may cause an increase in nighttime sympathetic activity, which elevates the risk of developing coronary heart disease. Melatonin is a suppressor of sympathetic activity at night. Low levels of melatonin can also lead to elevated levels of epinephrine and norepinephrine, which may damage vessel walls. Atherogenic uptake of LDL is increased by higher levels of epinephrine and norepinephrine.[85,136] Furthermore, patients who developed adverse effects after acute myocardial infarction (MI) were shown to have lower nocturnal melatonin levels.[230]

A medical trial found that melatonin supplementation inhibited platelet aggregation.[137] Melatonin can also be cardioprotective by reducing hypoxia and preventing reoxygenation-induced damage in patients with cardiac ischemia and ischemic stroke.[138,139] One study showed an inverse correlation between melatonin levels and CRP levels after acute MI.[141] Moreover, one trial showed that melatonin levels in patients undergoing coronary artery bypass grafting are disrupted during the procedure and for up to 48 hours after the procedure. Consider supplementing these patients with melatonin.[142]

The MARIA study was a prospective, randomized, double-blind, and placebo-controlled trial. It used IV melatonin in patients following an acute MI who were having angioplasty. The results of IV melatonin showed that it decreased CRP and IL-6. It also attenuated tissue damage from reperfusion and decreased V-tach and V-fib after reperfusion. Melatonin supplementation also attenuated cellular and molecular damage from ischemia.[143] Interestingly, one animal study showed that melatonin supplementation daily at middle age decreased abdominal fat and lowered plasma insulin to youthful levels.[144]

There are several reasons why one may have low melatonin levels. Alcohol and caffeine use can lower melatonin. Electromagnetic field exposure, some medications such as nonsteroidal anti-inflammatory drugs, and the use of tobacco can also lower melatonin levels. Melatonin levels can be measured by salivary testing and can be easily supplemented.

THYROID HORMONE

The link between dysfunction of the thyroid and cardiovascular disease has been known for more than 100 years.[100,101]

There are numerous signs and symptoms of hypothyroidism. They are listed here because some of them may not be as common or obvious to the practitioner who is considering hypothyroidism as a diagnosis. It is important to consider hypothyroidism in the differential diagnosis when you are seeing patients with the following signs and symptoms[71,146,147]:

- Depression
- Weight gain
- Constipation
- Headaches
- Brittle, ridged, striated, and thickened nails
- Rough, dry skin
- Menstrual irregularities
- Fluid retention
- Poor circulation
- Elbow keratosis
- Slow speech
- Nails that are easily broken
- Anxiety/panic attacks
- Decreased memory
- Inability to concentrate
- Muscle and joint pain
- Reduced heart rate
- Slow movements
- Morning stiffness
- Puffy face
- Swollen eyelids
- Decreased sexual interest
- Cold intolerance
- Cold hands and feet

- Swollen legs, feet, hands, and abdomen
- Insomnia
- Fatigue
- Low body temperature
- Hoarse, husky voice
- Low blood pressure
- Muscle weakness
- Agitation/irritability
- Sparse, coarse, and dry hair
- Dull facial expression
- Yellow discoloration of the skin due to the inability to convert β-carotene into vitamin A
- Muscle cramps
- Drooping eyelids
- Carpel tunnel syndrome
- Sleep apnea
- Endometriosis
- Hypercholesterolemia
- Infertility
- PMS
- Hyperinsulinemia
- Fibrocystic breast disease
- Nutritional imbalances
- Paresthesias
- Down-turned mouth
- Acne
- Allergies
- Tendency to develop allergies
- Loss of the lateral one-third of the eyebrows (Queen Anne's sign)
- "Fat pads" about the clavicles
- Hair loss in the front and back of the head
- Loss of hair in varying amounts from legs, axilla, and arms
- Poor night vision
- Loss of eyelashes, or eyelashes that are not thick
- Blepharospasm is more common
- Ear canal that is dry, is scaly, and may itch
- Iron deficiency anemia
- B12 deficiency
- Tinnitus
- Delayed deep tendon reflexes
- Low-amplitude theta and delta waves on electroencephalogram
- Bipolar disorders
- Schizoid or affective psychoses
- Dizziness/vertigo
- Congestive heart failure
- Coronary heart disease/acute MI
- Arrhythmias
- Increased risk of developing asthma
- Hypertension
- Mild elevation of liver enzymes
- Gallstones
- Bladder and kidney infections

- Eating disorders
- Increased appetite
- Deposition of mucin in connective tissues
- Muscular pain
- Arthralgias/joint stiffness
- Menorrhagia
- Recurrent miscarriage
- Nocturia

Many disease processes are associated with hypothyroidism, one of which is heart disease.[150] Elevated CRP levels have been found to be related to hypothyroidism.[148] Furthermore, homocysteine levels are commonly elevated in hypothyroid patients. The mean level of homocysteine in one medical trial was 16.3 in patients who were hypothyroid.[149] One study looked at the signs and symptoms of low T3 in patients with cardiovascular disease and found the following[151]:

- Bradycardia
- Dyslipidemia
- Endothelial dysfunction
- Narrowed pulse pressure
- Diastolic hypertension
- High CRP
- High homocysteine

Another study looked at T3 and cardiovascular disease. The results of that trial showed that cardiovascular disease may be associated with low T3 and that supplementation increased cardiac contractility and decreased systemic vascular resistance.[152] When looking specifically at congestive heart failure and thyroid function, a low ratio of T3 to reverse T3 is a predictor of mortality in patients with congestive heart failure. IV T3 was given, and it increased cardiac output and decreased systemic vascular resistance. It was well tolerated.[153–155] Another study showed that thyroid hormone dysfunction plays an important role in the progression to dilated heart failure. When thyroid hormone replacement was given, the patients showed improvements in remodeling, including beneficial changes in myocyte shape, microcirculation, and collagen.[156] In another study using IV T3 in individuals with dilated cardiomyopathy and congestive heart failure, the heart rate was decreased and improvement of B-type natriuretic peptide (BNP) was seen along with improvement of ventricular performance.[157] In patients with chronic congestive heart failure, one investigation found that if they developed V-tach it was commonly associated with low T3 or low T3 to T4 ratio and increased reverse T3.[158]

Thyroid function has also been evaluated in patients post coronary artery bypass grafting. If the patient had low T3, it was found to be predictive of an increased risk in the development of atrial fibrillation after surgery.[159] Low T3 was likewise shown in another study to be a strong predictor of death in cardiac patients.[160] Furthermore, when looking at reverse T3 levels elevated reverse T3 was the strongest predictor of mortality in the first year after a patient had an acute MI.[162] It is important to be judicious about the starting of thyroid medication after an acute MI. Thyroid replacement has been proved to aid in remodeling after the event. T3 supplementation was found to decrease inflammatory cytokines along with adrenergic signaling, which causes beta-like myosin expression. Thyroid supplementation in these patients also helped to normalize wall tension, and chamber geometry was found to improve.[163,164]

Thyroid hormone replacement when it is optimized has been shown to do the following:[165,166]

- Improves lipid levels
- Improves congestive heart failure

- Is vasodilatory
- Is a positive inotrope
- Normalizes QT interval
- Improves CRP levels
- Improves homocysteine levels
- Improves arterial stiffness and endothelial dysfunction
- Prevents abnormal cardiac remodeling after acute MI and help with repair
- Improves insulin sensitivity

Furthermore, serum thyroid hormone levels may not accurately reflect thyroid tissue levels and cardiac function in patients with mild hypothyroidism.[167] Therefore, it is important to look at optimal replacement along with factors that influence how thyroid hormones function. The body makes two active thyroid hormones: T3 and T4.

Factors that cause decreased production of T4 such as a deficiency of zinc; copper; and vitamins A, B2, B3, and B6 should be replaced. Sometimes the patient may just need to have a better eating program and/or take a multivitamin to help their thyroid function optimally. The body converts T4 to the more active T3 form. This conversion requires 5′-deiodinase production. The following elements negatively affect 5′-deiodinase production[168–172]:

- Selenium deficiency
- Cadmium, mercury, or lead toxicity
- Starvation
- Inadequate protein intake
- High carbohydrate diet
- Elevated cortisol levels/stress
- Chronic illness
- Decreased kidney or liver function
- Inflammation

Other factors can produce thyroid dysfunction by causing an inability to convert T4 to T3, which include the following nutritional deficiencies[173–175]:

- Iodine
- Iron
- Selenium
- Zinc
- Vitamins A, B2, B6, and B12

Medications can also negatively affect the conversion of T4 to T3[176–179]:

- β-Blockers
- Oral contraceptives
- Estrogen replacement
- Lithium
- Phenytoin
- Theophylline
- Chemotherapy
- Clomipramine
- Glucocorticoids
- IL-6

Even a diet that is not well balanced can affect the conversion of T4 to T3[180]:

- Too many cruciferous vegetables
- Low protein diet
- Low fat diet
- Low carbohydrate diet
- Excessive alcohol use
- Too many walnuts
- Excessive soy intake

In addition, the following entities can have an adverse effect on the conversion of T4 to T3[181–183]:

- Aging
- High α-lipoic acid supplementation (600 mg or more daily)
- Diabetes
- Fluoride
- Lead toxicity
- Mercury toxicity
- Pesticides
- Radiation
- Stress
- Surgery
- Copper excess
- Calcium excess
- Dioxins
- Polychlorinated biphenyls (PCBs)
- Inadequate production of DHEA and/or cortisol
- Phthalates

Furthermore, factors that are associated with low T3 or an increase in reverse T3 can affect thyroid function and increase the patient's risk of developing heart disease[184]:

- Increased epinephrine or norepinephrine levels
- Free radical production
- Aging
- Fasting
- Stress
- Prolonged illness
- Diabetes
- Toxic metal exposure
- Elevated levels of IL-6, TNF-α, and interferon (IFN)-2

The following factors increase the conversion of T4 to T3. Consequently, if the conversion is low, it may be possible to fix the etiology of the problem or to increase supplementation to enhance thyroid function[185–188]:

- Selenium
- Potassium
- Iodine
- Iron
- Zinc

- High protein diet
- *Ashwaganda*
- Vitamins A, B2, and E
- Growth hormone
- Testosterone (decreases the concentration of thyroid-binding globulin)
- Insulin
- Glucagon
- Melatonin
- Tyrosine

When ordering laboratory evaluations on a patient with expected hypothyroidism, it is paramount that an entire panel of studies is done:

- Thyroid-stimulating hormone (TSH)
- Free T3
- Free T4
- Reverse T3
- Thyroid antibodies (antithyroglobulin antibody, antimicrosomal antibody, and anti-TPO antibody)

Studies have shown that most patients have greater improvement when prescribed both T3 and T4 as thyroid replacement.[189–192] T3 and T4 can be given separately or they can be delivered as a combination drug such as desiccated thyroid. Most desiccated thyroid medications are close to four parts—T4 to one part T3. If this ratio is not the perfect thyroid replacement for the patient, then the practitioner can have the thyroid medication compounded. As a compound, thyroid can be any ratio that would be the perfect replacement for the patient's individual needs. It is also important when prescribing thyroid medication that optimal ranges are used. Studies have shown that a TSH of 2.0–2.5 as the upper limit of normal provides for optimal function along with decreasing the symptoms of hypothyroidism.[193–195] In a study performed on postmenopausal women, women with TSH levels in the upper reference range had increased arterial stiffness compared to women with lower but still normal TSH levels.[161] Furthermore, for optimal thyroid function free T3 and free T4 levels should be in the midrange of normal.

Also, other medications that the patient may be given should be taken into account when prescribing thyroid replacement. The following medications decrease the absorption of thyroid medications or increase their excretion[102]:

- Ferrous sulfate[210]
- Sucralfate[211]
- Bile acid sequestrants[212]
- Calcium carbonate[213,214]
- Aluminum hydroxide[215]
- Phenytoin[222]
- Carbamazepine
- Phenobarbital
- Tamoxifen used for more than 1 year[223]
- Rifampin[224]
- Ritonavir[225]
- Sertraline[226]
- Cation-exchange resins
- Proton pump inhibitors
- H$_2$ blockers[220]

Other medications can also negatively affect thyroid function:

- Oral contraceptives
- Clomiphene[221]
- Metoclopramide[219]
- Haloperidol[216]
- Lithium (blocks iodine transport)[217]
- Amiodarone[218]

In addition, the following medical conditions are associated with a decrease in absorption of thyroid medication[102]:

- Achlorhydria
- Malabsorption syndromes
- Jejunum-ileal bypass surgery
- Short bowel syndrome
- Cirrhosis

Likewise, a high fiber diet and excessive soy intake have also been associated with a decrease in absorption of thyroid drugs.[102]

Therefore, when prescribing thyroid medication make sure that you take into account any medication that the patient may be on, medical conditions, or dietary intake.

Pregnenolone

Pregnenolone is the precursor hormone for estrogen, progesterone, testosterone, DHEA, and cortisol. The body makes this hormone from cholesterol, and pregnenolone levels decline with age. By the age of 75 years, most people have 65% less pregnenolone than they had at the age of 35.[227] Pregnenolone has a number of functions in the body:

- Blocks the production of acid-forming compounds
- Enhances nerve transmission and memory
- Helps to repair nerve damage
- Improves energy
- Improves sleep
- Increases resistance to stress
- Modulates the neurotransmitter γ-aminobutyric acid (GABA)
- Modulates N-methyl-D-aspartate (NMDA) receptors (which regulate pain control, learning, memory, and alertness)
- Promotes mood elevation
- Reduces pain and inflammation
- Regulates the balance between excitation and inhibition in the nervous system

Pregnenolone also activates transient receptor potential melastatin-3 (TRPM3), which is a calcium-permeable ion channel. TRPM3 is positively coupled to insulin secretion in B cells. One study suggested that TRPM3 is functionally relevant in contractile and proliferating phenotypes of vascular smooth muscle cells, constitutive channel activity, and regulation of cholesterol. Human trials need to be done.[228]

The natural pathways to making pregnenolone are blocked when the patient eats too many saturated fats and intakes trans fats.[229] Furthermore, pregnenolone levels tend to decline when the patient is stressed because the body will preferentially convert pregnenolone into cortisol. Pregnenolone levels can be measured, and this hormone can be safely replaced in most patients provided that they do not have a hormonally related cancer.

CONCLUSION

There are many risk factors for heart disease that the practitioner is already aware of such as smoking, high blood pressure, diet, high cholesterol, diabetes, obesity, family history of early heart disease, physical inactivity, and stress. This chapter focuses on a lesser known but very important risk factor for heart disease, hormonal imbalance. All of the hormones in this chapter affect heart function and can be cardioprotective if replaced and balanced appropriately. It is paramount that the body maintains its perfect hormonal symphony.

TESTOSTERONE AND HEART DISEASE IN MALES: OPPOSING VIEWS AND A BRIEF LITERATURE REVIEW

INTRODUCTION

Two recent trials suggest that testosterone replacement therapy in men may increase the risk of heart disease and/or stroke.[231,232]

These were poorly designed studies that conflict with numerous previous medical trials that show the beneficial effects of testosterone on the heart and that low testosterone levels in males are associated with an increased risk in the development of heart disease.

The following is a comprehensive review of the medical literature on low testosterone being associated with an increased risk in the development of cardiovascular disease and that testosterone replacement at appropriate levels not only decreases the risk of heart disease but also can be used to treat coronary disease.

LOW TESTOSTERONE LEVELS AND INCREASED RISK OF HEART DISEASE

Men with coronary heart disease had a significantly lower total testosterone, free testosterone, and bioavailable testosterone.[233]

Low endogenous testosterone concentrations are related to mortality due to cardiovascular disease and other causes.[234,235]

One investigation showed a possible correlation between lower testosterone levels, erectile dysfunction, and conditions associated with a higher cardiovascular risk.[236]

Another study showed that men with coronary heart disease who were under the age of 45 years had total and free testosterone levels significantly lower than those of controls.[237]

Serum free testosterone levels were found to be inversely related to carotid IMT and plaque score.[238]

Low testosterone levels have been found to be associated with atherosclerosis in men.[239]

LOW TESTOSTERONE LEVELS AND INCREASED RISK OF DIABETES TYPE II AND METABOLIC SYNDROME

Low testosterone levels are associated with an increased risk for the development of type II diabetes and metabolic syndrome.[240–244]

Because low testosterone has been shown to impact blood sugar levels, the Endocrine Society now recommends the measurement of testosterone in all male patients with type II diabetes mellitus.[245]

LOW TESTOSTERONE LEVELS ARE ASSOCIATED WITH AN INCREASED RISK OF MORTALITY

Low testosterone predicts mortality from cardiovascular disease.[246]

Low testosterone levels were associated with an increased risk of all-cause mortality independent of numerous risk factors. Serum testosterone levels were inversely related to mortality due to cardiovascular disease and cancer.[247]

Low endogenous testosterone levels are associated with an increased risk of death from all causes and cardiovascular death.[248]

LOW TESTOSTERONE LEVELS AND INCREASED RISK OF HYPERTENSION

Low total testosterone concentrations are predictive of hypertension, suggesting total testosterone as a potential biomarker for increased cardiovascular risk.[249]

LOW TESTOSTERONE AND CONGESTIVE HEART FAILURE

In males with heart failure, low serum androgens were associated with an adverse prognosis.[250]

In men with chronic heart failure, anabolic hormone depletion is common and deficiency of each anabolic hormone is an independent marker of poor prognosis.[251]

TESTOSTERONE REPLACEMENT AND HEART DISEASE

For all-cause mortality, each increase of 6 ng/dl of testosterone per liter of serum was associated with an almost 14% drop in the risk of death.[252]

Testosterone replacement was associated with a decrease in HDL-C and lipoprotein(a).[253]

The mechanism of testosterone replacement decreasing lipids may be due to testosterone's positive effects on abdominal fat and insulin resistance.[254]

Short-term administration of testosterone induces a beneficial effect on exercise-induced myocardial ischemia in men with coronary heart disease. This effect may be related to a direct coronary-relaxing effect of testosterone.[255]

Short-term intracoronary administration of testosterone, at physiological concentrations, induces coronary artery dilatation and an increase in coronary blood flow in men with established coronary heart disease.[256]

Low-dose supplementation with testosterone in men with chronic stable angina reduced exercise-induced myocardial ischemia.[257]

Testosterone replacement has been shown to increase coronary blood flow in patients with coronary heart disease.[258,259]

Transdermal testosterone replacement has been shown to improve chronic stable angina by increasing the angina-free exercise tolerance versus controls that were getting placebos.[260]

Another study showed that testosterone replacement reduced exercise-induced myocardial ischemia.[261]

Testosterone is a coronary vasodilator by functioning as a calcium antagonistic agent.[262]

Testosterone replacement therapy in hypogonadism moderates metabolic components associated with cardiovascular risk.[263]

Testosterone replacement has been shown to decrease inflammation and lower total cholesterol.[264]

Testosterone replacement in patients with congestive heart failure has been shown to improve exercise capacity, improve insulin resistance, and improve muscle performance.[265]

Testosterone replacement has been shown to be helpful in patients with severe heart failure.[266,267]

In this review of the medical literature, one can see that numerous studies have shown that low testosterone levels are associated with an increased risk of heart disease and that testosterone replacement therapy is associated with a decreased risk of developing heart disease and is even beneficial in patients who already have coronary vascular disease.

So, why did the two recent studies (Vigen et al.[231] and Finkle et al.[232]) show that there was an increased risk of developing heart disease in male patients who were prescribed testosterone replacement therapy? There are five serious flaws associated with the two recent trials:

Firstly, estrone and estradiol levels were not measured in the subjects in the studies. High estrogen levels in males have been found to be associated with an increased risk in the development of heart disease and stroke. Estrogen levels may elevate due to an increase in aromatase activity, alteration in liver function, zinc deficiency, obesity, abuse of alcohol, drug-induced estrogen imbalance, and ingestion of estrogen-containing foods or environmental estrogens.

HIGH ESTROGENS ARE ASSOCIATED WITH AN INCREASED RISK OF HEART DISEASE AND STROKE

High estradiol in males was associated with an increased risk of stroke.[268]

Elevated circulating estradiol is a predictor of progression of carotid artery IMT in middle-aged men.[269]

High estradiol levels in men were associated with acute MIs.[270]

High estrone and low testosterone levels were associated with promoting the development of atherogenic lipid milieu in men with coronary heart disease.[271]

Low testosterone and elevated estradiol were associated in this study with lower extremity peripheral artery disease in older men.[272]

Men with MI had high estradiol and low testosterone levels.[273]

Elevated levels of estradiol in men were associated with an increased incidence of strokes, peripheral vascular disease, and carotid artery stenosis compared to subjects with lower estradiol levels.[274]

Elevated levels of estrogen in men are associated with an increased risk of heart disease.[275]

Secondly, having erythrocytosis is associated with an increased risk in the development of heart disease and thrombosis.[276] A major study on the risk and benefits of testosterone replacement suggests that a baseline hematocrit should be checked at 3 and 6 months and then every 6–12 months. If the hematocrit is more than 54%, then testosterone therapy should be stopped until the hematocrit is at a safe level.[277] Hematocrit levels were not measured in these two trials.

Thirdly, in both studies not all patients had follow-up testing of testosterone levels. Therefore, dosages of testosterone may have been higher than needed. Supraphysiologial levels of testosterone can induce nitric oxide production and cause oxidative stress, which induces endothelial dysfunction.[278]

Fourthly, some of the men in these trials were using testosterone injections, which are nonphysiological as they have peak and trough levels over the weekly or biweekly dosing. This issue was wonderfully discussed by Cappola in her review of Vigen's study.[279]

Lastly, testosterone can convert to dihydrotestosterone (DHT), which has been shown to enhance early atherosclerosis.[280] The conclusion of the author of this trial was that the findings highlighted a new androgen receptor–/nuclear factor-κB–mediated mechanism for vascular cell adhesion molecule-1 expression and monocyte adhesion operating in male endothelial cells that may represent an important unrecognized mechanism for the male predisposition to atherosclerosis. The higher the dose of testosterone prescribed, the more the testosterone converted by 5α-reductase into DHT. In these two recent trials (Vigen et al.[231] and Finkle et al.[232]) that suggest that testosterone replacement increases the risk of heart disease in men, DHT levels were not measured.

CONCLUSION

Given the plethora of medical studies indicating the beneficial effects of properly prescribed testosterone, one would have to conclude that these two recent medical trials are poorly designed and their conclusion is flawed. Some of the patients did not have repeat testosterone levels measured. Consequently, the patients may have had supraphysiological levels of testosterone. In addition, DHT, estrone, estradiol, and hematocrit (HCT) levels were not addressed. Furthermore, the medical literature has shown that hormones in the body are a symphony and this web of interconnection was not considered.

BIBLIOGRAPHY

Collins J. *What's Your Menopause Type*. Roseville, CA: Prima Health, 2000.

Ding EL, Song Y, Malik VS, Liu S. Sex differences of endogenous sex hormones and risk of type 2 diabetes: A systematic review and meta-analysis. *JAMA* 2006;295:1288–1299.

Duick DS, Warren DW, Nicoloff JT, Otis CL, Croxson MS. Effect of single dose dexamethasone on the concentration of serum triiodothyronine in man. *J Clin Endocrin Metab* 1974;39(6):1151–1154.

Gerhard M, Walsh BW, Tawakol A et al. Estradiol therapy combined with progesterone and endothelium-dependent vasodilation in postmenopausal women. *Circulation* 1998;98(12):1158–1163.

Guder G, Frantz S, Bauersachs J et al. Low circulating androgens and mortality risk in heart failure. *Heart* 2010;96:504–509.

Hak AE, Pols HA, Visser TJ, Drexhage HA, Hofman A, Witteman JC. Subclinical hypothyroidism is an independent risk factor for atherosclerosis and myocardial infarction in elderly women: The Rotterdam Study. *Ann Intern Med* 2000;132(4):270–278.

Kumar A, Chaturvedi PK, Mohanty BP. Hypoandrogenaemia is associated with subclinical hypothyroidism in men. *Int J Androl* 2007;30:14–20.

Laux M. Natural Woman, Natural Menopause. New York: HarperCollins, 1997.

Majewska MD, Harrison NL, Schwartz RD, Barker JL, Paul SM. Steroid hormone metabolites are barbiturate-like modulators of the GABA receptors. *Science* 1986;232:1004–1007.

Register TC, Adams MR, Golden DL, Clarkson TB. Conjugated equine estrogens alone, but not in combination with medroxyprogesterone acetate, inhibit aortic connective tissue remodeling after plasma lipoid lowering in female monkeys. *Arterioscler Thromb Vasc Biol* 1998;18(7):1164–1171.

Rizza RA. Androgen effect on insulin action and glucose metabolism. *Mayo Clin Proc* 2000; 75 (suppl): S61–S64.

Rouzier N. *Estrogen and progesterone replacement*. Longevity and Prevention Symposium 2002, p. 8.

Schlienger J, Kapfer MT, Singer L, Stephan F. The action of clomipramine on thyroid function. *Horm Metab Res* 1980;12(9):481–482.

Schreiner P, Morrisett JD, Sharrett AR et al. Lipoprotein[a] as a risk factor for preclinical atherosclerosis. *Arterioscler Thromb* 1993;13(6):826–833.

Stefanick ML. Estrogen, progestogens and cardiovascular risk. *J Reprod Med* 1999;44(2 suppl):221–226.

Torkler S, Wallaschofski H, Baumeister SE et al. Inverse association between total testosterone concentrations, incident hypertension and blood pressure. *Aging Male* 2011;14(3):176–182.

Torpy D, Tsigos C, Lotsikas AJ, Defensor R, Chrousos GP, Papanicolaou DA. Acute and delayed effects of a single-dose injection of interleukin-6 on thyroid function in healthy humans. *Metabolism* 1998;47(10):1289–1293.

REFERENCES

1. McCrohon J, Celermajer D. Effects of hormone replacement therapy on the cardiovascular system. In: Fraser J, editor. *Estrogens and Progestogens in Clinical Practice*. New York: Harcourt Publishers; 2000, pp. 711–725.

2. Miller V, Sieck G, Prakash Y, Fitzpatrick L. Vascular effects of estrogen and progesterone, In: Fraser J, editor. *Clinical Practice*. New York: Harcourt Publishers; 2000, pp. 215–223.

3. Miller V, Duckles SP. Vascular actions of estrogens: Functional implications. *Pharmacol Rev* 2008; 60(2):210–241.

4. Henderson B, Paganini-Hill A, Ross RK. Estrogen replacement therapy and protection from acute myocardial infarction. *Am J Obstet Gynecol* 1988;159:312–317.

5. Stampfer M, Colditz GA, Willet WC et al. Postmenopausal estrogen therapy and cardiovascular disease. Ten-year follow-up from the nurses' health study. *N Engl J Med* 1991;325:756–762.

6. Grodstein F, Stampfer MJ, Colditz GA et al. Postmenopausal hormone therapy and mortality. *N Engl J Med* 1997;336(25):1769–1775.

7. Bush T. Extraskeletal effects of estrogen and the prevention of atherosclerosis. *Osteoporos Int* 1991;2:5–11.

8. Nabulsi AA, Folsom AR, White A et al. Association of hormone-replacement therapy with various cardiovascular risk factors in postmenopausal women. *N Engl J Med* 1993;328:1069–1075.

9. Bush TL, Barrett-Connor E, Cowan LD et al. Cardiovascular mortality and non-contraceptive estrogen use in women: Results from the Lipid Research Clinics Program follow-up study. *Circulation* 1987;75:1102–1109.

10. Danesh J, Collins R, Peto R. Lipoprotein (a) and coronary heart disease. Meta-analysis of prospective. *Circulation* 2000;102(10):1082–1085.

11. Soma M, Fumagalli R, Paoletti R et al. Plasma Lp (a) concentration after oestrogen and progestogen in postmenopausal women. *Lancet* 1991;337:612.

12. Stevenson JC, Crook D, Godsland IF, Lees B, Whitehead MI. Oral versus transdermal hormone replacement therapy. *Int J Fertil Menopausal Stud* 1993;38(suppl 1):30–35.

13. Williams, JK, Adams MR, Herrington DM, Clarkson TB. Short-term administration of estrogen and vascular responses of artherosclerotic coronary arteries. *J Am Coll Cardiol* 1992;20:454–457.

14. Moriarty K, Kim KH, Bender JR. Minireview: Estrogen receptor-mediated rapid signaling. *Endocrinology* 2006;147:5557–5563.

15. Li L, Hisamoto K, Kim KH et al. Variant estrogen receptor-c Src molecular interdependence and c-Src structural requirement for endothelial NO synthase activation. *Proc Natl Acad Sci USA* 2007; 104:16468–16473.

16. Huber M, Poulin R. Post-transitional cooperativity of ornithine decarboxylase induction by estrogens and peptide growth factors in human breast cancer cells. *Mol Cell Endocrinol* 1996;117:211–218.

17. Ulloa-Aguirre A, Maldonado A, Damian-Matsumura P, Timossi C. Endocrine regulation of gonadotropin glycosylation. *Arch Med Res* 2001;32:520–532.

18. Wu Z, Maric C, Roesch DM, Zheng W, Verbalis JG, Sandberg K. Estrogen regulates adrenal angiotensin AT1 receptors by modulating AT1 receptor translation. *Endocrinology* 2003;144:3251–3261.

19. Wu H. Coordinated regulation of A181 transcriptional activity by SUMOylation and phosphorylation. *J Biol Chem* 2006;281:21848–21856.

20. Stirone C, Duckles SP, Krause DN, Procaccio V. Estrogen increases mitochondrial efficiency and reduces oxidative stress in cerebral blood vessels. *Mol Pharmacol* 2005;68:959–965.

21. Duckles SP, Krause DN, Stirone C, Procaccio V. Estrogen and mitochondria: A new paradigm for vascular protection? *Mol Interv* 2006;6:26–35.

22. O'Lone R, Knorr K, Jaffe IZ et al. Estrogen receptors alpha and beta mediate distinct pathways of vascular gene expression, including genes involved in mitochondrial electron transport and generation of reactive oxygen species. *Mol Endocrinol* 2007;21:1281–1296.

23. Strehlow K, Rotter S, Wassmann S et al. Modulation of antioxidant enzyme expression and function by estrogen. *Circ Res* 2003;93:170–177.

24. Juan SH, Chen JJ, Chen CH et al. 17beta-estradiol inhibits cyclic strain-induced endothelin-1 gene expression within vascular endothelial cells. *Am J Physiol Heart Circ Physiol* 2004;287:H1254–H1261.

25. Strumpf WE, Sar M, Aumuller G. The heart a target organ for estradiol. *Science* 1977;1:319–321.

26. Miller V, Mulvagh SL. Sex steroids and endothelial function: Translating basic science to clinical practice. *Trends Pharmacol Sci* 2007;28:263–270.

27. Vitale C, Mercuro G, Cerquetani E et al. Time since menopause influences the acute and chronic effect of estrogens in endothelial function. *Arterioscler Thromb Vasc Biol* 2008;28:348–352.

28. Ospina JA, Duckles SP, Krause DN. 17-estradiol decreases vascular tone in cerebral arteries by shifting COX-dependent vasoconstriction to vasodilation. *Am J Physiol Heart Circ Physiol* 2003;285:H241–H250.

29. Lieberman EH, Gerhard MD, Uehata A et al. Estrogen improves endothelium-dependent flow-mediated vasodilation in postmenopausal women. *Ann Intern Med* 1994;121:936–941.

30. Maddox Y et al. Endothelium-dependent gender differences in the response of the rat aorta. *J Pharmacol Exp Ther* 1980;40:452–457.

31. Ganger KF, Vyas S, Whitehead M, Crook D, Meire H, Campbell S. Pulsatility index in internal carotid artery in relation to transdermal oestradiol and time since menopause. *Lancet* 1991;338:839–842.

32. Prelevic GM, Beljic T. The effect of oestrogen and progestogen replacement therapy on systolic flow velocity in healthy postmenopausal women. *Maturitas* 1994;20:37–44.

33. Losordo DW, Kearney M, Kin EA, Jekanowski J, Isner JM. Variable expression of the estrogen receptor in normal and artherosclerotic coronary arteries of premenopausal women. *Circulation* 1994;89:1501–1510.

34. Foegh ML, Asotra S, Howell MH, Ramwell PW. Estradiol inhibition of arterial neointimal hyperplasia after balloon injury. *J Vasc Surg* 1994;19(4):722–726.

35. O'Keefe JH Jr, Kim SC, Hall RR, Cochran VC, Lawhorn SL, McCallister BD. Estrogen replacement therapy after coronary angioplasty in women. *J Am Coll Cardiol* 1997;29(1):1–5.

36. Caulin-Glaser T, Watson CA, Pardi R, Bender JR. Effects of 17 beta-estradiol on cytokine-induced endothelial cell adhesion molecule expression. *J Clin Invest* 1996;98:36–42.
37. Shi Y, O'Brien JE, Fard A, Mannion JD, Wang D, Zalewski A. Adventitial myofibroblasts contribute to neointimal formation in injured porcine coronary arteries. *Circulation* 1996;94:1655–1664.
38. Krasinski K, Spyridopoulos I, Asahara T, van der Zee R, Isner JM, Losordo DW. Estradiol accelerates functional endothelial recovery after arterial injury. *Circulation* 1997;95:1768–1772.
39. Horner S, Pasternak G, Hehlmann R. A statistically significant sex difference in the number of colony-forming cells from human peripheral blood. *Ann Hematol* 1997;74:259–263.
40. Mishra RG, Stanczyk FZ, Burry KA et al. Metabolite ligands of estrogen receptor-beta reduce primate coronary hyperreactivity. *Am J Physiol Heart Circ Physiol* 2006;290(1):H295–H303.
41. Sator MO, Joura EA, Gruber DM et al. The effect of hormone replacement therapy on carotid arteries: Measurement with a high frequency ultrasound system. *Maturitas* 1998;30:63–68.
42. Karim R, Hodis HN, Stanczyk FZ, Lobo RA, Mack WJ. Relationship between serum levels of sex hormones and progression of subclinical atherosclerosis in postmenopausal women. *J Clin Endocrinol Metab* 2008;93:131–138.
43. Feletou M, Vanhoutte PM. Endothelial dysfunction: A multifaceted disorder (The Wiggers Award Lecture). *Am J Physiol Heart Circ Physiol* 2006;291:H985–H1002.
44. Bush DE, Jones CE, Bass KM, Walters GK, Bruza JM, Ouyang P. Estrogen replacement reverses endothelial dysfunction in postmenopausal women. *Am J Med* 1998;104:552–558.
45. Dayas CV, Xu Y, Buller KM, Day TA. Effects of chronic oestrogen replacement on stress-induced activation of hypothalamic-pituitary-adrenal axis control pathways. *J Neuroendocrinol* 2000;12:784–794.
46. Lewis DA, Bracamonte MP, Rud KS, Miller VM. Selected contribution: Effects of sex and ovariectomy on responses to platelets in porcine femoral veins. *J Appl Physiol* 2001;91:2823–2830.
47. Proundler AJ, Ahmed AI, Crook D, Fogelman I, Rymer JM, Stevenson JC. Hormone replacement therapy and serum angiotensin-converting-enzyme activity in postmenopausal women. *Lancet* 1995;346:89–90.
48. Nickening C, Baumer AT, Grohe C et al. "Estrogen modulates AT1 receptor gene expression in vitro and in vivo. *Circulation* 1998;97:2197–2201.
49. Gallagher PE, Li P, Lenhart JR, Chappell MC, Brosnihan KB. Estrogen regulation of angiotensin-converting enzyme mRNA. *Hypertension* 1999;33:323–328.
50. Dubey RK, Jackson EK, Keller PJ, Imthurn B, Rosselli M. Estradiol metabolites inhibit endothelin synthesis by an estrogen receptor-independent mechanism. *Hypertension* 2001;37:640–644.
51. Herbison AE, Simonian SX, Thanky NR, Bicknell RJ. Oestrogen modulation of noradrenaline neurotransmission. *Novartis Found Symp* 2000;230:74–85, discussion 85–93.
52. Ball P, Knuppen R. Formation, metabolism and physiologic importance of catecholestrogens. *Am J Obstet Gynecol* 1990;163:2163–2170.
53. Budoff M, Chen GP, Hunter CJ et al. Effects of hormone replacement on progression of coronary calcium as measured by electron beam tomography. *J Womens Health* 2005;14:410–417.
54. Mackey RH, Kuller LH, Sutton-Tyrrell K, Evans RW, Holubkov R, Matthews KA. Hormone therapy, lipoprotein subclasses, and coronary calcification: The Healthy Women Study. *Arch Intern Med* 2005;165:510–515.
55. Manson JE, Allison MA, Rossouw JE et al. Estrogen therapy and coronary-artery calcification. *N Engl J Med* 2007;356:2591–2602.
56. Seed M, Sands RH, McLaren M, Krik G, Darko D. The effect of hormone replacement therapy and route of administration on selected cardiovascular risk factors in post-menopausal women. *Fam Pract* 2000;17:497–507.
57. Chen FP, Lee N, Soong YK, Huang KE. Comparison of transdermal and oral estrogen-progestin replacement therapy: Effects on cardiovascular risk factors. *Menopause* 2001;8:347–352.
58. Puder JJ, Freda PU, Goland RS, Wardlaw SL. Estrogen modulates the hypothalamic-pituitary-adrenal and inflammatory cytokine responses to endotoxin in women. *Clin Endocrinol Metab* 2001;86(6):2403–2408.
59. Os I, OS A, Abdelnoor M, Larsen A, Birkeland K, Westheim A. Insulin sensitivity in women with coronary heart disease during hormone replacement therapy. *J Womens Health (Larchmt)* 2005;14(2):137–145.
60. Kannel WB, Wolf PA, Castelli WP, D'Agostino RB. Fibrinogen and the risk of cardiovascular disease. The Framingham Study. *JAMA* 1987;258:1183–1186.
61. Philip KL, Hussain M, Byrne NF, Diver MJ, Hart G, Coker SJ. Greater antiarrhythmic activity of acute 17beta-estradiol in female than male anaesthetized rates: Correlation with Ca2+ channel blockade. *Br J Pharmacol* 2006;149(3):233–242.

62. Carmody B, Arora S, Wakefield MC, Weber M, Fox CJ, Sidawy AN. Progesterone inhibits human infragenicular arterial smooth muscle cell proliferation induced by high glucose and insulin concentrations. *J Vasc Surg* 2002;36(4):833–838.

63. Otsuki M, Saito H, Xu X et al. Progesterone, but not medroxyprogesterone, inhibits vascular cell adhesion molecule-1 expression in human vascular endothelial cells. *Arterioscler Thromb Vasc Biol* 2001;21(2):243–248.

64. Rosano GM, Webb CM, Chierchia S et al. Natural progesterone, but not medroxyprogesterone acetate, enhances the beneficial effect of estrogen on exercise-induced myocardial ischemia in postmenopausal women. *J Am Coll Cardiol* 2000;36(7):2154–2159.

65. L'hermite, M, Simoncini T, Fuller S, Genazzani AR. Could transdermal estradiol + progesterone be a safe postmenopausal HRT? A review. Maturitas 2008;60:185–201.

66. Sarrel PM. Cardiovascular aspects of androgens in women. *Semin Reprod Endocrinol* 1998;16(2):121–128.

67. Yue P, Chatterjee K, Beale C, Poole-Wilson PA, Collins P. Testosterone relaxes rabbit coronary arteries and aorta. *Circulation* 1995;91(4):1154–1160.

68. Rako S. Testosterone deficiency: A key factor in the increased cardiovascular risk to women following hysterectomy or with natural aging? *J Womens Health* 1998;7(7):825–859.

69. Albers JJ, Taggart HM, Applebaum-Bowden D, Haffner S, Chesnut CH 3rd, Hazzard WR. Reduction of lecithin-cholesterol acyltransferase, apolipoprotein D and the Lp(a) lipoprotein with the anabolic steroid stanozol. *Biochim Biophys Acta* 1984;795:293–303.

70. Collins J. *What's Your Menopause Type?* Roseville, CA: Prima Publishing, 2000.

71. Smith P. *What You Must Know About Women's Hormones.* Garden City Park, NY: Square One Publishing, 2010.

72. Aherne SA. Polycystic ovary syndrome. *Nurs Stand* 2004;18(26):40–44.

73. Atiomo W, El-Mahdi E, Hardiman P. Familial associations in women with polycystic ovary syndrome. *Fert Steril* 2002;89(1): 143–145.

74. Battaglia C, Regnani G, Mancini F, Iughetti L, Flamigni C, Venturoli S. Polycystic ovaries in childhood: A common finding in daughters of PCOS patients. A pilot study. *Hum Reprod* 2002;17(3):771–776.

75. Marantides D. Management of polycystic ovary syndrome. *Nurse Pract* 1997;22(12):34–8, 40–1.

76. Tsilchorozidou T, Honour JW, Conway GS. Altered cortisol metabolism in polycystic ovary syndrome: Insulin enhances 5 alpha-reduction but not the elevated adrenal steroid production rates. *J Clin Endocrinol Metab* 2003;88(12):5907–5913.

77. Pelusi B, Gambineri A, Pasquali R. Type 2 diabetes and the polycystic ovary syndrome. *Minerva Ginecol* 2004;56(1):41–51.

78. Talbott EO, Zborowski JV, Sutton-Tyrrell K, McHugh-Pemu KP, Guzick DS. Cardiovascular risk in women with polycystic ovary syndrome. *Obstet Gynecol Clin North Am* 2001;28(1):111–133.

79. Rajkhowa M, Glass MR, Rutherford AJ, Michelmore K, Balen AH. Polycystic ovary syndrome: A risk for cardiovascular disease. *BJOG* 2000;107(1):11–18.

80. Trent ME, Rich M, Austin SB, Gordon CM. Fertility concerns and sexual behavior in adolescent girls with polycystic ovary syndrome: Implications for quality of life. *J Pediatr Adolesc Gynecol* 2003;16(1): 33–37.

81. Hardiman P, Pillay OC, Atiomo W. Polycystic ovary syndrome and endometrial carcinoma. *Lancet* 2003;361(9371):1810–1812.

82. Wild S, Pierpoint T, Jacobs H, McKeigue P. Long-term consequences of polycystic ovary syndrome: Results of a 31-year study. *Hum Fertil (Camb)* 2000;3(2):101–105.

83. Gonzalez Centeno A, Hernandez Marin I, Mendoza R, Tovar Rodriguez JM, Ayala AR. Polycystic ovarian disease: Clinical and biochemical expression. *Ginecol Obstet Mex* 2003;71:253–258.

84. Shufelt C, Bretsky P, Almeida CM et al. DHEA-S levels and cardiovascular disease mortality in postmenopausal women: Results from the National Institutes of Health: National Heart, Lung, and Blood Institute (NHLBI) sponsored Women's Ischemia Syndrome Evaluation (WISE). *J Clin Endocrinol Metab* 2010;95(11):4985–4992.

85. Pizzorno JE, Murray M. Melatonin. In: *Textbook of Natural Medicine*, 3rd Ed. St. Louis: Elsevier, 2006.

86. Futterweit W. *A Patient's Guide to PCOS.* New York: Henry Holt and Company, 2006.

87. Fraser IS, Kovacs G. Current recommendations for the diagnostic evaluation and follow-up of patients presenting with symptomatic polycystic ovary syndrome. *Best Pract Res Clin Obstet Gynaecol* 2004; 18(5):813–823.

88. Solomon CG. The epidemiology of polycystic ovary syndrome: Prevalence and associated disease risks. *Endocrinol Metab Clin North Am* 1999;28(2):247–263.

89. Azziz R, Kashar-Miller MD. Family history as a risk factor for the polycystic ovary syndrome. *J Pediatr Endocrinol Metab* 2000;13:1303–1306.
90. Strauss JF 3rd. Some new thoughts on the pathophysiology and genetics of polycystic ovary syndrome. *Ann N Y Acad Sci* 2003;997:42–48.
91. Carey AH, Chan KL, Short F, White D, Williamson R, Franks S. Evidence for a single gene effect causing polycystic ovaries and male pattern baldness. *Clin Endocrinol* 1993:38(6):653–658.
92. Urbanek M, Legro RS, Driscoll DA et al. Thirty seven candidate genes for polycystic ovary syndrome: Strongest evidence of linkage is *follistatin*. *Proc Natl Acad Sci U S A* 1999;38(6):653–658.
93. Hopkinson ZE, Sattar N, Fleming R, Greer IA. Polycystic ovarian syndrome: The metabolic syndrome comes to gynecology. *BMJ* 1998;317:329–332.
94. Marchese M. *Environmental Medicine Update.* Townsend Letter Feb/March 2012, pp. 66–68.
95. Guzick D. Polycystic ovarian syndrome. *Obstet Gynecol* 2004;103(1):181–193.
96. Romm A. *Botanical Medicine for Women's Health.* St. Louis: Churchill Livingstone/Elsevier; 2010, pp. 175–185.
97. Wei AY, Pritts EA. Therapy for polycystic ovarian syndrome. *Curr Opin Pharmacol* 2003;3:678–682.
98. Ring M. Polycystic ovarian syndrome. In: Rakel D, editor. *Integrative Medicine*, 3rd Ed. Philadelphia: Elsevier; 2012, pp. 345–52.
99. Lindsay AN, Voorhess ML, MacGillivray MH. Multicystic ovaries in primary hypothyroidism. *Obstet Gynecol* 1983;61:433–437.
100. Franklyn JA, Gammage MD, Ramsden DB, Sheppard MC. Thyroid status in patients after acute myocardial infarction. *Clin Sci (Lond)* 1984;67:585–590.
101. Auer J, Berent R, Weber T, Lassnig E, Eber B. Thyroid function is associated with presence and severity of coronary atherosclerosis. *Clin Cardiol* 2003;26:569–573.
102. Wartofsky L, Van Nostrand D, editors. *Thyroid Cancer: A Guide for Patients*, 2nd Ed. Atlanta, GA: Keystone Press, 2010.
103. Rosengren A, Hawken S, Ounpuu S et al. Association of psychosocial risk factors with risk of acute myocardial infarction in 11,119 cases and 13, 648 controls in 52 countries (The INTERHEART study): Case-control study. *Lancet* 2004;364:953–962.
104. Barber DA, Sieck GC, Fitzpatrick LA, Miller VM. Endothelin receptors are modulated in association with endogenous fluctuations in estrogen. *Am J Physiol* 1996;271:H1999–H2006.
105. Wyss JM, Carlson SH. Effects of hormone replacement therapy on the sympathetic nervous system and blood pressure. *Curr Hypertension Rep* 2003;5:441–426.
106. Mercuro G, Podda A, Pitzalis L et al. Evidence of a role of endogenous estrogen in the modulation of autonomic nervous system. *Am J Cardiol* 2000;85:787–789.
107. Brosnan JF, Sheppard BL. Norris LA. Haemostatic activation in postmenopausal women taking low-dose hormone therapy: Less effect than with transdermal administration? *Thromb Haemost* 2007;97: 558–565.
108. Seed M, Sands RH, McLaren M, Krik G, Darko D. The effect of hormone replacement therapy and route of administration on selected cardiovascular risk factors in post-menopausal women. *Fam Pract* 2000;17:497–507.
109. Chen FP, Lee N, Soong YK, Huang KE. Comparison of transdermal and oral estrogen-progestin replacement therapy: Effects on cardiovascular risk factors. *Menopause* 2001;8:347–352.
110. Vehkavaara S, Silveira A, Hakala-Ala-Pietila T et al. Effects of oral and transdermal estrogen replacement therapy on markers of coagulation, fibrinolysis, inflammation and serum lipids and lipoproteins in postmenopausal women. *Thromb Haemost* 2001;85:619–625.
111. Strandberg TE, Ylikorkala O, Tikkanen MJ. Differing effects of oral and transdermal hormone replacement therapy on cardiovascular risk factors in healthy postmenopausal women. *Am J Cardiol* 2003;92:212–214.
112. Xing D, Feng W, Miller AP et al. Estrogen modulates TNF-alpha induced inflammatory responses in rat aortic smooth muscle cells through estrogen receptor-B activation. *Am J Physiol Heart Circ Physiol* 2007;292:H2607–H2612.
113. Wang D, Oparil S, Chen YF et al. Estrogen treatment abrogates neointima formation in human C-reactive protein transgenic mice. *Arterioscler Thromb Vasc Biol* 2005;25:2094–2099.
114. Puder JJ, Freda PU, Goland RS, Wardlaw SL. Estrogen modulates the hypothalamic-pituitary-adrenal and inflammatory cytokine responses to endotoxin in women. *J Clin Endocrinol Metab* 2001; 86(6):2403–2408.
115. Decensi A, Omodei U, Robertson C et al. Effect of transdermal estradiol and oral conjugated estrogen on C-reactive protein in retinoid-placebo trial in healthy women. *Circulation* 2002;106(10):1224–1228.

116. Speroff L Transdermal hormone therapy and the risk of stroke and venous thrombosis. *Climacteric* 2010;13(5):429–432.

117. Canonico M, Oger E, Plu-Bureau G et al. Hormone therapy and venous thromboembolism among postmenopausal women: Impact of the route of estrogen administration and progestogens: The ESTHER study. *Circulation* 2007;115:840–845.

118. Scarabin P, Alhenc-Gelas M, Plu-Bureau G, Taisne P, Agher R, Aiach M. Effects of oral and transdermal estrogen/progesterone regimens on blood coagulation and fibrinolysis in postmenopausal women. A randomized controlled trial. *Arterioscler Thromb Vasc Biol* 1997;17(11):3071–3078.

119. Christian RC, Dumesic DA, Behrenbeck T, Oberg AL, Sheedy PF2nd, Fitzpatric LA. Prevalence and predictors of coronary artery calcification in women with polycystic ovary syndrome. *J Clin Endocrinol Metab* 2003;88(6):2562–2568.

120. Wild S, Pierpoint T, McKeigue P, Jacobs H. Cardiovascular disease in women with polycystic ovary syndrome at long-term follow up: A retrospective cohort study. *Clin Endocrinol (Oxf)* 2000;52(5): 595–600.

121. Talbot EO, Zborowski JV, Sutton-Tyrrell K, McHugh-Pemu, Guzich DS. Cardiovascular risk in women with polycystic ovary syndrome. *Obstet Gynecol Clin North Am* 2001;28(1):111–133.

122. Orio F Jr, Palomba S, Spinelli L et al. The cardiovascular risk of young women with polycystic ovary syndrome: An observational, analytical, prospective case-control study. *J Clin Endocrinol Metab* 2004;89(8):3696–3701.

123. Chang RJ. A practical approach to the diagnosis of polycystic ovary syndrome. *Am J Obstet Gynecol* 2004;191:713–717.

124. Phelan N, O'Connor A, Kyaw-Tun T et al. Lipoprotein subclass patterns in women with polycystic ovary syndrome (PCOS) compared with equally insulin-resistant women without PCOS. *J Clin Endocrinol Metab* 2010;95(8):3933–3939.

125. Wild RA, Carmina E, Diamanti-Kandarakis E et al. Assessment of cardiovascular risk and prevention of cardiovascular disease in women with the polycystic syndrome: A consensus statement by the Androgen Excess and Polycystic Ovary Syndrome (AE-PCOS) Society. *J Clin Endocrinol Metab* 2010;95(3):1073–1079.

126. Ehrmann DA. Polycystic ovarian syndrome. *N Engl J Med* 2005;353:1223–1236.

127. Crook D, Seed M. Endocrine control of plasma lipoprotein metabolism: Effects of gonadal steroids. *Bailleres Clin Endocrinol Metabol* 1990;4(4):851–875.

128. Loverro G, Lorusso F, Mei L, Depalo R, Cormio G, Selvaggi L. The plasma homocysteine levels are increased in polycystic ovary syndrome. *Gynecol Obstet Invest* 2002;53(3):157–162.

129. Boulman N, Levy Y, Leiba R et al. Increased C-reactive protein levels in the polycystic ovary syndrome: A marker of cardiovascular disease. *J Clin Endocrinol Metabol* 2004;89(5):2160–2165.

130. Fenkci V, Fenkci S, Yilmazer M, Serteser M. Decreased total antioxidant status and increased oxidative stress in women with polycystic ovary syndrome may contribute to the risk of cardiovascular disease. *Fertil Steril* 2003;80(1):123–127.

131. Lefebvre P, Raingeard I, Renard E, Bringer J. Long-term risks of polycystic ovaries syndrome. *Gynecol Obstet Fertil* 2004;32(3):193–198.

132. Landsberg L. Insulin sensitivity in the pathogenesis of hypertension and hypertensive complications. *Clin Exp Hyper* 1996;18(3-4):337–346.

133. Robinson S, Chang SP, Spacey S, Anyaoku V, Johnston DG, Franks S. Postprandial thermogenesis is reduced in polycystic ovary syndrome and is associated with increased insulin resistance. *Clin Endocrinol (Oxf)* 1992;36(6):537–43.

134. Faloia E, Canibus P, Gatti C et al. Body composition, fat distribution and metabolic characteristics in lean and obese women with polycystic ovary syndrome. *J Endocrinol Invest* 2004;27(5):424–429.

135. Gambineri A, Pelusi C, Vicennati V, Pagotto U, Pasquali R. Obesity and the polycystic ovary syndrome. *Int J Obes Relat Metab Disord* 2002;26(7):883–896.

136. Brugger P, Marktl W, Herold M. Impaired nocturnal secretion of melatonin in coronary heart disease. *Lancet* 1995;345:1408.

137. Cardinali DP, Del Zar MM, Vacas MI. The effects of melatonin in human platelets. *Acta Physiol Pharmacol Ther Latinoam* 1993;43:1–13.

138. Reiter RJ, Tan DX. Melatonin: A novel protective agent against oxidative injury of the ischemic/reperfused heart. *Cardiovasc Res* 2003;58(1):10–19.

139. Reiter RJ, Tan DX, Leon J, Kilic U, Kilic E. When melatonin gets on your nerves: Its beneficial actions in experimental models of stroke. *Exp Biol Med* 2005;230(2):104–117.

140. Dominguez-Rodriguez A, Abreu-Gonzalez P, Garcia-Gonzalez M, Reiter RJ. Prognostic value of nocturnal melatonin levels as a novel marker in patients with ST-segment elevation myocardial infarction. *Am J Cardiol* 2006;97(8):1162–1164.

141. Dominguez-Rodriguez A, Garcia-Gonzalez M, Abreu-Gonzalez P, Ferrer J, Kaski JC. Relation of nocturnal melatonin levels to C-reactive protein concentration in patients with T-segment elevation myocardial infarction. *Am J Cardiol* 2006;97(1):10–12.

142. Guo X, Kuzumi E, Charman SC, Vuylsteke A. Perioperative melatonin secretion in patients undergoing coronary artery bypass grafting. *Anesth Analg* 2002;94:1085–1091.

143. Dominguez-Rodriguez A, Abreu-Gonzalez P, Reiter RJ. Clinical aspects of melatonin in the acute coronary syndrome. *Curr Vasc Pharmacol* 2009;7(3):367–373.

144. Wolden-Hanson T, Mitton DR, McCants RL et al. Daily melatonin administration to middle-aged rats suppresses body weight, intra-abdominal adiposity, and plasma leptin and insulin independent of food intake and total body fat. *Endocrinology* 2000;141(2):487–497.

145. Black PH, Garbutt LD. Stress, inflammation, and cardiovascular disease. *J Psychosom Res* 2002;51(1): 1–23.

146. Shomon M. *Living Well with Hypothyroidism*. New York: Avon Books, 2000.

147. Barnes B. *Hypothyroidism: The Unsuspected Illness*. Philadelphia: Harper and Row, 1976.

148. Christ-Crain M, Meier C, Guglielmetti M et al. Elevated c-reactive protein and homocysteine values: Cardiovascular risk factors in hypothyroidism? A cross-sectional and double-blind, placebo-controlled trial. *Atherosclerosis* 2003;166(2):379–386.

149. Nedrebo BG, Ericsson UB, Nygard O et al. Plasma total homocysteine levels in hyperthyroid and hypothyroid patients. *Metabolism* 1998;47(1):89–93.

150. Hak AE, Pols HA, Visser TJ, Drexhage HA, Hofman A, Witteman JC. Subclinical hypothyroidism is an independent risk factor for atherosclerosis and myocardial infarction in elderly women: The Rotterdam Study. *Ann Intern Med* 2000;132(4):270–278.

151. Fernandez-Real JM, Lopez-Bermejo A, Castro A, Casamitjana R, Ricart W. Thyroid function is intrinsically linked to insulin sensitivity and endothelium-dependent vasodilation in healthy euthyroid subjects. *J Clin Endocrinol Metab* 2006;91(9):3337–3343.

152. Danzi S, Klein I. Thyroid hormone and the cardiovascular system. *Minerva Endocrinol* 2004;29(3): 139–150.

153. Hamilton MA, Stevenson LW, Fonarow GC et al. Safety and hemodynamic effects of IV triiodothyronine in advanced congestive heart failure. *Am J Cardiol* 1998;81(4):443–447.

154. Hamilton MA, Stevenson LW. Thyroid hormonal abnormalities in heart failure: Possibilities for therapy. *Thyroid* 1996;6(5):527–529.

155. Danzi S, Klein I. Potential uses of T3 in the treatment of human disease. *Clin Cornerstone* 2005;7(suppl 2): S9–15.

156. Gerdes AM, Iervasi G. Thyroid replacement therapy and heart failure. *Circulation* 2010;122:385–393.

157. Pingitore A, Galli E, Barison A et al. Acute effects of triiodothyronine (T3) replacement therapy in patients with chronic heart failure and low-T3 syndrome: A randomized, placebo-controlled study. *J Clin Endocrinol Metab* 2008;93(4):1351–1358.

158. Shimoyama N, Maeda T, Inoue T, Niwa H, Saikawa T. Serum thyroid hormone levels correlate with cardiac function and ventricular tachyarrhythmia in patients with chronic heart failure. *J Cardiol* 1993; 23(2):205–213.

159. Cerillo AG, Bevilacqua S, Storti S et al. Free triiodothyronine: A novel predictor of postoperative atrial fibrillation. *Eur J Cardiothorac Surg* 2003;24(4):487–492.

160. Iervasi G, Pingitore A, Landi P et al. Low T3 syndrome, a strong prognostic predictor of death in patients with heart disease. *Circulation* 2003;107:708–713.

161. Lambrinoudaki I, Armeni E, Rizos D et al. High normal thyroid-stimulating hormone is associated with arterial stiffness in healthy postmenopausal women. *J Hypertens* 2012;30(3):592–599.

162. Friberg L, Drvota V, Bjelak AH, Eggertsen G, Ahnve S. Association between increased levels of reverse triiodothyronine and mortality after acute myocardial infarction. *Am J Med* 2001;111(9):699–703.

163. Klein I, Danzi S. Thyroid hormone treatment to mend a broken heart. *J Clin Endocrinol Metab* 2008; 93(4):1172–1174.

164. Pantos C, Mourouzis I, Cokkinos DV. Rebuilding the post-infarcted myocardium by activating 'physiologic' hypertrophic signaling pathways: The thyroid hormone paradigm. *Heart Fail Rev* 2010; 15(2): 143–154.

165. Razvi S, Shakoor A, Vanderpump M, Weaver JU, Pearce SH. The influence of age on the relationship between subclinical hypothyroidism and ischemic heart disease: A metaanalysis. *J Clin Endocrinol Metab* 2008;93(8):2998–3007.

166. Asvold BO, Vatten LJ, Nilsen TI, Bjoro T. The association between TSH within the reference range and serum lipid concentrations in a population-based study. The HUNT Study. *Eur J Endocrinol* 2007; 156(2):181–186.

167. Liu Y, Redetzke RA, Said S, Pottala JV, de Escobar GM, Gerdes M. Serum thyroid hormone levels may not accurately reflect thyroid tissue levels and cardiac function in mild hypothyroidism. *Am J Physiol Heart Circ Physiol* 2008;294:H2137–H2143.

168. Nishiyama S, Futagoishi-Suginohara Y, Matsukura M et al. Zinc supplementation alters thyroid hormone metabolism in disabled patients with zinc deficiency. *J Am Coll Nutr* 1994;13:62–67.

169. Meinhold H, Campos-Barros A, Behne D. Effects of selenium and iodine deficiency on iodothyronine diodinases in brain, thyroid, and peripheral tissues. *JAMA* 1992;19:8–12.

170. Berry MJ, Larsen PR. The role of selenium in thyroid hormone action. *Endocr Rev* 1992;13:207–220.

171. Kohrle J. The deiodinase family: Selenoenzymes regulating thyroid hormone availability and action. *Cell Mol Life Sci* 2000;57:1853–1863.

172. Jakobs TC, Mentrup B, Schmutzler C, Dreher I, Kohrle J. Proinflammatory cytokines inhibit the expression and function of human type I 5'deiodinase in HepG2 hepatocarcinoma cells. *Eur J Endocrinol* 2002;146(4):559–566.

173. Rouzier N. *Thyroid replacement therapy.* In: Longevity and Preventive Medicine Symposium, 2002; p. 2.

174. Contempre B, Duale NL, Dumont JE, Ngo B, Diplock AT, Vanderpas J. Effect of selenium supplementation on thyroid hormone metabolism in an iodine and selenium deficient population. *Clin Endocrinol* 1992;36:579–583.

175. St. Germain D. Selenium, deiodinases, and endocrine Function. In: Hatfield, editor. *Selenium Its Molecular Biology and Role in Human Health.* Boston: Kluwer; 2001, pp. 189–202.

176. DeGroot L. *Endocrinology.* 5th Ed. Philadelphia: Elsevier/Saunders, 2006.

177. Pansini F, Bassi P, Cavallini AR et al. Effect of the hormonal contraception on serum reverse triiodothyronine levels. *Gynecol Obstet Invest* 1987;23:133–134.

178. Cavalieri, R. Effects of Drugs on Human Thyroid Hormone Metabolism. In: Hennemann G, editor. *Thyroid Hormone Metabolism.* New York: Marcel Dekker; 1998, pp. 359–379.

179. Wiersinga WM. Propranolol and thyroid hormone metabolism. *Thyroid* 1991;1(3):273–277.

180. Divi, R, Chang HC, Doerge DR. Anti-thyroid isoflavones from soybean: Isolation, characterization, and mechanism of action. *Biochem Pharmacol* 1997;54(10):1087–1096.

181. Nishida M, Matsumoto H, Asano A, Umazume K, Yoshimura Y, Kawada J. Direct evidence for the presence of methylmercury bound in the thyroid and other organs obtained from mice given methylmercury; differentiation of free and bound methylmercuries in biological materials determined by volatility of methylmercury. *Chem Pharm Bull* 1990;38(5):1412,1413.

182. Brucker-David F. Effects of environmental synthetic chemicals on thyroid function. *Thyroid* 1998;8(9): 827–856.

183. Huseman C, Moriarty CM, Angle CR. Childhood lead toxicity and impaired release of thyroid stimulation hormone. *Environ Res* 1987;42:524–533.

184. Rachman B. Managing endocrine imbalance; autoimmune-induced thyroidopathy and chronic fatigue syndrome. In: *Functional Medicine Approaches to Endocrine Disturbances of Aging.* Gig Harbor Washington: The Institute for Functional Medicine; 2001, p. 226.

185. Portes E, Oliveira JH, MacCagnan P, Abucham J. Changes in serum thyroid hormones levels and their mechanisms during long-term growth hormone (GH) replacement therapy in GH deficient children. *Clin Endocrinol* 2000;53(2):183–189.

186. Jorgensen J, Pedersen SA, Laurberg P, Weeke J, Skakkebaek NE, Christiansen JS. Effects of growth hormone on thyroid function of growth hormone-deficient adults with and without concomitant thyroxine-substituted central hypothyroidism. *J Clin Endocrinol Metab* 1989;69(6):1127–1132.

187. Deyssig R, Weissel M. Ingestion of androgenic-anabolic steroids induces mild thyroidal impairment in male body builders. *J Clin Endocrinol Metab* 1993;76(4):1069–1071.

188. Glinoer D, Fernandez-Deville M, Ermans AM. Use of direct thyroxine-binding globulin measurement in the evaluation of thyroid function. *J Endocrinol Invest* 1978;1(4):329–335.

189. Bunevicius R, Kazanavicius G, Zalinkevicius R, Prange AJ Jr. Effect of thyroxine as compared with thyroxine plus triiodothyronine in patients with hypothyroidism. *N Engl J Med* 1994; 340(6): 424–429.

190. Adlin V. Subclinical hypothyroidism: Deciding when to treat. *Am Fam Physician* 1998;57(4):776–780.

191. Escobar-Morreale H, Botella-Carretero JI, Gómez-Bueno M, Galán JM, Barrios V, Sancho J. Thyroid hormone replacement therapy in primary hypothyroidism: A randomized trial comparing L-thyroxine plus liothyronine with L-thyroxine alone. *Ann Intern Med* 2005;142(6):412–424.

192. Baisier WV, Hertoghe J, Eeckhaut W. Thyroid insufficiency. Is thyroxine the only valuable drug? *J Nutr Environ Med* 2001;11:159–166.

193. Wartofsky L, Dickey RA. The evidence for a narrower thyrotropin reference range is compelling. *J Clin Endocrinol Metab* 2005;90(9):5483–5488.

194. Hollowell J, Staehling NW, Flanders WD et al. Serum TSH, T4 and thyroid antibodies in the United States population (1089 to 1994): National Health and Nutrition Examination Survey (NHAMES III). *J Clin Endocrinol Metab* 2002;87(2):489–499.

195. Woeber K. Levothyroxine therapy and serum free thyroxine and free triiodothyronine concentrations. *J Endocrinol Invest* 2002;25(2):106–109.

196. Nordestgaard BG, Chapman MJ, Ray K et al. Lipoprotein(a) as a cardiovascular risk factor: Current status. *Eur Heart J* 2010;31(23):2844–2853.

197. Kamstrup PR, Tybjærg-Hansen A, Nordestgaard BG. Lipoprotein(a) and risk of myocardial infarction—genetic epidemiologic evidence of causality. *Scand J Clin Lab Invest* 2011;71(2):87–93.

198. Schedlowski M, Wiechert D, Wagner TO, Tewes U. Acute psychological stress increases plasma levels of cortisol, prolactin, and thyroid stimulating hormone. *Life Sci* 1992;50:1201–1205.

199. [Unknown.] Drugs that cause sexual dysfunction: An update. *Med Lett Drugs Ther*1992;34(876):73–78.

200. Baghurst P, Carman JA, Syrette JA, Baghurst KI, Crocker JM. Diet, prolactin and breast cancer. *Am J Clin Nutr* 1992;56:943–939.

201. Panth M, Raman L, Ravinder P, Sivakumar B. Effect of vitamin A supplementation on plasma progesterone and estradiol levels during pregnancy. *Int J Vitam Nutr Res* 1991; p. 61.

202. Luck MR, Jeyaseelan I, Scholes RA. Ascorbic acid and fertility. *Biol Reprod* 1995;52:262–266.

203. Vliet E. *Women Weight and Hormones*. New York: M. Evans & Company, 2001.

204. Bland J. *Functional Medicine Approaches to Endocrine Disturbances of Aging*. Gig Harbor, Washington, DC: The Functional Medicine Institute, 2001.

205. Sinatra S. *Heart Sense for Women*. Washington, DC: LifeLine Press, 2000.

206. Ottoson U, Johansson BG, von Schoultz B. Subfractions of high-density lipo-protein cholesterol during estrogen replacement therapy: A comparison between progestogens and natural progesterone. *Am J Obstet and Gynecol* 1985;151:746–50.

207. Minshall RD, Stanczyk FZ, Miyagawa K et al. Ovarian steroid protection against coronary artery hyperreactivity in rhesus monkeys. *J Clin Endocrinol Metab* 1998;83(2):649–659.

208. Henderson B, Paganini-Hill A, Ross RK. Estrogen replacement therapy and protection from acute myocardinal infarction. *Am J Obstet Gynecol* 1988;159:312–317.

209. Melton L. Sex is all in the brain: Report of a Novartis Foundation Symposium on the Neuronal and Cognitive Effects of Oestrogens, London, UK, 7-9 September 1999. *Trends Endocrinol Metab* 2000; 11(2):69–71.

210. Campbell N, Hasinoff BB, Stalts H, Rao B, Wong NC. Ferrous sulfate reduces thyroxine efficacy in patients with hypothyroidism. *Ann Intern Med* 1992;117(12):1010–1013.

211. Sherman S, Tielens ET, Ladenson PW. Sucralfate causes malabsorption of thyroxine. *Am J Med* 1994; 96(6):531–535.

212. Northcutt RC, Stiel JN, Hollifield JW, Stant EG Jr. The influence of cholestyramine on thyroid absorption. *JAMA* 1969;208(10):1857–1861.

213. Singh N, Singh PN, Hershman JM. Effect of calcium carbonate on the absorption of levothyroxine. *JAMA* 2000;283(21):2822–2825.

214. Csako G, McGriff NJ, Rotman-Pikielny P, Sarlis NJ, Pucino F. Exaggerated levothyroxine malabsorption due to calcium carbonate supplementation in gastrointestinal disorders. *Ann Pharmacother* 2001;35(12):1578–1583.

215. Sperber A, Liel Y. Evidence for interference with the intestinal absorption of levothyroxine sodium by aluminum hydroxide. *Arch Intern Med* 1992;152(1):183,184.

216. Kirkegaard C, Bjørum N, Cohn D, Lauridsen UB. Thyrotropin-releasing hormone (TRH) stimulation test in manic depressive illness. *Arch Gen Pschiatr* 1978;35(8):1017–1021.

217. Lazarus J, John R, Bennie EH, Chalmers RJ, Crockett G. Lithium therapy and thyroid function: A long-term study. *Psychol Med* 1981;11(1):85–92.

218. Newman C, Price A, Davies DW, Gray TA, Weetman AP. Amiodarone and the thyroid: A practical guide to the management of thyroid dysfunction induced by amiodarone therapy. *Heart* 1998;79:121–127.

219. Kirkegaard C, Bjørum N, Cohn D, Faber J, Lauridsen UB, Nekup J. Studies on the influence of biogenic amines and psychoactive drugs on the prognostic value of TRH stimulation test in endogenous depression. *Psychoneuroendocrinology* 1977;2(2):131–136.

220. Nelis G, Van de Meene JG. The effect of oral cimetidine on the basal and stimulated values of prolactin, thyroid stimulating hormone, follicle stimulating hormone and luteinizing hormone. *Postgrad Med J* 1980;56(651):26–29.

221. Feidt-Rasmussen U, Lange AP, Date J, Hansen MK. Effect of clomiphene on thyroid function in normal men. *Acta Endocrinol* 1979;90(1):43–51.

222. Rootwelt K, Ganes T, Johannessen SI. Effect of carbamazepine, phenytoin and phenobarbital on serum levels of thyroid hormones and thyrotropin in humans. *Scand J Clin Lab Invest* 1978;38(8):731–736.

223. Anker G, Lønning PE, Aakvaag A, Lien EA. Thyroid function in post-menopausal breast cancer patients treated with Tamoxifen. *Scand J Clin Lab Invest* 1998;58:103–107.

224. Takasu N, Takara M, Komiya I. Rifampin-induced hypothyroidism in patients with Hashimoto's thyroiditis. *N Engl J Med* 2005;352(5):518,519.

225. Tseng A, Fletcher D. Interaction between ritonavir and levothyroxine. *AIDS* 1998;12(16):2235,2236.

226. McCowen K, Garber JR, Spark R. Elevated serum thyrotropin in thyroxine-treated patients with hypothyroidism given sertraline. *N Engl J Med* 1997;337(14):1010,1011.

227. Roberts E. Pregnenolone—from Selye to Alzheimer's and a model of the pregnenolone sulfate binding site on the GABA receptor. *Biochem Pharmacol* 1995;49(1):1–16.

228. Naylor J, Li J, Milligan CJ et al. Pregnenolone sulfate-and cholesterol-regulated TRPM3 channels couple to vascular smooth muscle secretion and contraction. *Cir Res* 2010;106(9):11507–11515.

229. Yanick P. *Prohormone Nutrition*. Montclair, NJ: Longevity Institute International; 1998, p. 358.

230. The role of melatonin in acute myocardial infarction, Frontiers in Bioscience, http://www.bioportfolio .com/resources/pmarticle (accessed January 11, 2014).

231. Vigen R, O'Donnell CI, Barón AE et al. Association of testosterone therapy with mortality, myocardial infarction, and stroke in men with low testosterone levels. *JAMA* 2013;310(17):1829–1836.

232. Finkle W, Greenland S, Ridgeway GK et al. Increased risk of non-fatal myocardial infarction following testosterone therapy prescription in men. *PLOS One* 2014;9(1):e85805.

233. English K, Mandour O, Steeds RP, Diver MJ, Jones TH, Channer KS. Men with coronary artery disease have lower levels of androgens than men with normal coronary angiograms. *Eur Heart J* 2000;21(11): 890–894.

234. Vermeulen A. Androgen replacement therapy in the aging male—a critical evaluation. *J Clin Endocrinol Metabol* 2001;86:2380–2390.

235. Malkin C, Pugh PJ, Morris PD et al. Low serum testosterone and increased mortality in men with coronary heart disease. *Heart* 2010;96:1821–1825.

236. Ma R, So WY, Yang X et al. Erectile dysfunction predicts coronary heart disease in type 2 diabetes. *J Am Coll Cardiol* 2008;51:2045–2050.

237. Turhan S, Tulunay C, Güleç S et al. The association between androgen levels and premature coronary artery disease in men. *Coron Artery Dis* 2007;18(3):159–162.

238. Fukui M, Kitagawa Y, Nakamura N et al. Association between serum testosterone concentration and carotid atherosclerosis in men with type 2 diabetes. *Diabetes Care* 2003;26:1869–1873.

239. Svartberg J, von Mühlen D, Mathiesen E et al. Low testosterone levels are associated with carotid atherosclerosis in men. *J Int Med* 2006;269(6):576–582.

240. Ding E, Song Y, Malik VS, Liu S. Sex differences of endogenous sex hormones and risk of type 2 diabetes: A systematic review and meta-analysis. *JAMA* 2006;295:1288–1299.

241. Laaksonen D, Niskanen L, Punnonen K et al. Testosterone and sex hormone-binding globulin predict the metabolic syndrome and diabetes in middle-age men. *Diabetes Care* 2004;27:1036–1041.

242. Pasquali R, Macor C, Vicennati V et al. Effects of acute hyperinsulinemia on testosterone serum concentrations in adult obese and normal-weight men. *Metabolism* 1997;46(5):526–529.

243. Rizza R. Androgen effect on insulin action and glucose metabolism. *Mayo Clin Proc* 2000;75(suppl): S61–S64.

244. Stellato R, Feldman HA, Hamdy O et al. Testosterone, sex hormone-binding globulin, and the development of type 2 diabetes in middle-aged men: Prospective results from the Massachusetts male aging study. *Diabetes Care* 2000;23(4):490–494.

245. Dardona P, Dhindsa S. Update: Hypogonadotropic hypogonadism in type 2 diabetes and obesity. *J Clin Endocrinol Metab* 2011;96(9):2643.

246. Hyde Z, Norman PE, Flicker L et al. Low free testosterone predicts mortality from CVD but not other causes: The Health in Men Study. *J Clin Endocrinol Metab* 2012;97(1):179–189.

247. Haring R, Völzke H, Steveling A et al. Low serum testosterone levels are associated with increased risk of mortality in a population-based cohort of men aged 20-79. *Eur Heart J* 2010;31(12):1494–1501.

248. Araujo AB, Dixon JM, Suarez EA, Murad MH, Guey LT, Wittert GA. Endogenous testosterone and mortality in men: A systematic review and meta-analysis. *J Clin Endocrinol Metab* 2011;90:3007–3019.

249. Torkler S, Wallaschofski H, Baumeister SE et al. Inverse association between total testosterone concentrations, incident hypertension and blood pressure. *Aging Male* 2011;14(3):176–182.

250. Guder G, Frantz S, Bauersachs J et al. Low circulating androgens and mortality risk in heart failure. *Heart* 2010;96:504–509.

251. Jankowska E, Biel B, Majda J et al. Anabolic deficiency in men with chronic heart failure: Prevalence and detrimental impact on survival. *Circulation* 2006;114:1829–1837.

252. Khaw K, Dowsett M, Folkerd E et al. Endogenous testosterone and mortality due to all causes, cardiovascular disease, and cancer in men: European Prospective Investigation into Cancer in Norfolk (EPIC-Norfolk) Prospective Population study. *Circulation* 2007;116(23):2694–2701.

253. Baum N, Crespi CA. Testosterone replacement in elderly men. *Geriatrics* 2007;62:15–18.

254. Marin P, Holmäng S, Gustafsson C et al. Androgen treatment of abdominally obese men. *Obes Res* 1993;1:245–248.

255. Rosano G, Leonardo F, Pagnotta P et al. Acute anti-ischemic effect of testosterone in men with coronary artery disease. *Circulation* 1999;99:166–170.

256. Webb C, McNeill JG, Hayward CS, de Zeigler D, Collins P. Effects of testosterone on coronary vasomotor regulation in men with coronary heart disease. *Circulation* 1999;100(16):1690–1696.

257. English K, Steeds RP, Jones TH, Diver MJ, Channer KS. Low dose transdermal testosterone therapy improves angina threshold in men with chronic stable angina. *Circulation* 2000;102:1906–1911.

258. Haffner J, Moss SE, Klein BE, Klein R. Sex hormones and DHEASO4 in relation to ischemic heart disease in diabetic subjects. The WESDR Study. *Diabetes Care* 1996;19:1045–1050.

259. Channer K, Jones TH. Cardiovascular effects of testosterone: Implications of the "male menopause?" *Heart* 2003;89(2):121–122.

260. Whitsel E, Boyko EJ, Matsumoto AM, Anawalt BD, Siscovick DS. Intramuscular testosterone esters and plasma lipids in hypogonadal men: A meta-analysis. *Am J Med* 2001;111:261–269.

261. English K, Steeds RP, Jones TH, Diver MJ, Channer KS. Low-dose transdermal testosterone therapy improves angina threshold in men with chronic stable angina: A randomized, double-blind, placebo-controlled study. *Circulation* 2000;102(16):1906–1911.

262. English K, Jones RD, Jones TH, Morice AH, Channer KS. Testosterone acts as a coronary vasodilator by a calcium antagonistic action. *J Endocrinol Invest* 2002;25(5):455–458.

263. Corona G, Rastrelli G, Monami M et al. Hypogonadism as a risk factor for CV mortality in men: A meta-analytic study. *Eur J Endocrinol* 2011;165:687–701.

264. Malkin C, Pugh PJ, Jones RD, Kapoor D, Channer KS, Jones TH. The effect of testosterone replacement on endogenous inflammatory cytokines and lipid profiles in hypogonadal men. *J Clin Endocrinol Metab* 2004;89(7):3313–3318.

265. Carminiti G, Volterrani M, Iellamo F et al. Effect of long-acting testosterone treatment on functional exercise capacity, skeletal muscle performance, insulin resistance, and baroreflex sensitivity in elderly patients with chronic heart failure a double-blind, placebo-controlled, randomized study. *J Amer Coll Cardiol* 2009;54(10):919–927.

266. Malkin C, Pugh PJ, West JN et al. Testosterone therapy in men with moderate severity heart failure: A double-blind randomized placebo controlled trial. *Eur Heart J* 2006;27:57–64.

267. Toma M, McAlister FA, Coglianese EE et al. Testosterone supplementation in heart failure: A meta-analysis. *Circulation* 2012;5:315–321.

268. Abbott R, Launer LJ, Rodriguez BL et al. Serum estradiol and risk of stroke in elderly men. *Neurology* 2007;68(8):563–568.

269. Tivesten A, Hulthe J, Wallenfeldt K et al. Circulating estradiol is an independent predictor of progression of carotid artery intima-media thickness in middle-aged men. *J Clin Endocrinol Met* 2006;91(11):4433–4437.

270. Mohamad M. Serum levels of sex hormones in men with acute myocardial infarction. *Neuro Endocrinol Lett* 2007;28(2):182–186.

271. Dunajska K, Milewicz A, Szymczak J. Evaluation of sex hormone levels and some metabolic factors in men with coronary atherosclerosis. *Aging Male* 2004;7(3):197–204.

272. Tivesten A, Mellström D, Jutberger H et al. Low serum testosterone and high serum estradiol associated with lower extremity peripheral arterial disease in elderly men. The MrOS Study in Sweden. *J Am Coll Cardiol* 2007;50(11):1070–1076.

273. Tripathi Y, Hegde BM. Serum estradiol and testosterone levels following acute myocardial infarction in men. *J Physiol Pharmacol* 1998;42(2):291–294.

274. Lerchbaum E, Pilz S, Grammer TB et al. High estradiol levels are associated with an increase in mortality in older men referred to coronary angiography. *Exp Clin Endocrinol Diabetes* 2011;119(8):490–496.

275. Sudhir K, Komesaroff PA. Clinical review 110: Cardiovascular actions of estrogens in men. *J Clin Endocrinol Metab* 1999;84(10):3411–3415.

276. Merchant S, Oliveira JL, Hoyer JD. Erythrocytosis. In: His E, editor. *Hematopathology*, 2nd Ed. Philadelphia, PA: Elsevier/Saunders; 2012.

277. Bassil, N, Alkaade S, Morley JE. The benefits and risk of testosterone replacement: A review. *Ther Clin Risk Manag* 2009;5:427–448.

278. Skogastiema C, Hotzen M, Rane A, Ekström L. A supraphysiological dose of testosterone induces nitric oxide production and oxidative stress. *Eur J Prev Cariol* 2013;21(8):1049–1054.

279. Cappola A. Testosterone therapy and risk of cardiovascular disease in men. *JAMA* 2013; 310(17): 1805–1806.

280. Death A, McGrath KC, Sader MA et al. DHT promotes vascular cell adhesion molecule-1 expression in male human endothelial cells via a nuclear factor-kappa-B-dependent pathway. *Endocrinology* 2004;145(4):1889–1897.

16 Consequences of Cardiovascular Drug-Induced Nutrient Depletion

James B. LaValle

CONTENTS

INTRODUCTION

One of the potential challenges facing health-care professionals today is the problem of drug-induced disease, especially drug-induced nutrient depletion (DIND). DIND in patients, including the cardiovascular (CV) patient, is a very important issue that the twenty-first-century clinician must become well versed in and consider implementing into practice. With approximately 48% of people in the United States taking prescription medications (up from 44% in the previous decade), patients with cardiovascular disease (CVD) are placed at a much higher risk for developing comorbid conditions and for increasing disease pathologies.[1] Polypharmacy prescribing is now occurring in younger and younger populations, so it is becoming increasingly important to assess nutrient depletion risks as they relate to increased drug side effects, future symptoms, comorbid condition development, or progression of the underlying disease itself.

In the medical management of individuals with CVD or comorbid conditions, several classes of prescription drugs may be employed with the potential for depletions of nutrients, which could induce metabolic changes, and further the progression of any component of the underlying CV problems or comorbidities.

It is of scientific interest and clinical concern that the reported side effects of some of these commonly used medications in patients are actually manifestations of drug-induced nutrient depletion of these same medications. Drugs can inhibit absorption, synthesis, transport, storage, metabolism, or excretion of essential nutrients. There are several factors that should be noted before discussing the relative impact of drug-induced depletions; whether a nutrient depletion will occur is a complex and multifactorial issue. Variations in diet, genetic differences, individual stress, and activity levels all contribute to the nutrition status of the individual before drug therapy is administered. Therefore, responses to drug therapy are highly individualized.

As an example, according to statistics over 22 million patients in the United States take β-blockers.[1] β-Blockers have been reported to reduce the production of melatonin via specific inhibition of β-1 adrenergic receptors.[2,3] Clinically, low levels of melatonin can lead to sleep disturbances, insulin resistance/impaired glucose tolerance, CV problems, increased CV events, immune imbalances, and increased oxidative stress and inflammation on various body systems.[4–6]

Several placebo-controlled studies have investigated the relationship between β-blocker-induced central nervous system (CNS) side effects and the nightly urinary excretion of melatonin via the inhibition of the release of the enzyme serotonin-N-acetyltransferase.[7,8] Results report that the CNS side effects (including sleep disorders and nightmares) during β-blocker therapy are related to a reduction of melatonin levels. Nighttime exogenous administration of melatonin as a dietary supplement is reported to reduce the incidence of β-blocker-induced sleep disturbances.[8,9]

It should be noted that melatonin is also reduced by the administration of nonsteroidal anti-inflammatory drugs (NSAIDs), commonly used in the CV patient with comorbid symptoms of joint/muscle pain. A recent cross-sectional, multicenter observational study of osteoarthritis patients reported that of the over 17,000 patients evaluated over 90% were at an increased risk of gastrointestinal (GI) and/or CV risk and that a large percentage of these patients (51%) were treated with an NSAID + a proton pump inhibitor (PPI).[10] It is of interest that PPI use, with PPIs being the most frequently prescribed drug in the United States, also is reported to increase the risk of hospitalization for a CV event by 51% and individual PPIs each significantly raise that risk as well, ranging from 39% to 61%.[11]

Coenzyme Q10 (ubiquinol) is also reported to be depleted by β-blocker therapy. β-Blocker use is reported to deplete CoQ10 by interfering with the production of this essential enzyme for energy production.[12] CoQ10 is important in CV function, including the production of cellular energy (adenosine triphosphate [ATP]) via the electron transport chain. Depletion of CoQ10 from the body is clinically associated with myopathy (including cardiomyopathy), rhabdomyolysis, hypertension, angina, stroke, cardiac dysrhythmias, fatigue, leg weakness, immune imbalances, neurodegenerative disease, and cognitive decline.[13] The use of β-blockers is also reported to increase the risk of hospitalization in the elderly (45% in those using propranolol) due to myopathy.[14]

It is also widely reported that CoQ10 levels are decreased in congestive heart failure (CHF) patients.[15,16] The use of β-blockers, although reported to deplete coenzyme Q10, is considered a standard of care in those with CHF. Use of oral CoQ10 is reported to improve functional capacity, endothelial function, and left ventricular (LV) contractility in CHF without side effects.[17] A 2013 meta-analysis reported that CoQ10 supplementation improved ejection fraction (EF) in those with CHF.[18] With the readmission rate of CHF patients within 6 months at approximately 30%–40%, supplementation with CoQ10 may be an appropriate choice for the clinicians and their patients.[19,20]

Also, genetic polymorphisms of substrates that metabolize CV medications may lead to specific nutrient depletions.[21] Only variations in vitamin K epoxide reductase complex subunit 1 (VKORC1) and CYP2C9 have consistently been associated with drug response (coumarins) that has clinical implications.

These polymorphisms include the following:

- Cyclooxygenase-1
- Vitamin D reductase complex subunit 1

- CYP2C9
- α-Adducin
- 3-Hydroxy-3-methylglutaryl-CoA reductase

POTENTIAL NUTRIENT DEPLETIONS: A REVIEW OF SIGNIFICANT FINDINGS

Rather than discussing the individual drugs used in the CV patient that may lead to nutrient depletion, a review of the principal nutrients depleted, their relationship to CVD and comorbid conditions, and the associated risks of nutrient depletion will be covered. Because these are chronic conditions, the drugs are used long term and patients are on several of these drug therapies for many years. It is important to remember that metabolic disturbances build over time with subtle disturbances in enzyme function leading to a cascade of metabolic disruption. Very often, patients display symptoms of a nutrient depletion. Rather than recommending the nutrients that may be depleted, polypharmacy-prescribing habits are often used, which can mask metabolic problems that have been brought about by drug therapy.

Part of patient management should be assessing the overall nutritional status of the individual. In assessing individuals for possible DINDs, the prescribed medications may have no known nutrient depletions; but signs and symptoms of nutrient deficiencies should always be assessed, regardless, because many lifestyle factors such as tobacco smoking and excessive and/or chronic alcohol intake can also influence nutrient depletions. Addressing nutritional deficiencies is a foundation to good health care and in a health-care environment where prevention is increasingly being mandated due to out of control health-care costs a very cost-efficient way to improve the overall health and well-being of the patient and to prevent further comorbidities.

Drugs commonly used in the CV patient that have the potential to lead to nutrient depletions are listed here. Table 16.1 further illustrates how these medications can affect the patient, with a listing of the drug's potential short- and long-term side effects, potential nutrient depletions, and some of the clinical effects often reported with the loss of one or more of these essential nutrients:

- Angiotensin II receptor blockers (ARBs) and angiotensin-converting enzyme (ACE) inhibitors
- Benzodiazepines
- β-Blockers
- Biguanides and sulfonylureas
- Cardiac glycosides
- Centrally acting antihypertensives
- Cholesterol management
- Diuretics (thiazide, loop, potassium sparing, etc.)
- GI management (antiulcer and antacids)
- Pain management (opiates, acetaminophen (APAP), salicylates, and NSAIDs)
- Potassium

MAGNESIUM

Magnesium is involved in over 300 enzymatic reactions in the body. It is needed for proper nerve transmission, production of energy, muscular activity, regulation of temperature, detoxification of cells, blood pressure regulation, regulation of blood sugar, and regulation of vasospasm, and it helps with the building of healthy bones and teeth. Appropriate magnesium levels are especially important for the CV patient, and low levels of magnesium are associated with an increased risk of heart disease.[80,81]

It is reported that the magnesium intake of approximately 75% of Americans is below the recommended dietary allowance (RDA).[82] In addition, many lifestyle factors such as stress and drinking alcohol can deplete magnesium, so it is easy to understand how with the addition of drug therapy a clinically significant low magnesium level can occur.

TABLE 16.1

Drugs Commonly Used in CV Patients that Have Reported Nutrient Depletions

Drug	Reported Potential Drug Side Effects (Short and Long Term)	Reported Potential Nutrient Depletion	Reported Potential Health Consequences of Nutrient Depletion
Cardiac glycosides[22,23] Digoxin (Lanoxin, Lanoxicap)	**Short term** Nausea/vomiting Diarrhea Fatigue Dry mouth Dizziness Visual disturbances Headache Low pulse rate **Long term** Rash Depression Irregular heart beat (arrhythmia) CV problems Gynecomastia (enlarging of breast in males) Increased bone fractures Increased risk for osteoporosis	Calcium Magnesium Phosphorus Vitamin B1 (Thiamine)	Osteoporosis, heart and blood pressure problems, back or leg pain, nervousness, tooth decay Muscle cramps, weakness, fatigue, insomnia, restless leg syndrome, irritability, anxiety, insulin resistance, depression, high blood pressure, CV problems, headaches Decreases calcium absorption, osteoporosis, brittle bones Depression, irritability, memory loss/confusion, indigestion, weight loss/anorexia, swelling, muscle weakness, irregular heartbeat, fatigue, numbness, and tingling
β-Blockers[12,8,9] Propranolol (Inderal, Inderal LA) Metolprolol (Lopressor, Toprol, Toprol XL) Atenolol (Tenormin) Pindolol (Visken) Bisoprolol (Monocor, Visken–w/HCTZ) Carvedilol (Coreg) Esmolol (Brevibloc) Labetelol (Normodyne) Naldolol (Corgard)	**Short term** Nausea/vomiting Diarrhea Fatigue Dry mouth Dizziness Visual disturbances Headache Sexual side effects Dyspnea Insomnia Nightmares	CoQ10	Hypertension CHF Muscular fatigue, weakness Joint and muscle aches Rhabdomyolysis Decreased cognitive function/memory loss Gingivitis Arrhythmia Imbalanced immunity Insulin resistance/impaired glucose tolerance

Drug	Nutrient depleted	Symptoms	Consequences
β-Blockers[1,8,9] (continued) Sotalol (Betapace) Timolol (Blocadren) Nebivolol (Bystolic) Nebivolol (Bystolic)	Melatonin	Arrhythmia **Long term** Depression Sexual side effects Decreased HDL Fatigue Blood glucose imbalances Increased risk of type II diabetes Increased risk of myocardial infarction/stroke	Sleep disturbances; insulin resistance/impaired glucose tolerance, CV problems, imbalanced immune system; increased cancer risk, increased oxidative stress in the brain, decreased seizure threshold
Thiazide diuretics[24–31] HCTZ, HydroDiuril Methclothiazide (Enduron) Indapamide (Lozol) Metolazone (Zaroxolyn)	CoQ10	**Short term** Nervousness/anxiousness Fatigue Increased urinary voiding Diarrhea Dizziness Loss of appetite Nausea/vomiting Headache Dry mouth and mucous membranes Constipation	High blood pressure CHF Muscular/joint fatigue/weakness Rhabdomyolysis Memory loss Gingivitis Irregular heartbeat Decreased immunity Insulin resistance
	Magnesium	**Long term** Arrhythmia	Muscle cramps Weakness Fatigue Insomnia Restless leg syndrome Irritability Anxiety Insulin resistance depression High blood pressure

(Continued)

Nutritional and Integrative Strategies in Cardiovascular Medicine

TABLE 16.1   (Continued)
Drugs Commonly Used in CV Patients that Have Reported Nutrient Depletions

Drug	Reported Potential Drug Side Effects (Short and Long Term)	Reported Potential Nutrient Depletion	Reported Potential Health Consequences of Nutrient Depletion
Thiazide diuretics[24-31] (continued) HCTZ, HydroDiuril Methclothiazide (Enduron) Indapamide (Lozol) Metolazone (Zaroxolyn)	Breathing difficulty Numbness/tingling in extremities Confusion Nervousness Fatigue Muscle cramps Mood changes Blurred vision Poor wound healing Lowered immunity Increased risk of osteoporosis CV problems Increased risk of birth defects	Phosphorus	CV problems, headaches Decreases calcium absorption, osteoporosis, brittle bones
		Potassium	Arrhythmia, poor reflexes, muscle weakness, fatigue, thirst, confusion, constipation, dizziness, nervousness
		Sodium	Muscle weakness, poor concentration, memory loss, dehydration, loss of appetite
		Zinc	Decreased immunity; decreased wound healing; smell and taste disturbances; anorexia; depression; night blindness; hair, skin, and nail problems; menstrual irregularities; joint pain; nystagmus (involuntary eye movements); insulin resistance
Loop diuretics[25,32-35] Bumetanide (Bumex) Ethacrynic acid (Edecrine) Furosemide (Lasix)		Calcium	Osteoporosis, heart and blood pressure problems, back or leg pain, nervousness, tooth decay
		Magnesium	Muscle cramps, weakness, fatigue, insomnia, restless leg syndrome, irritability, anxiety, insulin resistance, depression, high blood pressure, CV problems, headaches
		Potassium	Irregular heartbeat, poor reflexes, muscle weakness, fatigue, thirst, confusion, constipation, dizziness, nervousness
		Sodium	Muscle weakness, poor concentration, memory loss, dehydration, loss of appetite

Drug	Nutrient	
Loop diuretics[25,32-35] (continued) Bumetanide (Bumex) Ethacrynic acid (Edecrine) Furosemide (Lasix)	Vitamin B1 (thiamine)	Depression, irritability, memory loss/confusion, indigestion, weight loss/anorexia, swelling, muscle weakness, irregular heartbeat, fatigue, numbness, and tingling
	Vitamin B6 (pyridoxine)	Depression, sleep disturbances, nerve inflammation, premenstrual syndrome (PMS), lethargy, decreased alertness, anemia, altered mobility, elevated homocysteine, nausea, vomiting, and seborrheic dermatitis
	Vitamin C	Loss of antioxidant potential, increased capillary fragility, muscle weakness, poor wound healing, bleeding gums, anemia, poor appetite, tender and swollen joints
	Zinc	Decreased immunity; decreased wound healing; smell and taste disturbances; anorexia; depression; night blindness; hair, skin, and nail problems; menstrual irregularities; joint pain; nystagmus (involuntary eye movements); insulin resistance
Potassium-sparing diuretics[34,36] Triamterene (Diurenium) Triamterene and HCTZ (Dyazide, Maxide) Spironolactone (Aldactone)	Calcium	Osteoporosis, heart and blood pressure problems, back or leg pain, nervousness, tooth decay
	Folic acid	Birth defects, cervical dysplasia, anemia, heart disease, elevated homocysteine, headaches, fatigue, insomnia, diarrhea, nausea, increased cancer risk, decreased methylation
	Short term Nervousness/anxiousness Fatigue Increased urinary voiding Dizziness Loss of appetite Nausea/vomiting Headache Dry mouth and mucous membranes	

(Continued)

TABLE 16.1 (Continued)
Drugs Commonly Used in CV Patients that Have Reported Nutrient Depletions

Drug	Reported Potential Drug Side Effects (Short and Long Term)	Reported Potential Nutrient Depletion	Reported Potential Health Consequences of Nutrient Depletion
Potassium–sparing diuretics[34,36] (continued) Triamterene (Diurenium) Triamterene and HCTZ (Dyazide, Maxide) Spironolactone (Aldactone)	Constipation **Long term** Arrhythmia Breathing difficulty Numbness/tingling in extremities Confusion Nervousness Fatigue Muscle cramps Mood changes Blurred vision Poor wound healing Lowered immunity Increased risk of osteoporosis CV problems Increased risk of birth defects Diarrhea	Zinc	Decreased immunity; decreased wound healing; smell and taste disturbances; anorexia; depression; night blindness; hair, skin, and nail problems; menstrual irregularities; joint pain; nystagmus (involuntary eye movements); insulin resistance
Miscellaneous diuretics[29,37] Chlorthalidone (Hygroton, Thalidone)	**Short term** Nervousness/anxiousness Fatigue Increased urinary voiding Diarrhea Dizziness Loss of appetite Nausea/vomiting Headache Dry mouth and mucous membranes	Magnesium	Muscle cramps, weakness, fatigue, insomnia, restless leg syndrome, irritability, anxiety, insulin resistance, depression, high blood pressure, CV problems, headaches
		Phosphorus	Decreases calcium absorption, osteoporosis, brittle bones

Drug	Side effects	Nutrient depleted	Consequences of nutrient depletion
Miscellaneous diuretics[29,37] (continued) Chlorthalidone (Hygroton, Thalidone)	Constipation **Long term** Arrhythmia Breathing difficulty Numbness/tingling in extremities Confusion Nervousness Fatigue Muscle cramps Mood changes Blurred vision Poor wound healing Lowered immunity Increased risk of osteoporosis CV problems Increased risk of birth defects	Potassium	Arrhythmia, poor reflexes, muscle weakness, fatigue, thirst, confusion, constipation, dizziness, nervousness
		Sodium	Muscle weakness, poor concentration, memory loss, dehydration, loss of appetite
		Zinc	Decreased immunity; decreased wound healing; smell and taste disturbances; anorexia; depression; night blindness; hair, skin, and nail problems; menstrual irregularities; joint pain; nystagmus; insulin resistance
ACE inhibitors[38,39] Captopril (Capoten) Enalapril (Vasotec) Lisinopril (Zestril, Prinivil) Ramipril (Altace)	**Short term** Facial flushing Nausea/vomiting Headache Cough Insomnia Nasal congestion Sexual dysfunction **Long term** Edema Hypotension Kidney problems Increased potassium levels, which can lead to arrhythmias Immune imbalances	Zinc	Decreased immunity; decreased wound healing; smell and taste disturbances; anorexia; depression; night blindness; hair, skin, and nail problems; menstrual irregularities; joint pain; nystagmus (involuntary eye movements); insulin resistance
		Sodium	Muscle weakness, poor concentration, memory loss, dehydration, loss of appetite

(Continued)

TABLE 16.1 (Continued)
Drugs Commonly Used in CV Patients that Have Reported Nutrient Depletions

Drug	Reported Potential Drug Side Effects (Short and Long Term)	Reported Potential Nutrient Depletion	Reported Potential Health Consequences of Nutrient Depletion
ARBs (angiotensin II receptor antagonists)[40,41]		Zinc	Decreased immunity; decreased wound healing; smell and taste disturbances; anorexia; depression; night blindness; hair, skin, and nail problems; menstrual irregularities; joint pain; nystagmus (involuntary eye movements); insulin resistance
Losartan (Cozaar)	**Short term**		
Valsartan (Diovan)	Facial flushing		
Telmisartan (Micardis)	Nausea/vomiting		
Irbesartan (Avapro)	Headache		
Azilsartan (Edarbi)	Cough		
Olmesartan (Benicar)	Insomnia		
	Nasal congestion		
	Sexual dysfunction		
	Long term		
	Swelling (edema)		
	Low blood pressure (hypotension)		
	Kidney problems		
	Increased potassium levels, which can lead to irregular heartbeat (arrhythmias)		
	Immune imbalances		
Centrally acting antihypertensive drugs[24]	**Short term**	CoQ10	Hypertension, CHF, muscular fatigue, joint and muscle aches, rhabdomyolysis, memory loss, gingivitis, muscle weakness, arrhythmia, imbalanced immunity, insulin resistance
Clonidine (Catapres)	Nausea/vomiting		
Methyldopa (Aldomet)	Drowsiness		
	Sedation		
	Fatigue		
	Dry mouth		
	Sexual side effects		
	Nasal congestion		
	Long term		
	Fever		
	Blood sugar regulation problems		

Drug	Symptoms	Nutrient depleted	Consequences of depletion
Centrally acting antihypertensive drugs[24] (continued) Clonidine (Catapres) Methyldopa (Aldomet)	CV problems Psychotic reactions Depression Liver damage Anemia		
HMG-CoA reductase inhibitors[13,42–48] Atorvastatin (Lipitor) Lovastatin (Mevacor, Altocor) Fluvastatin (Lescol) Pravastatin (Pravachol) Simvastatin (Zocor)	**Short term** Nausea/vomiting Diarrhea Gas/bloating Blurred vision Constipation Heartburn Headache Dizziness **Long term** Elevated liver enzymes Muscle pain/weakness Memory loss Kidney failure	CoQ10	High blood pressure, CHF, fatigue, gingivitis, muscle weakness, irregular heartbeat, decreased immunity
		Vitamin E	Dry skin, dry hair, anemia, easy bruising, PMS, eczema, dermatitis, psoriasis, muscle weakness, decreased antioxidant capacity, poor wound healing/impaired immunity
		Vitamin D	Osteoporosis, increased risk of skeletal fractures, hearing difficulties, depression, hormonal imbalances, muscular weakness, hypertension, autoimmune diseases, multiple sclerosis, diabetes, schizophrenia, and decrease immunity
		Carnitine	Elevated blood lipids, abnormal liver function, muscle weakness, fatigue, blood sugar imbalances, increased risk of CVD
		Omega-3 fatty acids	Neurochemical imbalances, skin disorders, chronic inflammation, heart and blood vessel disorders, immune imbalances, autoimmune conditions, memory and cognitive impairment, joint and muscle pain, insulin resistance and increased risk of type II diabetes, increased risk of cancer
		Zinc	Decreased immunity; decreased wound healing; smell and taste disturbances; anorexia; depression; night blindness; hair, skin, and nail problems; menstrual irregularities; joint pain; nystagmus (involuntary eye movements); insulin resistance

(Continued)

TABLE 16.1 (*Continued*)
Drugs Commonly Used in CV Patients that Have Reported Nutrient Depletions

Drug	Reported Potential Drug Side Effects (Short and Long Term)	Reported Potential Nutrient Depletion	Reported Potential Health Consequences of Nutrient Depletion
HMG-CoA (*continued*) reductase inhibitors[13,42–48] Atorvastatin (Lipitor) Lovastatin (Mevacor, Altocor) Fluvastatin (Lescol) Pravastatin (Pravachol) Simvastatin (Zocor)		Selenium	Decreased antioxidant protection, muscle aches, decreased immunity, red blood cell fragility, fatigue, anemia, and decreased conversion of T4 to T3
		Copper	Hair color loss, anemia, fatigue, low body temperature, CV problems, nervous system disorders, decreased immunity
		Testosterone	Increased mortality in men with CHD Insomnia Insulin resistance/impaired glucose tolerance Obesity Type II diabetes Thyroid hormone imbalances Alzheimer's disease Osteoporosis/decreased bone mineral density Immune imbalances
Bile acid sequestrants[49,50] Cholestyramine (Questran)	**Short term** Nausea/vomiting Diarrhea Gas/bloating Blurred vision Constipation Heartburn Headache Dizziness Loss of appetite Anxiety/nervousness	β-Carotene (vitamin A)	Decreased immunity, night blindness, dry skin, brittle nails
		Calcium	Osteoporosis, heart and blood pressure problems, back or leg pain, nervousness, tooth decay
		Folic acid	Birth defects, cervical dysplasia, anemia, heart disease, elevated homocysteine, headaches, fatigue, insomnia, diarrhea, nausea, increased cancer risk, decreased methylation

	Long term		
Bile acid sequestrants[49,50] (continued) Cholestyramine (Questran)	Elevated liver enzymes Muscle pain/weakness Memory loss Kidney failure Increased risk of osteoporosis Increased risk of bleeding Increased risk of night blindness Increased tooth decay	Iron	Anemia, fatigue, hair loss, brittle nails, decreased thyroid hormone production
		Magnesium	Muscle cramps, weakness, fatigue, insomnia, restless leg syndrome, irritability, anxiety, insulin resistance, depression, high blood pressure, CV problems, headaches
		Phosphorus	Decreases calcium absorption, osteoporosis, brittle bones
		Vitamin B12	Fatigue, peripheral neuropathy, macrocytic anemia, depression, memory loss/confusion, easy bruising, loss of appetite, nausea, vomiting, increased CVD risk, increased homocysteine levels, decreased methylation
		Vitamin D	Osteoporosis, increased risk of skeletal fractures, hearing difficulties, depression, hormonal imbalances, muscular weakness, hypertension, autoimmune diseases, multiple sclerosis, diabetes, schizophrenia, and decrease immunity
		Vitamin E	Dry skin, dry hair, anemia, easy bruising, PMS, eczema, dermatitis, psoriasis, muscle weakness, decreased antioxidant capacity, poor wound healing/impaired immunity
		Vitamin K	Easy bleeding, osteoporosis, and brittle bones
		Zinc	Decreased immunity; decreased wound healing; smell and taste disturbances; anorexia; depression; night blindness; hair, skin, and nail problems; menstrual irregularities; joint pain; nystagmus (involuntary eye movements); insulin resistance

(Continued)

TABLE 16.1 (Continued)
Drugs Commonly Used in CV Patients that Have Reported Nutrient Depletions

Drug	Reported Potential Drug Side Effects (Short and Long Term)	Reported Potential Nutrient Depletion	Reported Potential Health Consequences of Nutrient Depletion
Colestipol (Colestid, Welchol)[51,52]	**Short term** Nausea/vomiting Diarrhea	β-Carotene (vitamin A)	Decreased immunity, night blindness, dry skin, brittle nails
	Gas/bloating Blurred vision Constipation Heartburn Headache Dizziness Fatigue Loss of appetite Anxiety/nervousness	Folic acid	Birth defects, cervical dysplasia, anemia, heart disease, elevated homocysteine, headaches, fatigue, insomnia, diarrhea, nausea, increased cancer risk
		Iron	Anemia, fatigue, hair loss, brittle nails
	Long term Anemia CV problems Irregular heartbeat (arrhythmia) Musculoskeletal pain	Vitamin B12	Fatigue, peripheral neuropathy, macrocytic anemia, depression, memory loss/confusion, easy bruising, loss of appetite, nausea, vomiting, increased CVD risk, increased homocysteine levels, decreased methylation
		Vitamin E	Dry skin, dry hair, anemia, easy bruising, PMS, eczema, dermatitis, psoriasis, muscle weakness, decreased antioxidant capacity, poor wound healing/impaired immunity
		CoQ10	High blood pressure, CHF, muscular fatigue, joint and muscle aches, rhabdomyolysis, memory loss, gingivitis, muscle weakness, irregular heartbeat, decreased immunity, insulin resistance

Drug	Nutrient	Consequences	Side effects
Fibrates[47,53] Fenofibrate (Tricor) Gemfibrozil (Lopid)	Vitamin E	Dry skin, dry hair, anemia, easy bruising, PMS, eczema, dermatitis, psoriasis, muscle weakness, decreased antioxidant capacity, poor wound healing/ impaired immunity	**Short term** Headache Abdominal pain Nausea/vomiting Muscle aches Flu-like symptoms Asthenia Diarrhea Constipation Abnormal liver function tests **Long term** Respiratory problems Albuminuria Pancreatitis Retinopathy Pulmonary embolism Anemia
	CoQ10	High blood pressure, CHF, muscular fatigue, joint and muscle aches, rhabdomyolysis, memory loss, gingivitis, muscle weakness, irregular heartbeat, decreased immunity, insulin resistance	
	Vitamin D	Osteoporosis, increased risk of skeletal fractures, hearing difficulties, depression, hormonal imbalances, muscular weakness, hypertension, autoimmune diseases, multiple sclerosis, schizophrenia, and decrease immunity	
	DHEA	Increased risk of developing type II diabetes, heart disease, cancer, osteoporosis, depression, obesity, decreased immune function, loss of strength and muscle mass and memory problems like Alzheimer's disease, high blood pressure, elevated cholesterol levels, increased platelet aggregation, increased risk of thrombosis	
Miscellaneous cholesterol-lowering drugs[54] Ezetimibe (Zetia)	Vitamin D	Osteoporosis, increased risk of skeletal fractures, hearing difficulties, depression, hormonal imbalances, muscular weakness, hypertension, autoimmune diseases, multiple sclerosis, schizophrenia, and decrease immunity	**Short term** Diarrhea Fatigue Joint pain Upper respiratory tract infections Sinus infection **Long term** Gallstones Muscle weakness Muscle breakdown/myopathy Liver problems

(Continued)

TABLE 16.1 (*Continued*)
Drugs Commonly Used in CV Patients that Have Reported Nutrient Depletions

Drug	Reported Potential Drug Side Effects (Short and Long Term)	Reported Potential Nutrient Depletion	Reported Potential Health Consequences of Nutrient Depletion
Salicylates[55]	**Short term**	Folic acid	Birth defects, cervical dysplasia, anemia, heart disease, elevated homocysteine, headaches, fatigue, insomnia, diarrhea, nausea, increased cancer risk, decreased methylation
Aspirin	GI ulcers		
Choline and magnesium salicylates (Tricosal, Trilisate)	Abdominal burning/pain/cramping		
	Nausea		
	Vomiting		
	Ringing in the ears (tinnitus)		
	Dizziness	Iron	Anemia, fatigue, hair loss, brittle nails, decreased thyroid hormone production
	Rash		
	Long term		
	Fatigue		
	Liver and kidney damage	Potassium	Irregular heartbeat, poor reflexes, muscle weakness, fatigue, thirst, confusion, constipation, dizziness, nervousness
	Black tarry stools		
	GI bleeding		
	Intestinal damage		
	Increased risk of birth defects		
		Sodium	Muscle weakness, poor concentration, memory loss, dehydration, loss of appetite
NSAIDs COX inhibitors[56–58]	**Short term**	Folic acid	Birth defects, cervical dysplasia, anemia, heart disease, elevated homocysteine, headaches, fatigue, insomnia, diarrhea, nausea, increased cancer risk, decreased methylation
Including Diclofenac (Cataflam, Voltaren)	GI ulcers		
Diflunisal (Dolobid)	Abdominal burning/pain/cramping		
Etodolac (Lodine, Lodine XL)	Nausea/vomiting		
Fenoprofen calcium (Nalfon)	Diarrhea		
Flurbiprofen (Ansaid)	Constipation		
Ibuprofen (Advil, Motrin)	Edema		

Drug	Side effects	Nutrient depleted	Consequences of depletion
Ketoprofen (Actron, Orudis, Orudis KT, Oruvail) Meclofenamate sodium (Meclomen) Mefenamic acid (Ponstel) Meloxicam (Mobic) Nabumetone (Relafen) Naproxen (Alleve, Naprosyn) Oxaprozin (Daypro) Piroxicam (Feldene) Sulindac (Clinoril) Tolmetin sodium (Tolectin)	Dizziness Sleep disturbances Rash Apnea (especially asthmatics) **Long term** Fatigue Liver and kidney damage GI bleeding Intestinal damage/dysbiosis Increased risk of birth defects	Melatonin	Sleep disturbances that may lead to insulin resistance and CV problems and a weakened immune system; increased cancer risk, increased oxidative stress in the brain, decreased seizure threshold
		Sodium	Muscle weakness, poor concentration, memory loss, dehydration, loss of appetite
		Zinc	Decreased immunity; decreased wound healing; smell and taste disturbances; anorexia; depression; night blindness; hair, skin, and nail problems; menstrual irregularities; joint pain; nystagmus (involuntary eye movements); insulin resistance
		DHEA	Fatigue, weight gain, depression, bone loss, musculoskeletal pain, immune imbalances, sleep disturbances
Opiate pain medications[59] Morphine Hydrocodone (Lortab, Vicodin) Oxycodone (Percocet, Percodan, Oxycontin) Meperidine (Demerol) Codeine	**Short term** Euphoria Fatigue Somnolence **Long term** Liver and kidney damage Sleep disturbances Musculoskeletal pain Immune imbalances Fatigue Bone loss	DHEA	Fatigue, weight gain, depression, bone loss, musculoskeletal pain, immune imbalances, sleep disturbances

(*Continued*)

TABLE 16.1 (*Continued*)
Drugs Commonly Used in CV Patients that Have Reported Nutrient Depletions

Drug	Reported Potential Drug Side Effects (Short and Long Term)	Reported Potential Nutrient Depletion	Reported Potential Health Consequences of Nutrient Depletion
Acetaminophen (Tylenol)[60,61]	**Short term** Liver toxicity Increased oxidative stress Increased sweating Nausea/vomiting Abdominal pain Gas/bloating **Long term** Liver damage Death from liver damage Anemia Fatigue Kidney damage CV problems Itching, dry skin Increased sweating Irritability/mood swings Confusion	Glutathione	Decreased antioxidant capacity, liver damage, sweating, fatigue, decreased immunity, hair loss, dry skin, itching
Biguanides[62–65] Metformin (Glucophage)	**Short-term** Diarrhea Dizziness Drowsiness Fatigue Anxiety Headache Nausea Weight gain/hunger increase	CoQ10	High blood pressure, CHF, muscle fatigue, joint and muscle aches, rhabdomyolysis, memory loss, gingivitis, muscle weakness, irregular heartbeat, decreased immunity, insulin resistance

Drug	Nutrient depleted	Consequences	Side effects
Biguanides[62-65] Metformin (Glucophage)	Folic acid	Birth defects, cervical dysplasia, anemia, heart disease, elevated homocysteine, headaches, fatigue, insomnia, diarrhea, nausea, increased cancer risk, decreased methylation	Fullness Heartburn Gas/bloating Hypoglycemia Edema (swelling) Long term Hypoglycemia Muscle weakness Tremor
	Vitamin B12	Fatigue, peripheral neuropathy, macrocytic anemia, depression, memory loss/confusion, easy bruising, loss of appetite, nausea, vomiting, increased CVD risk, decreased methylation	
Sulfonylureas[63] Glimepiride (Amaryl) Glipizide (Glucotrol) Glyburide (Diabeta, Glynase, Micronase) Tolbutamide (Orinase) Tolazamide (Tolinase)	CoQ10	Hypertension CHF, muscular and joint aches/fatigue Rhabdomyolysis Memory loss Gingivitis Imbalanced immunity insulin resistance/impaired glucose tolerance	**Short term** Dizziness Drowsiness Fatigue Anxiety Headache Nausea Weight gain/hunger increase Fullness Heartburn Gas/bloating Hypoglycemia Edema (swelling) **Long term** Hypoglycemia Muscle weakness Tremor Sleep disturbances Depression Arrhythmias CV problems

(Continued)

TABLE 16.1 (Continued)
Drugs Commonly Used in CV Patients that Have Reported Nutrient Depletions

Drug	Reported Potential Drug Side Effects (Short and Long Term)	Reported Potential Nutrient Depletion	Reported Potential Health Consequences of Nutrient Depletion
Potassium, timed release[66] Micro K, Klor-Con, Kaon CL, others	**Short term** Nausea/vomiting Gas/bloating Abdominal pain Diarrhea **Long term** Muscle cramps Weakness CV problems Swelling (edema) Dizziness Confusion	Vitamin B12	Fatigue, peripheral neuropathy, macrocytic anemia, depression, memory loss/confusion, easy bruising, loss of appetite, nausea, vomiting, increased CVD risk, elevated homocysteine levels, decreased methylation
Magnesium and aluminum antacids[67,68]	**Short term** Loss of appetite Diarrhea Constipation Nausea, vomiting **Long term** Mental confusion Osteoporosis, bone loss Weakness Irregular heartbeat Sleep disturbances Increased risk of birth defects	Calcium Folic acid Phosphorus	Osteoporosis, heart and blood pressure problems, back or leg pain, nervousness, tooth decay Birth defects, cervical dysplasia, anemia, heart disease, elevated homocysteine, headaches, fatigue, insomnia, diarrhea, nausea, increased cancer risk, decreased methylation Skeletal problems and anxiety or nervousness
H2 blockers[69–74] Cimetidine (Tagamet) Ranitidine (Zantac) Famotidine (Pepcid) Nizatidine (Axid)	**Short term** Diarrhea Constipation	Calcium	Osteoporosis, heart and blood pressure problems, back or leg pain, nervousness, tooth decay

Drug	Side effects	Nutrient depleted	Consequences of depletion
H2 blockers[69-74] *(continued)* Cimetidine (Tagamet) Ranitidine (Zantac) Famotidine (Pepcid) Nizatidine (Axid)	Dizziness Headaches Runny nose Weakness **Long term** Irregular heartbeat (arrhythmia) Depression Liver damage Swelling (edema) Sexual dysfunction Confusion	Folic acid	Birth defects, cervical dysplasia, anemia, heart disease, elevated homocysteine, headaches, fatigue, insomnia, diarrhea, nausea, increased cancer risk, decreased methylation
		Iron	Anemia, fatigue, hair loss, brittle nails, decreased thyroid hormone
		Vitamin B12	Fatigue, peripheral neuropathy, macrocytic anemia, depression, memory loss/confusion, easy bruising, loss of appetite, nausea, vomiting, increased CVD risk, decreased methylation
		Vitamin D	Osteoporosis, increased risk of skeletal fractures, hearing difficulties, depression, hormonal imbalances, muscular weakness, hypertension, autoimmune diseases, multiple sclerosis, type I diabetes, schizophrenia, and decrease immunity
		Zinc	Decreased immunity; decreased wound healing; smell and taste disturbances; anorexia; depression; night blindness; hair, skin, and nail problems; menstrual irregularities; joint pain; nystagmus (involuntary eye movements); insulin resistance
PPIs[75-78] Lansoprazole (Prevacid) Omeprazole (Prilosec) Pantoprazole (Protonix) Rabeprazole (Aciphex) Esomeprazole (Nexium)	**Short term** Diarrhea Constipation Dizziness Headaches Abdominal pain	Calcium	Osteoporosis, heart and blood pressure problems, back or leg pain, nervousness, tooth decay
		Folic acid	Birth defects, cervical dysplasia, anemia, heart disease, elevated homocysteine, headaches, fatigue, insomnia, diarrhea, nausea, increased cancer risk, decreased methylation

(Continued)

TABLE 16.1 (Continued)
Drugs Commonly Used in CV Patients that Have Reported Nutrient Depletions

Drug	Reported Potential Drug Side Effects (Short and Long Term)	Reported Potential Nutrient Depletion	Reported Potential Health Consequences of Nutrient Depletion
PPIs[75–78] (continued)	Nausea		
Lansoprazole (Prevacid)	**Long term**		
Omeprazole (Prilosec)	Increased risk of osteoporosis and bone fractures		
Pantoprazole (Protonix)	Depression		
Rabeprazole (Aciphex)	Weakness		
Esomeprazole (Nexium)	Numbness/tingling of hands/feet	Iron	Anemia, fatigue, hair loss, brittle nails, decreased thyroid hormone
	Increased risk of CVD	Sodium	Muscle weakness, poor concentration, memory loss, dehydration, loss of appetite
	Irregular heartbeat (arrhythmia)	Vitamin C	Loss of antioxidant potential, increased capillary fragility, muscle weakness, poor wound healing, bleeding gums, anemia, poor appetite, tender and swollen joints
	Immune imbalances	Vitamin D	Osteoporosis, increased risk of skeletal fractures, hearing difficulties, depression, hormonal imbalances, muscular weakness, hypertension, autoimmune diseases, multiple sclerosis, diabetes, schizophrenia, and decrease immunity
	Increased risk of insulin resistance/type II diabetes	Vitamin B12	Fatigue, peripheral neuropathy, macrocytic anemia, depression, memory loss/confusion, easy bruising, loss of appetite, nausea, vomiting, increased CVD risk, increased homocysteine levels, decreased methylation
	Increased risk of cancer	Magnesium	Muscle cramps, weakness, fatigue, insomnia, restless leg syndrome, irritability, anxiety, insulin resistance, depression, high blood pressure, CV problems, headaches

Benzodiazepines[79] Including Alprazolam (Xanax) Diazepam (Valium) Lorazepam (Ativan) Oxazepam (Serax)	**Short term** Loss of muscle coordination Dizziness Fatigue Drowsiness Blurred vision Upset stomach Mental fogginess Hangover effect Sleep disturbances Potential drug side effects **Long term** Tolerance and physical dependence Sleep disturbances Amnesia Vision changes Chest pain	Melatonin	Sleep disturbances that may lead to insulin resistance and CV problems and a weakened immune system; increased cancer risk, increased oxidative stress in the brain, decreased seizure threshold

Note: CHD, coronary heart disease; DHEA, dehydroepiandrosterone; HCTZ, hydrochlorothiazide.

Hypomagnesemia and low dietary intake of magnesium are strongly related to CV risk factors among known subjects with coronary artery disease, including increasing the proinflammatory/prooxidant status and an increased risk of ischemic heart disease.[83-86] Also, one of the most significant and least discussed nutrients depleted from first line drug therapy in hypertension is magnesium. A Japanese study of over 58,615 healthy men aged 40–79 years that lasted 14.7 years reported that increasing magnesium in the diet reduced CVD mortality risk by approximately 50%.[87]

In clinical practice, when patients are prescribed thiazide diuretics for hypertension typically only potassium depletion is addressed, with patients being advised to drink orange juice or eat a banana, which are rich sources of potassium. Often, no education in medical schools or allied health curriculums is given regarding the potential for magnesium depletion, despite the fact that many of the listed side effects of thiazide diuretics are also signs and symptoms of magnesium depletion. While this topic may be controversial in the literature,[88] enough studies have reported a magnesium-depleting effect from thiazides (one report in 2000 suggested that 20% of thiazide patients have hypomagnesemia[28]) to at least justify a screening for magnesium depletion symptoms among thiazide users.[30,89] This is especially true when it is considered that the clinical manifestations of hypomagnesemia can be so severe.

Deficiency of magnesium is associated with an increased incidence of atherosclerosis, hypertension, stroke, and myocardial infarction. Magnesium plays a role in inhibiting platelet aggregation, blood thinning, blocking calcium reuptake, relaxing blood vessels, and increasing oxygenation of the heart by improving contractility. Oral magnesium therapy is reported beneficial in patients with heart failure, in those undergoing cardiovascular surgery, in hypertensive patients needing improved endothelial function and in those needing improved myocardial function in general.[90-93]

It should be mentioned that serum magnesium is a poor measure of magnesium status because homeostatic mechanisms keep blood levels fairly constant by pulling magnesium from bone and other body tissues. It is often suggested that red blood cell (RBC) levels are a more reliable indicator of magnesium status.[94] However, some researchers state that midnormal magnesium levels could be indicative of an intracellular depletion. RBC levels of magnesium (RBC magnesium) should be 4.2–6.8 mg/dL for most individuals. Likewise, magnesium levels do not always correspond with magnesium utilization in the body. Serum magnesium levels of 1.7–2.2 mg/dL are appropriate for most individuals.

POTENTIAL SYMPTOMS OF MAGNESIUM DEFICIENCY

- Muscle cramps and spasms and vasomotor spasms
- Anxiousness, nervousness, and insomnia
- Hypertension and prehypertension
- Blood glucose imbalances/insulin resistance
- Depression/mood swings
- Fatigue
- Arrhythmias and dysrhythmias
- Migraines
- Constipation
- Osteoporosis/decreased bone density
- Kidney stones

CLINICAL MANIFESTATIONS OF MAGNESIUM DEFICIENCY

Even marginal magnesium deficiency can decrease myocardial magnesium, which can directly affect contractility and excitability of the heart. The mechanism of action of this result is primarily by the reduced regulation of calcium ion channel. Even perfusion of the heart can be easily compromised. Studies have reported that low magnesium can lead to coronary vasospasm, reduced energy metabolism, changes in potassium homeostasis, and excessive induction of free radical generation.[95] In an animal study demonstrating this principle, a diet low in magnesium and high in sucrose progressively induced elevations in triglycerides and a reduction of insulin binding to erythrocyte insulin receptors (increased insulin resistance) over a 3-month period.[96]

Many of the symptoms and conditions that develop, progress, and are prescribed for metabolic syndrome mimic the symptoms of magnesium depletion, primarily blood pressure regulation and blood sugar regulation. It should be noted that several of the listed side effects of thiazide diuretics are magnesium depletion symptoms, including arrhythmia, lower back pain, mood changes, muscle pain/weakness/cramps, constipation, headache, and fatigue.

An established potential consequence of long-term use of thiazide diuretics is development of type II diabetes and because of this their use is controversial in those predisposed to blood glucose dysregulation.[97] Medical literature is clearly establishing the role of magnesium in not only insulin regulation but also helping to control inflammatory chemistry.[98] Drug-induced intracellular depletion of magnesium could be playing a significant role in the rapid induction into the complications of metabolic syndrome. The clinical repletion dosage of magnesium as magnesium aspartate, citrate, or amino acid chelate is 300–800 mg/day. Larger dosages may induce loose stools, so titrate as magnesium aspartate, citrate, glycinate or amino acid chelate if needed.

COENZYME Q10 (COQ10)

One of the most frequently discussed depletions in DIND is the area of CoQ10 depletion and the use of statin (3-hydroxyl -3-methylglutaryl coenzyme A reductase inhibitors or HMG CoA reductase inhibitors) medications. This depletion can also occur in the use of HMG CoA reductase inhibitors, centrally acting antihypertensive agents, fibrates, diuretics, β-blockers, and second-generation sulfonylureas and biguanide drug therapies. It has been demonstrated that CoQ10 concentrations can fall as much as 54% in patients who are on HMG CoA reductase inhibitor therapy, with a dose-dependent drop in some patient populations.[99] Note that excessive and/or chronic alcohol consumption may also lead to CoQ10 depletion.[100]

CoQ10 is a cofactor in the electron transport chain, which is involved in cellular respiration and the generation of ATP. CoQ10 also plays an important role as an antioxidant and is a principal gene regulator in muscle tissue and plays a significant role in tissue metabolism. Clinical manifestations of CoQ10 depletion can include the following: myalgias, rhabdomyolysis, cardiomyopathy, hypertension, angina, stroke, cardiac dysrhythmias, fatigue, leg weakness, decline in immune function, increase in neurodegenerative diseases, and loss of cognitive function.

In one study, muscle fibers were examined in an elderly population preparing for hip surgery.[101] The findings were as follows: CoQ10-treated individuals had a lower proportion of type I (slow twitch) fibers and a higher concentration of type IIb (fast twitch) fibers compared to age-matched placebo-treated patients. This shift is consistent with fiber composition found in younger populations. In this study, significant change in gene expression of proteins was noted. The protective and regenerative effect of CoQ10 on skeletal muscle is promising, and it may be theorized that low CoQ10 status could accelerate aging and genetic changes in muscle tissue.

Another area of clinical concern in the metabolic syndrome patient is the increased risk for Alzheimer's disease. Disruption in mitochondrial ATP and an increase in hydrogen peroxide is one mechanism by which amyloid β-peptide toxicity can take place. Disruptions in both glucose metabolism and increased free radical damage have been implicated in the development of Alzheimer's disease. In a promising study, isolated brain mitochondria from diabetic rats were treated with CoQ10. Treatment with CoQ10 attenuated the decreased oxidative phosphorylation efficiency and halted the hydrogen peroxide production induced by neurotoxic peptides. This indicates that CoQ10 treatment changed the mitochondrial alterations in the peptide amyloid beta (1-40), suggesting that it could play a role in altering the cellular energy deficits correlated to diabetes and the progression of Alzheimer's disease.[102] These findings suggest that it does not make sense to administer drugs that deplete CoQ10 without repletion when clearly mitochondrial energy deficits are involved in the progression to Alzheimer's disease.

The value of CoQ10 in hypertension was reported in one clinical trial where supplementing CoQ10 decreased systolic and diastolic blood pressures, decreased total cholesterol, and increased high-density lipoprotein (HDL) cholesterol.[103] In another trial, supplementation of CoQ10 enabled hypertensive patients to reduce their medications. A mean dose of 225 mg in 109 patients led to discontinuation of one to three medications in 51% of patients within 6 months (average time, 4.4 months); 80% of the individuals had been diagnosed for 9.2 years. Only 3% required the addition of one more drug.[104] In another study, it was reported that drug-related myopathy, which is a complaint of CoQ10 therapy, was shown to be associated with a mild decrease in CoQ10 without presenting a histochemical or mitochondrial myopathy or even morphological evidence of apoptosis in most patients examined. The net meaning of this is that significant cellular pathology may not exist and yet symptom expression could be likely.[105] Even though there may be no evidence of changes via creatine kinase concentrations, metabolic disruption of ATP production and cellular energetics is probable.

With several of the most common drugs used in metabolic syndrome depleting CoQ10 (including statins, β-blockers, biguanides, sulfonylureas, and thiazide diuretics), clinicians should consider the implications of chronic mild decreases of CoQ10 and their impact on the progression of the metabolic pathology as it relates to the CV component.

CoQ10 serum optimal reference range greater than 2.5 μg/mL. Recommended clinical dosage range for repletion of CoQ10 ranges from 30 to 300 mg/day of a solubilized form of coenzyme Q10. It should be noted that concomitant administration of CoQ10 supplements with anticoagulants such as warfarin is reported in several case studies to lead to decreased levels of the anticoagulant.[106,107] CoQ10 is chemically similar to the K vitamins, which may explain the interaction with warfarin.

CONDITIONS AND SYMPTOMS ASSOCIATED WITH COENZYME Q10 DEPLETION

- Myalgia
- Arthralgia
- Rhabdomyolysis
- Hypertension
- Angina
- Mitral valve prolapse
- Stroke
- Arrhythmias
- Cardiomyopathy
- Poor insulin production
- Low energy
- Gingivitis
- Weakened immunity

ZINC

Marginal zinc deficiencies are thought to be common in the United States. Because of zinc involvement in over 300 enzymatic reactions, the symptoms of deficiency can present itself in a wide array of physiological dysfunctions.

Conditions and diseases associated with zinc deficiency can include the following:

- Loss of taste and smell
- Poor wound healing
- Anorexia
- Alterations in immunity including cytokine and T killer cell function

- Depression
- Photophobia
- Night blindness
- Frequent infections
- Disorders of skin, hair, and nails
- Arthralgia
- Alteration in hormones including leptin, thyroid, and insulin
- Kidney disease
- Celiac sprue and inflammatory bowel disorders
- Malignant melanoma
- Alcoholism
- Macular degeneration
- Prostate disorders

Zinc is depleted by several medications used in CV treatment, including ARB and ACE inhibitors, statins and bile acid sequestrants, H2 blockers, thiazide, K-sparing and loop diuretics, and NSAIDs. One of the more significant findings related to zinc deficiency is the influence on mRNA and levels of cytokines on cell lines. Zinc deficiency decreased expression of interleukin (IL)-2 and interferon (IFN)-γ in the Th1 cell gene expression and upregulated tumor necrosis factor (TNF)-α, IL-1β, and IL-8 gene expression.[108] This study clearly demonstrated the effects of zinc on genetic expression of cytokines and that the expression was specific to immune cells. Extrapolated to humans, this would mean that zinc deficiency could increase the production of TNF-α, IL-1β, and IL-8, which is associated with the development of chronic conditions such as CVD, metabolic syndrome, cancer, and Alzheimer's disease.[109]

In addition, it has been shown that increased TNF-α induces insulin resistance and increased oxidative stress. Alterations in TNF-α have been associated with decreased HDL, increased low-density lipoprotein (LDL) and triglycerides, and increases in C-reactive protein. As insulin resistance is increased by diet, mineral deficiencies including deficiencies of magnesium and chromium, deficiency of vitamin D, stress, lack of exercise, or other factors, the increase in adipocyte-driven TNF-α expression could be exacerbated by zinc-deficient chemistry.[110] The dosage for repletion of zinc is 10–50 mg of zinc glycinate daily.

B12/FOLIC ACID

Vitamin B12 (cyanocobalamin) and folate (folic acid) are often discussed together. While the value of B12 for reduction of anemia and regulation of DNA and neurologic changes is well understood, there are specific issues that relate to the depletion of B12 and the progression of metabolic syndrome.

Depletion of folate and B12 can elevate homocysteine levels. In a trial published in the *European Journal of Endocrinology*, folate and B12 therapy was reported to reduce homocysteine levels, ameliorate insulin resistance, and help resolve endothelial dysfunction in patients with metabolic syndrome.[111] In the treatment group, folate 5 mg and B12 500 mcg/day for 1 month led to striking results. There was a reported decrease in homocysteine of 27.8%, significant decrease in insulin levels along with an improvement in endothelial dysfunction as evidenced by hyperemic vasodilatation of 29.8% and a decrease of dimethylarginine levels by 21.7%. Plasma homocysteine is clearly elevated and is used as a biomarker in metabolic syndrome. It is also an independent marker for the development of atherosclerotic disease. It is thought that folic acid facilitates and restores endothelial nitric oxide by acting as a hydrogen donor and an electron donor to tetrahydrobiopterin and through the lowering of total homocysteine along with B12 by the enhancement of remethylation.[112]

Ironically, metformin, commonly used in metabolic syndrome to prevent progression to type II diabetes mellitus and hypertension, is reported to deplete vitamin B12 and folate.[113,114] A study of 122 patients (59 taking metformin and 63 not taking the drug) reported that metformin administration was associated with B12 depletion and an increase in homocysteine and an increase in peripheral neuropathy symptoms.[115] Metformin-treated patients had depressed cobalamin (Cbl) levels and elevated fasting methylmalonic acid (MMA) and homocysteine (Hcy) levels. Clinical and electrophysiological measures identified more severe peripheral neuropathy in these patients with the cumulative metformin dose correlated strongly with these clinical and paraclinical group differences.

Homocysteine, IL-6, and C-reactive protein can express more dramatically in a *677T* mutation (methylene tetrahydrofolate reductase [MTHFR]), and this shows that innate immunity is involved when this cascade of atherosclerosis occurs in patients with diabetes mellitus who are genetically predisposed.[116] Depletion of folic acid from drug therapy in an individual with the *677T* mutation could accelerate the cascade of elevated homocysteine, increased IL-6, and increased C peptide that is associated with metabolic syndrome, CVD, and type II diabetes. In these individuals who are homozygous for the TT genotype of *677T* (MTHFR), supplementation with 6-methyltetrahydrofolate (5-MTHF) (1–5 mg daily) may be necessary to overcome genotypic barrier for the absorption of folic acid.

Depression is a common comorbidity in CVD and in metabolic syndrome.[117] Studies are reporting low folate levels, low B12, and elevated homocysteine levels that correlated with depression.[118,119]

Folate and B12 status should be evaluated in CV patients. The dosage to replenish folate is 400–800 mcg of methylfolate daily. The dosage to replenish B12 is 500–1500 mcg/day (methylcobalamin is more readily absorbed and bioavailable with oral administration).

CONDITIONS ASSOCIATED WITH FOLIC ACID DEPLETION

- Elevated homocysteine
- Depression
- Cervical dysplasia
- Breast and colon cancer
- Anemia
- Fatigue
- CVD
- Birth defects

VITAMIN D

Vitamin D is a fat-soluble vitamin; it is also called the "sunshine vitamin." It is estimated that 1 billion people worldwide have vitamin D deficiency or insufficiency.[120]

Vitamin D is best known for its regulation, along with parathyroid hormone, of calcium and phosphorus metabolism. Vitamin D is primarily produced in the skin from 7-dehydrocholesterol through solar ultraviolet radiation.[121] Additional sources include diet and oral supplementation. Independent of source, all vitamin D is converted in the liver to 25-hydroxyvitamin D, which is the major circulating form in the blood. The kidneys produce the final step to the active form 1,25-dihydroxyvitamin D. Most vitamin D is stored in the body as 25-hydroxyvitamin D 25(OH)-D.[121] Vitamin D receptors have been identified in virtually every tissue, including bone/connective tissues, kidney, heart, adrenal, stomach, liver, skin, breast, pancreatic, immune, brain, prostate, ovaries, and testes.[122] Appropriate levels of vitamin D are necessary for the health of bones/teeth; CV system, including blood pressure and vascular health; insulin production; inflammatory balance; immune balance; and mood/cognitive function.[123–128]

A large study that looked at school children and adolescents in the United States found that approximately 50.8 million had low levels of vitamin D.[129] Age, season, northern latitudes, liver and kidney function, obesity, poor dietary intake, dark skin tone, and certain medications (corticosteroids and phenytoin) all contribute to low vitamin D levels.[130]

Vitamin D is deposited into fat stores, where it becomes less available for use in the body. This is a suggested mechanism leading to insulin resistance.[131] Vitamin D also helps to improve immunity and has anti-inflammatory effects that may indirectly help to improve insulin sensitivity.[124] Blood sugar control in people with type II diabetes has a seasonal variation, being worse in the winter, which is in part explained by variation in exposure to sunlight and vitamin D levels.[132] Research suggests that low levels of vitamin D may contribute to or be a cause of metabolic syndrome with associated hypertension, obesity, diabetes, and CVD.[133]

Research suggests that low levels of vitamin D may contribute to or be a cause of metabolic syndrome with associated hypertension, obesity, diabetes, and heart disease.[133] In humans, low vitamin D has been strongly linked to heart and vascular problems including high blood pressure,[134] blood vessel problems,[135] atherosclerosis, heart attack, and stroke.[136–139] In addition, low vitamin D is linked to death associated with heart problems.[140] In a prospective observational study of adults older than 65 years participating in NHANES III, the risk of death was 45% lower in those with 25(OH)-D values greater than 40 ng/mL compared with those with values less than 10 ng/mL (hazard ratio [HR], 0.55; 95% confidence interval [CI], 0.34–0.88).[120]

Vitamin D deficiency is also linked to poor bone mineral density.[141] As stated, vitamin D deficiency is prevalent in the United States, with 60% of nursing home residents and 57% of hospitalized patients being vitamin D deficient.[142,143] Vitamin D supplementation has been reported to reduce bone fractures by at least 20% in individuals aged 65 years and older.[144] 1000–5000 IU orally of vitamin D3 (25-hydroxyvitamin D) daily may help to improve vitamin D levels. Optimal laboratory levels of 25-hydroxyvitamin D are 30–50 ng/mL.

MELATONIN

Melatonin is an endogenous hormone synthesized from the amino acid tryptophan and secreted by the pineal gland. Melatonin is an antioxidant and is involved in the natural diurnal rhythm of the sleep/wake cycle. Chronic depletion of melatonin can directly influence daily rhythm of glucose, reduction in glucose transporter 4 (GLUT 4) (the insulin-sensitive glucose transporter) levels, and suppression of insulin secretion.[145] The correlation may be that melatonin deficits lead to disrupted sleep and disrupted sleep can lead to increased insulin resistance. Melatonin also has significant antioxidant effects as it stimulates glutathione peroxidase, superoxide dismutase (SOD), and catalase as well as NO synthase. Melatonin is reported to reduce oxidative stress in diabetic populations.

An evaluation of the NHANES Survey revealed that people who slept 5 hours a night had a 73% increased risk of becoming obese versus those who slept 7–9 hours per night.[146] Trials conducted at Stanford University found that people who slept an average of <5 hours per night had a 15.5% decrease in leptin, an increase of 14.9% of ghrelin, and higher body mass indexes (BMIs), regardless of the exercise and diet habits of the participants.[147] So with loss of sleep, the net effect was appetite centers were upregulated, BMI was increased, and there was a shift in metabolic dysfunction toward metabolic syndrome. When melatonin levels are low, rapid eye movement (REM) sleep cycles are disturbed, leading to increased wakefulness throughout the night, and studies have shown that administering melatonin in the late evening hours was significantly more effective than placebo at increasing REM sleep.[148,149]

Under conditions of high stress, cortisol levels increase, leading to a state of hyperarousal. Studies are showing that disturbed sleep as a result of hyperarousal can lead to its own effects on metabolic function (increased TNF-α, increased IL-6, increased visceral fat storage, increased insulin resistance, etc.)[30] Other nutrient depletions such as reduced magnesium status and low folate status (decreased serotonin synthesis) can also be simultaneously acting on the sleep center and inducing hyperarousal. All of these add up to increase the risk for obesity, diabetes, and CV risk. Melatonin may enhance insulin-receptor kinase and insulin receptor substrate (IRS)-1 phosphorylation, which may improve insulin signaling and may actually counteract TNF-α-induced insulin resistance in type II and metabolic syndrome populations.[89] Lastly, melatonin seems to have a direct effect on inhibiting tumorigenesis. Melatonin helps to inhibit cellular proliferation and stimulated differentiation and apoptosis.[90] This is particularly interesting as people with insulin resistance and sleep disturbances are more prone to cancer due to elevations of insulin-like growth factor (IGF)-1 and increases in the immunologic shift toward chronic inflammatory chemistry leading to reduced activity of NK cells.

Because of its potential to disrupt sleep and lead to further problems such as increased appetite, weight gain, insulin resistance, and increased inflammatory chemistry, melatonin is an important nutrient to assess and administer if disrupted sleep is present. Cortisol levels should also be evaluated to determine if steps may be necessary to downregulate cortisol to further address hyperarousal as an underlying cause of insomnia. It is noted that 3–15 mg of melatonin 1 hour before bedtime can help alleviate the symptoms of insomnia.

CONCLUSION

After reading this chapter, it should be evident that nutrient depletions from many drug therapies used in the CV patient can have a profound effect on the progression of the diseases and the development of new co-morbidities. Dysregulation of metabolic pathways should be evaluated to determine if nutrient depletions could be an underlying cause. This may help to resolve common comorbidities in CV patients, including restless leg syndrome, insomnia, low energy or depression, sexual dysfunction, and weight gain or to determine if medication side effects could be linked to a nutrient depletion. Because many of the marginal nutrient deficiencies do not show up on traditional laboratory tests, the patient is left with another prescription to fill and/or a decreased quality of life. Testing for nutrient deficiencies and then providing for these deficiencies in the form of vitamins, minerals, and other dietary supplements are relatively inexpensive and can provide significant margins of safety. They not only offer a solution to many of the comorbidities but also can reduce further progression of illness and improve patient quality of life.

As taught in didactic training, vitamins, minerals, amino acids, and essential fatty acids are needed by every cell of the body for proper function and maintenance of homeostasis. With depletion or genetic variation, metabolic consequences could lead to the initiation of chronic illness. Modern drug therapy and the emerging science of natural therapeutics together provide an integrative approach to management of chronic diseases as well as the best approach for prevention and wellness.

REFERENCES

1. Centers for Disease Control (CDC). www.cdc.gov (accessed March 2014).
2. Munoz-Hoyos A, Hubber E, Escames G et al. Effect of propranolol plus exercise on melatonin and growth hormone levels in children with growth delay. *J Pineal Res* 2001;30(2):75–81.
3. Stoschizky K, Sakotnik A, Lercher P et al. Influence of beta-blockers on melatonin release. *Eur J Clin Pharmacol* 1999;55(2):111–115.
4. Nishida S. Metabolic effects of melatonin on oxidative stress and diabetes. *Endocrine* 2005;27(2):131–136.
5. Dominguez-Rodriguez A. Melatonin in cardiovascular disease. *Expert Opin Investig Drugs* 2012; 21(11):1593–1596.
6. Dominguez-Rodriguez A, Abreu-Gonzalez IP, Sanchez-Sanchez JJ et al. Melatonin and circadian biology in human cardiovascular disease. *J Pineal Res* 2010;49(1):14–22.
7. Brismar K, Mogensen L, Wetterberg L. Depressed melatonin secretion in patients with nightmares due to beta-adrenoceptor blocking drugs. *Acta Med Scand* 1987;221:155–158.
8. Scheer FA, Morris CJ, Garcia JL et al. Repeated melatonin supplementation improves sleep in hypertensive patients treat with beta-blockers: A randomized controlled trial. *Sleep* 2012;35(10):1395–1402.
9. Fares A. Night-time exogenous melatonin administration may be a beneficial treatment for sleeping disorders in beta blocker patients. *J Cardiovasc Dis Res* 2011;2(3):153–155.

10. Lanas A, Garcia-Tell G, Armada B et al. Prescription patterns and appropriateness of NSAID therapy according to gastrointestinal risk and cardiovascular history in patients with diagnosis of osteoarthritis. *BMC Med* 2011;9:38.
11. Mahabaleshwarkar RK, Yang Y, Datar MV et al. Risk of adverse cardiovascular outcomes and all-cause mortality associated with concomitant use of clopidogrel and proton pump inhibitors in elderly patients. *Curr Med Res Opin* 2013;29(4):315–323.
12. Kishi T, Watanabe T, Folkers K. Bioenergetics in clinical medicine XV: Inhibition of coenzyme Q10-enzymes by clinically used adrenergic blockers of beta-receptors. *Res Commun Chem Pathol Pharmacol* 1977;17:157–164.
13. Potgieter M, Pretorius E, Pepper MS. Primary and secondary coenzyme Q10 deficiency: The role of therapeutic supplementation. *Nutr Rev* 2013;71(3):180–188.
14. Setoguchi S, Higgins JM, Mogun H et al. Propranolol and the risk of hospitalized myopathy: Translating chemical genomics findings into population-level hypotheses. *Am Heart J* 2010;159(3):428–433.
15. Fumagalli S, Fattirolli F, Guarducci L et al. Coenzyme Q10 terclatrate and creatinine in chronic heart failure: A randomized, placebo-controlled, double blind study. *Clin Cardiol* 2011;34(4):211–217.
16. Langsjoen PH, Langsjoen AM. Supplemental ubiquinol in patients with advanced congestive heart failure. *Biofactors* 2008;32(1–4):119–128.
17. Belardinelli R, Mucai A, Lacalaprice F et al. Coenzyme Q10 and exercise training in chronic heart failure. *Eur Heart J* 2006;27(22):2675–2681.
18. Fotino AD, Thompson-Paul AM, Bazzano LA. Effect of coenzyme Q10 supplementation on heart failure: A meta-analysis. *Am J Clin Nutr* 2013;97(2):268–275.
19. Hoyt R, Bowling LS. Reducing readmissions for congestive heart failure. *Am Fam Physician* 2001;63(8):1593–1599.
20. Molyneux SL, Florkowski CM, Richards AM et al. Coenzyme Q10: An adjunctive therapy for congestive heart failure? *N Z Med J* 2009;122(1305):74–79.
21. Johnson JA, Humma LM. Pharmacogenetics of cardiovascular drugs. *Brief Funct Genomic Proteomic* 2002;1(1):66–79.
22. Kupfer S, Kosovsky JD. Effects of cardiac glycosides on renal tubular transport of calcium, magnesium, inorganic phosphate and glucose in the dog. *J Clin Invest* 1965;44:1132–1143.
23. Crippa G, Sverzellati E, Giorgi-Piefrancehschi M et al. Magnesium and cardiovascular drugs: Interactions and therapeutic role. *Ann Ital Med Int* 1999;14(1):40–45.
24. Kishi H, Kishi T, Folkers K. Bioenergetics in clinical medicine. III. Inhibition of coenzyme Q0-enzymes by clinically used anti-hypertensive drugs. *Res Commun Chem Pathol Pharmacol* 1975;12(3):533–540.
25. Lindeman RD. Hypokalemia: Causes, consequences and correction. *Am J Med Sci* 1976;272(1):5–17.
26. Clayton JA, Rodgers S, Blakey J. Thiazide diuretic prescription and electrolyte abnormalities in primary care. *Br J Clin Pharmacol* 2006;61:87–95.
27. Khedun SM, Naicker T, Maharaj B. Zinc, hydrochlorothiazide and sexual dysfunction. *Cent Afr J Med* 1995;41:312–315.
28. Pak CY. Correction of thiazide-induced hypomagnesemia by potassium-magnesium citrate from review of prior trials. *Clin Nephrol* 2000;54:271–275.
29. Wester PO. Urinary zinc excretion during treatment with different diuretics. *Acta Med Scand* 1980;208(3):209–212.
30. Odvina CV, Mason RP, Pak CY. Prevention of thiazide-induced hypokalemia without magnesium depletion by potassium-magnesium-citrate. *Am J Ther* 2006;13(2):101–108.
31. Rastogi D, Pelter MA, Deamer RL. Evaluations of hospitalizations associated with thiazide-associated hyponatremia. *J Clin Hypertens (Greenwich)* 2012;14(3):158–164.
32. Sica DA. Loop diuretic therapy, thiamine balance, and heart failure. *Congest Heart Fail* 2007;13(4):244–247.
33. Hanze S, Seyberth H. Studies of the effect of the diuretics furosemide, ethacrynic acid and triamterene on renal magnesium and calcium excretion. *Klin Wochenschr* 1967;45(6):313–314.
34. Reyes AJ, Olhaberry JV, Leary WP, Lockett CJ, van der Byl K. Urinary zinc excretion, diuretics, zinc deficiency and some side-effects of diuretics. *S Afr Med J* 1983;64(24):936–941.
35. Cohen N, Alon I, Almoznino-Sarafian D et al. Metabolic and clinical effects of oral magnesium supplementation in furosemide-treated patients with severe congestive heart failure. *Clin Cardiol* 2000;23(6):433–436.
36. Schalhorn A, Siegert W, Sauer HJ. Antifolate effect of triamterene on human leucocytes and on human lymphoma cell line. *Eur J Clin Pharmacol* 1981;20(3):219–224.
37. Cocco G, Iselin HU, Strozzi C et al. Magnesium depletion in patients on long-term chlorthalidone therapy for essential hypertension. *Eur J Clin Pharmacol* 1987;32(4):355–358.

38. Golik A, Modai D, Averbukh Z et al. Zinc metabolism in patients treated with captopril versus enalapril. *Metabolism* 1990;39(7):665–667.

39. Chakithandy S, Evans R, Vyakarnam P. Acute severe hyponatremia and seizures associated with postoperative enalapril administration. *Anaesth Intensive Care* 2009;37(4):673–674.

40. Braun LA, Rosenfeldt F. Pharmaco-nutrient interactions – a systematic review of zinc and antihypertensive therapy. *Int J Clin Pract* 2013;67(8):717–725.

41. Park MH, Kim HN, Lim JS et al. Angiotensin II potentiates zinc-induced cortical neuronal death by acting on angiotensin II type 2 receptor. *Mol Brain* 2013;6(1):50.

42. Colquhoun DM, Jackson R, Walters M et al. Effects of simvastatin on blood lipids, vitamin E, coenzyme Q10 levels and left ventricular function in humans. *Eur J Clin Invest* 2005;35(4):251–258.

43. Harris JI, Hibbeln JR, Mackey RH et al. Statin treatment alters serum n-3 and n-6 fatty acids in hypercholesterolemic patients. Prostaglandins *Leukot Essent Fatty Acids* 2004;71(4):263–269.

44. Folkers K, Langsjoen P, Willis R et al. Lovastatin decreases coenzyme Q levels in humans. *Proc Natl Acad Sci USA* 1990;87(22):8931–8934.

45. Ghayour-Mobarhan M, Lamb DJ, Taylor A et al. Effect of statin therapy on serum trace element status in dyslipidemic subjects. *J Trace Elem Med Biol* 2005;19(1):61–67.

46. Ghirlanda, Oradei A, Manto AG et al. Evidence of plasma CoQ10-lowering effect by HMG-CoA reductase inhibitors: A double-blind, placebo-controlled study. *J Clin Pharmacol* 1993;33(3):226–229.

47. Sulcova J, Stulc T, Hill M et al. Decrease in dehydroepiandrosterone level after fibrate treatment in males with hyperlipidemia. *Physiol Res* 2005;54(2):151–157.

48. Schooling CM, Au Yeung SL, Freeman G et al. The effect of statins on testosterone in men and women, a systematic review and meta-analysis of randomized controlled trials. *BMC Med* 2013;11(1):57.

49. Knodel LC, Talbert RL. Adverse effects of hypolipidaemic drugs. *Med Toxicol* 2987;2(1):10–32.

50. West RJ, Lloyd JK. The effect of cholestyramine on intestinal absorption. *Gut* 1975;16(2):93–98.

51. Scwarz KB, Goldstein PD, Witztum JL et al. Fat soluble vitamin concentrations in hypercholesterolemic children treated with colestipol. *Pediatrics* 1980;65(2):243–250.

52. [No authors listed]. Colestipol therapy and selected vitamin and mineral levels in children. *Nutr Rev* 1980;38(7):236–237.

53. Wilczek H, Sobra J, Ceska R et al. Therapy with fibrates and vitamin D metabolism. *Cas Lek Cesk* 1993;132(20);630–632.

54. Liberopoulos EN, Makariou SE, Moutzouri E et al. Effect of Simvastatin/Ezetimibe 10/10 mg versus Simvastatin 40 mg on serum vitamin D levels. *J Cardiovasc Pharmacol Ther* 2013;18(3):229–233.

55. Temple AR. Pathophysiology of aspirin overdosage toxicity, with implications for management. *Pediatrics* 1978;65(Pt 2 suppl):873–876.

56. Wharam PC, Speedy DB, Noakes TD et al. NSAID use increases the risk of developing hyponatremia during an Ironman triathlon. *Med Sci Sports Exerc* 2006;38(4):618–622.

57. Baggott JE, Morgan SL, Ha T, Vaughn WH, Hine RJ. Inhibition of folate-dependent enzymes by non-steroidal anti-inflammatory drugs. *Biochem J* 1992;282(Pt 1):197–202.

58. Gates MA, Araujo AB, Hall SA et al. Non steroidal anti-inflammatory drug use and levels of oestrogens and androgens in men. *Clin Endocrinol (Oxf)* 2012;76(2):272–280.

59. Aloisi AM, Buonocore M, Merlo L et al. Chronic pain therapy and hypothalamic-pituitary-adrenal axis impairment. *Psychoneuroendocrinology* 2011;36(7):1032–1039.

60. McGill MR, Yan HM, Ramachandran A et al. HepaRG cells; a human model to study mechanisms of acetaminophen hepatotoxicity. *Hepatology* 2011;53(3):974–982.

61. Anoush M, Eghbal MA, Fathiazad F et al. The protective effects of garlic extract against acetaminophen-induced oxidative stress and glutathione depletion. *Pak J Biol Sci* 2009;12(10):765–771.

62. Adams JF, Clark JS, Ireland JT, Kesson CM, Watson WS. Malabsorption of vitamin B12 and intrinsic factor secretion during biguanide therapy. *Diabetologia* 1983;24(1):16–18.

63. Kishi T, Kishi H, Watanabe T, Folkers K. Bioenergetics in clinical medicine. XI. Studies on coenzyme Q and diabetes mellitus. *J Med* 1976;7(3–4):307–321.

64. Ting RZ, Szeto CC, Chan MH et al. Risk factors of vitamin B12 deficiency in patients receiving metformin. *Arch Int Med* 2006;166(18):1975–1979.

65. De Jager J, Kooy A, Lehert P et al. Long term treatment with metformin in patients with type 2 diabetes and risk of vitamin B-12 deficiency: Randomized placebo controlled trial. *BMJ* 2010;340:c2181.

66. Palva IP, Salokannel SJ, Timonen T, Palva HL. Drug-induced malabsorption of vitamin B12. IV. Malabsorption and deficiency of B12 during treatment with slow-release potassium chloride. *Acta Med Scand* 1972;191(4):355–357.

67. MacKenzie JF, Russell RI. The effect of pH on folic acid absorption in man. *Clin Sci Mol Med* 1976;51: 363–368.
68. O'Neil-Cutting MA, Crosby WH. The effect of antacids on the absorption of simultaneously ingested iron. *JAMA* 1986;255(11):1468–1470.
69. Belaiche J, Zittoun J, Marquet J, Nurit Y, Yvart J. [Effect of ranitidine on secretion of gastric intrinsic factor and absorption of vitamin B12]. *Gastroenterol Clin Biol* 1983;7(4):381–384.
70. Bo-Linn GW, Davis GR, Buddrus DJ, Morawski SG, Santa Ana C, Fordtran JS. An evaluation of the importance of gastric acid secretion in the absorption of dietary calcium. *J Clin Invest* 1984;73(3):640–647.
71. Ghishan FK, Walker F, Meneely R, Patwardhan R, Speeg KV Jr. Intestinal calcium transport: Effect of cimetidine. *J Nutr* 1981;111(12):2157–2161.
72. Odes HS. Effect of cimetidine on hepatic vitamin D metabolism in humans. *Digestion* 1990;46(2):61–64.
73. Russell RM, Golner BB, Krasinski SD, Sadowski JA, Suter PM, Braun CL. Effect of antacid and H2 receptor antagonists on the intestinal absorption of folic acid. *J Lab Clin Med* 1988;112(4):458–463.
74. Sturniolo GC, Montino MC, Rossetto L et al. Inhibition of gastric acid secretion reduces zinc absorption in man. *J Am Coll Nutr* 1991;10(4):372–375.
75. Gau JT, Heh V, Acharya U et al. Uses of proton pump inhibitors and serum potassium levels. *Pharmacoepidemiol Drug Saf* 2009;18(9):865–871.
76. Danziger J, William JH, Scott DJ et al. Proton-pump inhibitor use is associated with low serum magnesium concentrations. *Kidney Int* 2013;83(4):692–699.
77. Marcuard SP, Albernaz L, Khazanie PG. Omeprazole therapy causes malabsorption of cyanocobalamin (vitamin B12). *Ann Intern Med* 1994;120:211–215.
78. Long AN, Atwell CL, Yoo W et al. Vitamin B12 deficiency associated with concomitant metformin and proton pump inhibitor use. *Diabetes Care* 2012;35(12):e84.
79. Wakabayashi H, Shimada K, Aizawa Y, Satoh T. Effect of psychotropic drugs on the contents of melatonin, serotonin and N-acetylserotonin in rat pineal gland. *Jpn J Pharmacol* 1989;49(2):225–234.
80. Alon I, Gorelik O, Berman S et al. Intracellular magnesium in elderly patients with heart failure: Effects of diabetes and renal dysfunction. *J Trace Elem Med Biol* 2006;20(4):221–226.
81. Gao XR, Wang MD, He XY et al. Decreased intralymphocytic magnesium content is associated with diastolic heart dysfunction in patients with essential hypertension. *Int J Cardiol* 2011;147(2):331–334.
82. Alaimo K, McDowell MA, Briefel RR et al. Dietary intake of vitamins, minerals and fiber of persons age 2 months and over in the United States: Third National Health and Nutrition Examination Survey, phase 1, 1988–91. *Advance Data from Vital and Health Statistics* 1994;258:1–26.
83. Chakraborti S, Chakraborti T, Mandal M et al. Protective role of magnesium in cardiovascular disease: A review. *Mol Cell Biochem* 2002;238(1–2):163–179.
84. Tejero-Taldo MI, Kramer JH, Mak Iu T et al. The nerve-heart connection in the pro-oxidant response to Mg-deficiency. *Heart Fail Rev* 2006;11(1):35–44.
85. Joosten MM, Gansevoort RT, Mukamai KJ et al. Urinary and plasma magnesium and risk of ischemic heart disease. *Am J Clin Nutr* 2013;97(6):1299–1306.
86. Del Gobbo LC, Song Y, Poirier P et al. Low serum magnesium concentrations are associated with a high prevalence of premature ventricular complexes in obese adults with type 2 diabetes. *Cardiovasc Diabetol* 2012;11:23.
87. Zhang, W, Iso H, Ohira T, Date C, Tamakoshi A; JACC Study Group. Associations of dietary magnesium intake with mortality from cardiovascular disease: The JACC study. *Atherosclerosis* 2012;221(2):587–595.
88. Atsmon J, Dolev E. Drug-induced hypomagnesaemia: Scope and management. *Drug Saf* 2005; 28(9):763–788.
89. Palmer BF, Naderi AS. Metabolic consequences associated with thiazide diuretics. *J Am Soc Hypertens* 2007;1(6):381–392.
90. Kass L, Weekes J, Carpenter L. Effect of magnesium supplementation on blood pressure: A meta analysis. *Eur J Clin Nutr* 2012;66(4):411–418.
91. Dorman B, Sade RM, Burnette JS et al. Magnesium supplementation in the prevention of arrhythmias in pediatric patients undergoing surgery for congenital heart defects. *Am Heart J* 2000;139(3):522–528.
92. Shechter M, Sharir M, Labrador MJ et al. Oral magnesium therapy improves endothelial function in patients with coronary artery disease. *Circulation* 2000;102(7):2353–2358.
93. Pokan R, Hofmann P, von Duvillard SP et al. Oral magnesium therapy, exercise heart rate, exercise tolerance and myocardial function in coronary artery disease patients. *Br J Sports Med* 2006;40(9):773–778.
94. Bralley JA, Lord RS. *Laboratory Evaluations in Molecular Medicine.* Norcross, GA: The Institute for Advances in Molecular Medicine, 2001.

95. Nair RR, Nair P. Alteration of myocardial mechanics in marginal magnesium deficiency. *Magnes Res* 2002;15(3–4):287–306 (ISSN:0953–1424).

96. Chaudhar DP, Boparai RK, Sharma R et al. Studies on the development of an insulin resistant rat model by chronic feeding of low magnesium high sucrose diet. *Magnes Res* 2004;17(4):293–300.

97. Shafi T, Appel LJ, Miller ER 3rd et al. Changes in serum potassium mediate thiazide-induced diabetes. *Hypertension* 2008;52(6):1022–1029.

98. Nadler JL, Buchanan T, Natarajan R, Antonipillai I, Bergman R, Rude R. Magnesium deficiency produces insulin resistance and increased thromboxane synthesis. Hypertension 1993;21;1024–1029.

99. Kamikawa T, Kobayashi A, Yamashita T, Hayashi H, Yamazaki N. Effects of coenzyme Q10 on exercise tolerance in chronic stable angina pectoris. *Am J Cardiol* 1985;56:247–251.

100. Vidyashankar S, Nandakumar KS, Patki PS. Alcohol depletes coenzyme-Q10 associated with increased TNF-alpha secretion to induce cytotoxicity in HepG2 cells. *Toxicology* 2012;302(1):34–39.

101. Linnane AW, Kopsidas G, Zhang C et al. Cellular redox activity of coenzyme Q10 effect of CoQ10 supplementation on human skeletal muscle. *Free Radic Res* 2002;36(4):445–453.

102. Moreira PL, Santos MS, Sena C, Nunes E, Seiça R, Oliveira CR. CoQ10 therapy attenuates amyloid beta-peptide toxicity in brain mitochondria isolated from aged diabetic rats. *Exp Neurol* 2005;196(1):112–119.

103. Digiesi V, Cantini F, Oradei A et al. Coenzyme Q10 in essential hypertension. *Mol Aspects Med* 1994;15 suppl:s257–263.

104. Langsjoen P, Langsjoen P, Willis R, Folkers K. Treatment of essential hypertension with CoQ10. *Mol Aspectsf Med* 1994;15 suppl:265–272.

105. Lamperti C, Naini AB, Lucchini V et al. Muscle coenzyme Q10 level in statin related myopathy. *Arch Neurol* 2005;62(11):1709–1712.

106. Spigset O. Reduced effect of warfarin caused by ubidecarenone. *Lancet* 1994;344(8933):1372–1373.

107. Landbo C, Almdal TP. [Interaction between warfarin and coenzyme Q10]. *Ugeskr Laeger* 1998;160 (22):3226–3227.

108. Bao B, Prasad AS, Beck FW, Godmere M. Zinc modulates mRNA levels of cytokines, *Am J Physiol Endocrinol Metab* 2003;285(5):E1095–1102.

109. Foster M, Samman S. Zinc regulation of inflammatory cytokines: Implications for cardiometabolic disease. *Nutrients* 2012;4(7):676–694.

110. Beletate V, El Dib RP, Atallah AN. Zinc supplementation for the prevention of type 2 diabetes mellitus. *Cochrane Database Syst Rev* 2007;(1):CD005525.

111. Setola E, Monti LD, Galluccio E et al. Insulin Resistance and endothelial function are improved after folate and vitamin B12 therapy in patients with metabolic syndrome: Relationship between homocysteine levels and hyperinsulinemia. *Eur J Endocrinol* 2004;151(4):483–489.

112. Hayden MR, Tyagi SC. Homocysteine and reactive oxygen species in metabolic syndrome, type 2 diabetes mellitus, and atheroscleropathy: The pleiotropic effects of folate supplementation. *Nutr J* 2004;3:4.

113. Derosa G, Cicero AF, Gaddi AV et al. Long-term effects of glimepiride or rosiglitazone in combination with metformin on blood pressure control in type 2 diabetic patients affected by the metabolic syndrome: A 12-month, double-blind, randomized clinical trial. *Clin Ther* 2005;27(9):1383–1391.

114. Peterson JL, McGuire DK. Impaired glucose tolerance and impaired fasting glucose—A review of diagnosis, clinical implications and management. *Diab Vasc Dis Res* 2005;2(1):9–15.

115. Wile DJ, Toth C. Association of metformin, elevated homocysteine, and methylmalonic acid levels and clinically worsened diabetic peripheral neuropathy. *Diabetes Care* 2010;33(1):156–161.

116. Akai A, Hosoi T, Ito H. Association of plasma homocysteine with serum interleukin 6 and C-peptide levels in patients with type 2 diabetes. *Metabolism* 2005;54(6):809–810.

117. Bonnet F, Irving K, Terra JL, Nony P, Berthezène F, Moulin P. Depressive symptoms are associated with unhealthy lifestyle in hypertensive patients with the metabolic syndrome. *J Hypertens* 2005;23(3):611–617.

118. Sachdev PS, Parslow RA, Lux O et al. Relationship of homocysteine, folic acid and vitamin B12 with depression in a middle-aged community sample. *Psychol Med* 2005;35(4):529–538.

119. Tiemeier H, van Tuijl HR, Hofman A, Meijer J, Kiliaan AJ, Breteler MM. Department of Epidemiology and Biostatistics, Erasmus Medical Centre, The Netherlands. Vitamin B-12, folate, and homocysteine in depression: The Rotterdam Study. *Am J Psychiatry* 2002;159(12):2099–2101.

120. Holick MF. Vitamin D deficiency. *N Engl J Med* 2007;357:266–281.

121. Vieth R. Vitamin D supplementation, 25-hydroxyvitamin D concentrations, and safety. *Am J Clin Nutr* 1999;69(5):825–826.

122. Nagpal S, Na S, Rathnachalam R. Noncalcemic actions of vitamin D receptor ligands. *Endocr Rev* 2005;26:662–687.

123. Shoji T, Shinohara K, Kimoto E et al. Lower risk for cardiovascular mortality in oral 1alpha-hydroxy vitamin D3 users in a haemodialysis population. *Nephrol Dial Transplant* 2004;19:179–184.

124. Palomer X, Gonzalez-Clemente JM, Blanco-Vaca F, Mauricio D. Role of vitamin D in the pathogenesis of type 2 diabetes mellitus. *Diabetes Obes Metab* 2008;10:185–197.

125. Mezawa H, Sugiura T, Watanabe M et al. Serum vitamin D levels and survival of patients with colorectal cancer: Post-hoc analysis of a prospective cohort study. *BMC Cancer* 2010;10(1):347.

126. Holmøy T, Moen SM. Assessing vitamin D in the central nervous system. *Acta Neurol Scand Suppl* 2010;(190):88–92.

127. Murphy PK, Wagner CL. Vitamin D and mood disorders among women: An integrative review. *J Midwifery Womens Health* 2008;53(5):440–446.

128. Prince RL, Austin N, Devine A et al. Effects of ergocalciferol added to calcium on the risk of falls in elderly high-risk women. *Arch Intern Med* 2008;168(1):103–108.

129. Kumar J, Muntner P, Kaskel FJ, Hailpern SM, Melamed ML. Prevalence and associations of 25-hydroxyvitamin D deficiency in US children: NHANES 2001-2004. *Pediatrics* 2009;124:e362–370.

130. Webb AR, Kline L, Holick MF. Influence of season and latitude on the cutaneous synthesis of vitamin D3: Exposure to winter sunlight in Boston and Edmonton will not promote vitamin D3 synthesis in human skin. *J Clin Endocrinol Metab* 1988;67:373–378.

131. Liel Y, Ulmer E, Shary J et al. Low circulating vitamin D in obesity. *Calcif Tissue Int* 1998;43(4):199–201.

132. Dasgupta K, Chan C, Da Costa D et al. Walking behaviour and glycemic control in type 2 diabetes: Seasonal and gender differences—study design and methods. *Cardiovasc Diabetol* 2007;6:1.

133. Beydoun MA, Boueiz A, Shroff MR et al. Associations among 25-hydroxyvitamin D, diet quality, and metabolic disturbance differ by adiposity in United States adults. *J Clin Endocrinol Metab* 2010;95(8):3814–3827.

134. Scragg R, Sowers MF, Bell C. Serum 25-hydroxyvitamin D, ethnicity, and blood pressure in the third national health and nutrition examination survey. *Am J Hypertens* 2007;20:713–719.

135. Sugden JA, Davies JI, Witham MD, Morris AD, Struthers AD. Vitamin D improves endothelial function in patients with type 2 diabetes mellitus and low vitamin D levels. *Diabet Med* 2008;25:320–325.

136. Melamed ML, Muntner P, Michos ED et al. Serum 25-hydroxyvitamin D levels and the prevalence of peripheral arterial disease: Results from NHANES 2001 to 2004. *Arterioscler Thromb Vasc Biol* 2008;28:1179–1185.

137. Targher G, Bertolini L, Padovani R et al. Serum 25-hydroxyvitamin D3 concentrations and carotid artery intima-media thickness in type 2 diabetic patients. *Clin Endocrinol* 2006;65:593–597.

138. Lindén V. Vitamin D and myocardial infarction. *Br Med J* 1974;3:647–650.

139. Pilz S, Marz W, Wellnitz B et al. Association of vitamin D deficiency with heart failure and sudden cardiac death in a large cross-sectional study referred for coronary angiography. *J Clin Endocrinol Metab* 2008;93:3927–3935.

140. Dobnig H, Pilz S, Scharnagl H et al. Independent association of low serum 25-hydroxyvitamin D and 1,25-dihydroxyvitamin D levels with all-cause and cardiovascular mortality. *Arch Intern Med* 2008;168:1340–1349.

141. Harwood RH, Sahota O, Gaynor K et al. A randomised, controlled comparison of different calcium and vitamin D supplementation regimens in elderly women after hip fracture: The Nottingham Neck of Femur (NONOF) Study. *Age Ageing* 2004;33(1):45–51.

142. Hoeck HC, Li B, Qvist P. Changes in 25-hydroxyvitamin D3 to oral treatment with vitamin D3 in postmenopausal females with osteoporosis. *Osteoporos Int* 2009;20(8):1329–1335.

143. Elliott ME, Binkley NC, Carnes M et al. Fracture risks for women in long-term care: High prevalence of calcaneal osteoporosis and hypovitaminosis D. *Pharmacotherapy* 2003;23(6):702–710.

144. Bischoff-Ferrari HA, Willett WC, Wong JB et al. Prevention of nonvertebral fractures with oral vitamin D and dose dependency: A meta-analysis of randomized controlled trials. *Arch Intern Med* 2009;169(6):551–561.

145. Picinato MC, Haber, EP, Carpinelli AR et al., Daily rhythm of glucose-induced secretion by isolated islets from the intact and pinealectomized rat. *J Pineal Res* 2002;33(3):172–177.

146. NHANES I Data. Findings reported at the annual scientific meeting of North American Society for the Study of Obesity, November 2004.

147. Spiegel K, Tasali E, Penev P, Van Cauter E. Brief communication: Sleep curtailment in healthy young men is associated with decreased leptin levels, elevated ghrelin levels, and increased hunger and appetite. *Ann Intern Med* 2004;141(11):846–850.

148. Kunz D, Mahlberg R, Müller C, Tilmann A, Bes F. Melatonin in patients with reduced REM sleep duration: Two randomized controlled trials. *J Clin Endocrinol Metab* 2004;89(1):128–134.
149. Rajaratnam SM, Middleton B, Stone BM, Arendt J, Dijk DJ. Melatonin advances the circadian timing of EEG sleep and directly facilitates sleep without altering its duration in extended sleep opportunities in humans. *J Physiol* 2004;561(Pt 1):339–351.

Index

Printed in the United States
by Baker & Taylor Publisher Services